# Coercion and Violence in Mental Health Settings

Nutmeg Hallett • Richard Whittington
Dirk Richter • Emachi Eneje
Editors

# Coercion and Violence in Mental Health Settings

## Causes, Consequences, Management

Second Edition

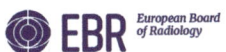

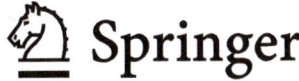

*Editors*
Nutmeg Hallett
Risk, Abuse and Violence Research
Programme
School of Nursing and Midwifery
University of Birmingham
BIRMINGHAM, UK

Dirk Richter
Division of Nursing
Department of Health Professions
Bern University of Applied Sciences
Bern, Switzerland

Richard Whittington
Centre for Research and Education in
Security
Prison and Forensic Psychiatry.
St. Olavs hospital
Trondheim University Hospital
Trondheim, Norway

Department of Mental Health
Norwegian University of Science
and Technology (NTNU)
Trondheim, Norway

Emachi Eneje
School of Nursing and Midwifery
University of Birmingham
Birmingham, UK

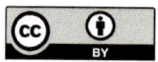

ISBN 978-3-031-61223-7    ISBN 978-3-031-61224-4   (eBook)
https://doi.org/10.1007/978-3-031-61224-4

St. Olavs hospital HF, Postboks 3250 Torgarden, 7006 Trondheim, Norway

This work was supported by St. Olavs hospital HF, Postboks 3250 Torgarden, 7006 Trondheim, Norway.

# Acknowledgements

This publication is based upon work from the COST Action FOSTREN (Fostering and Strengthening Approaches to Reducing Coercion in European Mental Health Services, CA19133) supported by COST (European Cooperation in Science and Technology).

COST (European Cooperation in Science and Technology) is a funding agency for research and innovation networks. COST Actions help connect research initiatives across Europe and enable scientists to grow their ideas by sharing them with their peers. This boosts their research, career and innovation. www.cost.eu.

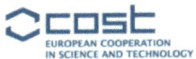 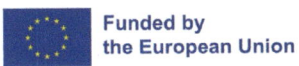

# Introduction

## Introduction

Mental health services around the world are, by definition, designed to provide care and treatment for people experiencing severe distress in their lives or those who are living with long-term disability. Many, if not most, services successfully provide a place of safety where equanimity can be regained and therapeutic growth can take place. Such recovery requires an environment which values human dignity at all times and in which the person's basic right to autonomy and respect is fostered as much as it can be in everyday life. This is the ideal.

Most services sometimes, and some services often, encounter violence, suicidality and self-harm in the course of providing care—both initiated by and directed towards patients—and then rely on coercion to extinguish the perceived threat against staff, service users and those who risk harm to themselves. Violence and coercion can therefore quickly contaminate the therapeutic environment for both service users and care staff and thus can prevent mental health services from doing the very job they have been set up to do. Unintended harm on either side can be the result, as coercion can breed violence and violence often breeds coercion. This book seeks to explore some ways out of this conundrum.

Our focus is timely as both coercion and workplace violence in mental health services are now high up on the international health policy agenda. With regard to coercion, representatives of both the United Nations and the Council of Europe have called for its abolition as something incompatible with human rights and the World Health Organization has established a global training initiative to facilitate the achievement of this goal (United Nations, 2008; Council of Europe, 2019; World Health Organization, 2019). At the same time, the evidence base for interventions that might enable professionals and their employing organisations to move away from coercion has grown enormously since the start of the century (Gooding et al., 2018). There is also a growing understanding of how such interventions might be successfully implemented into everyday practice (Lantta et al., 2023). In parallel, healthcare violence, the flipside of coercion, has been and remains a high priority for the World Health Organization and other influential entities with extensive evidence of widespread harm across many settings (Mento et al., 2020; World Health Organization, 2024). The time is right therefore to draw together knowledge on these twin topics and to consider some ways forward over the next decade.

## A(nother) New Look at an Old Problem

This book is a new edition of a text that was published nearly twenty years ago (Richter and Whittington 2006). It retains the basic philosophy that underpinned its predecessor with an emphasis on the interactional nature of violence and coercion in mental health settings, a focus on practice in real-world settings informed by theoretical and empirical insights, and the need for a systems-based approach to understanding and breaking the cycle. However, in the years since the first edition, our understanding of the dynamics within mental health settings has significantly evolved. This updated edition attempts to reflect a substantial shift in our understanding of the issues from a sole focus on patient-related violence to a broader examination of coercion in mental health settings and its intricate relationship with violence.

Mental health care has long grappled with the challenge of balancing patient autonomy with the need for effective treatment, particularly in cases involving involuntary admissions and interventions. The use of coercion, whether in the form of physical restraints, compulsory medication or involuntary confinement, raises critical ethical and practical questions. It is a complex phenomenon that exists in a tension-filled space between therapeutic intent and the lived experience of being disrespected as a person.

This book examines the complex nature of coercion in mental health care, analysing its causes, consequences and management. It explores coercive practices, examining how they can lead to violence and, conversely, be a response to violent behaviours. The interaction between patient and staff perspectives on coercion is a central theme, highlighting the tensions between conflicting rights and responsibilities inherent in mental health care.

Our focus extends to the legal, ethical and practical ramifications of coercion, with an eye towards developing strategies that minimise its use while maintaining safety and therapeutic integrity. Through a comprehensive review of recent research and practice, we aim to illuminate the complex dynamics at play and offer guidance for mental health professionals and service users navigating these challenging waters. As we move forward, the mental health professional community must continue to critically evaluate and enhance its approaches to coercion and violence through both dialogue with service users and self-reflection. By understanding the interconnectedness of these issues, we can strive for what we all want to achieve: more humane, effective and ethical mental health care systems worldwide.

Since the publication of the first edition of this book, understandings of inpatient violence in mental health settings have undergone a significant expansion and, in places, transformation. Until relatively recently, the focus was predominantly on the incidence and management of incidents construed simply as violence perpetrated by service users within psychiatric institutions and individual risk factors for such aggression. Recently, there has been a significant shift towards integrating the concept of coercion more directly into discussions about violence. This concept encompasses the use of force, threat or manipulation to compel individuals with mental health conditions to comply with treatments, confinement or interventions against their will. Coercion, always a complex and controversial issue at the intersection of healthcare and individual autonomy, raises profound ethical and human rights concerns. We have aimed to reflect this shift in focus in this new edition; the title now includes coercion explicitly alongside violence, and ethical and human rights concerns are interwoven throughout the book in line with contemporary international policy and guidance (World Health Organization, 2019).

Empirical research on coercion in psychiatry was basically non-existent before the 1990s (Lidz, 1998), so any criticism of it was based more on ethical and philosophical grounds (Szasz, 1963, 1997). Ground-breaking empirical research can be traced back to key studies like the EUNOMIA project, which ran from 2002 to 2006, providing the first systematic comparative insights into coercive measures in psychiatric treatment across 12 European countries (Kallert et al., 2005). Since then, the literature on coercion has expanded exponentially.

## Causes, Consequences and Management

Our subtitle highlights three main areas which the chapters consider in various ways. As we have already noted, the *causes* of coercion and violence in mental health inpatient settings are complex and deeply intertwined with each other. Coercion, often arising implicitly in both the management and creation of aggressive behaviour (Hassiotis et al., 2022), is influenced by various factors. These include not only direct practices like seclusion, restraint or involuntary treatment but also systemic elements such as the built environment, organisational culture and social milieu. Importantly, perceptions and expectations of coercion can begin even before a person enters hospital and then continue through their treatment experience. Therefore, addressing these comprehensive issues is crucial for reducing both coercion and violence, emphasising the significant role played by systems, environments and interpersonal interactions in influencing these dynamics.

Although the wellbeing of the person against whom coercion is used must be ensured from an ethical perspective (the beneficence principle), the *consequences* of coercion are almost always negative for the person subjected to it with the constant risk of both psychological trauma and sometimes physical injury. These consequences have been systematically uncovered particularly in the last 15 years and several chapters in this book highlight the many issues. There are also undoubtedly psychological and physical risks for the staff implementing the restrictive practice and indeed for those who witness it on the ward or in the neighbourhood. If used appropriately and genuinely as an intervention of last resort, the safety of all can be preserved and the therapeutic relationship can be maintained, at least in principle. This is, however, not always possible in reality. This recognition of the full reality of coercion is considered at various points below.

The therapeutic *management* and prevention of violence in mental health services is a key set of skills for professionals which have been evolving since at least the 1990s and is a constant topic in the chapters below as it was in the first edition. A new theme now though is the idea of managing and preventing coercion itself.

Just as violence was once seen merely as an individual pathology, coercion is now seen increasingly as an organisational pathology with the same implied need for treatment. Perhaps the most notable feature of the past twenty years since the first edition of the book is the development and testing of a range of comprehensive system-level interventions such as Safewards (Al-Wandi et al., 2023) designed to minimise and ideally (some would say idealistically) eradicate the use of coercion. The optimism generated by these and other interventions as the basis for a truly human-rights based approach to mental care underpins much of the work discussed in this book.

It is also worth noting briefly what we mean here specifically by a *mental health service*. The emphasis in the book is very much on in-patient services where the most intrusive and forceful physical interventions are repeatedly imposed on a small but significant proportion of service users. Looking across the whole phenomenon, most coercive incidents occur in hospital settings and the bulk of the research on coercion is undoubtedly focused on the use of physical restraint (manually and/or mechanically), seclusion and, to a lesser extent, forced medication with in-patients. But of course, coercion is frequently applied in community settings as well either at the moment of involuntary admission to hospital or in the prolonged regime of compulsory community treatment after discharge. We consider coercion across all these phases below but with an emphasis on the hospital phase because, as noted above, this is where most of the research has been conducted.

## Zero Tolerance for Coercion?

A fervent debate is currently ongoing about the feasibility of the goal sought by some for mental health services based entirely on autonomy and voluntariness with the total eradication of coercion in any form. The clash, best exemplified in contradictory statements on human rights by two bodies within the United Nations, has been dubbed the Geneva Impasse (Martin and Gurbai, 2019). As individuals, we have certain attitudes towards this debate. As editors of the book, however, we have taken no specific position on this debate but we welcome it as a question that inevitably runs through several chapters. We hope that some of the discussions here will inform the debate and perhaps contribute to its resolution.

In this updated edition of the book, we have attempted to embed lived experience voices into our exploration of coercion and violence in mental health settings, with a lived experience editor participating in the construction of the text and co-authors on many of the individual chapters. This inclusion is designed to amplify a unique and still frequently overlooked perspective. We recognise that professionals working within these settings have their own lived experiences, which inform their understanding and approach to care, bridging the gap between professional practice and personal insight. This is also reflected in the book but the emphasis throughout, where possible, is more on the personal experiences of individuals who have both experienced mental ill health and been subjected to coercion and violence in these environments. These individuals bring first-hand knowledge of how coercive practices affect their lives, offering critical insights into the current system's deficiencies, oversights and biases. Incorporating these voices allows for a more thorough understanding of the issues, facilitating our aim of contributing to the creation of mental health systems that are both empathetic and effective.

In addition to the lived experience perspective, the contributors to this book represent a wide range of professional viewpoints including authors who are mental health nurses, psychologists, psychiatrists, educationalists, psychotherapists and researchers. Many of the contributors here are linked to an active research network, the European Violence in Psychiatry Research Group (EViPRG, www.eviprg.eu), which was also a key platform for the production of the first edition of the book. This new edition has been further enhanced by other connections forged through the work of a collaboration funded by the European Commission COST (Co-operation in Science and Technology) programme. This collaboration, called FOSTREN (Fostering and Strengthening Approaches to Reducing Coercion in European Mental Health Services), has met regularly since 2020 and brought together many people with relevant expertise and commitment to the goal of moving away from coercive practice. This book has directly grown out of the work of these networks.

In this book, it is particularly important to present the perspectives of those who have directly experienced coercion and/or violence, as their unique insights are instrumental in identifying and addressing the limitations of current practice, steering efforts towards a more compassionate and efficient approach to mental health care. This, incidentally, includes our avoidance of imposing any requirement on authors here to adopt a consistent terminology in contested areas. In particular, there have long been divergent views among people who receive mental health services on the relative degrees of stigma and empowerment attached to the terms 'patient', 'service user', etc. (Dickens and Picchioni 2011). All of these terms are used interchangeably throughout this book with no judgement here on their merits.

In this context, our ethical and legal understanding of coercion in psychiatry has also changed. Whereas in earlier years the use of coercion was generally accepted reluctantly but ultimately uncritically, the question of legitimacy is now central. Recent studies have looked at the consequences of coercive measures and tend to assume that the majority of patients affected do not benefit from the use of coercion. It is therefore predominantly not in the best interests of the patients—which is the central ethical justification for measures against a person's will. In addition, as noted above, the United Nations Convention on the Rights of Persons with Disabilities has since 2006 given rise to a new perspective that views coercive measures as (potential) human rights violations. This view, which has led to considerable controversy between United Nations bodies and psychiatric associations, questions the use of coercion on legal grounds.

Overall, the dynamic between mental health professionals, patients and the broader societal context is now a critical subject of examination. By exploring the various dimensions of coercion and its impact on individuals' experiences and outcomes, researchers aim to deepen our understanding of this complex issue. This shift in focus reflects a broader recognition of the need to balance safety within mental health settings with respecting the autonomy and dignity of those receiving care, while considering the role of systems, environments and interpersonal interactions in situations leading to distress, challenging behaviours and sometimes violence.

## The Structure of the Book

This book is structured into four parts. The first, 'Diverse Voices', seeks to amplify perspectives that are often marginalised within the Western-centric, professionally dominated discourse about coercion and mental health more broadly. This part highlights a range of perspectives, with an example of a non-Western viewpoint and insights from individuals with lived experience. Our aim is not to homogenise the different ways in which coercion and violence experiences in mental health are articulated but rather to render the diversity of these experiences and voices as inclusively as possible. It is beyond our scope, and possibly our ability, to capture the full array of potential voices, but this inclusion should enrich the dialogue and hopefully provide a more nuanced view of the challenges and complexities in mental health care.

Incorporating a non-Western perspective in discussions of coercion and violence in mental health settings introduces an angle that challenges dominant Western-centric views. This enriches the conversation and can facilitate a more holistic, globally relevant understanding of the issues. Of course, the broader dialogue on coercion in mental health noted earlier, and the inclusion of lived experience voices in research, policy and practice, are closely interrelated. This inclusion points to the personal impact of, and ethical considerations arising from coercion, which can be overlooked in traditional narratives which attribute violence almost exclusively to patients. Hearing directly from those who have experienced coercion highlights its complexities, calling into question the desirability of even well-intentioned practices that effectively deny patients their autonomy and dignity. This can be challenging for professionals, but it inevitably fosters a more comprehensive approach to both research and clinical practice, emphasising again the complexity of interactions in mental health care.

'Key Concepts' is the second part, and it aims to set out the foundational ideas related to coercion and violence within mental healthcare. It seeks to do this by explaining the terminology and establishing a theoretical basis for understanding the topic. It also examines how these concepts intersect with ethical concerns, human rights issues and practical interventions like reducing involuntary admissions. This information is essential for professionals as well as service users who aim to deal effectively with these difficult, complex issues.

The 'Human and Physical Context' part of the book addresses the environments and conditions that shape experiences and actions within psychiatric settings. It addresses how the design and layout of physical spaces, the implementation of safety and security measures, the prevailing ward culture and atmosphere, and the systemic responses to aggressive behaviours contribute to the therapeutic milieu for better or worse. Furthermore, it discusses trauma-informed care as a crucial approach that recognises and responds to the role of trauma in the lives of individuals receiving mental health care.

The final part of the book discusses 'Interventions' in response to violence and how these can aim to reduce reliance on coercion as well as the violence itself. While it acknowledges the widespread use of coercive measures, taken together the chapters collectively advocate for a reduction in their use. They explore a range of strategies including aggression management training, de-escalation techniques, pharmacological interventions and alternative approaches that should minimise the need for coercion. The part also emphasises the importance of providing support after incidents, advocating for practices that uphold patient dignity and promote safety.

## Science, Evidence and the Future

In mental healthcare, staying current with knowledge and practices is necessary for anyone in a professional role. The mental health landscape is constantly evolving. It is influenced by new research, shifting societal norms and a deeper understanding of the human psyche. Mental health professionals must be perpetually inquisitive, seeking out the latest information and integrating it into their practice. This commitment to ongoing education is not only about basing care on the most current understanding—though this is particularly crucial in a time of rapidly developing neuroscience and psychology. It reflects a commitment to the highest ethical standards and to offering care that serves patients best. In mental health, the understanding of conditions—and treatments—can shift dramatically. Clinging to outdated or discredited methods can be not only ineffective but also actively harmful. And so, mental health professionals must constantly tack across a shifting sea of knowledge, adapting to new theories, therapeutic techniques and ethical considerations. Mapping this ever-evolving landscape of learning allows practitioners to offer the most effective treatments, respond with genuine empathy to their patients, and contribute to the study and practice of mental health with full awareness of innovations. The continual renovation of knowledge and practice in mental health in this way is not a matter only of 'staying current', but of demonstrating respect for the complexity of the challenges in mental health. It also requires acknowledgment of the trust that people who are seeking help from mental health professionals place in them.

When it comes to our topic here—coercion and violence in mental health settings—the urgency of continually updating our knowledge and practices becomes even greater. The field is rapidly evolving with new insights into the causes and prevention of violence and the ethical implications of coercion. Staying current with these developments is crucial for reducing reliance on coercive measures and enhancing patient care. Updating knowledge and practices in this area involves integrating new research findings, reassessing risk assessment tools, refining intervention strategies and understanding patient perspectives better. This continuous evolution has as its aim the creation of a safer, more humane therapeutic environment that respects the rights and dignity of our patients and, ultimately, allows for

more effective, humane treatment. We hope that this book will help the next generation of scientist-practitioners and experts by experience to grapple with these issues
more effectively and to formulate the principles which make human rights-based
services a reality.

Risk, Abuse and Violence Research Programme                    Nutmeg Hallett
School of Nursing and Midwifery
University of Birmingham,
Birmingham, UK

Centre for Research and Education                           Richard Whittington
in Security, Prisons and Forensic
Psychiatry, Forensic Department Østmarka
St. Olav's Hospital, Trondheim, Norway

Department of Mental Health
Norwegian University of Science
and Technology (NTNU)
Trondheim, Norway

Division of Nursing, School of Health Professions               Dirk Richter
Berner Fachhochschule
Bern, Switzerland

Risk, Abuse and Violence Research Programme,                   Emachi Eneje
School of Nursing and Midwifery
University of Birmingham
Birmingham, UK

School of Nursing and Midwifery
University of Birmingham
Birmingham, UK

## References

Al-Wandi, M. S. I., Baumgardt, J., Jäckel, D., Helber-Böhlen, H., Voigt, A., McCutcheon, A. K.,
    et al. (2023). [Long term evaluation of the implementation of the safewards model—Results of
    a follow-up-study among patients and staff in acute psychiatric wards]. *Psychiatrische Praxis,
    50*(2), 98–102. https://doi.org/10.1055/a-1961-1486
Council of Europe (2019). *Ending coercion in mental health: The need for a human rights-based
    approach.* https://pace.coe.int/en/files/28038/html
Dickens, G., & Picchioni, M. (2011). A systematic review of the terms used to refer to people
    who use mental health services: User perspectives. *International Journal of Social Psychiatry,
    58*(2), 115–122. https://doi.org/10.1177/0020764010392066.
Gooding, G., McSherry, B., Roper, C., & Grey, F. (2018) *Alternatives to coercion in mental health
    settings: A literature review.* Melbourne Social Equity Institute. https://socialequity.unimelb.
    edu.au/__data/assets/pdf_file/0012/2898525/Alternatives-to-Coercion-Literature-Review-
    Melbourne-Social-Equity-Institute.pdf

Hassiotis, A., Almvik, R., & Fluttert, F. (2022). Coercion as a response to violence in mental health-care settings. *The Lancet Psychiatry, 9*(1), 6–8. https://doi.org/10.1016/S2215-0366(21)00476-4

Kallert, T. W., Glöckner, M., Onchev, G., Raboch, J., Karastergiou, A., Solomon, Z., et al. (2005). The EUNOMIA project on coercion in psychiatry: study design and preliminary data. *World Psychiatry, 4*(3), 168–172.

Lantta, T., Duxbury, J., Haines-Delmont, A., Björkdahl, A., Husum, T., Lickiewicz, J., et al. (2023). Models, frameworks and theories in the implementation of programs targeted to reduce formal coercion in mental health settings: A systematic review. *Frontiers in Psychiatry, 14*, 1158145.

Lidz, C. W. (1998). Coercion in psychiatric care: What have we learned from research? *Journal of the American Academy of Psychiatry and the Law, 26*(4), 631.

Martin, W., & Gurbai, S. (2019). Surveying the Geneva impasse: Coercive care and human rights. *International Journal of Law and Psychiatry, 64*, 117–128. https://doi.org/10.1016/j.ijlp.2019.03.001.

Mento, C., Silvestri, M. C., Bruno, A., Muscatello, M. R. A., Cedro, C., Pandolfo, G., et al. (2020). Workplace violence against healthcare professionals: A systematic review. *Aggression and Violent Behavior, 51*, 101381. https://doi.org/10.1016/j.avb.2020.101381.

Richter, D., & Whittington, R. (Eds.) (2006). *Violence in mental health settings: Causes, consequences and management.* Springer.

Szasz, T. (1963). *Law, liberty, and psychiatry: An inquiry into the social uses of mental health practices.* Macmillan.

Szasz, T. (1997). The case against psychiatric coercion. *The Independent Review, 1*(4), 485–498. http://www.jstor.org/stable/24560781.

United Nations (2008). *Convention on the rights of persons with disabilities.* United Nations General Assembly. https://www.ohchr.org/en/instruments-mechanisms/instruments/convention-rights-persons-disabilities

World Health Organization (2019). *Quality rights materials for training, guidance and transformation.* https://www.who.int/publications/i/item/who-qualityrights-guidance-and-training-tools

World Health Organization (2024). *Violence and harassment.* https://www.who.int/tools/occupational-hazards-in-health-sector/violence-harassment

# Contents

**Part III   Human and Physical Context**

**Part IV   Interventions**

# Part I

# Diverse Voices

# The Lived Experience of Coercion

Chris Munt and Brian Littlechild

## 1    Introduction

This chapter is the culmination of sensitively paced and carefully structured work, coordinated by myself and Prof Brian Littlechild, and crucially guided by the contributions of our cohort of co-authors with Lived Experience allies, coming together in a collective effort to state, categorically, that violence towards patients, and deliberate and premeditated coercion, though rare, does exist in the UK Mental Health system. We believe this happens more frequently than we would care to contemplate. These vulnerable patients are no different to you and me. They are indeed parents, siblings, partners, colleagues and neighbours, who in the midst of a mental health crisis, reach out for help in places that fall short of the maxim, 'places of safety'. The fact that these incidents do not routinely result in criminal or disciplinary proceedings against the alleged perpetrators, perhaps says more about ill-informed and malign attitudes to mental health patients and the lack of understanding in society of mental illness, than about the perceived probity of provider services and their practitioners. The common misconception of people with a mental illness being chaotic, disordered, and unreliable may lead some to conclude that when an incident is reported, the victim's account is considered unsound. The shared experience gleaned from consultation with our co-authors is

---

*NB—when the terms 'I', 'me' or 'myself' are used in the chapter, this refers to the first author, Chris Munt.*

C. Munt (✉)
Letchworth Garden City, UK

B. Littlechild
School of Health and Social Work, University of Hertfordshire, Hatfield, UK
e-mail: b.littlechild@herts.ac.uk

© The Author(s) 2024                                                                    3
N. Hallett et al. (eds.), *Coercion and Violence in Mental Health Settings*,
https://doi.org/10.1007/978-3-031-61224-4_1

that the cards are stacked so heavily against the victim, that violence is endured, left unchecked, and is often repeated.

Our lived experience co-author colleagues have been at pains to state and restate that the vast majority of mental health practitioners do not present a direct threat towards their patients. However, as many of our lived experience colleagues testified in what they wished to have represented in this chapter, at least some of the incidents they have experienced, were witnessed by the perpetrator's colleagues, and the perpetrator encountered little or no challenge, formally or informally.

Illustrative quotes from our lived experience colleagues are presented throughout this chapter, and tell their own story:

> Who will believe me, a nutter, rather than a trusted member of staff?
> They have all the authority, and I have no rights.

For the purpose of gathering the experiences of our cohort, we have defined violence as physical and sexual assault, threat and implied threat, explicit coercion, aggression and bullying. We are aware of how incongruous this appears when applied to what many of us hold dear- that being our National Health Service (NHS). However, we ignore the reality of what goes on, both hidden and in plain sight, at our peril. We should reflect on the statistic that one in eight people will experience an episode of significant mental illness in their lifetime (World Health Organization, 2022). The challenge for us all is to illuminate the good, bad and indifferent experiences of those using mental health services, and not potentially exacerbate the problems. Our cohort wishes only to present their lived experiences, for meaningful and measurable improvements to follow, and a more trusting dialogue to emerge. People should no longer experience the guilt and shame of feeling that it is they who are the problem.

> Staff were trying to do their best, but even they did nothing when other staff behaved badly.

## 1.1 Research Evidence and How It Relates to the Work for This Chapter

As previously noted, there has been very little attention paid to the area of violence and abuse towards patients/service users from staff in mental health services, whilst there have been many studies and publications relating to violence and abuse from patients/service users to staff. In one Southern German multicentre study, which included 20 community mental health care facilities, Rossa-Roccor et al. (2020) commented on how people with a mental health disorder have significantly higher risks of becoming victims of violence in the community compared to the general population, an issue noted by others (e.g. Bhavsar et al., 2019; Dean et al., 2018; Kamperman et al., 2014; Khalifeh et al., 2015; Latalova et al., 2014; Maniglio, 2009). In addition, violence and abuse towards patients/service users from staff has attracted much less attention than violent behaviour by the patients even though one study found violent victimisation of patients occurs more frequently than violent offending by the patient and found it ironic 'that the discipline's focus on perpetration among inpatients may contribute to negative stereotypes' (Choe et al., 2008, p. 1).

Rossa-Roccor et al. (2020, p. 1) note that within mental health provision, for example, inpatient units and community-based treatment, 'data on victimization is scarce and the prevalence of crimes against patients in the mental health care setting remains largely unknown', indicating that agencies' greater effective recording of such data, and availability of such data on incidents when they are recorded on patient victimisation is needed.

The National Institute for Health and Care Excellence (NICE), serving the English and Welsh NHS, have produced guidance on managing short-term violence (NICE, 2015), and it includes several points relevant to the current discussion. For example, it sets out how 'Treatment and care should take into account individual needs and preferences' (NICE, 2015, p. 12), by setting out that staff should work as a team in a therapeutic, positive and encouraging way, with good leadership, whilst maintaining staff emotional regulation and self-management. It also states that when prescribing p.r.n. (pro re nata) medication in order to prevent or de-escalate situations that are at risk of ending in violence and/or aggression, the p.r.n. medication should be prescribed based upon 'individual need and include discussion with the service user if possible' (NICE, 2015, p. 13). In relation to using restrictive interventions in inpatient psychiatric settings, it directs staff to 'not use restrictive interventions to punish, inflict pain, suffering or humiliation, or establish dominance' (NICE, 2015, p. 14).

Another key area regarding the inclusion of service users in the NICE guideline in this area is covered by a recommendation which applies to violence and aggression against staff but applies equally to our current concern of staff violence against patients/service users, where it advises that formal external post-incident review should take place through a service user experience monitoring unit or equivalent service user group as soon as possible after the incident, led by a service user and includes staff from outside the ward where the incident took place. This might include, it suggests, interviews with staff, the service user involved and any witnesses if further information is needed. This would be valuable, the guideline suggests, in identification of what led to the incident and what might possibly have been done differently.

The book *Men in White Coats: Treatment under Coercion* by George Szmukler (2018) examines the current justifications for involuntary treatment of patients/service users with mental disorders and argues that existing laws and procedures are discriminatory and morally unacceptable, and they should be replaced by a completely different approach for over-riding treatment refusals.

Against this background, we know we have the challenge of winning over hearts and minds that reject any inference that there is something very wrong with existing provisions, but we are emboldened by our collective desire for positive change and reform. Health services must be as willing to embrace those who are critical of its performance, as those who resoundingly approve.

*I offered to get involved with the book, because I want other people to be treated better than I was.*
    *I wanted to help, but I do have trust issues, and it took me a long time to be able to share what happened.*
    *We all helped each other.*
    *A part of me still worries that someone from services will find out what I've said.*
    *I want to be believed.*

The final section of our chapter also sets out an agenda for change, providing services, practitioners and politicians with a set of key challenges and establishing a pathway towards more consistently humane environments, practices, values and principles.

## 2    Representing the Views of Service User Colleagues

As the lead author of this chapter, I spent many months talking, building trust and facilitating an open dialogue with people who have been profoundly affected by violence perpetrated by staff, without individuals or services being held to account. The cohort is made up of individual patients with similar lived experiences, known to me by way of established peer networks and other related forums. We, myself and Brian Littlechild, recognised the need to approach individuals and groups with both sensitivity and probity. I have the advantage of having achieved a certain profile and recognition in peer circles, and initially this helped in bringing this project to people's attention. However, we realised that to win people's trust and goodwill, we would need tangible protocols to fully deliver our desired outcomes. Through a series of individual and group participation virtual meetings, we agreed to a binding term of reference that fully supported their need for unconditional anonymity, and for my expectation of reliable and consistent testimony. Initially, such meetings were scheduled every week to facilitate the right conditions for each member of the cohort to move at a pace that met their requirements. I made it clear from the outset that our chapter would focus on presenting themes, rather than in-depth case histories with considered and detailed examination. Over time, we achieved a certain rhythm that seemed to generate the testimony whilst at the same time not exposing them to the risk of being retraumatised. Over time, there was less need for frequent 'checking' in with people and updating our evidence, but after every thousand words were written, this was shared for feedback, comments and agreement. Whilst some discretion for myself as the main author was agreed to by the expert by experience (EBE) co-authors, for myself to develop the text as a composite of all co-authors' comments, all changes and the final version to the text were agreed to by all.

The co-authors' primary concern from the outset was establishing and maintaining their anonymity, for fear of future harassment and mistreatment, as a direct result of their disclosing their adverse and traumatic experiences. These deeply impactful disclosures have not been tested, corroborated or investigated. It was never our intention to interrogate their testimony. However, though I found some variation in what someone might share from one interview to another, it is the contention here that the core factual detail remained relatively intact. If this was not the case, I would explain that for reasons of consistency, we would have to exclude the incident and press on.

In exploring the prevalence of violence in our services, we were almost overwhelmed with research papers looking into violence towards staff, perpetrated by service users and patients. However, our search generated only a handful of references focusing specifically on institutional violence within UK mental health services (e.g. Macdonald, 2021; Joyes et al., 2021; Kumar et al., 2001; Liberati et al., 2023).

It might appear that we are swimming against the tide of opinion, outside of formal and informal service user networks. At this point, I must reveal my hand. I have a lived experience of serious mental illness. On multiple occasions, I have found myself on acute wards, and have used community services for many years. Though I have avoided serious acts of violence on my person, there are far too many occasions when I've witnessed my peers suffering at the hands of professionals. I have witnessed people forcibly restrained, secluded and sedated. I've had to listen to practitioners defame, threaten and intimidate people. I can recount multiple occasions when I have been subject to implied and covert threats as well as attempts at coercion.

One key feature in relation to effective responses to institutionalised violence across health, mental health and care facilities is the perceived lack of credibility of litigants and complainants, and this deserves further investigation (Cremin et al., 2009; Mahomed et al., 2022). These studies and investigations conclude how the power differential can render people who believe that they are somehow complicit in the harm they have suffered and demonstrate just how powerless they feel about seeking redress. Those who are beset by mental illness and the very real impact of stigma are, it can be argued from this, ready subjects for abuse and exploitation.

My lived experience is one thing, but I've also held numerous senior positions in health and social care, and academia. By instinct, I'm not a 'fire starter' for the sake of it, my instinct is to extinguish the blaze and shine a light on the subject instead, but I have not, and will not, avoid my responsibility in articulating the testimony, selflessly shared by our cohort of lived experience colleagues, no matter how conflicted I might feel, or worried about any personal or professional consequences. The narrative I have been privileged to scribe has left an indelible impression on me. I was no stranger to the themes presented here, but I have been shocked by the number of incidents and similarity of the offending behaviours the length and breadth of the country.

It is hoped our efforts to communicate our work will be viewed as being a largely rounded, informed and progressive perspective, building a bridge between ourselves, and those who feel moved to strive for services that routinely meet the expectations of all stakeholders, with patients' experiences, safety and wellbeing first and foremost.

What you will read here is written in my (Chris's) hand, but the pen is guided by those people who make up our cohort and details the narrative of each and every one. This is their story, purely and simply, and without embellishment or attempts to re-author a story that must be heard, if we are to finally overturn the dominant discourse that it is only staff who are the victims of violence within our services. It is important to reiterate here that at all points of progress, each person in the cohort has reviewed what has been written, and their consent has been sought to move forward to the next phase, and the final wording.

I'm challenged every time I enter a mental health unit, and am confronted by a large poster, with bold lettering, stating the organisation's determination that they will not tolerate violence against members of staff. Why is it beyond our wit to simply have a statement that the organisation doesn't tolerate violence, full stop? To commission and develop services that are safe for everyone.

An agreed plan to invite those who had experienced violence within the UK mental health sector was issued in the summer of 2021. Our plan was to identify patient/service user-led organisations and invite people to contribute their testimony, via their databases. It was notable that a number of leading organisations declined to become involved. Most cited that projects such as ours do not correspond with their present strategy and priorities. It might be that these large organisations are significantly dependent on secondary and core commissioning at both a national and local level, and see potential tensions to these funding streams, by aligning themselves too closely with this endeavour. We fully accept such conclusions are difficult to evidence, and that many will take a view that such a hypothesis is merely conjecture. Yet many patients and service users share concerns that such organisations have shifted from their original constitutions and have lost sight of the need for autonomy when working in partnership with Mental Health providers. I recognise the value of partnership working, but such arrangements should not get in the way of patient-led groups adhering to their primary purpose. Despite the lack of official support and engagement from some quarters, we managed to engage 21 motivated service user colleagues and 2 carers. All had observed or had experienced violence within acute and community provision.

All were extremely worried that their involvement might lead to adverse consequences and a threat to their ongoing care needs. We had anticipated this, and I spent several weeks, reassuring the cohort, that their identities were secure and would never be shared, even with other colleagues associated with our project.

As they began to detail and share their experiences with me, it became clear that these concerns of reprisals were too great, and some simply could not be sufficiently reassured, and they withdrew from the process, but wished the rest of us every success. I still maintain informal contact with them and keep them appraised of our progress. The cohort continues to have access to me and is very much a live influence on our collaborative efforts, in the shaping and writing of this chapter.

*Why do they employ people like that?*
*Why should you need to teach staff to be nice?*

When presenting both the individual and collective themes, it is incumbent on me to not become embedded in statistics. Each and every notation captures an individual's pain, suffering and trauma. Some testimony has been spoken for the very first time and required a great deal of care and safeguarding on our part. We were most careful not to re-traumatise people and derail their recovery. Most stories were gathered over multiple interviews and conducted in a patient and gradual process.

Invariably, their motivation wasn't to lambast services engaged in supporting people with complex needs, with finite resources. Rather they wished to inform, that sometimes, in some places, some practitioners can carry out acts of violence. The impact on the individual is profound with enduring and debilitating consequences.

Post-incident, the majority did not make a formal complaint, for fear of reprisals. Those that did complain were confronted with a rather crude and overly officious complaints procedure, which appeared to not advocate for them as victims. Of the four cases where formal complaints were levelled against services, not one was partially or wholly upheld.

This is indeed a conundrum, concerning whether the alleged acts of violence are significantly unfounded or malicious, or whether it is the case that services are so preoccupied with protecting their reputations, that get to a situation where they cannot/will not admit that sometimes, in some places, some practitioners do carry out acts of violence on persons who are vulnerable where they were in the care of those very services who were mandated to support them. This is not entirely anecdotal, and there have been notable examples where health and social care staff and institutions have been found responsible for inflicting acts of violence and coercion on their patients and service users. These events have been present in institutional 'care' for vulnerable people for many years (Foucault, 1961), with abusive care highlighted in NHS hospitals by official government inquiries in the 1960s and 1970s—for example, Ely (Department of Health, 1969) and Normansfield (Department of Health, 1978) hospitals—and continue until today. In 2011, the abuse of people with learning disabilities by staff of people with learning disabilities detained at the private Winterbourne View Hospital in South Gloucestershire was exposed by a BBC television programme (Department of Health, 2013; McKitterick, 2016). Even more recently, exposures by the BBC have included patient abuse within an NHS Trust in Essex in the East of England, with a public inquiry being set into place in 2022. This inquiry was set up after the Trust was prosecuted by the Health and Safety Executive and fined £1.5m by the courts over the deaths of 11 patients between 2004 and 2015 in the care of one of its predecessor NHS Trusts (Precey & Fox, 2022) and convictions of four staff over abuse within a private residential facility, Whorlton Hall, in North East England (Holt, 2023).

The likelihood is that false accusations do occur (see Lester, 2021; Safe Workers, 2023). However, mental health patients who allege they are victims of violence perpetrated by staff are disadvantaged by the fact that they have a diagnosis of mental illness. The institutional and sometimes judicial conjecture is that they either feel aggrieved about their treatment, that they are delusional or confused, or that they have malign motives. For example, Lester (2021) in the *Handbook for Judicial Officers* states that:

> Difficult complainants may… suffer from a major psychiatric illness, most often schizophrenia. These complainants are easily identified as they have the general signs of the illness, are aggrieved primarily by feelings of persecution and victimisation, and the content of their complaints arises totally from their delusional beliefs, which are often bizarre and in a constant state of flux. As a result, it is often impossible to define, let alone resolve, their complaints. Their pre-existing major psychiatric illness requires treatment, rather than the complaint being initially addressed.

Within the current group of co-authors, we agreed that I would only represent incidents that had common features of reliability. That being the individual demonstrated a contextual account of each and every incident. We agreed that where memories and recall were limited to feelings or intuitions, for the purpose of articulating testimony that carried a reasonable threshold of detail, we would not detail these in this chapter.

> *I'm confused sometimes, but I'm not a liar.*
> *It's my word against his, and we know how that works out.*

Between us, we assembled a combined 754 accounts of individual acts of violence and coercion. This involved many hours of interviewing those individuals so terribly impacted by their experiences. It required a great deal of time, patience and empathy, whilst at the same time adhering to rigour to ensure consistency and efficacy. Individuals generated multiple occasions when they were subject to violent behaviour. The range of multiple incidents ranged from 4 to 17 separate incidents. Eight individuals identified one or two practitioners being the perpetrators of the violence they endured. Eighteen individuals stated the acts were witnessed by other patients/members of staff.

We agreed on the following classifications of incidents.
1. Physical restraint
2. Medication administered by force
3. Being moved with force and against their will
4. Verbal abuse
5. Implied threat and coercion
6. Deliberately ignoring a patient
7. Threats to alter and tamper with care notes and records

## 3      Physical Restraint

We agreed that physical restraint involves being pinned down to the ground by multiple members of staff. Eight of our cohort experienced this a total of 37 times over a period of 5–19 years. Only three felt that restraint was avoidable, not because the behaviour posed a significant threat to themselves or others, but because experience informed them the service has a very low threshold for outbursts of any kind. All agreed that the majority of incidents could have been de-escalated satisfactorily through a more timely and considered response to their distress and frustrations.

The use of physical restraint on patients has rightly undergone great analysis and study. It is important to record just how upsetting it can be for someone to find themselves a patient in a mental health unit. You find yourself in an environment that is often at odds with your normal experience. You are subject to regimes that can often challenge your normal conduct and behaviour. You are expected to share a living space with complete strangers who may exhibit strange and difficult behaviours. Staff can appear to be agents of authority, who wish to do things you don't want to comply with. All normal routines, social contacts and references are suspended. These factors can contribute to feelings of anger and distress. If this isn't recognised early by staff, it can result in patients having violent outbursts. The cohort strongly believes that rather than focusing on the questionable efficacy of physically restraining someone, a greater emphasis should be placed on creating safer, more therapeutic environments to accommodate people in crisis. These places of safety and treatment should be resourced with well-trained and motivated staff, who share a common goal of delivering a high-quality service that is both audited and constructively tested whenever something doesn't reach the threshold of humane and therapeutic engagement.

Those who had undergone physical restraint received no obvious aftercare, and each of them lived with significant and ongoing emotional trauma. Even those in our cohort who had observed incidents of physical restraint reported feelings of distress and helplessness. Indeed, victims and observers stated that such incidents had a significant, enduring and traumatising impact on both the victim and witnesses, and also creates a divide between patients and services, one of fear, caution and mistrust physical. Restraint should always be the last option when every other intervention has been deployed and has failed. However, there is a shared concern that it is employed too soon, and with the wrong motives. Some believe that such unacceptability occurs when staff numbers, training and experience are not where they should be.

*People kept telling me to calm down, then I was on the floor with staff holding me down. I was so scared.*

*I saw the staff telling her to stop it, she kept shouting at them to go away, this went on till they forced her to the floor, and injected her, I was so scared.*

*Some staff seemed to enjoy confronting people, especially pinning them down.*

*How can hurting someone be helpful?*

## 4    Forcibly Medicated

We have included both sedatives administered intravenously at the time when an individual has been physically restrained, and other medications that come under Community Treatment Orders, legislation. The cohort had personal experience with both, and had strong feelings on the matter. Many talked about medication regimes being associated with feelings of fear and uncertainty. It is vital to begin at this point of origin, to establish how the benefits of medication are sometimes overstated and the side effects are not fully presented or explained; members of the group have had a range of medications imposed, with little or no context about their positive and negative effects. Psychiatric medication is both powerful in its formulation, and significant in its often-dramatic impact. The cohort was as one in its support of medication but under the following preconditions.

1. That it is evidenced to be effective for the right person, at the right time, and kept under both scrutiny and review.
2. Before a medication is prescribed, there should be a full and fair account of its evidenced benefits along with its potential risks and side effects. This information should not only be shared with the patient but with due consideration with their carer. Independent evaluations of its impact should be included in this discourse.
3. The relationship between prescriber and patient should be established on the principle of concordance rather than compliance.
4. Normal, everyday functioning should be impacted as little as possible by the introduction of medications.

The exact nature and properties of medication are not routinely and fully shared with patients, so when it becomes problematic for the patient, any historical concerns about the efficacy of some or all medications can become more certain, and resistance can take hold. When the patient enters a crisis period in their illness, the resistance can spill over into covert or overt rejection of medications. We spent a great deal of time exploring the dilemmas and concerns surrounding the pros and cons of medication. We also explored tensions that exist when treatment options are loaded heavily on the side of pharmacology. The consensus was that even with the very best intentions and full transparency some patients will not cooperate with taking certain medications. When this occurs, the right of the patient's self-determination should prevail, unless a lack of capacity can be established. Many members of the cohort shared personal insights that where compliance is promoted, patients will invariably find ways to undermine the intentions of the prescriber. When matters of fertility, impotence, obesity and insomnia are the very real consequences of certain medications, it is perfectly reasonable to withdraw your cooperation. We believe that a more trusting relationship between patient and prescriber would be mutually beneficial and an opportunity to resolve issues that might otherwise result in non-compliance.

*They tell you not to do drugs cause they're dangerous, then pump you full of weird stuff.*
*You know if you refuse meds, they'll find a way to make sure you take it.*
*I'm like a zombie on meds, and my family don't recognise me.*

## 5      Being Moved Forcibly and Against Your Will

The cohort contributed 31 incidents of being forcibly removed from an area or being physically compelled to move somewhere else. The extent of the force ranged from being assertively propelled by physical force, or by being shouted out to move from one location to another, for example, from a communal area to their bedroom, or from their bedroom to a review meeting or activity group on the ward. Once again this would often occur in the presence of other patients, and with staff observing the interaction. The cohort agreed that such incidents establish and underpin the power differential that permeates through many aspects of life in a unit. Furthermore, it serves to undermine the key importance of doing things with people rather than doing things to people. A sense of 'us' and 'them' can flourish in what those in the cohort characterised as a 'toxic environment'. These incidents were so commonplace that many accounts aren't detailed here because of a lack of quality recall and detail. The cohort supported our principle of only recording incidents that could be recalled with some accuracy. If we had not already agreed on this threshold the number of incidents would be very much higher. There was a consensus that such behaviours prevent the formation of relationships between patients built on mutual trust, consent and respect.

> If you found yourself in their way, they would just shove you out of the way, or barge past you, without asking you to move.
>
> When I was agitated, staff would surround me like a stray animal and get hold of me, moving me into my room.
>
> It felt like I was trespassing on their property, and rather than politely asking you to move out of the way, they would force me to get out of their way.
>
> It felt like I was an item of furniture in the wrong place all the time.
>
> I accept that there are times when staff need to get physically, but sometimes more force is used than is justified.
>
> Staff should have CCTV and body cameras, then you'd see a drop in complaints made about them, because they wouldn't get away with their abusive behaviour anymore.

## 6      Verbal Abuse

Our cohort was united in disclosing that they suffered verbal abuse both as inpatients and receiving services in the community, and perpetrated by a range of mental health practitioners. In total, they detailed 107 incidents that met our threshold for inclusion in this chapter. However, so common is the use of verbal abuse by practitioners, that our cohort had in the main become conditioned to it, and so it became just another background detail, which could not be reliably detailed. We agreed that verbal abuse for our purposes should capture:

> Humiliating patients through the use of dehumanising language. Using words that would reference their sexual orientation, body type, race, religion, social class, gender, sex, and weaponise them to inflict maximum harm.

The cohort recounted times when the presence or absence of family and friends was the motivation for some staff to mock them. If they had a network of supporters, they might be accused of being needy or manipulative. If they had no such support, some staff would say they were undeserving of love and care, that nobody was concerned about them, and that people were better off without them.

There was a consensus among the cohort that verbal abuse was a litmus test for other types of violence, as detailed in this chapter. It is its commonplace presence on wards and within community services, which is so concerning, so commonplace, that many patients would simply accept its everyday presence without challenge.

'Otherism' is a term more commonly used when exploring issues of race and religion. That we denigrate certain groups by consciously and unconsciously rationalising and justifying that not only are they significantly different to ourselves, but also they are inferior. If we view people as inferior or different, we are complicit in the harm this causes others, directly and indirectly.

Many reported that when they suffered verbal abuse, it was often explained away as a joke and that the victim should just lighten up and should not be so sensitive. This tactic that verbal abuse is just casual and victimless banter, is in itself evidence to support why other incidents of violence do not result in formal complaints, or indeed in satisfactory conclusions.

It is most important to detail how often staff will verbally abuse patients as malingerers, who are using and manipulating the system and casting doubt on the probity of their condition. Our cohort reports how hurtful and injurious such speculation can be.

The irony is that when patients sometimes verbally abuse staff, there is usually an assertive, timely and formal response by the service, often resulting in some sanction or penalty. However, our cohort's experience is that they do not benefit from the same fulsome and swift action.

> It costs nothing to be nice.
> Try saying please and thank you.
> I didn't think staff could get away with being so hurtful.
> They don't even make eye contact with you.
> If we talked to them like that, they'd soon have a go.

## 7    Implied Threat and Coercion

Again, using our very specific threshold measure for including incidents in this chapter, we gathered 83 incidents of implied threat and coercion. The use of coercion is in our experience endemic both in acute care and the community. Staff will seek to enforce the routines and processes that permeate institutions by bluntly or more subtly illustrating to the patient that refusal to follow instructions will be met with sanctions. We have experienced ourselves that such threats of sanctions are routinely disproportionate.

The cohort was as one in agreeing that it was often sometime after the incident, after some considerable period of reflection, that they were in a space to better judge whether they had experienced implied threat or coercion. Again, many events did not reach our threshold criteria, as the passage of time has taken its toll in terms of recall. If in this and our other subsets, incidents were investigated and assessed at the time, we would be presented with many more cases of violent actions and behaviour.

*They always get their own way.*
*If you don't do what you're told, they will make life very difficult for you.*
*I took my rights for granted until I became mentally ill.*
*You don't want to do it, but they have a way of working on you, until you think it's the best thing to do for everyone.*

## 8    Deliberately Ignoring Patients

Our cohort of co-authors shared multiple incidents of staff ignoring their questions, and requests for assistance. This appears to be so routine that it is impossible to quantify beyond being an almost default position of many practitioners. Readers might question how such behaviour equates to an act of violence, but our cohort believes that such basic disregard for someone's right to a timely answer or response, causes a great deal of harm, and inflicting unnecessary harm is in itself an act of violence. The cohort gave examples of staff not passing on routine messages from family and friends, meetings with clinicians being cancelled, referrals, benefits queries, and unspecified medication changes individually and collectively, we maintain that distrust of institutions is centred on such failures to be helpful, courteous and make difficulties just a little easier to endure, and failure to carry this out to a satisfactory standard can lead to stress, anxiety, justified paranoia and distress, all of which can reinforce people's feelings of powerlessness and alienation. In turn, this worsened people's mental state, at a time when practitioners and services should be focused on healing people.

## 9    Threats to Alter or Misrepresent Incidents or Events in Medical Records

This was in itself an extremely rare occurrence, but its importance is crucial to better understand the lengths that some practitioners and services will go to in order to present themselves in a better light, discredit the patient and undermine the efficacy of legally binding medical records. Our cohort believes strongly that though rare, it is a most sinister misuse of institutional power and authority.

Those affected in this manner reported threats to record non-compliance with medication regimes, portray the patient's behaviour and conduct unfavourably and not truthfully, and to detain or discharge for non-clinical reasons. They feel the motivations for such misconduct were grievances towards certain patients, retaliation for challenging someone's authority, and not complying with their care plans. Our cohort believes that the threshold to challenge this and all misuses of power that inflict harm is far too high. Recorded untruths, in medical records that are permanent in nature, are a prescient concern for each and every patient.

*He told me that what was recorded could make or break me.*
*How do they get away with it?*
*They're my records, not theirs.*
*I hate to think what's been written about me?*

## 10   Barriers and Obstacles Precluding Patient and Service User Involvement

When our cohort was assembled, I enquired why they hadn't availed themselves of the opportunity to represent, and attempt to resolve their traumatic experiences, through the many widely available co-production vehicles. The unanimous response was a lack of faith and trust that anything meaningful would come of it and that they might face adverse consequences. It is also worth noting how many were suspicious of patients who participated in such programmes. They believe these patients had 'betrayed' themselves and their peers, had become 'part of the problem' and were being 'manipulated'.

In this regard, it is of interest to consider the work of Flanders et al. (2016). They consider co-production as a high-risk method of social enquiry, being ethically complex, emotionally demanding and inherently unstable. Its attempts to bring together often conflicting expectations and agendas can take their toll. Consequentially, processes looking to reduce risk, use of force and conflict resolution remain underdeveloped and struggle to achieve lasting traction. These are factors that prevent past and present patients from working with institutions that have failed them. The promise of full and equal collaboration in reality becomes messy and unsatisfactory with the status quo largely unchanged. Those of our cohort who have attempted to bring about change from within have been frustrated and obstructed in their attempts to document their unedited, authentic and intact truth.

We are mindful that this chapter is in itself not a research paper, based on established protocols and methodology. However, I would like to draw your attention to a recent study by Macdonald (2021) titled 'Therapeutic Institutions of Violence'. My motive for doing so is that it provides an interesting context as to how the culture that prevailed before the 1983 Mental Health Act has survived many attempts to reform a controversial culture that attracted so much popular criticism.

Long-stay hospitals were routinely located in semi-rural communities, where secure and well-paid jobs were hard to find. These institutions gave opportunities for the populous to transition from insecure and low-paid manual labour, and into white-collar jobs that offered training and development. However, though some had a genuine desire to help and support their patients, because of a low qualification entry point, all and sundry could apply for these very desirable jobs, and some were not driven by such altruistic motives. They were afforded a level of power, influence and autonomy, which would previously have been out of their reach in traditional employment. Some flourished, and when their places of work began to close from the 1980s onwards, they moved to the next generation of mental health community-located resources, with some of the mindsets and behaviours that precipitated the closure of their former places of work. Many achieved senior roles and positions of influence. The old culture that had made so many negative headlines, and led to well-intentioned reforms, has had to bend and accommodate to fit this new more enlightened age, but some commentators believe the core values and principles of care through control are still largely in place.

I have been involved in the development of numerous strategies to make mental health organisations, future-facing, caring and compassionate, and patient-centred. The NHS has initiated a raft of strategic and operational initiatives specifically to impact more positively on the patient experience. Like many colleagues and peers, I happily participated in many of them. Disappointingly few achieved any real traction and were sidelined by institutional inertia.

As I have stated previously, I believed the system was open and ready for change and worked hard in leadership roles to implement these new approaches. I was optimistic that I and my colleagues were acting in mutual good faith. I trusted that we recognised the same inherent failings in the status quo that often place patients at risk and were as one in wanting to bring about lasting change. Over time, it emerged that the organisation wanted only superficial change that required minimal effort on their part to assimilate. Wholesale changes appear under present conditions beyond the acceptance of the most senior professionals and decision-makers.

For our cohort, it is most important that our desire to bring about these changes and reforms has not dampened. Though I now choose to focus my efforts outside of the mainstream, colleagues such as Ron Coleman, Glenn Roberts, Jeff Shepard, Len Bowers, Karen Taylor, Clare Shaw, Helen Glover, the National Survivor User Network (NSUN),[1] and Implementing Recovery through Organisational Change (ImROC)[2] remain dedicated to the process, and we are supported by the thousands of patients and survivors, who also desire change but are yet to find their voice and platform. Any incident of institutional violence is one too many and so we continue to campaign for zero tolerance.

---

[1] https://www.nsun.org.uk/

[2] https://imroc.org/

My career in health and social care has proved to me just how hard it is to challenge colleagues about things you observe firsthand and behaviours that you hear about thirdhand. Though absolute incidents of malpractice and criminality require a great deal of personal and professional courage to manage and deal with, it is the lower-level, nuanced indifference that proves to be the greater challenge. In health and social care, there have been all too many inquiries looking at the tragic realities of institutional violence. Overwhelmingly, they reveal a toxic culture characterised by the underreporting of malpractice, a lack of dignity and respect towards patients, with poor training, supervision, leadership, independent scrutiny and record keeping. All these individual and collective elements give staff-perpetrated violence the oxygen to flourish.

From the very outset, our intention and purpose have been to shine a light on the violence that is carried out by some practitioners representing some organisations towards some patients, some of the time. We do not claim these incidents typify the millions of interactions that take place on wards and in the community each year, but neither do we accept these actions are so rare, that they don't justify greater scrutiny. Many of the violent acts and behaviours perpetrated by practitioners are enabled by systemic, structural and cultural failings in the organisations themselves. We believe it is reasonable to say that central and local government, communities and society, and the media are culpable to some extent.

Central government sets the tone in respect of its policy commitments to health and social care. Irrespective of political philosophy, incumbent parties have set out grand plans for mental health, yet for decades it has been underfunded and resourced, and as a result, it has underperformed against the expectations of the end user. The Covid-19 inquiry has established that the UK has significantly fewer hospital beds when compared with many of our Western counterparts. In mental health, we have observed incremental declines in bed numbers. This is explained by pointing to the community being the best place to support the majority of patients. However, community services have also undergone the self-same steady decline in provision and funding. We are told the patient is at the centre of commissioning decisions, yet we receive less and less. Sanctions for poorly performing service providers seem too little and often too late. Parts of the media are yet to catch up with developments in understanding mental illness and demystifying the human emotional struggle. As a direct consequence of lurid media headlines, many people still perceive people in mental crisis as mad, bad and dangerous to know. For the past two decades, we have seen a reluctance to acknowledge mental illness, and a readiness to engage with all sorts of things titled mental health. There are many of us who consider this to be a deliberate move to make up and dress up what for many is a deeply distressing and enduring condition that is dangerous to simply glamourise and make entertaining.

The cohort is keen to communicate the indifference we see towards mental health from those who have the power to craft a meaningful way forward, resort to lurid or salacious headlines, or overly romanticised notions about how creative and inspiring mental illness can be. This paradoxical preoccupation serves only to hide the real experiences of everyday people. We believe there exists an enormous divide between intentions and deeds. This is best illustrated by the corporate response to public inquiries into institutional harm and violence, which is that lessons will be learned. Those same organisations end up repeating the very same incidents. The question is when will the learning end and lasting reforms begin? What is required to assure patients that they will be safe and treated with unconditional high regard? People should have complete confidence in their care provider being caring, compassionate and competent. We have been cognisant throughout to not label all professionals and services as falling short against this measure. Many of us have interacted with services and members of staff who have an unfailing positive demeanour and have been active supporters of the struggle to be as well as we can be. As we have previously stated, there are many real and momentous challenges to making a complaint about individual and institutional violence and a huge amount of good fortune in reaching the right outcome.

Our experience is that if you really want to understand the routine performance and efficacy of an organisation, don't restrict yourself to scanning their in-house surveys to determine quality and satisfaction, get yourself an invite to a patient drop-in, there you will encounter some compelling accounts that may test the organisations own findings. Surveys and questionnaires are a conundrum indeed. They seek honest and reliable feedback, yet the simple truth is that though anonymised, they carry a perceived jeopardy that all might not be as confidential as stated. Therefore, the resulting data might not be reliable or untainted. There exists a weight of evidence illustrating how victims can be manipulated into believing that they are wholly or partly inculcated and responsible in what has happened to them. Research in this field will validate our beliefs and experience and has been conducted with an objectivity and neutrality that we do not possess. We do accept that our position, though constructive, is deeply subjective, in as much as it is profoundly personal. This should not discredit or undermine the value of the collective breadth of experiences, much of it confirmed by one another. We propose that enough subjective lived experience coalesces around a set of themes, that in itself can be viewed as having the same currency as objectivity.

The typical surveys and questionnaires to determine patient/service user experiences here in the UK, tend to invite binary responses to set questions. These questions will have undergone little if any scrutiny from individual patients or patient groups. We accept that those setting the questions in the main are not setting out to deliberately manipulate the process, but it is probable that this methodology has some inherent flaws. The process should for efficacy and fidelity reasons be conducted by a third party in order to convey confidence in its delivery. The old saying, that 'he who pays the piper calls the tune', resonates with many patients, and so attracts only superficial attention from the respondent, which harvests unreliable data. I and many others would be more likely to commit to a process that is independent and more configured to qualitative data.

If we, as patients, find the complaints process and practice audits, ill-prepared and conceived to highlight the violent actions that are prevalent in our services, where else can the patient turn to for validation? I have always believed that a public-facing organisation should embrace both critique and even open dissent on occasion, just as readily as it absorbs and assimilates compliments. This standard has been my default position throughout my long and relatively successful career. Over time this principle underwent a great deal of attrition. My work in mental health strategy and operation has afforded me influence, but only on the periphery and in the margins. My achievements were no more than incremental and relatively easy wins. My original ambitions of transformation and reform remained unfulfilled. This inertia carried with it a great deal of frustration, and so I abandoned my attempts to bring about change from within and to work for change externally. I am not alone, and many have tried to work with the system in good faith. We wanted many of the same things: honesty, transparency, easy-to-access care and support, and compassionate staff. It isn't a matter of us failing against our brief, but not being allowed to succeed by an institution that is inconsistent in its strategy, operation and responsiveness. The tension is that on the inside you run the risk of being co-opted and 'professionalised' and becoming part of the problem you set out to challenge. On the outside, you are open to judgements that label you as militant, unrealistic and unhelpful. We are on the outside and still campaigning for change because we have tried working within the system and finding the whole experience unfulfilling. At no time have we chosen to place ourselves outside, looking in, it is simply a case of the institution failing in its invitation of full and meaningful collaboration. We propose that any public acceptance that an organisation has a problem with practitioner-perpetrated violence carries with it far too much jeopardy to its reputation and Care Quality Commission rating. We do not have all the answers and accept that to break out from this pragmatic lack of progress, we do need to cooperate, but on equal terms and with mutually agreed terms of reference.

## 11   Recommendations for Change

At the outset of this chapter, we were clear about a readiness to be candid and a desire to be constructive. To this end, we wish to craft a way forward with a manifesto, which we believe can eliminate harm and violence in our places of safety.

We believe this manifesto to be ambitious yet to secure its full implementation it will require a reconfiguration of present funding and initial capital spending. We accept that though some points are relatively easy wins, some will require a paradigm shift in respect of priorities. We run the risk of being labelled naïve in our proposals, yet we believe that it is vital for change to take place, for the reasons set out in this chapter. It is our intention to challenge decision-makers, not alienate them. We believe many from the patient community would be prepared to set aside their scepticism and match the goodwill which will be a prerequisite for engagement.

1. A prominent sign in every setting stating: 'Violence and aggression from staff or patients will not be tolerated, and any harm inflicted will result in a swift and proportionate response'.
2. Policies should include a statement of intent such as: 'Institutional violence will be treated as a serious breach of duty of care, and dealt with as criminal matter where apropriate, as well as being subject to disciplinary proceedings'.
3. Trials should take place to see if body worn cameras can positively impact patient and indeed staff safety and to see if it might have a benefit in moderating conduct in general.
4. As a matter of urgency, there should be an independent review of the use and application of restraint in our care settings. In the meantime, we must have more transparency regarding the decision-making process, the leadership role and intervention/action to establish what post-incident support was required, and finally post-incident debriefs with the full involvement of peer colleagues.
5. A multi-disciplinary review of the routines and protocols in our inpatient units. The review should publish its full findings with mandatory recommendations within a timely period.
6. Medication regimes should be used not to render patients compliant and malleable. Medications should only be prescribed for therapeutic purposes.
7. Florid outbursts should be viewed as symptoms and not simply as threats. We accept the real need to protect everyone, but individuals should not endure punitive sanctions, as a hastily formulated response.
8. A great deal of work must take place, to foster and secure better interpersonal relations on the ward. The environment should reflect a place where staff look forward to coming to work, patients feel they can begin to feel better, and carers and friends are welcome visitors.
9. All sides need to commit to being the best version of themselves and treat one another with dignity and respect.
10. Service provider organisations, as a matter of urgency, need to commission an independent group to review and reform complaints procedures. They need to be easy to navigate, the burden of proof needs to be realistic, and not discourage complainants.

This list should become the priority for us all. There is much to be done but the solutions are out there and do exist, but in isolation. This type of silo working must cease, and best practices should reach every point of the compass.

## 12  Postscript

As we were carrying out final pieces of work on the chapter, our feelings of having achieved something that we could all take some pride in, despite the distressing nature of the subject matter, we were hit by the undercover investigation into inhumane treatment in a leading NHS mental health unit discussed above.[3] Once again whistleblowers and undercover journalists uncovered an establishment that operated outside of the law and ignored policies, professional standards, duty of care and safeguarding. Service users and patients are often made to feel that they are to blame for failures of standards of care; either they are making up the incident, or inflating it for nefarious motivations.

During my social work training, we students were encouraged to avoid absolutes, but listening to the despairing accounts shared by our cohort, reinforced by the documentary exposing yet another unit that had failed to honour the trust placed in their hands, 'evil' and 'cruel' seem entirely proportionate adjectives to apply to such abhorrent behaviours. That establishment had been awarded a 'Good' rating by the UK Government's inspection service Care Quality Commission (CQC).

> *They will take it on the chin, promise that lessons will be learned, move on and repeat the same crimes in five years' time.*
>
> *It's not the first case of whistleblowing and exposing brutal staff and uncaring services, I hope this is the one that will lead to change, but I'm not holding my breath.*
>
> *We are collateral damage for a service that no one really cares about. In a week from today, most people will have forgotten about it, unless they are unfortunate to find themselves as a patient.*
>
> *It needs dismantling and redesigned by us, the patients.*

These sentiments carry with them a certain cynicism, but it is well founded. In my working life, I've witnessed one tragic failure of care, being replaced by another, then another and so on. There is fatigue regarding the platitudes forthcoming from service leaders and politicians following every inquiry. The number one default response is that lessons will be learned. If lessons are being learned, why are we witnessing one incident after another? When will we reach a point of competent, safe practitioners and safe services ensuring that we have finally learned those lessons once and for all?

We have to challenge the ways in which patients are involved in projects to improve patient safety and the patient experience. These patients must not be co-opted by the organisation. Instead, their independence and autonomy should be viewed as their strength and an active asset to the task at hand. We might consider the merits of organisations having to devolve their patient involvement activities to stand-alone patient-led and external consultancies. Practitioners, politicians and organisations have had so many opportunities to advance patient safety, yet the evidence would suggest that all too often their efforts have little or no positive impact. We must place those with lived experience front and centre of any future transformation plans. We propose that patients are not just patients; they have diverse employment backgrounds that might bring a more objective vision of where we need to be and how to get there. These peer colleagues must however resist the often subtle attempts by institutions to bring them into the fold and see things their way. This I believe isn't our primary purpose. It is

---

[3] West Lane Hospital: Review finds 'deteriorating spiral' of care in months before teenagers' deaths: https://www.itv.com/news/tyne-tees/2023-03-20/review-finds-deteriorating-spiral-of-care-at-mental-health-hospital

possible to be collegiate and collaborative whilst maintaining an authentic critique of both resistance and pragmatism. In my work experience, a patient involvement team, held within the service provider's structure, for all the goodwill in the world, has a challenge to both articulate the patient narrative and the service's own operational and strategic priorities. Many of my peers don't want minimal tweaking at the margins of the service; rather, we propose that fulfilling the mission statements of some organisations requires a root and branch transformation.

Unless all stakeholders commit to an honest assessment of the structural and systemic flaws that allow violence to be perpetrated by staff against vulnerable people, we will all be complicit in another plan that has no radical centre. It is a radical plan that is required. The discourse that occurs in Board rooms and across conference tables doesn't reflect the stories that take place in virtual and in-person patient forums. Don't judge a service by a glossy brochure on its own merits. Instead, go along unannounced and sit in a patient coffee drop-in, then compare and contrast the two worlds. What we need is an ongoing 'sea change' of questioning service performance, patient safety and accountability. We need to test orthodoxy and demonstrate an ability to look beyond and underneath what is presented to us as being 'factual'.

If we are not to let yet another watershed moment pass into historical ignominy, we must demand a paradigm shift away from the status quo, and in the direction of meaningful, measurable and patient-led reform. All these salient points relate to our 'agenda for change' detailed earlier in the chapter. It's about shining a light into every facet of patient care, where nowhere is off limits. We desperately need far more unannounced monitoring inspections. Staff in these units need to feel that eyes and ears are upon them at all times. Transparency and a culture of openness must replace environments that evoke fear and suspension. Patients, staff, carers and friends, and visitors should be able to enter a unit with a sense of hope even optimism and leave with a sense of accomplishment and shared progress.

Finally, I must thank all those in our cohort, for their consistent support and valuable critique. They tasked me to write a journal of sorts spanning the multiple failings that lead to institutional violence. They asked me to be brave, consistent and unwavering, and not to deliver a textbook. On all these points, I hope I have fulfilled their expectations.

## References

Bhavsar, V., Dean, K., Hatch, S. L., MacCabe, J. H., & Hotopf, M. (2019). Psychiatric symptoms and risk of victimisation: A population-based study from Southeast London. *Epidemiology and Psychiatric Sciences, 28*(2), 168–178. https://doi.org/10.1017/S2045796018000537

Choe, J. Y., Teplin, L. A., & Abram, K. M. (2008). Perpetration of violence, violent victimization, and severe mental illness: Balancing public health concerns. *Psychiatric Services, 59,* 153–164.

Cremin, K. M., Philips, J., Sickinger, C., & Zelhof, J. (2009). Ensuring a fair hearing for litigants with mental illnesses: The law and psychology of capacity, admissibility, and credibility assessments in civil proceedings. *Brooklyn Journal of Law and Policy, 17*(2). Retrieved February 12, 2024 from https://brooklynworks.brooklaw.edu/jlp/vol17/iss2/2.

Dean, K., Laursen, T. M., Pedersen, C. B., Webb, R. T., Mortensen, P. B., & Agerbo, E. (2018). Risk of being subjected to crime, including violent crime, after onset of mental illness: A

Danish National Registry study using police data. *JAMA Psychiatry, 75*(7), 689–696. https://doi.org/10.1001/jamapsychiatry.2018.0534

Department of Health. (1969). *Report of the Committee of Inquiry into allegations of ill-treatment of patients and other irregularities at the Ely Hospital, Cardiff, Cmnd 3975.* HMSO.

Department of Health. (1978). *Report of the Committee of Inquiry into Normansfield Hospital, Cmnd 7357.* HMSO.

Department of Health. (2013). *Winterbourne view: Transforming care one year on.* HMSO.

Flanders, M., Wood, M., & Cunningham, M. (2016). The politics of co-production: Risks, limits and pollution. *Evidence & Policy, 12*(2), 261–279. https://doi.org/10.1332/174426415X14412037949967

Foucault, M. (1961). *Madness and civilization: A history of insanity in the age of reason.* Routledge.

Holt, A. (2023, April 28). Whorlton Hall verdicts: Can further scandals be prevented? *BBC News.* Retrieved February 12, 2024, from https://www.bbc.co.uk/news/uk-65388035.

Joyes, E. C., Jordan, M., Winship, G., & Crawford, P. (2021). Inpatient institutional care: The forced social environment. *Frontiers in Psychology.* https://doi.org/10.3389/fpsyg.2021.690384

Kamperman, A. M., Henrichs, J., Bogaerts, S., Lesaffre, E. M. E. H., Wierdsma, A. I., Ghauharali, R. R. R., Swildens, W., Nijssen, Y., Gaag, M., Theunissen, J. R., Delespaul, P. A., Weeghel, J., van Busschbach, Y. T., Kroon, H., Teplin, L. A., van de Mheen, D., & Mulder, C. L. (2014). Criminal victimisation in people with severe mental illness: A multi-site prevalence and incidence survey in The Netherlands. *PLoS One, 9*(3), e91029. https://doi.org/10.1371/journal.pone.0091029

Khalifeh, H., Johnson, S., Howard, L. M., Borschmann, R., Osborn, D., Dean, K., Hart, C., Hogg, J., & Moran, P. (2015). Violent and non-violent crime against adults with severe mental illness. *British Journal of Psychiatry, 206*(4), 275–282. https://doi.org/10.1192/bjp.bp.114.147843

Kumar, S., Guite, H., & Thornicroft, G. (2001). Service users' experience of violence within a mental health system: A study using grounded theory approach. *Journal of Mental Health, 10*(6), 597–611. https://doi.org/10.1080/09638230120041353

Latalova, K., Kamaradova, D., & Prasko, J. (2014). Violent victimization of adult patients with severe mental illness: A systematic review. *Neuropsychiatric Disease and Treatment, 10,* 1925–1939. https://doi.org/10.2147/NDT.S68321.2014

Lester, G. (2021). Handbook for Judicial Officers: The querulant litigant. Retrieved February 12, 2024, from https://www.judcom.nsw.gov.au/publications/benchbks/judicial_officers/querulant_litigant.html#ftn.d5e18731.

Liberati, E., Richards, N., Ratnayake, S., Gibson, J., & Martin, G. (2023). Tackling the erosion of compassion in acute mental health services. *BMJ, 382,* e073055. https://doi.org/10.1136/bmj-2022-073055

Macdonald, S. J. (2021). Therapeutic institutions of violence: Conceptualising the biographical narratives of mental health service users/survivors accessing long term "treatment" in England. *Journal of Criminological Research, Policy and Practice, 7*(2), 179–194. https://doi.org/10.1108/JCRPP-02-2020-0027

Mahomed, F., Stein, M. A., Sunkel, C., Restivo, J. L., & Patel, V. (2022). Mental health, human rights, and legal capacity. *Lancet Psychiatry, 9*(5), 341–342. https://doi.org/10.1016/S2215-0366(21)00463-6

Maniglio, R. (2009). Severe mental illness and criminal victimization: A systematic review. *Acta Psychiatrica Scandinavica, 119*(3), 180–191. https://doi.org/10.1111/j.1600-0447.2008.01300

McKitterick, B. (2016). The Winterbourne View Hospital scandal "vanishing pact". *International Journal of Public Leadership, 12*(1), 2–13.

Mental Health Act. (1983). Retrieved February 12, 2024 from https://www.legislation.gov.uk/ukpga/1983/20/contents.

National Institute for Health and Care Excellence. (2015). *Violence and aggression: Short-term management of violent and physically threatening behaviour in mental health, health and community settings.* National Institute for Health and Care Excellence. Retrieved February 12, 2024, from https://www.nice.org.uk/guidance/ng10.

Precey, M. & Fox, N. (2022, April 28). Essex mental health services inquiry probes 1,500 deaths. BBC News. Retrieved February 12, 2024, from https://www.bbc.co.uk/news/uk-england-essex-60865519.

Rossa-Roccor, V., Schmid, P., & Steinert, T. (2020). Victimization of people with severe mental illness outside and within the mental health care system: Results on prevalence and risk factors from a multicenter study. *Frontiers in Psychiatry, 11*, 563860. https://doi.org/10.3389/fpsyt.2020.563860

Safe Workers. (2023). Defending yourself against false accusations at work in 7 steps. Retrieved February 12, 2024, from https://www.safeworkers.co.uk/employment-law/false-allegations-work/.

Szmukler, G. (2018). *Men in white coats: Treatment under coercion*. Oxford University Press.

World Health Organization. (2022). *Mental disorders*. World Health Organization.

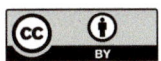

# Eastern and Western Approaches to Coercion in Mental Health

B. N. Raveesh, Peter Lepping, and Tom Palmstierna

## 1    Introduction

Coercion is a global reality in caring for people with psychiatric illnesses. Its history goes back to the earliest known mental health systems and remains present as psychiatric care moves beyond mental health institutions and into the community. Despite its global prevalence, coercion, both as a concept and practice, has remained understudied in the context of this discipline. Researchers, carers and psychiatrists have only recently begun to turn a critical eye on the mental healthcare systems that have long maintained coercive practices and started raising questions about the long-term consequences of coercion, whether it is avoidable and how.

However, the answers to these questions are as varied as there are psychiatric practices around the world. Coercion is a complex phenomenon and the forms it takes are inextricably linked to cultural and social norms. For instance, individual autonomy is valued in most European and North American cultures, whereas Indian, Arab, African and Japanese cultures are more community and family-centred. This difference may affect involuntary admission and informed consent in family-centred versus individualist societies (Shah & Basu, 2010), although all societies undergo constant changes and developments that change attitudes about coercion over time. Soft medical paternalism ('the doctor knows best') may be more acceptable to the

B. N. Raveesh (✉)
Department of Psychiatry, Mysore Medical College and Research Institute, Mysuru, Karnataka, India

P. Lepping
Centre for Mental Health and Society, Wrexham Academic Unit, Bangor University, Bangor, Wales, UK
e-mail: peter.lepping@wales.nhs.uk

T. Palmstierna
Department of Clinical Neuroscience, Karolinska Institute, Huddinge, Sweden
e-mail: tom.palmstierna@ki.se

© The Author(s) 2024                                                                                    27
N. Hallett et al. (eds.), *Coercion and Violence in Mental Health Settings*,
https://doi.org/10.1007/978-3-031-61224-4_2

patient in less individualistic societies. However, that does not imply the right of the treating agent to assume the role of a benign decision-maker in the form of involuntary treatment and coercion. Due to this complexity and cultural dependency, straightforward directions about ethical considerations and normative claims about what should or should not be done cannot be expected. Even in high-income countries where substantial research has been conducted on the subject in the past 20 years, there are no conclusive answers, and debates are still ongoing. It took European researchers three decades to get from an initial starting point of general curiosity when each other's practices were deemed barbaric to start to appreciate that staff in different countries have developed coercive measures for specific cultural and practical reasons. In lower-income countries, on the other hand, much research is still needed. To understand how mental health institutions and community care systems can be designed, considering the culture-specific issues surrounding coercion, we need to understand the causes and consequences of coercion in different settings and the roles and perceptions of various stakeholders. In the following sections of this chapter, we explore some of these debates to understand the different perspectives and analyse their implications for practice. We first discuss some of the key elements of the concept of coercion and then consider its application in one specific non-Western country, India. In this way, we hope to broaden the debate about this issue to ensure that voices outside of the standard perspective are considered.

## 2    Definitions of Coercion

Despite the long history of the concept of coercion and its existence within nearly every discipline of thought, such as philosophy, medicine (including psychiatry), law, sociology and literature, a comprehensive understanding of the full implications of coercion within a given context still prompts debate and discussion. Coercion is the act of exercising power, defined as an agent intentionally influencing the behaviour of others (Lee, 2014). The agent could do this by persuasion, but if this fails, they may make the other person do something or act against their will by trickery, intimidation, threats, force or extortion. It may involve the infliction of physical or psychological pain to enhance the threat's credibility, as in extreme torture cases (Rhodes, 2000). Coercion is closely related to exercising power. Power can be exercised in a threefold fashion: (a) immanently as a felt essence that is used to overcome resistances; (b) by implying the possible use of persuasion, manipulations, coercion, compulsion, pressures or constraints; or (c) by resorting to the actual use of duress, force and violence (Arboleda-Flórez, 2005).

In law, being coerced is akin to acting 'under duress' or because of 'undue influence'. It is also seen as equivalent to an 'extortion' crime. In the case of a victim, if the threat is substantial, coercion can be used as a defence with two possible meanings: when the victim was compelled by force of authority to do something, or when actual power was used to cause the victim to do something (compulsion) they would not otherwise do. Coercion could also be conceived as exerting social influence via international power exercised through authoritative requests, persuasion, induce-ments, threats, offers or actual use of force (Albrecht, 2016).

These definitions merely scrape the surface of the variety of questions that the issue of coercion raises in actuality. How does pressure affect its victims? What ethical concerns need to be presented when normative statements about force are made in theory? How do people experience coercion? What necessitates coercion in any given circumstance? How can we begin to address the conflicts of interest that arise? In many ways, the focus of this chapter is an attempt to move towards a deeper understanding of the reasons behind coercion in medical practice, specifi-cally psychiatry, and how such an understanding can inform ongoing and future techniques, policies and research.

## 3     Current Understandings of Coercion

Coercive measures are seen internationally as human rights issues, and internation-ally binding documents like the United Nations Convention on the Rights of Persons with Disabilities (UNCRPD) emphasise this. The effects of protecting human rights in providing mental health care to ensure good outcomes are an area of interest for this research.

International studies have shown that from 3% (Portugal) to 30% (Sweden) of all psychiatric inpatient episodes consist of involuntary hospital admission of general psychiatric patients (Salize & Dressing, 2004). These figures are rising across Europe, for example, in England where 60% of all psychiatric admissions were involuntary in 2019–2020. As shown in another European multi-site study using 2012/2013 data, about 5% of all inpatients (Lepping et al., 2016) and approximately one-third of involuntarily admitted patients were subjected to individual coercive measures such as mechanical restraint, seclusion or forced medication within the first 4 weeks after admission; again, variation across clinical sites is enormous, and rates can be as high as 60% (Raboch et al., 2010). There is no broad and robust empirical knowledge base on such service provision elements (Kallert et al., 2008). Ethical issues associated with clinical practice and research on coercive measures have become important. They range from exploring undue influences on research and adequately assessing the ability to give informed consent to professionals' atti-tudes towards coercive measures (Steinert, 2007).

There is a lack of data on the effectiveness of coercive measures. The literature on coercive measures includes a long list of possible adverse effects and complica-tions of being restrained. This includes complications such as pneumonia, circula-tory obstruction, cardiac stress, skin damage, poor appetite, dehydration, thrombosis and accidental death. Other complications reported are injuries whilst getting out of restraints, vomiting, self-harm, injuring others and hostility or increased agitation (Mohr, 2006). Studies from outside India on this topic often conclude that the rela-tionship between subjective and reported coercive incidents and care outcomes is not yet fully understood and should be investigated (Kjellin & Wallsten, 2010). A recent systematic review concluded that the data on whether compliance improves after compulsory admissions are inconclusive (Cossu et al., 2023).

Developing and critically analysing strategies to reduce coercive measures in different settings are areas of significant relevance for public mental health care and research. Coercive measures are not only essential in shaping public opinion regarding psychiatry, they are also the main area in which this medical discipline faces increasing criticism, particularly from a human rights perspective (Dudley et al., 2012), voiced by users of mental health services and prominent international political bodies such as the Council of Europe. Furthermore, coercive measures constitute and symbolise a core element of the relationship between mental health professionals and their patients and dialogue with professional bodies. A variety of interventions have been identified to be useful in reducing coercion in psychiatric settings in high-income countries. These can be divided into seven different types of content: organisation, staff training, risk assessment, environment, psychotherapy, debriefings and advance directives (Hirsch & Steinert, 2019). It requires sustained efforts and clear leadership focus on all of these types of interventions to achieve reduced coercion over a sustained period of time.

## 4 Coercion on a Spectrum of Treatment Pressure

Szmukler and Appelbaum (2009) have conceptualised a hierarchical framework of 'treatment pressures' commonly encountered in clinical practice. The lowest level of pressure is persuasion, in which the benefits and risks of treatment are debated, and the patient's arguments are respected. A higher level of force may be exerted by using an interpersonal relationship between a clinician and a patient to exert 'leverage', perhaps by expressing disapproval or withdrawing emotional support. 'Inducement' describes the exertion of positive pressure on the patient by offering financial or other benefits in exchange for cooperation. For example, a threat could be made to withdraw services on which the patient relies (which is typically more coercive than simply failing to offer inducements over and above standard services) or to detain the patient in the hospital. Finally, at the highest level of the hierarchy, patients may be compelled to take treatment against their will by detention in the hospital and, if necessary, by using physical force.

## 5 Coercion in Healthcare

There has been growing attention paid to coercion in both Eastern and Western health services among health professionals, managers, service users/patients, researchers, policymakers and society at large. 'Coercion' in health care refers to formal, informal and perceived coercion. Legal coercion is regulated by legislation, and can include physical restraint, seclusion and forced medication; other interventions, often called informal coercion, are less regulated. Perceived coercion is the subjective perception of the intervention received. Healthcare professionals have different opinions about the use of coercion. A study from New Zealand conducted by Bigwood and Crowe (2008) describes moral injury and fear among health workers due to physically restraining patients. The nurses said restraint 'is part of the job, but it spoils the job' (Bigwood & Crowe, 2008). The ambiguity connected to their role could easily lead to feelings of moral distress. Vatne and Fagermoen (2007) reported conflicting personal feelings concerning the ambiguity created by balancing safety, acknowledging dignity, and facilitating treatment. To cope with using coercion in their work, some employees tend to defend the need to use it. A newer study in India amongst psychiatrists shows the ambivalence in clinicians' attitudes towards coercion (Gowda et al., 2019). Whilst two-thirds of psychiatrists perceived physical and chemical restraint (sedation) as necessary and acceptable in acute emergency care, one-third felt their patients lost autonomy, dignity and the possibility of interpersonal contact. One-third also agreed that some patients could have been treated with less restriction and fewer coercive measures. But whilst coercion can have deleterious effects on patients and staff, the problems related to coercion are complex, making it difficult to discontinue its use. There are justifications for coercion which are articulated in mental health laws in all democratic states and confirmed by High or Constitutional Courts and Ethical Bodies.

Debates surrounding definitions of coercion are further intensified in psychiatry, where coercive treatment, although controversial, is legally sanctioned under limited conditions (Szmukler & Appelbaum, 2009). Coercive measures always involve a conflict of medico-ethical principles. Medical professionals need to balance beneficence ('doing good') and non-maleficence (avoiding harm) with the requirement to respect the patient's autonomy to justify coercion in extreme situations (Beauchamp & Childress, 2001), and requirements to provide safe environments for staff and visitors.

In the context of health care, an exploration of the issue of coercive treatment concentrates on diverse settings amongst patients who are highly vulnerable to the use of coercive measures, such as general hospitals, nursing homes and long-term care homes for chronically and severely ill or disabled persons (Kallert, 2008). Acknowledgment of practices as coercive varies widely in those settings, and data collection and reporting are usually concentrated on psychiatric wards only. As a result, it is difficult to gauge a comprehensive picture of the actual situation of coercion in health care, even in a single country, let alone globally, and even though health workers and patients are among the most likely to experience aggression and subsequent coercive interventions (Lepping & Raveesh, 2013) and should therefore be highly invested in the subject matter.

## 5.1 Coercion in Mental Health Care

In a psychiatric context, the term 'coercive measures' usually refers to coercive interventions occurring during hospitalisation in psychiatric wards (Kalisova et al., 2007). However, with the expansion of community care, coercion can also be experienced outside hospital settings (usually legalised with Community Treatment

Orders). Increasingly, implied pressure to comply with treatment plans can be perceived as coercive (Burns et al., 2011). Szmukler (2015) points out that coercion covers both compulsion and threats, in contrast to Wertheimer (1993) who contrasts threats and offers, with the latter not being considered coercive. When a patient is at imminent risk of harming themselves or others, the need for coercion is less disputed (Swartz et al., 2002). The question is more difficult in non-emergency situations, but where aspects of safety or harm to health are the primary consideration. Such problems commonly occur in geriatric medicine and psychiatry. In these cases, it can be unclear whether the principle of acting in the patient's best interest justifies the restriction of the patient's autonomy.

Coercion has been part of medical interventions in India and Europe since antiquity. In psychiatry, they are partly related to outdated prevailing beliefs about the nature and prognosis of mental illnesses. People with mental disorders across the world were usually placed at the state's mercy in person or imprisoned, chained or banished from their homes and towns (Colin, 2014). This put the responsibility for care firmly into the arms of the detaining authorities. However, modern research into psychiatric illness and into violence in healthcare settings has not confirmed ancient assumptions that violence in healthcare settings is always illness-related and that patients always lack capacity and thus have diminished responsibility for their actions. To know when an action is related to illness has profound legal implications for the patient, especially in cases of severe violence against staff and members of the public.

Perceived coercion in mental health is defined as an individual's perception of being pressured by internal or external sources to accept containment and treatment for mental illness (Lee & Seo, 2021). It is a challenging clinical issue. Compulsory admission and other coercive interventions are complex and stressful experiences for patients and family carers. Whether coercion damages the patient's autonomy, liberty and dignity must be understood from the perspectives of the service provider, clinicians and service users. In a study undertaken by Theodoridou et al. (2012), investigating the relationship between perceived coercion and the therapeutic relationship, they found that 'perceived coercion predicts the patients' appraisal of the therapeutic relationship'. Their findings suggest that perceived coercion is related to a more negative patient–therapist relationship, whilst a perceived loss of autonomy is closely linked to a negative relationship between the clinician and the patient. van den Hooff and Goossensen (2014) found that whether or not patients are listened to stand out as a core experience in determining whether they feel respected as human beings in the case of involuntary admission. Thus, the simple question of how to relate positively in an interaction may sometimes be just as important as determining what treatment to start. It indicates the importance of communication between clinician and patient. Indeed, the qualities allowing clinicians to be effective in helping patients (clinical skills, knowledge and attitudes) overlap with the qualities that make them morally good (Liberto, 2021).

Coercive interventions in mental health care do not come exclusively from mental health services (Sashidharan et al., 2019). Pressure to accept treatment can arise from family and carers who are often intimately involved in treating and caring for someone with a severe mental illness. The family's role is vital and worthy of note. Family members often deal with crises and are interested in good outcomes. In addition, a person can feel coerced to accept treatment because of social and cultural expectations (Canvin et al., 2013). There are distinct differences between Western countries and India regarding the practical importance of relatives. In India, all psychiatric and medical admissions usually require a member of the family to look after the patient whilst they are an inpatient. In Western countries, this is almost never the case, despite recent attempts to allow relatives of dementia patients to remain present during hospital admissions. Autonomy principles may make it impossible for staff to discuss patient progress with their family if patients do not wish this to happen. In both settings, however, relatives want to be engaged with treatment decisions and aftercare. In India, having extended family support decreased the perception of coercion whilst a psychiatric inpatient (Raveesh et al., 2016b).

The expectations and experiences of family members about working with mental health professionals and services can be unclear (Gowda et al., 2018). A potential discrepancy between the wishes of family members and patients can present an additional complication. The role of family members in decisions and services regarding treatment tends to be poorly recognised in involuntary admissions and other coercive practices. A hospital stay will be stressful for the family members caring for a patient. A better understanding of family carers' attitudes may help to address their needs more effectively and improve their involvement in care during and after involuntary hospital admission for the patient's benefit. In India, where family members are always present during the patient's hospital admission, they have been shown to be a trigger of patient aggression and part of managing aggression, exemplifying the complexity of the carer experience.

## 5.2  Coercion in Indian Mental Health Services

Coercive experiences are associated with several socio-demographic and clinical variables, especially concerning perceived coercion and negative pressure. An Indian study on perceived coercion found that perceived coercion was higher amongst women than men, higher amongst Muslims and Christians than Hindus, and higher amongst those from lower-income groups (Raveesh et al., 2016a). Perceived coercion decreased with past experiences of coercion, forensic history and more prolonged illness duration. It showed that despite India being a more community-oriented society than most high-income countries, coercion is a reality for Indian patients. The factors that increase perceived coercion include poor insight, poor global functioning and the persistent severity of illness (Gowda et al., 2018). In keeping with studies from the UK, 87% of patients reported that their admission was justified even though many felt coerced during their hospital stay (Raveesh et al., 2016a).

In an Indian study on perceived coercion, it was found that most psychiatrists feel that coercion violates the patients' integrity and may harm therapeutic relationships. Psychiatrists have more significant experience with various treatment interventions than family caregivers. They may also internalise different normative ethical attitudes during their medical education (Raveesh et al., 2016b). The Indian psychiatrists' attitudes align with the findings (Raveesh et al., 2016b) in European samples and an Australian survey (Kinner et al., 2017). In two Dutch studies, a staff mix of more and less experienced staff (Janssen et al., 2007) and the availability and application of clear treatment protocols (Verlinde et al., 2017) predicted less use of coercion. This emphasises the need for a clear non-coercive treatment protocol in Indian mental health care settings. The staff's attitude may be influenced by knowledge of the hospital resources, their training in coercive practices, locally supervised operating procedures for coercive interventions, and cultural factors, such as accepting doctors' decisions (Viswanath & Chaturvedi, 2012).

When mental illness is associated with aggressive behaviour, staff and caregivers are commonly the targets of such aggression (Danivas et al., 2016). Democratic countries tend to have legal frameworks regulating the use of coercion in healthcare, usually sanctioned and amended by High Court decisions. Employers have a legal duty to provide safe environments for staff. This is the background to staff and caregivers' attitudes towards coercion. Psychiatrists in our Indian study (Raveesh et al., 2016b) agreed more often than family caregivers with the statements regarding coercion for safety reasons. Both psychiatrists and family caregivers agreed that coercion should not be used more frequently in treatment. However, almost half of all family caregivers wanted to see more coercion as an intervention, probably because they face difficulty bringing a person with a mental disorder to the hospital. Agreement existed only in the judgement about the necessity of coercion in cases of aggression and lack of insight. Staff and family caregivers agreed that coercion could be reduced significantly, given more time and personal contact. These findings are similar to a Norwegian study (Wynn et al., 2011). Researchers have found a significant relationship between staff attitudes and the use of restraint. The nursing staff who were not actively involved in coercion had more negative attitudes towards using it and more knowledge about the regulations regarding its use (Janssen et al., 2007).

In the Indian context family, caregivers' attitudes towards patients may differ from clinicians' and patients' attitudes because caregivers are often confronted first and for some time with a patient's symptoms. In addition, they need fast recovery as the costs associated with the illness may lead to significant financial distress. The family caregivers' perception of outward- or inward-directed aggression or suicidal tendencies may differ from psychiatrists', as they are emotionally involved. The general education of family caregivers is by and large less than that of staff, and in some areas, family caregivers may have hardly any experience with mental illness and associate it with adverse outcomes.

Vast differences exist between the likelihood of being coerced in European psychiatric wards compared to Indian psychiatric wards. Whilst in European settings, this risk is about 5% (Lepping et al., 2016), in an Indian setting, one or more types of restraint were used in 63% of admitted patients, of whom 27% were subjected to intravenous injections when the target of the aggression was a doctor or nurse (Danivas et al., 2016). We understand that coercion is a dynamic state, changing with treatment and care. Clinical care may result in improved global functioning, insight and a reduction in the severity of illness, and consequently, less coercion. This gives scope for developing a standard clinical guideline in mental health care in India focusing on the variables mentioned, without any coercive measures, especially as recent studies have indicated that restraint can exacerbate mental health issues and, ironically, increase behaviours of concern (Webber et al., 2011).

Conversely, when discharged, most patients who regained insight into their illness reported in India and the UK that their admission and treatment were justified, even though they felt coerced during their hospital stay and agreed to treatment against their will within a safe, standardised coercive practice. A possible explanation for the decrease in coercive severity and frequency at discharge may be due to effective inpatient treatment and insight facilitation as part of the treatment program (Gowda et al., 2018).

The evidence to date emphasises the importance of the attitudes of mental health workers towards their patients as a critical factor that may be amenable to change. A combination of listening and respecting the patient's views is likely to minimise any experience of coercion, even if the outcome is compulsory treatment (Newton-Howes, 2010). Although mental health professionals have worked hard to minimise the negative attitudes towards mental ill-health in the community, these negative attitudes remain present even within services, suggesting a need to stay focused on the interactions of all clinicians (Newton-Howes et al., 2008). They must reflect on how they can work with individuals to maximise a positive outcome from a patient's perspective and eliminate coercion in day-to-day care. In the context of involuntary admission and care in mental health, communication is pivotal, whether before, during or after coercion or pressure. In the existing situation in Indian mental health care, no agreements are made beforehand with patients with a mental disorder. When force or pressure is used, the family caregiver and the patient often hold different views (Raveesh et al., 2016b).

## 6      Mysore Declaration

A number of high-profile incidents in which psychiatric patients were shown to have been mistreated made a wider Indian public aware of the situation in some chronic patient facilities back in the 1990s. These incidents also highlighted problems with coercion, and an opportunity arose to start more formal discussions about coercion in medical settings in India. In February 2013, experts from India and Europe came together in Mysore, India, for an international symposium on coercion. As a result, a declaration was drafted, discussed and ratified, which defined coercive measures in the Indian context and outlined aims and possible ways to minimise coercion in medical settings in India. The declaration asserted that:

There is an urgent need for the recognition and implementation of the rights of persons with mental illness, following principles about equality, security, liberty, health, integrity and dignity of all people, with a mental illness or not. All parties responsible for treating mental illness should eliminate all forms of discrimination, stigmatisation, violence, cruelty, and inhumane, or degrading treatment. We affirm that disproportionate, unsafe, or prolonged coercion or violence against persons with mental illness violates human rights and fundamental freedoms and impairs or nullifies their enjoyment of those rights and freedoms. (Lepping & Raveesh, 2013).

The declaration recognises the potential tension between the rights of patients who refuse medication and the benefits of possible restoration to normal functioning through involuntary treatment, as well as the wishes of family members, who often play an essential role in the treatment of mental illness in India (Lepping & Raveesh, 2013).

## 7    Conclusion

In Western and Eastern cultural contexts, coercion in mental health is approached and viewed differently, although there are also some significant similarities. In Western cultures, coercion in mental health is generally associated with legal frameworks and ethical conflicts.

Strict legal requirements are in place in many Western nations for involuntary treatment; these requirements usually involve proof that the individual presents a serious risk to themselves or others. A robust legal framework is in place to safeguard individual rights and autonomy, which are frequently prioritised. The effectiveness and morality of involuntary treatment are frequent topics of discussion, as is how to strike a balance between a person's rights and the safety of their community.

In Eastern cultures, distinct societal beliefs and customs can have an impact on the way coercion is approached with regard to mental health. Family decision-making and group well-being are frequently given more weight than individual rights. Mental health concerns may be more stigmatised in certain Eastern cultures, where family members are frequently heavily involved in decisions about how to care for and support their relatives who are mentally ill. This can occasionally result in more paternalistic treatment philosophies when the patient's family or caregivers make choices on their behalf. On the other hand, there is a high likelihood of significant family support for those who are ill.

It is crucial to remember that there is substantial diversity within these broad categories, and that Eastern and Western cultures are not monolithic. Global trends also impact many countries' practices, such as the growing focus on patient autonomy and human rights. In the field of mental health, across cultural boundaries, striking a balance between upholding individual rights and guaranteeing appropriate care for those in need continues to be a major concern.

## References

Albrecht, H. J. (2016). Legal aspects of the use of coercion measures in psychiatry. In B. Völlm & N. Nedopil (Eds.), *The use of coercive measures in forensic psychiatric care: Legal, ethical and practical challenges* (pp. 31–48). Springer.

Arboleda-Flórez, J. (2005). The ethics of biomedical research on prisoners. *Current Opinion in Psychiatry, 18*(5), 514–517.

Beauchamp, T., & Childress, J. (2001). *Principles of biomedical ethics* (5th ed.). Oxford University Press.

Bigwood, S., & Crowe, M. (2008). It's part of the job, but it spoils the job': A phenomenological study of physical restraint. *International Journal of Mental Health Nursing, 17*(3), 215–222.

Burns, T., Yeeles, K., Molodynski, A., Nightingale, H., Vazquez-Montes, M., Sheehan, K., & Linsell, L. (2011). Pressures to adhere to treatment ('leverage') in English mental health care. *British Journal of Psychiatry, 199*, 145–150.

Canvin, K., Rugkasa, J., Sinclar, J., & Burns, T. (2013). Leverage and other informal pressures in community psychiatry in England. *International Journal of Law and Psychiatry, 36*, 100–106.

Colin, B. (2014). Coercion and public justification. *Politics, Philosophy and Economics, 13*, 189–214.

Cossu, G., Gyppaz, D., Kalcev, G., Manca, A. R., Angermeyer, M., Zreik, T., & Carta, M. G. (2023). Systematic review of involuntary hospitalisation and long-term compliance. *International Review of Psychiatry, 35*(2), 209–220.

Danivas, V., Lepping, P., Punitharani, S., Gowrishree, H., Ashwini, K., Raveesh, B. N., & Palmstierna, T. (2016). Observational study of aggressive behaviour and coercion on an Indian acute ward. *Asian Journal of Psychiatry, 22*, 150–156.

Dudley, M., Silove, D., & Gale, F. (2012). *Mental health and human rights: Vision, praxis, and courage.* Oxford University Press.

Gowda, G. S., Lepping, P., Noorthoorn, E. O., Ali, S. F., Kumar, C. N., Raveesh, B. N., & Suresh, B. M. (2018). Restraint prevalence and perceived coercion among psychiatric inpatients from South India: A prospective study. *Asian Journal of Psychiatry, 36*, 10–16.

Gowda, G. S., Lepping, P., Ray, S., Noorthoorn, E., Nanjegowda, R. B., Kumar, C. N., Naveen, C., & Math, S. B. (2019). Clinician attitude and perspective on the use of coercive measures in clinical practice from tertiary care mental health establishment—A cross-sectional study. *Indian Journal of Psychiatry, 61*(2), 151–155.

Hirsch, S., & Steinert, T. (2019). Measures to avoid coercion in psychiatry and their efficacy. *Deutsches Ärzteblatt International, 116*(19), 336–343.

Janssen, W. A., Noorthoorn, E., Linge, R., & Lendemeijer, B. (2007). The influence of staffing levels on the use of seclusion. *International Journal of Law and Psychiatry, 30*(2), 118–126.

Kalisova, L., Raboch, J., Kitzlerova, E., & Kallert, T. W. (2007). Coercive measures used during hospitalization. Eunomia—Final results in the Czech Republic. *European Psychiatry, 22*(S1), S309.

Kallert, T. W. (2008). Coercion in psychiatry. *Current Opinion in Psychiatry, 21*, 485–489.

Kallert, T. W., Glockner, M., & Schutawhol, M. (2008). Involuntary vs. voluntary hospital admission—A systematic review on outcome diversity. *European Archives of Psychiatry and Clinical Neuroscience, 258*, 195–209.

Kinner, S. A., Harvey, C., Hamilton, B., Brophy, L., Roper, C., McSherry, B., & Young, J. T. (2017). Attitudes towards seclusion and restraint in mental health settings: Findings from a large, community-based survey of consumers, carers and mental health professionals. *Epidemiology and Psychiatric Sciences, 26*(5), 535–544.

Kjellin, L., & Wallsten, T. (2010). Accumulated coercion and short-term outcome of inpatient psychiatric care. *BMC Psychiatry, 10*, 53.

Lee, A. Y. K. (2014). Legal coercion, respect & reason-responsive agency. *Ethical Theory and Moral Practice, 17*, 847–859.

Lee, M. H., & Seo, M. K. (2021). Perceived coercion of persons with mental illness living in a community. *International Journal of Environmental Research and Public Health, 18*(5), 2290.

Lepping, P., & Raveesh, B. N. (2013). The Mysore declaration. *International Psychiatry, 10*, 98–99.

Lepping, P., Masood, B., Noorthoorn, E. O., & Flammer, E. (2016). Comparison of restrain data from four countries. *Social Psychiatry and Psychiatric Epidemiology, 51*(9), 1301–1309.

Liberto, H. (2021). Coercion, consent, and the mechanistic question. *Ethics, 131*, 210–245.

Mohr, W. (2006). *Psychiatric-mental health nursing* (6th ed.). Lippincott Williams & Wilkins.

Newton-Howes, G. (2010). Coercion in psychiatric care: Where are we now, what do we know, where do we go? *The Psychiatrist, 34*, 217–220.

Newton-Howes, G., Tyrer, P., & Weaver, T. (2008). The attitudes of mental health workers towards patients with personality disorders in community mental health settings. *Australian and New Zealand Journal of Psychiatry, 42*, 572–577.

Raboch, J., Kališová, L., Nawka, A., Kitzlerová, E., Onchev, G., Karastergiou, A., Magliano, L., Dembinskas, A., Kiejna, A., Torres-Gonzales, F., Priebe, S., & Kallert, T. (2010). Use of coercive measures during involuntary hospitalization: Findings from ten European countries. *Psychiatric Services, 61*(10), 1012–1017.

Raveesh, B. N., Pathare, S., Lepping, P., Noorthoorn, E. O., Gowda, G. S., & Bunders-Aelen, J. (2016a). Perceived coercion in persons with mental disorder in India: A cross-sectional study. *Indian Journal of Psychiatry, 58*, 210–220.

Raveesh, B. N., Pathare, S., Noorthoorn, E. O., Gowda, G. S., Lepping, P., & Bunders-Aelen, J. (2016b). Staff and caregiver attitude to coercion in India. *Indian Journal of Psychiatry, 58*, 221–229.

Rhodes, M. (2000). The nature of coercion. *The Journal of Value Inquiry, 34*, 369–381.

Salize, H. J., & Dressing, H. (2004). Epidemiology of involuntary placement of mentally ill people across the European Union. *British Journal of Psychiatry, 184*, 163–168.

Sashidharan, S. P., Mezzina, R., & Puras, D. (2019). Reducing coercion in mental healthcare. *Epidemiology and Psychiatric Sciences, 28*, 605–612.

Shah, R., & Basu, D. (2010). Coercion in psychiatric care: Global and Indian perspective. *Indian Journal of Psychiatry, 52*, 203–206.

Steinert, T. (2007). Ethical attitudes towards involuntary admission and involuntary treatment of patients with schizophrenia. *Psychiatrische Praxis, 34*, S186–S190.

Swartz, M. S., Wagner, H. R., Swanson, J. W., Hiday, V. A., & Burns, B. J. (2002). The perceived coerciveness of involuntary outpatient commitment: Findings from an experimental study. *Journal of the American Academy of Psychiatry and the Law, 30*(2), 207–217.

Szmukler, G. (2015). Compulsion and "coercion" in mental health care. *World Psychiatry, 14*, 259–261.

Szmukler, G., & Appelbaum, P. S. (2009). Treatment pressures, coercion, and compulsion in mental health care. *Journal of Mental Health, 17*(3), 229–231.

Theodoridou, A., Schlatter, F., Ajdacic, V., Rössler, W., & Jäger, M. (2012). Therapeutic relationship in the context of perceived coercion in a psychiatric population. *Psychiatry Research, 200*(2–3), 939–944.

van den Hooff, S., & Goossensen, A. (2014). How to increase quality of care during coercive admission? A review of literature. *Scandinavian Journal of Caring Sciences, 28*(3), 425–434.

Vatne, S., & Fagermoen, M. S. (2007). To correct and to acknowledge: Two simultaneous and conflicting perspectives of limit-setting in mental health nursing. *Journal of Psychiatric and Mental Health Nursing, 14*, 41–48.

Verlinde, L., Noorthoorn, E. O., Snelleman, W., van den Berg, H., van der Plas, M. S., & Lepping, P. (2017). Seclusion and enforced medication in dealing with aggression: A prospective dynamic cohort study. *European Psychiatry, 39*, 86–92.

Viswanath, B., & Chaturvedi, S. K. (2012). Cultural aspects of major mental disorders: A critical review from an Indian perspective. *Indian Journal of Psychological Medicine, 34*(4), 306–312.

Webber, L., Mcvilly, K., & Chan, J. (2011). Restrictive interventions for people with a disability exhibiting challenging behaviours: Analysis of a population database. *Journal of Applied Research in Intellectual Disabilities, 24*, 495–507.

Wertheimer, A. (1993). A philosophical examination of coercion for mental health issues: Some basic distinctions: Analysis and justification. *Behavioral Sciences and the Law, 11*, 239–258.

Wynn, R., Kvalvik, A. M., & Hynnekleiv, T. (2011). Attitudes to coercion at two Norwegian psychiatric units. *Nordic Journal of Psychiatry, 65*, 133–137.

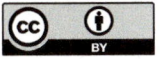

# The Experience of Coercion and Violence: Service User, Professional and Informal Caregiver Perspectives

Sabine Hahn, Melina Hasler, Sabine Rühle Andersson, Yvonne D. B. Bonner, and Dirk Richter

## 1    Introduction

This chapter is a revision of the fourth chapter 'Users' Perceptions and Views on Violence and Coercion in Mental Health' published in the first edition of this book. We thank the authors of the first edition, Christoph Abderhalden (1954–2013) and Gian Maria Galeazzi, for their profound work, which is the basis of this revised chapter.

Professional workers in medicine and psychiatry are usually considered clinical experts and thus are entitled to deal with service users. However, in most countries, social, attitudinal and legal changes in medical treatment now underline the right of opinion and self-determination of each service user. Service users—encouraged and empowered by the recovery movement—ask to be involved in the decision-making process of their therapy and the choice of the pathway to recovery (Slade et al., 2012; von Peter, 2017). These changes have led to the development of coop-eration-based medical and social services (World Health Organization (WHO), 2021; Gooding, 2023). Furthermore, informal caregivers (relatives, friends or neighbours) want to be heard and involved. They would like their opinion and experience to be taken into account and ask to be involved in the treatment process and caring system.

On the other hand, shifts in the attitudes of professionals towards violence and coercion occur slowly. Coercion and restraint are still considered useful clinical

S. Hahn (✉) · M. Hasler · S. Rühle Andersson · D. Richter
School of Health Professions, Division of Nursing, Bern University of Applied Sciences, Bern, Switzerland
e-mail: sabine.hahn@bfh.ch; melina.hasler@bfh.ch; sabine.ruehleandersson@bfh.ch; dirk.richter@bfh.ch

Y. D. B. Bonner
Psychotherapist, Private Practice, Reggio Emilia, Italy

© The Author(s) 2024
N. Hallett et al. (eds.), *Coercion and Violence in Mental Health Settings*,
https://doi.org/10.1007/978-3-031-61224-4_3

responses in acute emergency situations to protect society, service users and staff and to guarantee the safety of the persons involved.

The paternalistic model (in which decision-making authority is reserved for the professionals, because they know what is best for the patient) may be considered useful by some professionals as it side-steps the complex task of informing, explaining, negotiating and reaching an agreement with the service user, who might even dissent from the recommended treatment. Moreover, the paternalistic model of interaction generally reinforces the mental health professional's position.

The main argument in favour of a paternalistic approach is that psychiatric patients lack insight into their illness and sometimes have to be (or are) treated against their will. Therefore, from the viewpoint of the paternalistic approach, measures such as involuntary admission and forced medication are considered unavoidable. Today, the view that some service users lack insight into their illness is complemented by the view that some service users lack capacity to consent. This has led to some services being based on voluntary informed consent and the assessment of the service user's capacity to consent. This in turn has led to the development of tools to systematically assess service users' capacity to consent. It has also led to coercion not being seen as coercion in the absence of capacity and objectifiable service user resistance, for example in psychogeriatric care where service users are fixed to their chairs by tables and do not appear to resist this fixation (Hofmann & Hahn, 2013).

In most European countries, this intricate situation is regulated by a law that allows psychiatrists to hospitalise service users against their will when assessed as dangerous to themselves and others (Wasserman et al., 2020; Dressing & Salize, 2004). Sociological studies have drawn researchers' attention to the link between the description of mental illness in the media (that often emphasises the risk of violence) and its impact on subsequent social and recovery policies that support coercive practices (Rose, 1998; Philo, 1996). Public concern for the perceived risk of violence caused by the presence of psychiatric patients in the community has led some countries to expand the setting of involuntary treatment from the hospital to community services (Rugkåsa, 2016). Research has examined the relationship between media information and hospitalisation rates. These studies suggest that political decisions and media information on crimes committed by psychiatric patients in the community increase the rate of involuntary admissions to inpatient forensic psychiatric services (Brophy & McDermott, 2003; Cutcliffe & Hannigan, 2001). As a result, psychiatrists are increasingly responsible for risk assessment, despite the lack of standardised and clinically feasible instruments (Whiting et al., 2021). Consequently, this development does not encourage a flexible approach towards service users but reinforces the paternalistic model of care (Gowda et al., 2019b) and the opinion that some service users represent a danger to themselves and others. Hence, mental health services have the responsibility of protecting service users from themselves and others, e.g. in circumstances such as suicidality, self-harm, acute psychosis or dementia. In other words, service users who show signs of serious behavioural disorganisation, confusion and extreme agitation.

These developments in mental health services can promote violence and coercion, but they can also empower service users and informal caregivers. Likewise, reflective professionals are increasingly questioning current practices and the negative impact they can have on service users' feelings of dignity and therapeutic relationships (Gowda et al., 2019b). This chapter reviews the current literature on service users', informal caregivers' and professionals' views towards aggression, violence and coercive practices and examines their impact on mental health practices and future research.

## 1.1    Public Response to Violence and Coercion

The civil and service user rights movements have, for decades, condemned the use of force and coercion in psychiatry, questioned the legitimacy of paternalism and authoritarianism in mental health care (Szasz & Alexander, 1968) and, consequently, generated a shift in psychiatric perspectives. Thus, laying the foundation for a novel ethical approach, i.e. respect for the individual as a person, and not simply as a patient, with his/her subjective experiences, choices, values and rights. This change empowers service users by placing them at the centre of therapy, scientific research and care (Funk et al., 2022). The public, however, is on the whole not that critical towards the use of coercion in mental health care. Current research has shown that coercive measures are accepted when the public recognises potential benefits from their use (Steiger et al., 2022a, 2022b). Nevertheless, stigmata do reinforce the social perception of the danger caused by mentally ill people (Schomerus et al., 2023).

## 1.2    Research on the Views of Service Users and Informal Caregivers

Historically, service users' perceptions of mental health care were ignored. Some decades ago, thanks to the quality assurance approach—first developed in the industrial field and next in the health sector—brought forth an increasing interest in service users' perceptions of the healthcare sector and also of mental health services. This approach underlined that the 'user satisfaction criterion' could be an outcome measure for assessing the quality of a treatment plan (Ruggeri et al., 2004). It also highlighted the need to explore the subjective determinants of a patient's satisfaction, focusing on the entire care process (including informal caregivers) and not only on the psychopathological outcomes. This shift in perspective emphasises the importance of involving psychiatric service users in their care. It is also useful to include service users and/or informal caregivers as experts in all the stages of service planning.

Moreover, there is a current ongoing discussion on the meaningful involvement of service users and informal caregivers as active collaborators in research projects, and on the advantages of such partnerships in all stages of a scientific project.

Efforts are needed to develop recruitment and training strategies to support this type of active participation of service users (Hahn & Wolfensberger, 2022; Trivedi & Wykes, 2002; Bird et al., 2020). Incorporating the perceptions and personal experiences of service users and informal caregivers into research opens new avenues for studying violent incidents, prevention, and the reduction of violence and restraint. Although an increasing number of studies examine service users' perspectives and include them in studies on aggression, violence and coercion in health care, the perspective of informal caregivers is still rarely analysed (Hotzy et al., 2019).

## 2 Instruments to Measure the Experience and Perception of Aggression, Violence and Coercion

### 2.1 Instruments to Measure the Experience of Aggression and Violence

According to a systematic review of studies on the perception of aggression and violence prevention in mental health care, there are no instruments available to measure the perceptions of violence and foster prevention in a psychometrically sound manner (Hallett et al., 2014). The only scale—the Perception of Aggression Scale (POAS) (Jansen et al., 1997)—that is supposed to do so, is in reality an instrument that measures attitudes, rather than experiences and perceptions.

### 2.2 Instruments to Measure the Perception of Coercion

However, there are several instruments available that measure the perception of coercion from the different stakeholders' perspectives. The most frequently used scale for service users is the MacArthur Perceived Coercion Scale (MPCS). It is a five-item scale that measures perceived coercion on hospital admission (Gardner et al., 1993). It was built on the MacArthur Admission Experience Interview (AEI), a semi-structured interview, and the MacArthur Admission Experience Survey (AES), a 15-item instrument (Gardner et al., 1993). Each item of the MPCS comprises a different aspect of perceived coercion. The items are 'influence' ('What had more influence on your being admitted: what you wanted, or what other people wanted?'), 'control' ('How much control did you have?'), 'choice' ('You chose' or 'Somebody made you choose'), 'freedom' ('How free did you feel to do what you wanted?'), and finally 'idea' or 'perceived initiative' ('Whose idea was it to come to hospital?'). The MPCS has demonstrated several psychometric qualities, leading to its adoption by numerous research teams—initially in North America, where it was developed, and subsequently in Europe and New Zealand.

The AEI and the AES also measure other relevant dimensions of coercion in psychiatric treatment, i.e., 'coercion related behavior' (experienced by users during hospital admission) and 'procedural justice'. 'Coercion related behavior' is categorised by the MacArthur Collaboration in three clusters: 'positive pressure' (persuasion, inducements and asking for preferences), 'negative pressure' (threats, giving orders, deception and exhibition of force), and 'force' (legal and physical forces that impede the patient to refuse what is imposed by staff) (Lidz, 1998). As for 'procedural justice', research highlights that the degree of procedural justice (or process inclusion) perceived by the service user is linked to their likelihood to be heard, have their opinions been taken into account and also to their perception of fairness in the decision-making process, in other words, up to what point they feel treated with respect and dignity by the decision-maker (Poythress et al., 2002).

The MacArthur Experience Survey has recently been adapted to assess antipsychotic medication related to involuntary treatment (Horvath et al., 2018). Further instruments have been developed to measure coercion experiences such as informal coercion, including the Experienced Coercion Scale (ECS) (Nyttingnes et al., 2017) and the Coercion Experience Scale (CES) (Bergk et al., 2010). Additionally, the Staff Attitude to Coercion Scale (SACS) has been developed to study staff attitudes towards coercion (Husum et al., 2022).

## 2.3    Instruments to Measure Involuntary Admission

Only one instrument, as far as we know, measures the perception of involuntary admissions (Gabriel, 2017). This 21-item instrument was developed by people who have experienced involuntary admission and by clinical experts in Canada. However, this instrument should be adapted to the different influencing factors due to differences in legislation and practical implementation in different countries.

## 3    View on Violent Incidents from Service User, Staff and Informal Caregivers

### 3.1    Service Users' Views on Violent Incidents

Some studies examine participants' perceptions of violent incidents in a broad sense, revealing thus the multiple and complex components of aggression. Benson et al. (2003), for example, emphasise that one of the central concerns of service users is the discourse of the mutual attribution of blame about reasons for violent incidences. Kumar et al. (2001), using the grounded theory approach, revealed from the viewpoint of experienced service users that the power imbalance observed in the mental health system fosters institutional violence against service users.

When service users are interviewed on the causes of aggressive behaviour, they mention various aspects of the hospital environment (Johnson et al., 1997; Love & Hunter, 1999), institutional, interpersonal or procedural factors, lack of communication, unmet needs, interpersonal conflicts and personal factors (Välimäki et al., 2022b). However, further research underlines that service users often describe staff behaviour as provocative and disrespectful, and therefore the main trigger for violence (Duxbury, 2002; Duxbury & Whittington, 2005; Fagan-Pryor et al., 2003;

Ilkiw-Lavalle & Grenyer, 2003; Fletcher et al., 2021). For example, Omérov et al. (2004), studying 41 violent incidents, found that service users considered staff behaviour provocative in 75% of the episodes analysed. The findings are confirmed by a systematic review of qualitative studies and examine the service users' opinion about the reason for patients' violent behaviour (Gudde et al., 2015). Another systematic review has also linked these impressions of service users' about staffs' provocative behaviour to the occurrence of coercive treatment practices in the mental health care system (Tingleff et al., 2017).

## 3.2    Staff Views on Violent Incidents

Current research underlines the fundamental differences in perspective on aggression and violence between staff and service users. While service users consider staff behaviour as a potential trigger for violence, staff often highlight organisational policies, staffing levels and/or patients' personalities and diagnoses (Fletcher et al., 2021). A survey revealed clear differences in the attitudes of nurses ($n = 782$), service users ($n = 886$) and informal caregivers ($n = 765$) towards aggression in psychiatric hospitals (Välimäki et al., 2022a). Nurses had a significantly lower tolerance and more negative perceptions towards violent behaviour than service users and informal caregivers. Nurses were significantly more likely to perceive violence as unpleasant, repulsive, unnecessary and unacceptable behaviour that causes mental or physical harm than the other participants.

## 3.3    Informal Caregivers' Views on Violent Incidents

There is little research on informal caregivers' perspectives on aggression and violence. Informal caregivers agreed with staff and service user view that illness itself can be a reason for violent patient behaviour. Also, problems with communication and relationships on the ward can lead to social conflicts as a reason for violence. Informal caregivers identified sudden change in treatment without a clear explanation as trigger for service user violence. Staff and relatives sometimes also see no reason for violent behaviour (Välimäki et al., 2022b) As an intervention, informal caregivers described comforting service users after an event (Välimäki et al., 2022a, 2022b; Duxbury et al., 2013). In dementia care, Duxbury et al. (2013) found that both informal caregivers of individuals with dementia and nurses attribute aggressive behaviours observed in these individuals to the condition of dementia itself.and they support the person-centred approach of nurses in the prevention and non-coercive approaches in dealing with aggression.

# 4 View on Coercion from Service User, Staff and Informal Caregivers

## 4.1 Service Users' Views on Coercion

Service users tend to have a negative view of the coercive measures they have experienced (Tingleff et al., 2017). Systematic reviews have highlighted that the majority of service users, subjected to coercive measures, do not consider them positive (Chieze et al., 2019; Aguilera-Serrano et al., 2018; Akther et al., 2019) chiefly because their rights are not respected (Allison & Flemming, 2019; Hawsawi et al., 2020). The most common emotions triggered by coercive incidents are anger, discontentment, feeling powerless or overwhelmed, depression, fear, anxiety, humiliation, desperation and a feeling of dependency. Most service users are convinced of not being heard, nor taken seriously (Krieger et al., 2018; Armgart et al., 2013; Thøgersen et al., 2010; Hawsawi et al., 2020; Fugger et al., 2016; Ling et al., 2015).

In situations of restraint and/or seclusion, service users often feel bored and/or unsettled by the absence of stimuli (Kontio et al., 2012). Even if restraint might appear necessary from the viewpoint of service users, this psychiatric practice remains a distressing and dehumanising experience for the patient (Wilson et al., 2017; Wong et al., 2020). During seclusion, some service users feel neglected, powerless, fearful, anxious or even punished (El-Badri & Mellsop, 2008), while others feel safe, protected, more at ease and in control (Van Der Merwe et al., 2013).

Service users' level of perceived coercion is influenced by experienced coercive incidents, from personal attitudes towards prescribed medication or from their capacity to reflect and gain insight into their own mental state (Hirsch et al., 2021; Horvath et al., 2018). The perception of coercive incidents can also derive from the type of hospital admission: voluntary or involuntary. Service users who have experienced involuntary hospitalisation tolerate less coercive measures (Reisch et al., 2018).

Informal coercion (positive motivational influence, imposing threats of negative penalties) is also associated with a broader sense of coercion but is perceived by service users as unfair treatment. However, the treatment fidelity of service users who have experienced this form of coercion does not seem to differ from those who have not (Jaeger & Rossler, 2010).

The personal experience of coercion will, however, influence the choice of coercive treatment (Georgieva et al., 2012). For example, physical and/or mechanical restraint may be perceived as more violent than forced medication or seclusion (Mielau et al., 2016; Guzmán-Parra et al., 2019; Vishnivetsky et al., 2013).

It is not surprising that these negative experiences of coercive practices—which should not be overlooked—can generate feelings of rejection and a loss of trust between service users and health professionals (Ling et al., 2015; Sheehan & Burns, 2011). Negative experiences impact both the patient's quality of life and level of satisfaction with the therapeutic setting (Lee & Seo, 2021). Furthermore, it is probable that a recurring experience of coercive measures increases a service user's resistance towards coercion and lowers his or her confidence in the benefits of such a practice (Brady et al., 2017). Coercive measures are considered unproductive when other less drastic measures could solve the problem and they can also be interpreted as a violation of the service user's freedom of choice and autonomy (Norvoll & Pedersen, 2018).

In brief, service users are more critical of hospitalisation if they have already suffered coercive measures (Guzmán-Parra et al., 2019; Stanhope et al., 2009). The more psychologically stable the service user is, the more negatively she or he will regard coercive treatment. However, now and again, some service users understand why such coercive clinical measures are taken (Armgart et al., 2013). However, service users usually prefer other treatment options to coercion. To bear in mind service users' opinions could result in a qualitative improvement in the mental health care system (Norvoll & Pedersen, 2018).

## 4.2    Staff Views on Coercion

Staff views on coercive incidents derive from the wish to feel safe at work. Coercion is thus considered necessary to ensure a safe working environment and to contain the fear of losing control when a patient becomes violent or suicidal (Doedens et al., 2020; Gowda et al., 2019a; Gerace & Muir-Cochrane, 2019) or when the personnel has to deal with violent or suicidal behaviours. Therefore, staff view the use of coercion as safeguard against violence and as protection of the service user, rather than a therapeutic measure (Wilson et al., 2017; Molewijk et al., 2017; Morandi et al., 2021; Doedens et al., 2020). However, coercion can also be seen from staff's view as a therapeutical intervention rather than violence and suicide prevention, e.g. seclusion can be viewed as a treatment and a benefit for the service users—the seclusion room or restraint can calm the service user down and allow them to regain control of their behaviour through less irritation from the environment (Larsen & Terkelsen, 2014; Van Der Merwe et al., 2013; Kinner et al., 2017). Therefore, some staff tend to believe that institutions could not function effectively without seclusion (Van Der Merwe et al., 2013).

In brief, professionals view the following indicators as reasons to consider seclusion or restraint: violence and physical aggression, self-harm, sexualised behaviour, vandalism, drug abuse, intoxication, as well as a history of coercion and uncooperative behaviour (Gerace & Muir-Cochrane, 2019; Happell & Koehn, 2011; Muir-Cochrane et al., 2015; Vedana et al., 2018).

The work environment and conditions also influence staff decision-making regarding the use of coercive measures. Clinical professionals at times feel compelled to use coercion, feeling as though they have no other option. Several factors influence decisions such as low staff-to-patient ratio, employee restrictions for an intervention, low job satisfaction, stressful work conditions, the gender composition of the team, the absence of planning options, a lack of consensus when deciding on coercion, and finally, insufficient opportunities for professional training (Hawsawi et al., 2020; Krieger et al., 2021; Muir-Cochrane et al., 2015; Happell & Koehn, 2011; Raveesh et al., 2016b).

Attitudes, behaviour and personal traits can also influence the way coercion is implemented. Optimistic or more experienced staff members may use seclusion less frequently, adopting a more pragmatic and critical approach towards coercive measures (Happell & Koehn, 2011; Krieger et al., 2021). Furthermore, male staff tend to use more coercion than female staff, and also more often with male patients (Al-Maraira & Hayajneh, 2020; Bregar et al., 2018). Other factors such as low self-esteem or doubts about their professional skills, lack of professional models in the team, little or no supervision, and poor clinical management all increase the use of coercive practices (Gandhi et al., 2018; Gerace & Muir-Cochrane, 2019). Furthermore, the more often coercive practices are used, the less staff perceive the negative aspects of coercion (Doedens et al., 2020).

It is not clear which coercive measures clinical staff are more willing to use. Some professionals consider seclusion the most useful restraint procedure, some prefer physical or mechanical restraint (Gerace & Muir-Cochrane, 2019), and others consider restraint and seclusion too restrictive and would prefer using less ruthless measures (Doedens et al., 2020). Chemical restraint is usually depicted as the least harmful practice (Kinner et al., 2017).

In short, staff consider coercion the last resort after having tried out all other interventions that either did not work or were unsatisfactory. Clinical professionals underline that many different interventions can be put into practice before using coercion. Moreover, the decision to use coercive measures is not an easy decision to take (Gerace & Muir-Cochrane, 2019; Morandi et al., 2021; Moran et al., 2009), as problems usually arise when coercion is used (Muir-Cochrane et al., 2015; Vedana et al., 2018).

Staff have difficulty justifying the use of coercive practice as safety measures, because care is seen as engaging, compassionate, calming, comfortable and free from coercion. Staff can also consider coercion potentially risky for patients and team members (Hawsawi et al., 2020; Vedana et al., 2018). The impact of coercive episodes can be traumatic for both service users and staff (Bigwood & Crowe, 2008; Hawsawi et al., 2020; Krieger et al., 2021). Staff are also aware that coercion can harm the service user's feeling of integrity and influence negatively the therapeutic relationship (Raveesh et al., 2016b).

In a nutshell, staff are aware of the harm coercive measures can cause to the relationship between service users and staff, for instance, producing a lack of regard for the service user's opinion (Gerace & Muir-Cochrane, 2019; Gowda et al., 2019b). Seclusion and restraint are deemed stressful, for they generate anxiety and feelings of guilt (Moran et al., 2009). Staff hence try to cope by suppressing emotions, without always being successful. This unsuccessful suppression of emotions can provoke an emotional distance between staff and service users that can disrupt communication between them and hamper their relationship (Morandi et al., 2021). Staff can also consider coercive measures an offence against service users' rights (Morandi et al., 2021) and feel ethically in the wrong when using them. Staff, as a rule, endeavour to keep the patient situation under control, and can occasionally understand the service user's resistance against coercive practices (Hawsawi et al., 2020; Larsen & Terkelsen, 2014; Happell & Harrow, 2010; Bigwood & Crowe,

2008; Gerace & Muir-Cochrane, 2019; Haugom et al., 2019). This can also lead to resistance to coercion if staff do not see the need for restriction. They raise their voices against coercive interventions and against a superior ordering this measure (Gandhi et al., 2018). Also, staff agree that it is necessary to be transparent with the service user about the use of coercive interventions and the reasons behind it, and meeting with patients after the incident is seen as important, but it does not always happen (Krieger et al., 2021).

## 4.3    Informal Caregivers' Views on Coercion

Informal caregivers, mainly in acute and emergency situations, consider it necessary that the staff use coercion (Gowda et al., 2019a), even if they criticise this type of treatment (Reisch et al., 2018). Compared to other coercive measures, chemical restraint is the most accepted in these acute situations (Gowda et al., 2019a). Coercion is seen as a way to help service users with the difficulties they experience as a result of their mental health problems. Coercion can also reduce stress for informal caregivers, for example by relieving them of the 24-h care they have been providing. Other positive effects of coercion can be seen as building structure and control in a challenging situation within the family, which can lead to a better quality of life for the family members involved (Norvoll et al., 2018). Sometimes informal caregivers use coercion (such as threats or forced persuasion) to convince the service user to be hospitalised (Gowda et al., 2019a).

However, informal caregivers also perceive coercive measures as inconsiderate when they feel excluded by the healthcare team and are uncertain about the measures' beneficial outcomes (Norvoll et al., 2018). In coercive situations, informal caregivers often feel responsible and anxious, even if the professionals carry responsibility for the treatment (Førde et al., 2016). Informal carers may have little social support, and feel lonely and uneasy when disclosing their negative experiences (Førde et al., 2016). Therefore, coercive incidents often put informal caregivers in an uneasy situation (Norvoll et al., 2018). So, it is not surprising that informal caregivers often disapprove of coercive measures, even if they object slightly less than service users. They clearly don't have the same opinion as staff on this topic (Reisch et al., 2018; Raveesh et al., 2016a). Norvoll et al. (2018) used qualitative interviews with 36 family members of adult and adolescent people with mental health problems and experiences of coercion and describe that informal caregivers have a different level and type of responsibility (Norvoll et al., 2018). Parents of hospitalised teenagers, for instance, worry mostly about the harm coercion could do to their children now or in the future (Norvoll et al., 2018). They fear the negative impact of coercive interventions on their family member (Norvoll et al., 2018). Hence, it is crucial to reassure a family that the patient will be well looked after and receive good care. After coercive incidents, informal caregivers usually feel more positive having been helped thanks to the compulsory admission of their family member. However, after some time, they usually feel guilty and disheartened by the course of events. They notice that coercive incidents can harm their relationship with the service user. Coercion, threats of coercion, or not disclosing health-related information can foster mistrust, damage relations and trigger conflicts in a family system (Norvoll et al., 2018).

According to informal caregivers, low quality of care, lack of alternatives or concrete interventions, staff shortages and negative attitudes are all factors that foster the use of coercion (Norvoll et al., 2018). Informal caregivers do agree with the idea of eliminating coercion (Kinner et al., 2017; Brophy et al., 2016) and believe that coercion would be less needed if health workers could spend more time with the patients (Raveesh et al., 2016a). Finally, they have little knowledge of the risks and consequences of coercive measures (Shrestha, 2018).

## 4.4    Summary

There are many areas in which the views of service users, staff and informal carers on coercion in mental health care do not coincide. These sometimes divergent views highlight the challenges that all parties face in preventing, using and following up coercive interventions in mental health care. In all mental health care settings, service users disapprove of coercive practices that, in their opinion, violate the patient's rights and trigger past traumas. Informal coercion is perceived as unfair and interferes with relationships with professionals, leading to feelings of rejection. In contrast, staff and informal caregivers consider coercion necessary to react to aggressive behaviour of service users to ensure a safe environment. However, staff usually consider coercion a last resort as it fosters ethical dilemmas and preferences for types of coercion vary according to the ward's style of work, working conditions and staff attitudes. Informal caregivers often maintain a critical attitude towards coercive measures. They consider coercion as an extreme practice that generates among informal caregivers feelings of exclusion and insecurity. Service user, staff and informal caregiver view the impact of coercion on the service user as distressing and as having the potential to disrupt the therapeutic relationship. The importance of being explicit with the service user when coercion is needed is supported by staff and informal caregivers. Informal caregivers do understand the complexities of coercive measures but advocate for its elimination, requesting more staff to allow more personal contact between personnel and patient.

## 5    Service User, Staff and Informal Caregivers Perspectives on Coercion in the Community

Involuntary admission and Community Treatment Orders (CTO) are commonly used coercive practices in the community. Service users' perceptions of coercion, involuntary hospitalisation and treatment have received attention on a global scale, at least in part due to the United Nations Convention on the Rights of Persons with Disabilities (UN-CRPD) (United Nations, 2006). The convention has been signed by 182 states. The UN-CRPD emphasises 'respect for inherent dignity, individual autonomy including the freedom to make one's own choices, and independence of persons; non-discrimination; full and effective participation and inclusion in society; respect for differences and acceptance of persons with disabilities as part of human diversity and humanity; equality of opportunity; accessibility […]' (United Nations, 2006, Article 3). Article 15, in particular, addresses the use of coercion and its ties with torture: 'No one shall be subjected to torture or to cruel, inhuman or degrading treatment or punishment'. By international legal standards and UN bodies, compulsory treatment is considered a form of torture (UN General Assembly, 2013). Even so, countries are still not reducing hospitalisations, nor do they propose to ban involuntary hospitalisation. Quite the opposite, a trend of increasing rates of coercive admissions is becoming a serious cause of concern (Sheridan Rains et al., 2019; de Stefano & Ducci, 2008; Dressing & Salize, 2004). This is happening even though research provides evidence that shared decision-making interventions (including advance directives, crisis cards and patient-held information strategies), CTOs, adherence-enhancement interventions and integrated care interventions can reduce involuntary hospitalisation (Barbui et al., 2021).

In brief, forced admission to hospital with deprivation of autonomy is an extreme, but commonly used, practice in psychiatry. The widespread opinion, that persons suffering from psychiatric disorders represent a danger to themselves and the community, legitimises the policy of involuntary hospitalisation, often used as a preventive measure against social disturbances (Georgieva et al., 2019). Laws on this issue vary from country to country, but usually also prescribe the provision of impartial information and a legal procedure to appeal against compulsory measures (Wasserman et al., 2020).

## 5.1   Service Users' Views on Involuntary Hospitalisation and Community Treatment Orders

Service users of mental health services have conflicting opinions on involuntary hospitalisation. Opponents of coercive treatment argue that these laws violate basic human rights—i.e. autonomy and freedom of movement—and should simply be withdrawn (Sugiura et al., 2020). Other service users agree that involuntary hospitalisation may be helpful in extreme situations of crisis (i.e. as a last resort if serious hazards are feared), provided that other options in less restrictive environments have been attempted first and legal or advocacy support have been guaranteed. Service users recognise that involuntary treatment can have some positive aspects, as they appreciate that they could have experienced more problems if they had not been hospitalised (Allison & Flemming, 2019). Involuntary hospitalisation can generate positive feelings, including emotional states of comfort and safety (Krieger et al., 2018).

In brief, service users' views on compulsory hospitalisation vary. For some, hospitalisation can be considered necessary. Moreover, a service user can change opinions and feelings towards coercion (Sibitz et al., 2011; Larsen & Terkelsen, 2014; Verbeke et al., 2019). Finally, a service user who has suffered involuntary admission tends to report higher levels of coercion than a patient admitted voluntarily to hospital (Hirsch et al., 2021). This is probably related to higher acceptance of the illness model and the entire mental health care system.

Most service users view the Community Treatment Order (CTO), recently introduced in several countries, as an alarming increase in social control. Recommended for emergency situations or to address simple everyday events, CTOs risk severely limiting people's rights and freedoms. The UN-CRPD recommends that member states ensure that people with mental disabilities enjoy the same rights and bear the same duties as the rest of the population. Therefore, disabled persons have the right to set their priorities and choose what treatments to receive (United Nations, 2006). This convention has strengthened the rights of service users and has restricted the possibilities for clinical care services to use compulsory commitment. Now and again however some clinicians are concerned that they will no longer be able to protect service users (Scholten & Gather, 2017) or follow service user's preferences (Dawson, 2015).

Service users on the whole consider CTO coercion less aggressive than other coercive measures, and on occasion, even consider it helpful and supportive, i.e. when it offers access to local mental health care services (Pridham et al., 2016). Nonetheless, service users still have mixed feelings about CTOs. They acknowledge that CTOs can consider personal needs, yet they emphasise that it remains a stressful experience due to the loss of the right to decide (Riley et al., 2014). The absence of a shared decision-making process during CTOs represents a substantial problem. In brief, even if service users are not physically coerced, they still feel coerced as they are not free to live how they want to (Riley et al., 2014).

## 5.2    Staff Views on Involuntary Hospitalisation and Community Treatment Orders

Health professionals consider involuntary hospitalisation necessary when they feel threatened or misunderstood by a patient and in need of help from their colleagues. They have a desire for better communication and coordination among team members (Sugiura et al., 2020). CTOs are primarily viewed as medication-oriented by psychiatrists who have been interviewed about this (Canvin et al., 2014). However, the establishment of a therapeutic relationship with the patient under CTO seems to be challenging for staff, but of paramount importance (Jansson & Fridlund, 2016).

## 5.3    Informal Caregivers' View on Involuntary Hospitalisation and Community Treatment Orders

Informal caregivers often struggle with the issue of involuntary admission of family members. Involuntary hospitalisation can however also produce distressing feelings, for instance when informal caregivers worry that their family member may suffer coercive practices (Norvoll et al., 2018). They may feel responsible for the hospitalisation of their family member and fear the disruption of their relationship (Sugiura et al., 2020). Often, professional help and support are sought prior to involuntary hospitalisation, but at times informal caregivers do not receive, or do not know how to get the help they need (Jankovic et al., 2011). Also, from the informal caregivers' perspective, alarming changes in the patient's behaviour reinforce the decision to ask for involuntary hospitalisation (Gowda et al., 2019a). When a service user is admitted involuntarily, informal caregivers often feel anxious and guilty, but also relieved (Jankovic et al., 2011).

Informal caregivers have mixed feelings towards CTOs context (Canvin et al., 2014). They feel responsible for having asked for the treatment but do not consider themselves a member of the health team. The CTO gives them a feeling of security: the patient is looked after in a steady context. However, in some cases, family members feel excluded and that their personal experience is not taken into consideration.

Coercion is accepted by informal caregivers, when they believe that the patient is suffering and the available medical help does not solve the informal caregivers' problems in dealing with the entire situation (Stensrud et al., 2015). In the caregiver's opinion, CTOs should have a more integrated approach and should be more specific when responding to the patient's needs. Hence, informal caregivers can have conflicting ideas, either they want to help the service user to make personal decisions, or they choose to assist the professional in medical treatment. Yet, informal caregivers usually do not consider CTOs hazardous.

## 5.4 Summary

Many service users support the proposed ban of coercive measures as expressed in the UN-CRPD. Even if the principles of dignity, autonomy and inclusion are underlined, many countries still struggle to reduce involuntary hospitalisation. Research suggests interventions such as shared decision-making, CTOs and integrated care can reduce involuntary admissions. However, challenges are still on the agenda as national health policies and professional associations often do not support the proposed abolition of coercion.

Service users have varied perspectives on involuntary hospitalisation and CTOs. Some people disagree with involuntary hospitalisation, others consider it useful in situations of extreme crises, if less restrictive options have been tried, and legal advocacy and support have been given.

Health professionals consider involuntary hospitalisation as necessary when a service user, from a professional perspective, becomes a risk to others or to himself or herself. Under these circumstances, there is an increasing demand for improved coordination among staff and services.

For informal caregivers, involuntary hospitalisation remains a challenge even when it represents a last effort in developments that often result in difficult family tensions. Informal caregivers can express concern and internal conflicts feeling responsible for the hospitalisation. While seeking professional assistance is common, informal caregivers frequently encounter difficulties in accessing appropriate support. The changes in the patient's mental state and the alleged danger provide a rationale for the request for involuntary admission. The informal caregiver initially feels anxious, but afterwards relief. Informal caregivers have mixed feelings about CTOs. They appreciate the feeling of safety and its stabilising effect, and welcome the return of a sense of security, but also feel excluded and psychologically unsettled by the medical intervention. They live in a contradictory way as they are upholding the service user's autonomy, but at the same time also assisting with medical treatment. However, they are convinced that the CTO does not deal with everyday problems. In brief, informal caregivers generally do not consider CTOs to be problematic.

## 6    Conclusion

The original chapter, published in the first edition, concluded that service users' perspectives should be taken into consideration in the research and the present state of research has indeed advanced in this direction. Service users' views of coercion and violence have not however led to significant changes in legal and clinical practices, which are still underpinned by formal and informal coercion. While service users' views have been included in research recently, informal carers' perspectives have not. Furthermore, few studies have been led, or co-led by service users. Nevertheless, research on this topic has become much clearer and, in some ways, more stable.

Service users, staff and informal caregivers often have differing views about violence and coercion. Although no stakeholder group agrees with today's clinical practices, staff and informal caregivers still see the root cause of violence in the service user's mental disorder and behaviour. This fundamental belief explains why coercion is seen as necessary more by staff and informal caregivers than by patients. Service users, however, often do not attribute the reasons for problems and conflicts to a mental illness.

A key conclusion is to challenge the conventional view on aggression and coercion that prioritised the service providers' perspective. Clinical practice will not advance in the direction of minimisation or abolition of violence and coercion as long as service users are not involved as active participants in research, teaching and service provision. While shared decision-making in mental health care has been promoted by official bodies such as the US Substance Abuse and Mental Health Services Administration for some years (SAMHSA, 2010), research has highlighted that shared decision-making usually does not work even in non-risk situations in everyday practice (Gurtner et al., 2022; Huang et al., 2020). In many situations, service users' views are not taken into account, let alone followed. This is particularly true in the case of conflicts between patients and staff and when there is a risk of self-harm or harm to others from a staff perspective.

## 6.1    Next Steps

As the UN-CRPD has explicitly stated, the issue of decision-making is central to the use of coercion in mental health care. Clinicians should be aware of the political and legal discussions around decision-making in mental health care, that currently go beyond shared decision-making, in order to promote supported decision-making (ENNHRI/MHE, 2020; Gooding, 2013). Supported decision-making leaves the final decision on health matters to the service user exclusively, while the service provider's role is to support the client with information, but not to instruct on the best ways of being treated. The legal and political discussions mentioned above increasingly support the transformation to supported decision-making.

As shared decision-making has not yet been fully implemented in clinical routine, there is still a long way to go to achieve supported decision-making. Based on our knowledge and experience and to advance the next steps into this direction, the involvement of stakeholders' perspectives on violence and coercion prevention could be organised practically as follows:

- Involving service users in mental health care management, providing training and service provisions.
- Involving informal caregivers in advisory boards of service providers.
- Training mental health professionals to interpret aggressive incidents in care settings not solely from a pathological viewpoint, but additionally sensitising them to be aware of their own role in escalating aggression.
- Take into consideration and explore, if possible, the service user's perspective after an aggressive and/or coercive incident in order to learn from it.
- Explore possible traumatic or fear-inducing consequences after service users have experienced a coercive incident directly or indirectly.
- Prevent aggressive and/or coercive incidents by utilising advance directives.
- Utilise shared decision-making or even supported decision-making, in risk-prone situations.

## References

Aguilera-Serrano, C., Guzman-Parra, J., Garcia-Sanchez, J. A., Moreno-Küstner, B., & Mayoral-Cleries, F. (2018). Variables associated with the subjective experience of coercive measures in psychiatric inpatients: A systematic review. *Canadian Journal of Psychiatry, 63*(2), 129–144. https://doi.org/10.1177/0706743717738491

Akther, S. F., Molyneaux, E., Stuart, R., Johnson, S., Simpson, A., & Oram, S. (2019). Patients' experiences of assessment and detention under mental health legislation: Systematic review and qualitative meta-synthesis. *BJPsych Open, 5*(3), e37. https://doi.org/10.1192/bjo.2019.19

Allison, R., & Flemming, K. (2019). Mental health patients' experiences of softer coercion and its effects on their interactions with practitioners: A qualitative evidence synthesis. *Journal of Advanced Nursing, 75*(11), 2274–2284. https://doi.org/10.1111/jan.14035

Al-Maraira, O. A., & Hayajneh, F. A. (2020). Correlates of psychiatric staff's attitude toward coercion and their sociodemographic characteristics. *Nursing Forum, 55*(4), 603–610. https://doi.org/10.1111/nuf.12476

Armgart, C., Schaub, M., Hoffmann, K., Illes, F., Emons, B., Jendreyschak, J., et al. (2013). Negative Emotionen und Verständnis—Zwangsmaßnahmen aus Patientensicht [Negative emotions and understanding—Patients' perspective on coercion]. *Psychiatrische Praxis, 40*(5), 278–284. https://doi.org/10.1055/s-0033-1343159

Barbui, C., Purgato, M., Abdulmalik, J., Caldas-de-Almeida, J. M., Eaton, J., Gureje, O., et al. (2021). Efficacy of interventions to reduce coercive treatment in mental health services: Umbrella review of randomised evidence. *British Journal of Psychiatry, 218*(4), 185–195. https://doi.org/10.1192/bjp.2020.144

Benson, A., Secker, J., Balfe, E., Lipsedge, M., Robinson, S., & Walker, J. (2003). Discourses of blame: Accounting for aggression and violence on an acute mental health inpatient unit. *Social Science and Medicine, 57*(5), 917–926. https://doi.org/10.1016/s0277-9536(02)00460-4

Bergk, J., Flammer, E., & Steinert, T. (2010). "Coercion experience scale" (CES)—Validation of a questionnaire on coercive measures. *BMC Psychiatry, 10*(1), 5. https://doi.org/10.1186/1471-244X-10-5

Bigwood, S., & Crowe, M. (2008). It's part of the job, but it spoils the job': A phenomenological study of physical restraint. *International Journal of Mental Health Nursing, 17*(3), 215–222. https://doi.org/10.1111/j.1447-0349.2008.00526.x

Bird, M., Ouellette, C., Whitmore, C., Li, L., Nair, K., McGillion, M., et al. (2020). Preparing for patient partnership: A scoping review of patient partner engagement and evaluation in research. *Health Expectation, 23*(3), 523–539. https://doi.org/10.1111/hex.13040

Brady, N. S., Spittal, M. J., Brophy, L. M., & Harvey, C. A. (2017). Patients' experiences of restrictive interventions in Australia: Findings from the 2010 Australian Survey of Psychosis. *Psychiatric Services, 68*(9), 966–969. https://doi.org/10.1176/appi.ps.201600300

Bregar, B., Skela-Savič, B., & Kores Plesničar, B. (2018). Cross-sectional study on nurses' attitudes regarding coercive measures: The importance of socio-demographic characteristics, job satisfaction, and strategies for coping with stress. *BMC Psychiatry, 18*(1), 171. https://doi.org/10.1186/s12888-018-1756-1

Brophy, L. M., & McDermott, F. (2003). What's driving involuntary treatment in the community? The social, policy, legal, and ethical context. *Australasian Psychiatry, 11*, 84–88.

Brophy, L. M., Roper, C. E., Hamilton, B. E., Tellez, J. J., & McSherry, B. M. (2016). Consumers' and their supporters' perspectives on barriers and strategies to reducing seclusion and restraint in mental health settings. *Australian Health Review, 40*(6), 599–604. https://doi.org/10.1071/AH15128

Canvin, K., Rugkåsa, J., Sinclair, J., & Burns, T. (2014). Patient, psychiatrist and family carer experiences of community treatment orders: Qualitative study. *Social Psychiatry and Psychiatric Epidemiology, 49*(12), 1873–1882. https://doi.org/10.1007/s00127-014-0906-0

Chieze, M., Hurst, S., Kaiser, S., & Sentissi, O. (2019). Effects of seclusion and restraint in adult psychiatry: A systematic review. *Frontiers in Psychiatry, 10*, 491. https://doi.org/10.3389/fpsyt.2019.00491

Cutcliffe, J. R., & Hannigan, B. (2001). Mass media, 'monsters' and mental health clients: The need for increased lobbying. *Journal of Psychiatry and Mental Health Nursing, 8*(4), 315–321. https://doi.org/10.1046/j.1365-2850.2001.00394.x

Dawson, J. (2015). A realistic approach to assessing mental health laws' compliance with the UNCRPD. *International Journal of Law and Psychiatry, 40*, 70–79. https://doi.org/10.1016/j.ijlp.2015.04.003

de Stefano, A., & Ducci, G. (2008). Involuntary admission and compulsory treatment in Europe: An overview. *International Journal of Mental Health, 37*(3), 10–21. https://doi.org/10.2753/IMH0020-7411370301

Doedens, P., Vermeulen, J., Boyette, L. L., Latour, C., & de Haan, L. (2020). Influence of nursing staff attitudes and characteristics on the use of coercive measures in acute mental health services—A systematic review. *Journal of Psychiatry and Mental Health Nursing, 27*(4), 446–459. https://doi.org/10.1111/jpm.12586

Dressing, H., & Salize, H. J. (2004). Compulsory admission of mentally ill patients in European Union member states. *Social Psychiatry and Psychiatric Epidemiology, 39*(10), 797–803.

Duxbury, J. (2002). An evaluation of staff and patient views of and strategies employed to manage inpatient aggression and violence on one mental health unit: A pluralistic design. *Journal of Psychiatry and Mental Health Nursing, 9*(3), 325–337. https://doi.org/10.1046/j.1365-2850.2002.00497.x

Duxbury, J., & Whittington, R. (2005). Causes and management of patient aggression and violence: Staff and patient perspectives. *Journal of Advanced Nursing, 50*(5), 469–478. https://doi.org/10.1111/j.1365-2648.2005.03426.x

Duxbury, J., Pulsford, D., Hadi, M., & Sykes, S. (2013). Staff and relatives' perspectives on the aggressive behaviour of older people with dementia in residential care: A qualitative study. *Journal of Psychiatry and Mental Health Nursing, 20*(9), 792–800. https://doi.org/10.1111/jpm.12018

El-Badri, S., & Mellsop, G. (2008). Patient and staff perspectives on the use of seclusion. *Australasian Psychiatry, 16*(4), 248–252. https://doi.org/10.1080/10398560802027302

ENNHRI/MHE. (2020). *Implementing supported decision-making*. European Network of National Human Rights Institutions/Mental Health Europe.

Fagan-Pryor, E. C., Haber, L. C., Dunlap, D., Nall, J. L., Stanley, G., & Wolpert, R. (2003). Patients' views of causes of aggression by patients and effective interventions. *Psychiatric Services, 54*(4), 549–553. https://doi.org/10.1176/appi.ps.54.4.549

Fletcher, A., Crowe, M., Manuel, J., & Foulds, J. (2021). Comparison of patients' and staff's perspectives on the causes of violence and aggression in psychiatric inpatient settings: An integrative review. *Journal of Psychiatry and Mental Health Nursing, 28*(5), 924–939. https://doi.org/10.1111/jpm.12758

Førde, R., Norvoll, R., Hem, M. H., & Pedersen, R. (2016). Next of kin's experiences of involvement during involuntary hospitalisation and coercion. *BMC Medical Ethics, 17*(1), 76. https://doi.org/10.1186/s12910-016-0159-4

Fugger, G., Gleiss, A., Baldinger, P., Strnad, A., Kasper, S., & Frey, R. (2016). Psychiatric patients' perception of physical restraint. *Acta Psychiatrica Scandinavica, 133*(3), 221–231. https://doi.org/10.1111/acps.12501

Funk, M., Drew, N., & Robertson, P. (2022). *WHO quality rights: Act, unite and empower for mental health*. World Health Organisation. Retrieved from January 15, 2023.

Gabriel, A. (2017). Development of an instrument to measure patients' attitudes towards involuntary hospitalization. *World Journal of Psychiatry, 7*(2), 89–97. https://doi.org/10.5498/wjp.v7.i2.89

Gandhi, S., Poreddi, V., Nagarajaiah, Palaniappan, M., Reddy, S. S. N., & BadaMath, S. (2018). Indian nurses' knowledge, attitude and practice towards use of physical restraints in psychiatric patients. *Investigacion y Educacion en Enfermeria, 36*(1), e10. https://doi.org/10.17533/udea.iee.v36n1e10

Gardner, W., Hoge, S. K., Bennett, N., Roth, L. H., Lidz, C. W., Monahan, J., et al. (1993). Two scales for measuring patients' perceptions for coercion during mental hospital admission. *Behavioral Sciences and The Law, 11*(3), 307–321.

Georgieva, I., Mulder, C. L., & Wierdsma, A. (2012). Patients' preference and experiences of forced medication and seclusion. *Psychiatric Quarterly, 83*(1), 1–13. https://doi.org/10.1007/s11126-011-9178-y

Georgieva, I., Whittington, R., Lauvrud, C., Steinert, T., Wikman, S., Lepping, P., et al. (2019). International variations in mental-health law regulating involuntary commitment of psychiatric patients as measured by the Mental Health Legislation Attitudes Scale. *Medicine, Science and the Law, 59*, 104–114.

Gerace, A., & Muir-Cochrane, E. (2019). Perceptions of nurses working with psychiatric consumers regarding the elimination of seclusion and restraint in psychiatric inpatient settings and emergency departments: An Australian survey. *International Journal of Mental Health Nursing, 28*(1), 209–225. https://doi.org/10.1111/inm.12522

Gooding, P. (2013). Supported decision-making: A rights-based disability concept and its implications for mental health law. *Psychiatry, Psychology and Law, 20*(3), 431–451. https://doi.org/1 0.1080/13218719.2012.711683

Gooding, P. (2023). *Compendium report: Good practices in the Council of Europe to promote Voluntary Measures in Mental Health Services* (p. 103). Council of Europe Committee on Bioethics. Retrieved from https://www.coe.int/en/web/bioethics/compendium-report-good-practices-in-the-council-of-europe-to-promote-voluntary-measures-in-mental-health-

Gowda, G. S., Kumar, C. N., Ray, S., Das, S., Nanjegowda, R. B., & Math, S. B. (2019a). Caregivers' attitude and perspective on coercion and restraint practices on psychiatric inpatients from South India. *Journal of Neurosciences in Rural Practice, 10*(2), 261–266. https://doi.org/10.4103/jnrp.jnrp_302_18

Gowda, G. S., Lepping, P., Ray, S., Noorthoorn, E., Nanjegowda, R. B., Kumar, C. N., et al. (2019b). Clinician attitude and perspective on the use of coercive measures in clinical practice from tertiary care mental health establishment—A cross-sectional study. *Indian Journal of Psychiatry, 61*(2), 151–155. https://doi.org/10.4103/psychiatry.IndianJPsychiatry_336_18

Gudde, C. B., Olsø, T. M., Whittington, R., & Vatne, S. (2015). Service users' experiences and views of aggressive situations in mental health care: A systematic review and thematic synthesis of qualitative studies. *Journal of Multidisciplinary Healthcare, 8*, 449–462. https://doi.org/10.2147/jmdh.S89486

Gurtner, C., Lohrmann, C., Schols, J. M. G. A., & Hahn, S. (2022). Shared decision making in the psychiatric inpatient setting: An ethnographic study about interprofessional psychiatric consultations. *International Journal of Environmental Research and Public Health, 19*(6), 3644. Retrieved from https://www.mdpi.com/1660-4601/19/6/3644

Guzmán-Parra, J., Aguilera-Serrano, C., García-Sanchez, J. A., García-Spínola, E., Torres-Campos, D., Villagrán, J. M., et al. (2019). Experience coercion, post-traumatic stress, and satisfaction with treatment associated with different coercive measures during psychiatric hospitalization. *International Journal of Mental Health Nursing, 28*(2), 448–456. https://doi.org/10.1111/inm.12546

Hahn, S., & Wolfensberger, P. (2022). Enhancing the quality of care through participatory generation of evidence. In A. Higgins, N. Kilkku, & G. Kort Kristofersson (Eds.), *Advanced practice in mental health nursing* (pp. 449–466). Springer. https://doi.org/10.1007/978-3-031-05536-2_19

Hallett, N., Huber, J. W., & Dickens, G. L. (2014). Violence prevention in inpatient psychiatric settings: Systematic review of studies about the perceptions of care staff and patients. *Aggression and Violent Behavior, 19*(5), 502–514. https://doi.org/10.1016/j.avb.2014.07.009

Happell, B., & Harrow, A. (2010). Nurses' attitudes to the use of seclusion: A review of the literature. *International Journal of Mental Health Nursing, 19*(3), 162–168. https://doi.org/10.1111/j.1447-0349.2010.00669.x

Happell, B., & Koehn, S. (2011). Seclusion as a necessary intervention: The relationship between burnout, job satisfaction and therapeutic optimism and justification for the use of seclusion. *Journal of Advanced Nursing, 67*(6), 1222–1231. https://doi.org/10.1111/j.1365-2648.2010.05570.x

Haugom, E. W., Ruud, T., & Hynnekleiv, T. (2019). Ethical challenges of seclusion in psychiatric inpatient wards: A qualitative study of the experiences of Norwegian mental health professionals. *BMC Health Services Research, 19*(1), 879. https://doi.org/10.1186/s12913-019-4727-4

Hawsawi, T., Power, T., Zugai, J., & Jackson, D. (2020). Nurses' and consumers' shared experiences of seclusion and restraint: A qualitative literature review. *International Journal of Mental Health Nursing, 29*(5), 831–845. https://doi.org/10.1111/inm.12716

Hirsch, S., Thilo, N., Steinert, T., & Flammer, E. (2021). Patients' perception of coercion with respect to antipsychotic treatment of psychotic disorders and its predictors. *Social Psychiatry and Psychiatric Epidemiology, 56*(8), 1381–1388. https://doi.org/10.1007/s00127-021-02083-z

Hofmann, H., & Hahn, S. (2013). Characteristics of nursing home residents and physical restraint: A systematic literature review. *Journal of Clinical Nursing, 11*, 1–13.

Horvath, J., Steinert, T., & Jaeger, S. (2018). Antipsychotic treatment of psychotic disorders in forensic psychiatry: Patients' perception of coercion and its predictors. *International Journal of Law and Psychiatry, 57*, 113–121. https://doi.org/10.1016/j.ijlp.2018.02.004

Hotzy, F., Jaeger, M., Buehler, E., Moetteli, S., Klein, G., Beeri, S., et al. (2019). Attitudinal variance among patients, next of kin and health care professionals towards the use of containment measures in three psychiatric hospitals in Switzerland. *BMC Psychiatry, 19*(1), 128. https://doi.org/10.1186/s12888-019-2092-9

Huang, C., Plummer, V., Lam, L., & Cross, W. (2020). Perceptions of shared decision-making in severe mental illness: An integrative review. *Journal of Psychiatric and Mental Health Nursing, 27*(2), 103–127. https://doi.org/10.1111/jpm.12558

Husum, T. L., Ruud, T., Lickiewicz, J., & Siqveland, J. (2022). Measurement properties of the staff attitude to coercion scale: A systematic review (systematic review). *Frontiers in Psychiatry, 13*. https://doi.org/10.3389/fpsyt.2022.744661

Ilkiw-Lavalle, O., & Grenyer, B. F. (2003). Differences between patient and staff perceptions of aggression in mental health units. *Psychiatric Services, 54*(3), 389–393. https://doi.org/10.1176/appi.ps.54.3.389

Jaeger, M., & Rossler, W. (2010). Enhancement of outpatient treatment adherence: Patients' perceptions of coercion, fairness and effectiveness. *Psychiatry Research, 180*(1), 48–53. https://doi.org/10.1016/j.psychres.2009.09.011

Jankovic, J., Yeeles, K., Katsakou, C., Amos, T., Morriss, R., Rose, D., et al. (2011). Family caregivers' experiences of involuntary psychiatric hospital admissions of their relatives—A qualitative study. *PLoS One, 6*(10), e25425. https://doi.org/10.1371/journal.pone.0025425

Jansen, G., Dassen, T., & Moorer, P. (1997). The perception of aggression. *Scandinavian Journal of Caring Sciences, 11*(1), 51–55. https://doi.org/10.1111/j.1471-6712.1997.tb00430.x

Jansson, S., & Fridlund, B. (2016). Perceptions among psychiatric staff of creating a therapeutic alliance with patients on community treatment orders. *Issues in Mental Health Nursing, 37*(10), 701–707. https://doi.org/10.1080/01612840.2016.1216207

Johnson, B., Martin, M. L., Guha, M., & Montgomery, P. (1997). The experience of thought-disordered individuals preceding an aggressive incident. *Journal of Psychiatric and Mental Health Nursing, 4*(3), 213–220. https://doi.org/10.1046/j.1365-2850.1997.00041.x

Kinner, S. A., Harvey, C., Hamilton, B., Brophy, L., Roper, C., McSherry, B., et al. (2017). Attitudes towards seclusion and restraint in mental health settings: Findings from a large, community-based survey of consumers, carers and mental health professionals. *Epidemiology and Psychiatric Sciences, 26*(5), 535–544. https://doi.org/10.1017/S2045796016000585

Kontio, R., Joffe, G., Putkonen, H., Kuosmanen, L., Hane, K., Holi, M., et al. (2012). Seclusion and restraint in psychiatry: Patients' experiences and practical suggestions on how to improve practices and use alternatives. *Perspectives in Psychiatric Care, 48*(1), 16–24. https://doi.org/10.1111/j.1744-6163.2010.00301.x

Krieger, E., Moritz, S., Weil, R., & Nagel, M. (2018). Patients' attitudes towards and acceptance of coercion in psychiatry. *Psychiatry Research, 260*, 478–485. https://doi.org/10.1016/j.psychres.2017.12.029

Krieger, E., Moritz, S., Lincoln, T. M., Fischer, R., & Nagel, M. (2021). Coercion in psychiatry: A cross-sectional study on staff views and emotions. *Journal of Psychiatric and Mental Health Nursing., 28*(2), 149–162. https://doi.org/10.1111/jpm.12643

Kumar, S., Guite, H., & Thornicroft, G. (2001). Service users' experience of violence within a mental health system: A study using grounded theory approach. *Journal of Mental Health, 10*(6), 597–611. https://doi.org/10.1080/09638230120041353

Làrsen, I. B., & Terkelsen, T. B. (2014). Coercion in a locked psychiatric ward: Perspectives of patients and staff. *Nursing Ethics, 21*(4), 426–436. https://doi.org/10.1177/0969733013503601

Lee, M. H., & Seo, M. K. (2021). Perceived coercion of persons with mental illness living in a community. *International Journal of Environmental Research and Public Health, 18*(5), 2290. https://doi.org/10.3390/ijerph18052290

Lidz, C. W. (1998). Coercion in psychiatric care: What have we learned from research? *Journal of the American Academy of Psychiatry and the Law, 26*(4), 631–637.

Ling, S., Cleverley, K., & Perivolaris, A. (2015). Understanding mental health service user experiences of restraint through debriefing: A qualitative analysis. *Canadian Journal of Psychiatry (Revue Canadienne de Psychiatrie), 60*(9), 386–392. https://doi.org/10.1177/070674371506000903

Love, C. C., & Hunter, M. (1999). The Atascadero State Hospital experience. Engaging patients in violence prevention. *Journal of Psychosocial Nursing and Mental Health Services, 37*(9), 32–36. https://doi.org/10.3928/0279-3695-19990901-10

Mielau, J., Altunbay, J., Gallinat, J., Heinz, A., Bermpohl, F., Lehmann, A., et al. (2016). Subjective experience of coercion in psychiatric care: A study comparing the attitudes of patients and healthy volunteers towards coercive methods and their justification. *European Archives of Psychiatry and Clinical Neuroscience, 266*(4), 337–347. https://doi.org/10.1007/s00406-015-0598-9

Molewijk, B., Kok, A., Husum, T., Pedersen, R., & Aasland, O. (2017). Staff's normative attitudes towards coercion: The role of moral doubt and professional context-a cross-sectional survey study. *BMC Medical Ethics, 18*(1), 37. https://doi.org/10.1186/s12910-017-0190-0

Moran, A., Cocoman, A., Scott, P. A., Matthews, A., Staniuliene, V., & Valimaki, M. (2009). Restraint and seclusion: A distressing treatment option? *Journal of Psychiatric and Mental Health Nursing, 16*(7), 599–605. https://doi.org/10.1111/j.1365-2850.2009.01419.x

Morandi, S., Silva, B., Mendez Rubio, M., Bonsack, C., & Golay, P. (2021). Mental health professionals' feelings and attitudes towards coercion. *International Journal of Law and Psychiatry, 74*, 101665. https://doi.org/10.1016/j.ijlp.2020.101665

Muir-Cochrane, E. C., Baird, J., & McCann, T. V. (2015). Nurses' experiences of restraint and seclusion use in short-stay acute old age psychiatry inpatient units: A qualitative study. *Journal of Psychiatric and Mental Health Nursing, 22*(2), 109–115. https://doi.org/10.1111/jpm.12189

Norvoll, R., & Pedersen, R. (2018). Patients' moral views on coercion in mental healthcare. *Nursing Ethics, 25*(6), 796–807. https://doi.org/10.1177/0969733016674768

Norvoll, R., Hem, M. H., & Lindemann, H. (2018). Family members' existential and moral dilemmas with coercion in mental healthcare. *Qualitative Health Research, 28*(6), 900–915. https://doi.org/10.1177/1049732317750120

Nyttingnes, O., Rugkåsa, J., Holmén, A., & Ruud, T. (2017). The development, validation, and feasibility of the Experienced Coercion Scale. *Psychological Assessment, 29*(10), 1210–1220. https://doi.org/10.1037/pas0000404

Omérov, M., Edman, G., & Wistedt, B. (2004). Violence and threats of violence within psychiatric care—A comparison of staff and patient experience of the same incident. *Nordic Journal of Psychiatry, 58*(5), 363–369. https://doi.org/10.1080/08039480410005918

Philo, G. (1996). *Media and mental distress*. Longman.

Poythress, N. G., Petrila, J., McGaha, A., & Boothroyd, R. (2002). Perceived coercion and procedural justice in the Broward mental health court. *International Journal of Law and Psychiatry, 25*(5), 517–533.

Pridham, K. M., Berntson, A., Simpson, A. I., Law, S. F., Stergiopoulos, V., & Nakhost, A. (2016). Perception of coercion among patients with a psychiatric community treatment order: A literature review. *Psychiatric Services, 67*(1), 16–28. https://doi.org/10.1176/appi.ps.201400538

Raveesh, B. N., Pathare, S., Lepping, P., Noorthoorn, E. O., Gowda, G. S., & Bunders-Aelen, J. G. (2016a). Perceived coercion in persons with mental disorder in India: A cross-sectional study. *Indian Journal of Psychiatry, 58*(Suppl 2), S210–S220. https://doi.org/10.4103/0019-5545.196846

Raveesh, B. N., Pathare, S., Noorthoorn, E. O., Gowda, G. S., Lepping, P., & Bunders-Aelen, J. G. (2016b). Staff and caregiver attitude to coercion in India. *Indian Journal of Psychiatry, 58*(Suppl 2), S221–S229. https://doi.org/10.4103/0019-5545.196847

Reisch, T., Beeri, S., Klein, G., Meier, P., Pfeifer, P., Buehler, E., et al. (2018). Comparing attitudes to containment measures of patients, health care professionals and next of kin. *Frontiers in Psychiatry, 9*, 529. https://doi.org/10.3389/fpsyt.2018.00529

Riley, H., Høyer, G., & Lorem, G. F. (2014). 'When coercion moves into your home'—a qualitative study of patient experiences with outpatient commitment in Norway. *Health & Social Care in the Community, 22*(5), 506–514. https://doi.org/10.1111/hsc.12107

Rose, D. (1998). Television, madness and community care. *Journal of Community and Applied Social Psychology, 8*(3), 213–228.

Ruggeri, M., Lasalvia, A., Tansella, M., Bonetto, C., Abate, M., Thornicroft, G., et al. (2004). Heterogeneity of outcomes in schizophrenia. 3-year follow-up of treated prevalent cases. *British Journal of Psychiatry, 184*, 48–57. https://doi.org/10.1192/bjp.184.1.48

Rugkåsa, J. (2016). Effectiveness of community treatment orders: The international evidence. *Canadian Journal of Psychiatry, 61*(1), 15–24. https://doi.org/10.1177/0706743715620415

SAMHSA. (2010). *Shared decision-making in mental health care: Practice, research, and future directions.* Center for Mental Health Services, Substance Abuse and Mental Health Services Administration. HHS Publication No. SMA-09-4371.

Scholten, M., & Gather, J. (2017). Adverse consequences of article 12 of the UN Convention on the Rights of Persons with Disabilities for persons with mental disabilities and an alternative way forward. *Journal of Medical Ethics, 44*, 226. https://doi.org/10.1136/medethics-2017-104414

Schomerus, G., Sander, C., Schindler, S., Baumann, E., & Angermeyer, M. C. (2023). Public attitudes towards protecting the human rights of people with mental illness: A scoping review and data from a population trend study in Germany. *International Review of Psychiatry, 35*(2), 167–179. https://doi.org/10.1080/09540261.2022.2087494

Sheehan, K. A., & Burns, T. (2011). Perceived coercion and the therapeutic relationship: A neglected association? *Psychiatric Services, 62*(5), 471–476. https://doi.org/10.1176/ps.62.5.pss6205_0471

Sheridan Rains, L., Zenina, T., Dias, M. C., Jones, R., Jeffreys, S., Branthonne-Foster, S., et al. (2019). Variations in patterns of involuntary hospitalisation and in legal frameworks: An international comparative study. *Lancet Psychiatry, 6*(5), 403–417. https://doi.org/10.1016/S2215-0366(19)30090-2

Shrestha, Y. (2018). Knowledge and attitude of family member of mentally ill patient regarding restraint, 2016. *Archives of Psychiatric Nursing, 32*(2), 297–299. https://doi.org/10.1016/j.apnu.2017.11.018

Sibitz, I., Scheutz, A., Lakeman, R., Schrank, B., Schaffer, M., & Amering, M. (2011). Impact of coercive measures on life stories: Qualitative study. *British Journal of Psychiatry, 199*(3), 239–244. https://doi.org/10.1192/bjp.bp.110.087841

Slade, M., Adams, N., & O'Hagan, M. (2012). Recovery: Past progress and future challenges. *International Review of Psychiatry, 24*(1), 1–4. https://doi.org/10.3109/09540261.2011.644847

Stanhope, V., Marcus, S., & Solomon, P. (2009). The impact of coercion on services from the perspective of mental health care consumers with co-occurring disorders. *Psychiatric Services, 60*(2), 183–188. https://doi.org/10.1176/ps.2009.60.2.183

Steiger, S., Moeller, J., Sowislo, J. F., Lieb, R., Lang, U. E., & Huber, C. G. (2022a). Approval of coercion in psychiatry in public perception and the role of stigmatization. *Frontiers in Psychiatry, 12*, 819573. https://doi.org/10.3389/fpsyt.2021.819573

Steiger, S., Moeller, J., Sowislo, J. F., Lieb, R., Lang, U. E., & Huber, C. G. (2022b). Corrigendum: Approval of coercion in psychiatry in public perception and the role of stigmatization. *Frontiers in Psychiatry, 13*. https://doi.org/10.3389/fpsyt.2022.881898

Stensrud, B., Høyer, G., Granerud, A., & Landheim, A. S. (2015). 'Responsible, but still not a real treatment partner': A qualitative study of the experiences of relatives of patients on outpatient commitment orders. *Issues in Mental Health Nursing, 36*(8), 583–591. https://doi.org/10.3109/01612840.2015.1021939

Sugiura, K., Pertega, E., & Holmberg, C. (2020). Experiences of involuntary psychiatric admission decision-making: A systematic review and meta-synthesis of the perspectives of service users, informal carers, and professionals. *International Journal of Law and Psychiatry, 73*, 101645. https://doi.org/10.1016/j.ijlp.2020.101645

Szasz, T. S., & Alexander, G. J. (1968). Mental illness as an excuse for civil wrongs. *The Journal of Nervous and Mental Disease, 147*(2), 113–123.

Thøgersen, M. H., Morthorst, B., & Nordentoft, M. (2010). Perceptions of coercion in the community: A qualitative study of patients in a Danish assertive community treatment team. *Psychiatric Quarterly, 81*(1), 35–47. https://doi.org/10.1007/s11126-009-9115-5

Tingleff, E. B., Bradley, S. K., Gildberg, F. A., Munksgaard, G., & Hounsgaard, L. (2017). "Treat me with respect". A systematic review and thematic analysis of psychiatric patients' reported perceptions of the situations associated with the process of coercion. *Journal of Psychiatric and Mental Health Nursing, 24*(9–10), 681–698. https://doi.org/10.1111/jpm.12410

Trivedi, P., & Wykes, T. (2002). From passive subjects to equal partners: Qualitative review of user involvement in research. *British Journal of Psychiatry, 181*, 468–472. https://doi.org/10.1192/bjp.181.6.468

UN General Assembly. (2013). Report of the Special Rapporteur on torture and other cruel, inhuman or degrading treatment or punishment, Juan E. Méndez. A/HRC/22/53.

United Nations. (2006). *United Nations convention on the rights of persons with disabilities.* United Nations. Retrieved April 20, 2023, from https://www.un.org/development/desa/disabilities/convention-on-the-rights-of-persons-with-disabilities.html

Välimäki, M., Lam, J., Bressington, D., Cheung, T., Wong, W. K., Cheng, P. Y. I., et al. (2022a). Nurses', patients', and informal caregivers' attitudes toward aggression in psychiatric hospitals: A comparative survey study. *PLoS One, 17*(9), e0274536. https://doi.org/10.1371/journal.pone.0274536

Välimäki, M., Lantta, T., Lam, Y. T. J., Cheung, T., Cheng, P. Y. I., Ng, T., et al. (2022b). Perceptions of patient aggression in psychiatric hospitals: A qualitative study using focus groups with nurses, patients, and informal caregivers. *BMC Psychiatry, 22*(1), 344. https://doi.org/10.1186/s12888-022-03974-4

Van Der Merwe, M., Muir-Cochrane, E., Jones, J., Tziggili, M., & Bowers, L. (2013). Improving seclusion practice: Implications of a review of staff and patient views. *Journal of Psychiatric and Mental Health Nursing, 20*(3), 203–215. https://doi.org/10.1111/j.1365-2850.2012.01903.x

Vedana, K. G. G., da Silva, D. M., Ventura, C. A. A., Giacon, B. C. C., Zanetti, A. C. G., Miasso, A. I., et al. (2018). Physical and mechanical restraint in psychiatric units: Perceptions and experiences of nursing staff. *Archives of Psychiatric Nursing, 32*(3), 367–372. https://doi.org/10.1016/j.apnu.2017.11.027

Verbeke, E., Vanheule, S., Cauwe, J., Truijens, F., & Froyen, B. (2019). Coercion and power in psychiatry: A qualitative study with ex-patients. *Social Science & Medicine, 1982*(223), 89–96. https://doi.org/10.1016/j.socscimed.2019.01.031

Vishnivetsky, S., Shoval, G., Leibovich, V., Giner, L., Mitrany, M., Cohen, D., et al. (2013). Seclusion room vs. physical restraint in an adolescent inpatient setting: Patients' attitudes. *Israel Journal of Psychiatry and Related Sciences, 50*(1), 6–10.

von Peter, S. (2017). Partizipative und kollaborative Forschungsansätze in der Psychiatrie. *Psychiatrische Praxis, 44*(08), 431–433. https://doi.org/10.1055/s-0043-120241

Wasserman, D., Apter, G., Baeken, C., Bailey, S., Balazs, J., Bec, C., et al. (2020). Compulsory admissions of patients with mental disorders: State of the art on ethical and legislative aspects in 40 European countries. *European Psychiatry, 63*(1), e82. https://doi.org/10.1192/j.eurpsy.2020.79

Whiting, D., Lichtenstein, P., & Fazel, S. (2021). Violence and mental disorders: A structured review of associations by individual diagnoses, risk factors, and risk assessment. *Lancet Psychiatry, 8*(2), 150–161. https://doi.org/10.1016/S2215-0366(20)30262-5

Wilson, C., Rouse, L., Rae, S., & Kar Ray, M. (2017). Is restraint a 'necessary evil' in mental health care? Mental health inpatients' and staff members' experience of physical restraint. *International Journal of Mental Health Nursing, 26*(5), 500–512. https://doi.org/10.1111/inm.12382

Wong, A. H., Ray, J. M., Rosenberg, A., Crispino, L., Parker, J., McVaney, C., et al. (2020). Experiences of individuals who were physically restrained in the emergency department. *JAMA Network Open, 3*(1), e1919381. https://doi.org/10.1001/jamanetworkopen.2019.19381

World Health Organization (WHO). (2021). *Hospital-based mental health services: Promoting person-centred and rights-based approaches*. Policy, Law and Human Rights, Department of Mental Health and Substance Use, World Health Organization.

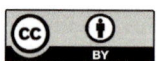

# Coercion in Contemporary Mental Health Services: Key Concepts, Historical Development and Contextual Factors

Deborah Oyine Aluh, José Miguel Caldas de Almeida, Dirk Richter, and Richard Whittington

Note: This chapter reproduces some material that was previously published under a CC-BY licence in the following sources:
Whittington, R., Aluh, D. O., & Caldas-de-Almeida, J.-M. (2023). Zero tolerance for coercion? Historical, cultural and organisational contexts for effective implementation of coercion-free mental health services around the world. *Healthcare, 11*, 2834. https://doi.org/10.3390/healthcare11212834
Richter, D. (2023). *Menschenrechte in der Psychiatrie: Prinzipien und Perspektiven einer psychosozialen Unterstützung ohne Zwang.* Psychiatrie Verlag. https://doi.org/10.1486/9783966052504

D. O. Aluh (✉)
Lisbon Institute of Global Mental Health, Comprehensive Health Research Centre, Nova Medical School, Lisbon, Portugal

Department of Clinical Pharmacy and Pharmacy Management, University of Nigeria Nsukka, Nsukka, Nigeria
e-mail: do.aluh@ensp.unl.pt

J. M. C. de Almeida
Lisbon Institute of Global Mental Health, Comprehensive Health Research Centre, Nova Medical School, Lisbon, Portugal

D. Richter
School of Health Professions, Division of Nursing, Bern University of Applied Sciences, Bern, Switzerland
e-mail: dirk.richter@bfh.ch

R. Whittington
Centre for Research and Education in Security, Prison and Forensic Psychiatry, St. Olav's hospital, Trondheim University Hospital, Trondheim, Norway

Department of Mental Health, Norwegian University of Science and Technology (NTNU), Trondheim, Norway
e-mail: richard.whittington@ntnu.no

## 1    Terminology

Contemporary international health policy envisions a move towards reducing and eventually eradicating the use of coercion in mental health services around the world (Council of Europe, 2019). The World Health Organization (WHO) Quality Rights Initiative, for example, sets out a framework which places an obligation on all WHO member states to appraise their services and transform them in such a way that respect for human rights is at the core of their practice principles (World Health Organization, 2019). Such a shift requires a credible approach to monitoring coercion as the fundamental basis for national and international benchmarking which can, in turn, act as a baseline for measuring change over time. Setting up such monitoring is very much a work in progress internationally with huge variation in the quality of recording systems and currently little scope for meaningful international comparisons between rates using even the most robust national systems (Reid & Price, 2022; Savage et al., 2024). While it is easy to recognise coercion when you are the person being subjected to it, establishing international consensus on definitions that would enable valid benchmarking and monitoring against international standards is very difficult.

Various national initiatives have taken place since the first edition of this book was published to remedy this situation. In particular, national guidelines have become a key mechanism for standardising and improving many aspects of healthcare, including the minimisation of coercion in mental health services. Such guidelines usually attempt to specify key terms as a starting point for a shared understanding of the problem and its potential solutions. Two examples of such attempts within Europe (Germany and England & Wales) are given in Table 1.

These definitions are drawn from the national guidelines for clinical practice when encountering violence especially (although not exclusively) in mental health services in Germany and the UK (England & Wales) (NICE, 2015; German Psychiatric Association (DGPPN), 2018). Together they provide both a basis for understanding the concepts which will be discussed throughout this book, but they also illustrate some subtle differences between two near-neighbour countries in the same global region. It can be seen firstly that the overall concept of coercion in both countries specifies the core idea of restriction applied with force and without consent. With regard to particular types of coercion, there is also some clear consensus alongside some variation. It is noteworthy, for example, that manual restraint is not considered to be a technique suitable for inclusion in the German guideline. Such manual restraint must be used in Germany, as elsewhere, as a first response before other coercive interventions can be implemented but it is not defined here. The terms 'isolation' and 'seclusion' are conflated in the German guideline but isolation is not named at all in the UK document. The policy of locking the door and the level of contact with the patient when secluding is also emphasised differently with a slightly softer tone in the UK definition. With regard to forced medication, the German guideline is explicit about the lack of consent whereas in the UK this is, at most, implied.

These key coercive interventions are well-known and sometimes referred to collectively as formal coercion to distinguish them from other types of coercion designated as 'informal' (Hotzy & Jaeger, 2016). This designation as formal coercion

**Table 1** Selected definitions of key coercive measures in two European countries (note: abbreviated in places)

| | Germany[a] | England & Wales[b] |
|---|---|---|
| General terminology and definitions of coercion | **Freedom-depriving and restricting measures** Mechanical, spatial or chemical measures that restrict freedom of movement against the will of the person concerned and are of a certain intensity, for example, isolation, restraint, including with bed rails, chair tables, net beds | **Restrictive interventions** Interventions that may infringe a person's human rights and freedom of movement |
| Involuntary hospitalisation | Transfer to a (psychiatric) hospital under application of a legal provision | |
| Physical immobilisation | **Restraint** Restraining a mentally ill person with wide leather or fabric straps | **Manual restraint** A skilled, hands-on method of physical restraint used by trained healthcare professionals to prevent service users from harming themselves, endangering others or compromising the therapeutic environment **Mechanical restraint** A method of physical intervention involving the use of authorised equipment, for example, handcuffs or restraining belts, applied in a skilled manner by designated healthcare professionals |
| Isolation/ seclusion | Transfer of a mentally ill person to a locked room without direct contact with staff | The supervised confinement of a patient in a room, which may be locked |
| Involuntary medication | **Forced medication** The administration of medication against the expressed or even only unarticulated (natural) will of the mentally ill person | **Rapid tranquillisation** Use of medication by the parenteral route (usually intramuscular or exceptionally intravenous) if oral medication is not possible or appropriate and urgent sedation with medication is needed |

[a] German Psychiatric Association (DGPPN) (2018). S3-Guideline prevention of coercion: Prevention and therapy of aggressive behaviour in adults. https://register.awmf.org/de/leitlinien/detail/038-022. Accessed 7-2-2024. Deepl Pro Translation
[b] NICE Guideline (NG10) (2015). Violence and aggression: short-term management in mental health, health and community settings. Accessed 7-2-2024

means that their use is almost always based on a legal decision which has been informed by a medical assessment under the relevant mental health legislation operating in the country. This requirement of a formal procedure for permission to deploy these types of coercion (e.g. paperwork, public hearings) ensures that effective monitoring should be feasible and therefore any gaps in knowledge are likely to be due to inadequate recording systems rather than difficulties in definition.

In contrast, informal coercion, also known as 'soft coercion' (Allison & Flemming, 2019) is not accompanied by explicit medical or legal measures. Here, communicative pressure is usually exerted on a person by professionals or legal representatives in order to achieve a certain behaviour or outcome (Hotzy & Jaeger, 2016). This pressure may be exerted verbally or non-verbally through body postures or simply exposure to a gathering of staff on a ward. But such pressure is largely subjective in the minds of both patients and staff and can be manifested in many different ways that, unlike formal coercion, are hard to capture. Many hospital admissions that begin voluntarily can subsequently involve such informal, and indeed formal, coercion. Threats of physical violence by staff have also occasionally been observed (BBC, 2022), but such behaviour crosses the line from informal coercion to illegality and thus makes the individual and their employer liable to criminal proceedings. Overall, informal coercion occupies a grey zone between formal coercion and autonomy.

Alongside attempts to clarify the language of coercion, there have been recent efforts to build a consensus on the main provisions designed to prevent coercion. The UK guidelines cited above in Table 1 (NICE, 2015, pp. 18–19) specify positive engagement, for example, as an 'intervention that aims to empower service users to actively participate in their care' though negotiation; and de-escalation as the 'use of techniques (including verbal and non-verbal communication skills) aimed at defusing anger and averting aggression' that do not include restraint. In an alternative approach, a recent international consensus exercise drew upon the expertise of clinicians and researchers across Europe with the aim of clarifying the terminology of both coercion itself and coercion-prevention. This led to an agreed taxonomy with 32 concepts in six domains: general concepts, involuntary inpatient care, involuntary outpatient care, spatial isolation, restraint practices and rights protection and administrative tools (FOSTREN, 2023). An extract from the last section is provided in Table 2.

These and other consensus efforts are all a work in progress driven by the hope that they will eventually lead to international best practice standards. But it is

**Table 2** Items from the FOSTREN Glossary Section 6: rights protection and administrative tools (FOSTREN 2023). NB: PMHC refers to a 'person with a mental health condition'

| Term | Definition |
|---|---|
| Supported decision-making | The PMHC is supported by others in making decisions. This can be structured support by clinical staff or others to facilitate that the person's will and preferences are respected in treatment decisions |
| Advance directives | Refers to a written statement by a PMHC when well, which sets out the way in which they want to be treated and/or treatment they do not want for their mental health condition should they deteriorate |
| CRPD | Convention on the Rights of Persons with Disabilities. A United Nations Human Rights Treaty to protect the rights and dignity of people with disabilities, including disability resulting from mental health conditions |
| Decision-making-capacity | In some jurisdictions, the lack of decision-making capacity is a legal requirement for involuntary care. Decision-making capacity means the ability to make (treatment) decisions, and this is usually assessed by checking that the person is able to understand and retain information, weigh it up to make a choice and express this |

important as well to consider this phenomenon within its historical context. Mental illness, medical treatment, care and coercion are all complex social processes that have challenged societies around the world and attitudes have evolved substantially but differently over time. An understanding of the changing narratives in this area is important to remind us that we are at one particular moment in history now and current approaches are only a temporary arrangement which may or may not provide the basis for future improvements.

## 2  Coercion in the History of Psychiatry

Throughout history, and into the present day, attitudes towards the use of coercive measures in the treatment of persons with mental disorders have always been closely associated with the prevailing cultural, religious and political context. In most of Europe, for centuries, persons with mental disorders were isolated, chained and victims of all kinds of violence and abuse (Shorter, 1997). It was in Classical Greece that madness was viewed for the first time as a strange phenomenon but nevertheless, one determined by natural causes and therefore part of the human condition (Thumiger, 2017). Different disorders were described, natural explanations were advanced for these disorders, and various therapeutic interventions were developed to mitigate the effects of the disorders. However, in Greece as well as in the Roman Empire, this medical interpretation always co-existed with magical and religious interpretations from the past. Those primarily responsible for caring for these persons were their families, who often limited themselves to isolating them and locking them up in their homes. The use of chains and other coercive instruments was common practice (Gonzalez de Chavez, 1980).

As early as the thirteenth and fourteenth centuries, there were examples of places in Europe where people with mental disorders were treated humanely and integrated into the community. In Geel, Belgium, persons with mental disorders began, in those days, to be accepted into the homes of farmers, where they lived as members of the family and participated in work and community activities, a practice that has survived until the present day (van Bilsen, 2016). In Granada, Spain, in the fourteenth century, at the Maristan hospital, the first European hospital created for the mentally ill, the patients were treated in a setting of tolerance and inclusion, which reflected the context that prevailed in that city at the time, marked by a peaceful and harmonious coexistence between Arabs, Christians and Jews that ushered a period of great progress in arts and science (Pérez et al., 2012).

In the Middle Ages, however, care for most persons with mental disorders continued to depend on families, except in the most serious cases. Then, if they were not abandoned and doomed to wander along with other beggars, they were locked up in cells located in hospices managed by monasteries and churches or in prisons administered by civil authorities (Gonzalez de Chavez, 1980). The growing influence of the Christian faith in this period also explains the occurrence of regular pilgrimages, involving thousands of mentally ill every year, to shrines believed to have miraculous powers in healing people with mental illnesses.

At the beginning of industrialisation, only patients with a lot of resources were treated in small private institutions, known in England then as 'madhouses'. The poor did not have access to such specialised institutions. The vast majority were locked up in their homes, or placed in rooms of general hospitals or asylums, together with physically ill patients, elderly persons and persons with disabilities, in subhuman living conditions. Others wandered aimlessly or ended up in workhouses.

The increase in the influx of patients to these institutions and the growing denunciations of the terrible conditions in which they lived led to the creation, from the eighteenth century onwards, of new general hospitals in many cities in Europe and the appearance of institutions specially dedicated to various types of illnesses (Porter, 2002). Asylums for the 'insane' (as persons with mental disorders were designated) began to emerge in the eighteenth century and the first attempts to change attitudes towards mental illness were part of this movement (Gonzalez de Chavez, 1980). These changes, however, would not have been possible without the new ideas of the philosophers of the Enlightenment. It was these new ideas that contributed to lessening the grip of superstition and emphasising a rational approach to natural phenomena, thus making possible the dissemination of new ways of understanding mental disorders and their treatment.

## 2.1    Pinel and Moral Treatment

François Pinel, freeing the patients from the chains in Bicêtre in 1793, went down in history as the symbol of a new attitude towards the mentally ill and the author of the so-called moral treatment. However, similar innovations were at the same time being developed in other countries, and the concept of moral treatment was, in fact, first formulated by William Tuke in the UK, where he created The Retreat in 1792, an institution where the mentally ill were treated using moral management and with a minimum of mechanical restraint (Raad & Makari, 2010). At the Lincoln Hospital, Robert Gardiner Hill also managed patients without the use of mechanical restraint. John Connolly, at the Hanwell Hospital, not only abolished the use of restraint but also introduced many other ideas, then quite innovative, such as improving facilities and food and promoting occupational activities; and, in Italy, Chiarugi also promoted the abolition of chains at the Ospedale Bonifazio in 1788 (Shorter, 1997).

Pinel had the merit of having defended in a very clear way that 'the insane, far from being persons guilty of something which should be punished, are patients whose painful condition deserves all the consideration that is due to the humanity that suffers and for whom one must seek by the simplest means to restore the "deviated reason"' (Pinel, 1801). The 'moral treatment' proposed by Pinel was based on the conviction that it would be possible to introduce significant changes in the behaviour of patients via humane, though firm, attitudes on the part of the caregivers. Pinel's innovation, however, did not consist only of a therapeutic approach to patients but also in the association of a humanist stance with, on the one hand, the effort to study the phenomenon of madness rationally and methodically and, on the other hand, the recognition of the importance of the patient's subjectivity (Pereira, 2004).

The new therapeutic approaches based on moral treatment played a fundamental role in the development of the psychiatric asylum model that would form the basis of psychiatric care throughout the world since the beginning of the nineteenth century. At the same time, the recognition of the need to study mental illnesses from a scientific perspective would allow the birth of psychiatry as a medical discipline and contribute to the developments that would come to be verified in the understanding of the causes of mental illnesses at a biological, psychological and social level.

Although this new approach had a significant impact in many countries, the discontinuation of shackles and the prohibition of systematic punishment did not imply the abandonment of compulsion and other forms of coercion. All people hospitalised in asylums continued to be committed involuntarily and had to be certified as mentally ill, which explains why most European countries began to create legislation to regulate psychiatric hospitalisation during the nineteenth century.

## 2.2  Post-War Health Service Reforms

The truth is that it took more than a century and two world wars for the understanding to develop that asylums also had important limitations in effectively responding to the needs of people with mental disorders. The main drivers for this move towards deinstitutionalisation were a growing awareness of overcrowding, financial shortages due to worsening economic conditions, reduced government expenditure and the availability of new pharmaceutical treatments. Governments and professionals realised that, to end the marginalisation and exclusion of persons with mental disorders, it was necessary to develop new models of care, better respond to the various needs of the mentally ill and promote their access to equal rights.

In terms of human rights, World War II and the impact of the Holocaust (Levav et al., 1998; Strous, 2007), responsible for the killing of hundreds of thousands of mentally ill persons in psychiatric hospitals, were the great turning point in this evolution. It was this impact born out of the horrors of the war and the experiences of solidarity with its victims that created the conditions for the emergence of a new recognition of the importance of respecting the political, social and economic rights of all individuals, including the ones belonging to the most vulnerable and excluded groups. This impact was also fundamental for the emergence of two movements that would constitute, and continue to do so until today, an essential driver of the fight against the use of coercion: the reform of mental health services and the international human rights mechanisms.

In both Europe and the USA, the argument against psychiatric asylums grew significantly after the war, contributing to the implementation of mental health service reforms based on three common elements: deinstitutionalisation and development of services in the community; involvement of primary health care; and protection of the human rights of persons with mental disorders.

These reforms were inseparable from other social movements that sprung up at the same time with the objective of fighting for the emancipation of groups that had been discriminated against and excluded until then because of their gender, sexual orientation or ethnicity. As Franco Basaglia, the leader of the Italian psychiatric reform, said, 'When we say no to the asylum, we say no to the world's misery, and we join all the people in the world who fight for the emancipation of human beings' (Basaglia, 2000). It was not by chance that the first mental health services reforms were initiated in countries that were engaged in political processes aiming at improving the social and economic conditions of their populations and ensuring better access to healthcare. Similar Reforms later developed in other countries (e.g. in Southern Europe, Latin America and Eastern Europe) when they experienced processes of democratisation. This could be seen in Spain (Vázquez-Barquero et al., 2001), Brazil and Chile (Caldas-de-Almeida & Horvitz-Lennon, 2010) and the Czech Republic (Pec, 2019). More recently, mental health reforms also developed in other parts of the world, among others, in Lebanon (Chammay et al., 2016), India (Gupta & Sagar, 2022) and South Africa (Kleintjes & Schneider, 2023).

## 2.3    Key Statements on Human Rights Since 1945

The Universal Declaration of Human Rights (UDHR), adopted by the United Nations General Assembly in 1948 in response to the atrocities committed during World War II, marked the beginning of a movement that led to the creation of a comprehensive set of international human rights mechanisms, which had, and still have, a key role in attitudes towards the use of coercion in mental health services. The UDHR does not mention mental health, but Article 25 says that 'Everyone has the right to a standard of living adequate for the health and well-being of themselves and of their family, including food, clothing, housing and medical care and necessary social services, and the right to security in the event of unemployment, sickness, disability, widowhood, old age or other lack of livelihood in circumstances beyond his control' (UN General Assembly, 1948).

The first official document that directly and explicitly refers to mental health is the WHO definition of health in 1948 as 'a state of complete physical, mental and social well-being [which] is not just the absence of illness or infirmity' (World Health Organization (WHO), 1946). The International Covenant on Economic, Social and Cultural Rights (United Nations, 1966) is especially important because it recognises the right of all persons to enjoy the 'best possible physical and mental health status', and because, for the first time, the right to health was recognised in a legally binding pact.

Another document relating to the rights of persons with mental disorders is the UN General Assembly Resolution 'Principles for the protection of people with mental illness and the improvement of mental health care' (United Nations, 1991). Approved on 17 December 1991, it describes fundamental freedoms and basic rights—access to quality care, internationally recognised rights, protection of dignity and prohibition of discrimination—as well as principles related to consent, involuntary treatment regulation (decision, review, procedural safeguards), community life and access to information, among others.

The most recent and most important international treaty that is relevant to the use of coercion is the Convention for the Rights of Persons with Disabilities (CRPD), approved in 2008 (United Nations, 2008). The purpose of the Convention 'is to promote, protect and ensure the full and equal enjoyment of all human rights and fundamental freedoms for all persons with disabilities,' which includes persons with serious mental disorders.

The approval of the CRPD represents a great advance in the promotion of the rights of persons with mental disorders, as it is based on a consensus of the international community (governments, NGOs and citizens) on the need to effectively ensure respect for the integrity, dignity and individual freedoms of persons with mental disabilities and to strengthen the prohibition of discrimination against these citizens via laws, policies and programmes that specifically meet their needs and promote their participation in society. It includes several articles especially relevant to the reduction of coercion. Article 12, on equal recognition before the law, places the legal capacity of persons with disabilities on an equal footing with others. According to this article, people with disabilities have the right to maintain and exercise their legal right to make decisions and should have access to the support they may need in their decision-making process from people they trust who may be legally recognised or informally designated. Consequently, this could mean that people with disabilities can legally reject coercive measures that are justified by a mental disorder.

According to the CRPD Committee's interpretation, any form of substitute decision-making is considered a violation of the Convention's guarantee of legal capacity on an equal basis, meaning that involuntary treatment is prohibited. This position is supported by some UN bodies and not by others, a split that is also found among users and professionals (Freeman et al., 2015; Caldas de Almeida, 2019) who, although believing that supported decision-making is, in general, the best way of respecting the rights of persons with mental conditions, consider that, with the mental health services currently available in most countries, it is impossible to completely rule out the use of substitute decision-making in every circumstance. However, despite these differences of interpretation on this specific point, there is now a broad consensus on the importance of joining efforts on concrete actions that may contribute to effectively reducing coercion in mental health services—at the policy and legislation level, the incorporation of evidence-based interventions in clinical practice, the reform of mental health systems, and research.

## 3    Are Coercive Measures Ever in the Best Interest of the Person Being Coerced?

A key ethico-legal justification for the utilisation of coercive measures in healthcare settings is that the intervention is in the best interests of the person subjected to it. This means that, in hindsight, people who have experienced coercion should provide consent and should be able to report that they benefited from the intervention (Taylor, 2016).

Numerous studies deal primarily with the effects of direct coercion and many of these have been summarised in various systematic reviews. A qualitative meta-synthesis examined the experiences of people who were initially hospitalised against their will and then had to experience further coercive measures such as isolation and fixation (Akther et al., 2019). The authors concluded that 'patients…believed that their involuntary admission had kept them safe at a time when they could not recognise the severity of their illness, but negative experiences were commonly described' (Akther et al., 2019, p. 7).

Additionally, this review found physical interventions, such as restraint and seclusion, were experienced particularly negatively by many patients and played an important role in the negative experiences reported in the majority of studies. This review also highlights the lasting impact of detention with patients across studies reporting feelings of shame and marginalisation, particularly those in forensic settings who had also committed an offence (Akther et al., 2019).

Another systematic review analysed the consequences of restraint and seclusion for the people affected (Chieze et al., 2019). These authors concluded that.

> The identified literature strongly suggests that seclusion and restraint have deleterious physical or psychological consequences. The incidence of PTSD after seclusion or restraint ranges from 25% to 47% which is not negligible…Subjective perception has high interindividual variability and can be positive, with feelings of safety, help, clinical improvement or evaluation as necessary. However, seclusion and restraint are mainly associated with negative emotions, particularly feelings of punishment and distress. Conclusions on protective or therapeutic effects of seclusion and restraint are more difficult to draw. Our results provide little evidence for these outcomes, but further research is clearly necessary (Chieze et al., 2019, p. 13; citations not reproduced here)

Another review looked at the experiences of people who have had to undergo coercive measures (Aguilera-Serrano et al., 2018). These authors come to a similar conclusion, that the experiences associated with coercive measures are predominantly negative, regardless of the type of measure. The described experiences include anxiety and post-traumatic stress; powerlessness, neglect, mistrust and loneliness; punishment, abuse and pain; anger, rage and bitterness; depression, powerlessness and sadness; humiliation and shame; loss of freedom and coercion. However, according to the study, positive experiences such as help, necessity, reassurance, time for reflection, safety, control and the prevention of violence were also reported in a few original studies. Furthermore, it should not be forgotten that physical restraint not only has psychological consequences but can also lead to physical harm and—albeit rarely—even death (Kersting et al., 2019; Steinberg, 2021). The latter are usually caused by cardiac arrest as well as by pulmonary and thromboembolism.

Other reviews on individual aspects of the experience of coercion largely point in the same direction (Tingleff et al., 2017; Cusack et al., 2018; Sugiura et al., 2020; Modini et al., 2021; Muir-Cochrane & Oster, 2021). The majority of people affected do not experience psychiatric coercion as benevolent. However, there is a minority who view coercive measures as positive in retrospect, and there are certain situations in which people experience hospitalisation as a form of security.

It must be noted that all of these conclusions relate to direct and ultimately physical coercion. However, there is some evidence that the situation is similar to informal coercion, and there is also a feeling of inferiority when those affected are granted fewer rights and less freedom of choice than other people (Allison & Flemming, 2019).

## 4     The International Epidemiology of Coercion

With an awareness of both this historical context and the difficulties of benchmarking due to the terminological issues noted above, it is important to establish where we are now in terms of estimating the frequency with which coercion is used in mental health services around the world. Over the past 15 years, there has been a series of international studies on this topic which enable some meaningful, although imperfect, international comparisons. This enables us to identify some international averages and outliers in terms of both best practice and over-use of coercion.

There has been substantial progress made in estimating the proportion of patients exposed to inpatient coercion worldwide with a series of studies (Steinert et al., 2010; Lepping et al., 2016; Gowda et al., 2018; Savage et al., 2024). The most comprehensive review (Belayneh et al., 2024) estimates the following rates for the proportion of inpatients subjected to each type of inpatient coercion: 0.14 (95% CI: 0.13–0.16) for physical/mechanical restraint; 0.15 (0.14–0.16) for seclusion; and 0.25 (0.18–0.31) for chemical restraint. The latter term is roughly synonymous with the descriptions of forced medication and rapid tranquillisation in Table 1. These estimates were based on more than 70 studies published in just over a decade after 2010, which indicates the concerted recent international efforts in this area to establish the prevalence of inpatient coercion as a baseline for mounting reduction strategies.

However, a key finding of this and most other reviews is the huge variability between rates in different samples. Physical/mechanical restraint ranged from 0.3% in one sample from the USA to 54% in Italy; seclusion rates from 0.2% in one service in the USA to 56% in Japan; and chemical restraint from 2% in Norway to 58% in India (Belayneh et al., 2024). It is important to note that these are not nationally representative samples so conclusions about the overall national profile in any country cannot be deduced from these figures. Such deductions require a standardised data-collection process within countries, and international comparisons also require a population denominator for meaningful comparisons. Savage et al. (2024) achieve the latter goal by reporting a median figure across nine countries of 29 restrictive practice interventions per 100,000 population per year with the highest rate in the Netherlands (42/100,000) and the lowest in the UK (England; 18/100,000).

Looking beyond the hospital inpatient setting the same variability phenomenon arises with involuntary admissions (Salize & Dressing, 2004) and compulsory community treatment. With regard to involuntary hospitalisation, Sheridan Rains et al.

(2019) report a median rate of 106 compulsory admissions per 100,000 population across 22 countries in Europe and Australasia but the rate was 20 times higher in the country with the highest rate, Austria, than it was in neighbouring Italy which had the lowest rate. There was also some variation over time with rates increasing year-on-year—between 2008 and 2017—on average by more than 5% in the Netherlands and Spain and decreasing by 3–4% in Italy and Finland.

Community Treatment Orders (CTOs) are ambiguous in the context of debates about the meaning of coercion as they are both a coercive intervention per se and an alternative to the arguably more severe coercive interventions related to hospitalisation. As such they have been developed and evaluated as an intervention which is deemed successful if it is associated with reductions in compulsory admissions, and there are mixed results on this question (Rugkåsa, 2016). Notwithstanding the debate on effectiveness, a variable pattern in the use of CTOs, similar to that observed with other coercive measures, has been observed within and between countries. Relatively high rates of CTO use have been reported in Australia and New Zealand compared to samples in Canada, Israel, the USA and the UK (Scotland) (O'Brien, 2014), but once again caution is advised due to the reliance on unstandardised data across studies, which complicates any attempt to make meaningful comparisons.

## 5    Contextual Factors Influencing Coercion

These global variations in rates of coercion indicate the importance of considering the social, political and economic factors that may impact the decision to use coercion. The prevalence of coercion in mental health care is influenced by various contextual factors that are interrelated and not necessarily associated directly with service users. Although clinical and sociodemographic features of patients are well-established risk factors for the use of coercion (Aguilera-Serrano et al., 2018; Walker et al., 2019; Beames & Onwumere, 2021), contextual factors such as service-related characteristics and the characteristics of mental healthcare professionals appear to be influential as well (Wierdsma & Mulder, 2009; Beghi et al., 2013; Dahan et al., 2018; Barnett et al., 2019; Walker et al., 2019; Newton-Howes et al., 2020; Mann et al., 2021). Factors such as economic conditions and the impact of COVID-19 have the potential to augment the demand for mental health services. Additionally, the design, efficiency and staffing levels of these services play a crucial role in determining their ability to meet increased demands. Staff attitudes have been associated with the use of coercion, and these attitudes usually reflect the prevailing mental health laws (Brooks, 2006), policies and public perceptions towards individuals with mental health conditions. (Brooks, 2006) It is crucial to recognise contextual factors since they could guide the development and implementation of interventions to reduce coercion in specific settings. Contextual factors are particularly important to note since the strategies aimed at minimising coercive practices in mental health settings are often developed and tested in relatively controlled, idealised environments that do not fully mirror the complexities of many mental health systems. Consequently, the recommendations that arise from these studies are often too generic to effectively address the specific practical barriers that mental health professionals encounter when attempting to adapt these strategies to their particular organisational contexts. Moreover, they fail to account for changes that affect services, such as the effects of austerity measures and regulatory changes on public services (Fletcher et al., 2019). Few studies have specifically assessed the influence of contextual factors on the use of coercion (Schön et al., 2018).

## 5.1   Service Design

Considering that involuntary legal status at the time of admission predicts the use of other coercive measures (Korkeila et al., 2002; Bilanakis et al., 2010; Raboch et al., 2010), it seems reasonable to assume that contextual factors that influence involuntary admission indirectly contribute to the use of additional coercive measures such as restraints and seclusion. The organisation of mental health services influences the quality of mental health care, and since the use of coercive measures is an indication of the quality of mental health treatment (Hermann, 2005), the same variable should indirectly influence it. The recommended approach for organising mental health care services is to close large, independent psychiatric hospitals and instead establish psychiatric departments within general hospitals and community-based mental health services (World Health Organization, 2022). This model is preferred as it promotes continuity of care, increases user satisfaction, enhances human rights protection and decreases the stigma surrounding mental health (World Health Organization, 2022).

Deinstitutionalisation is a sensitive process that needs to be managed with caution to avoid negative consequences on the quality of care, including the use of coercive measures. Decreasing psychiatric beds without a corresponding development of community resources could lead to adverse outcomes, such as a rise in involuntary admissions. An ecological study in England found a synchronous increase in the rate of involuntary admissions with decreasing available beds between 1988 and 2008 (Keown et al., 2011). Smith et al. (2020) also found that a decreased availability of psychiatric beds amplified the impact of austerity measures on the rates of involuntary admissions and 'Place of Safety' detentions in England. In Italy, however, a reduction of psychiatric beds led to a reduction in the rates of involuntary admissions within the 18 years following the implementation of the new Mental Health Law in 1979 (Guaiana & Barbui, 2004). The parallel expansion of community mental health care, the legal framework and the nationwide movement for the rights of people with mental health conditions in Italy may explain the disparity in the impact of reducing psychiatric beds.

The availability of alternative services to inpatient care has been shown to significantly reduce the rates of involuntary admission in a given location (Gandré et al., 2017), especially in intensive crisis teams in the community (McGarvey et al., 2013; Aagaard et al., 2017). The extent to which available mental health services are utilised has significant effects on the risk of involuntary admissions (van der Post et al., 2009). The importance of a functional primary care network that is adequately integrated into the mental health care system is highlighted by the association between referrals from general practitioners and a decreased incidence of involuntary admissions (van der Post et al., 2009). To meet the non-clinical needs of people with mental health conditions, social services that are complementary to the services offered by psychiatric care are required and have been reported to have a protective effect on acute psychiatry (Emons et al., 2013).

The use of seclusion and restraint are also known to be influenced by organisational factors, such as ward characteristics. Wards located in metropolitan areas have been reported to use more isolation and restraint (Husum et al., 2010), possibly due to a higher demand for services. Ward size, male-to-female staff ratio and staff experience have also been linked to the use of seclusion (Janssen et al., 2007, 2013; van der Schaaf et al., 2013) with mixed results (Doedens et al., 2020). In addition, factors like staffing levels, staff training and attitudes are connected to the use of coercive measures. Nurses from countries with a varying range of resources report how insufficient resources, especially human resources, contribute to the use of coercive measures (Gagnon et al., 2013; Wilson et al., 2018; Krieger et al., 2021; Navarro et al., 2021; Aluh et al., 2023). Staffing levels have been reported to be related to perceived concerns about the causes and responses to conflict and aggression (McKeown et al., 2019). However, it is possible that increasing staffing levels in a ward may not necessarily lead to a reduction in the use of coercion, as a recent study reported that both seclusion and mechanical restraint were utilised more frequently in wards with more nurses (Fukasawa et al., 2018).

## 5.2    National Legislation and Policy

The use of coercive measures in mental health care can also be viewed as an indicator of the underlying characteristics of mental health legislation and policies in a specific jurisdiction. Studies on the impact of legislation on rates of involuntary admission have shown mixed results. The most effective legal framework that can safeguard the rights of people with mental health conditions and the general public while also minimising coercion is yet to be determined. In Italy, a new mental health legislation was associated with a lower proportion of involuntary admissions (Guaiana & Barbui, 2004), while the reverse was the case in China (Zhang et al., 2016). The increase in involuntary admission rates after a change in mental health legislation in China was attributed to the comparatively low number of psychiatric beds and the cultural stigma there. A review of the mental health laws in European countries revealed that those that demanded the participation of independent legal representatives had lower involuntary admission rates (Salize & Dressing, 2004). However, a more recent comparison of involuntary admission rates in 22 countries found no association with any characteristics of the legal framework (Sheridan Rains et al., 2019). Cultural norms have an impact on the laws regulating coercive measures, which may explain why some restrictive practices are legally regulated and monitored in some countries but not in others.

While involuntary admissions are regulated by mental health legislation in most European countries, the use of mechanical restraints, seclusion and other coercive measures is not regulated by law in some countries and is left to the discretion of hospitals and regional authorities (Navarro et al., 2021). An international evaluation of restraints conducted more than 10 years ago indicated that there was insufficient information available and that national databases were necessary (Steinert et al., 2010). Differences in the prevalence of restraints used in Dutch and British services were attributed to Dutch psychiatric professionals' opinion of involuntary medication being more invasive and threatening to personal integrity to a higher degree than the application of seclusion or mechanical restraint. This is reflected by the Dutch mental health legislation, which is very restrictive regarding involuntary medication, permitting its use only in cases of acute emergency (Steinert et al., 2010). In traditional acute settings in the UK, physical restraints tend to be preferred over mechanical restraints, which are rarely used. However, if mechanical restraints are used, they are carefully observed and recorded (Nijman et al., 2005; Steinert et al., 2010). This has important implications since mandatory review of all mechanical restraint episodes has been reported to be associated with low rates of use (Bak et al., 2014), and hospitals using detailed guidelines for seclusion and restraint have been reported to use fewer of these coercive measures (Steinert et al., 2007).

## 5.3   Economic Factors

Economic recessions and austerity measures often lead to an increased need for mental health care. A study conducted in Florida confirmed that declining regional economies reduce community tolerance for people seen as a threat to others, leading to an increase in involuntary psychiatric admissions (Kessell et al., 2006). Similarly, in the UK, the recent rise in involuntary admissions has been attributed to the economic recession, legislative changes and the impact of austerity measures on health and social care services (Smith et al., 2020). Previous studies have highlighted the two opposing trends of funding reductions with ensuing staff shortages and growing demand to minimise the use of coercive measures notwithstanding these insufficiencies (McKeown et al., 2017, 2019). These pressures have been linked to the emergence of 'defensive psychiatry', a term coined to describe the practice of healthcare professionals making decisions to reduce their legal liability while ensuring the safety of patients and others. This phenomenon has been reported among both psychiatrists and nurses (Sattar et al., 2006; Bifarin et al., 2022).

## 5.4   COVID-19

The impact of the COVID-19 pandemic on the use of coercive measures has been contradictory across different countries, as some have documented changes during lockdowns while others have reported no changes. In Portugal, although there was a decrease in overall psychiatric admissions, the proportion of involuntary admissions increased during the pandemic (Rodrigues et al., 2022). In Italy, all psychiatric admission rates significantly decreased in the 40 days after the start of the pandemic, but involuntary admission rates remained unchanged (Clerici et al., 2020). In Canada, a reduction in the use of restraints and seclusion was reported during the COVID-19 pandemic due to organisational changes that were made to foster service users' well-being (Martin et al., 2022), while in Germany, an increase in these coercive measures was reported during the pandemic due to rules made to prevent infection (Flammer et al., 2022).

## 5.5    Staff Attitudes and Training

The duration and frequency of restrictive practices vary across countries, organisations, and individuals and this cannot be explained solely by differences in legislation (Husum et al., 2011; Boumans et al., 2012; Laiho et al., 2014). Evidence increasingly suggests that staff attitudes, particularly those of nurses, could have a direct impact on the prevalence and continued use of restrictive practices (Husum et al., 2010; Bregar et al., 2018). The variation in the thresholds for using restrictive practices among staff members (Price et al., 2018) implies that there are differences in how staff perceive violence (Happell & Koehn, 2010) and how much agitation and disturbed behaviour they are willing to tolerate (Jalil et al., 2017). It is challenging to determine the actual need for restrictive practices when they are used routinely rather than as a last resort for safety purposes (Slemon et al., 2017). Nurses often have to make decisions about restrictive practices, which can result in inconsistency and an underestimation or exaggeration of risk, leading to unnecessary or prolonged seclusion or restraint (Looi et al., 2014). These individual differences were highlighted as reasons to avoid using ward culture as an explanation for the adoption of restrictive measures in psychiatric wards (Laiho et al., 2014). Since each staff member has a unique perspective on aggressiveness, training for dealing with aggression or violent occurrences should be done, at least in part, on an individual basis. A lack of training on the alternative approaches to coercion is also implicated in the use of coercion, as many mental health professionals tend to perceive coercion as an inherent part of care (Husum et al., 2011). This argument is supported by evidence highlighting the effectiveness of training in reducing the occurrence of coercion (Barbui et al., 2020).

## 5.6    Public Attitudes

Public attitudes towards coercive measures in psychiatric care are important in understanding the context of their use. These attitudes can range from stigmatising and fear-based perceptions of people with mental health conditions to more empathetic and supportive attitudes that prioritise human rights and recovery-oriented care. Cultural factors can also play a role, as collectivist cultures often emphasise family involvement in decision-making, while individualistic cultures may prioritise individual autonomy and self-determination (Erez, 1993). Increasingly, there is a reduced tolerance for deviant behaviours, which can lead to pressure for inpatient care and the subsequent use of other coercive measures (Gravier & Eytan, 2011). Empirical evidence suggests that public attitudes towards coercive measures vary by country and are influenced by existing laws and regulations. In Norway and France, the majority of participants agreed that involuntary hospitalisation was acceptable in certain circumstances (Guedj et al., 2012; Joa et al., 2017). From 1993 to 2011 in Germany, the percentage of individuals who endorsed involuntary admissions remained steady despite the presence of mental health awareness initiatives and anti-stigma campaigns during that time. However, there was a decrease in opposition to involuntary admissions for reasons not aligned with legal criteria, suggesting a shift towards a more liberal perspective on patient rights while displaying reduced tolerance for inappropriate behaviour (Angermeyer et al., 2014). These findings highlight the necessity of incorporating specific elements pertaining to the rights of people with mental health conditions into stigma reduction campaigns. Similarly, a US study found that support for involuntary admissions increased steadily over the 22 years from 1996 to 2018 for various mental health conditions (Pescosolido et al., 2019).

Measuring the impact of contextual factors is challenging; nonetheless, they play a significant role in the problem and present possibilities for long-term interventions. Since contextual factors do not act independently and often reinforce one another, effective strategies to reduce coercion must address these contextual factors using multiple approaches. Given the involvement of various stakeholders, it is crucial not to leave the responsibility for reducing coercion in mental health care solely to mental health professionals. The complexity of the problem calls for collaborative efforts involving various stakeholders, such as policymakers, mental health professionals, service users and the broader community.

## 6    Some Promising Innovations

The growth in knowledge on contextual factors in coercion has led to a step-change in ideas and initiatives to tackle the issue. Many new initiatives recognise the need, noted above, to locate change at the team and organisational level rather than leaving it to individual staff to change their practice regardless of the larger culture in which they are operating. We are still nowhere near possessing a road map towards the ultimate goal of services that are entirely free of coercion, but there has been a noticeable shift in how much attention and money society as a whole is willing to pay to address the problem in the past decade. It is too soon to say that there is zero tolerance for coercion in services but judging by the growing attention devoted to considering the problem, there is certainly significant discomfort among many decision-makers, which differs from earlier widespread obliviousness. People with lived experience of mental disorders who have suffered more than discomfort when subjected to coercion may be frustrated by the slow pace of change, but there are grounds for optimism now that did not exist 20 years ago.

Three recent systematic reviews, in combination, provide an indication of the state of the art in this area which can support decision-makers in the task of choosing innovative interventions to reduce coercion in their service (Gooding et al., 2018; Barbui et al., 2020; Baker et al., 2021). All three reviews adopted a systematic approach to gathering relevant empirical evidence and focused on interventions to reduce inpatient coercion and/or community-based coercion (i.e. involuntary admission) in mental health services. Each had distinctive aims and adopted a different approach to analysing their included studies, but taken together, their conclusions on certain key aspects are in harmony and provide a credible basis for the next stage of clinical development and research. A summary of their combined conclusions is reported in Table 3.

It should be noted that inclusion in this table indicates that an intervention has, at the very least, been widely implemented based on relevant publications reporting on the intervention. Inclusion here does not, however, on its own indicate that the intervention has been found to be effective or that it has even necessarily been tested in a trial.

It can be seen here that two specific organisational and/or team-level interventions—Six Core Strategies and Safewards (Huckshorn, 2006; Bowers et al., 2015)—have been extensively tested and have shown promising results for inpatient services. In the community, joint crisis plans and shared decision-making also have evidence of effectiveness. Several of these interventions are discussed elsewhere in this book.

**Table 3** Promising interventions that have been implemented to reduce coercive practice in mental health services

| Community services | Inpatient services | Both |
|---|---|---|
| Advance directives/planning[a] | **Six core strategies**[b,c] | Medication discontinuance[c] |
| **Joint crisis plans**[a] | **Safewards**[b,c,d] | Peer support[c] |
| Crisis plan/card[a] | Talk First[b] | Recovery models[c] |
| Early warning symptoms[a] | ResTrain Yourself[b] | Representation agreements[c] |
| Community treatment order[a] | Scottish Patient Safety Programme[b] | **Shared decision-making**[a,c,d] |
| Treatment adherence therapy[a] | Seclusion Reduction Programme[b] | Trauma-informed[c] |
| Financial incentives[a] | Sensory Modulation[b] | |
| Crisis resolution team[a] | **Restraint education**[a] | |
| Integrated treatment[a] | | |
| Club house[c] | | |
| Hearing voices network[c] | | |
| Respite houses[c] | | |
| Soteria house[c,d] | | |
| Trialogue[c] | | |

**Bold**: Intervention with evidence of effectiveness in at least one RCT
[a] Cited as an intervention tested in at least one RCT reported by Barbui et al. (2020)
[b] Cited as an 'intervention family' in four or more empirical studies analysed by Baker et al. (2021)
[c] Cited as a 'prominent measure or approach' which has been implemented 'internationally' or in at least five countries by Gooding et al. (2018)
[d] Intervention implemented at least once in a low- or middle-income country

# 7    Conclusions

In the last few decades, there have been important conceptual developments in the way we approach the nature and causes of mental illness, the factors involved in disabilities and the organisation of services. Important paradigm shifts took place and are still occurring, moving from a custodial paradigm to a care paradigm, then to a recovery paradigm and now to a human rights paradigm. The goal of reducing coercion continues to face important obstacles. However, because of the increasing awareness of the risks involved in using coercive practices, the increasing knowledge of the current availability of alternatives to coercion, and the challenges associated with implementation, never have there been such favourable and fertile conditions to reach these goals. The project of a more humane and multi-faceted conception of mental health patients and their care continues to advance and is going through a particularly exciting phase.

## References

Aagaard, J., Tuszewski, B., & Kølbæk, P. (2017). Does assertive community treatment reduce the use of compulsory admissions? *Archives of Psychiatric Nursing, 31*(6), 641–646. https://doi.org/10.1016/J.APNU.2017.07.008

Aguilera-Serrano, C., Guzman-Parra, J., Garcia-Sanchez, J. A., Moreno-Küstner, B., & Mayoral-Cleries, F. (2018). Variables associated with the subjective experience of coercive measures in psychiatric inpatients: A systematic review. *The Canadian Journal of Psychiatry, 63*(2), 129–144. https://doi.org/10.1177/0706743717738491

Akther, S. F., Johnson, S., Molyneaux, E., Oram, S., Simpson, A., & Stuart, R. (2019). Patients' experiences of assessment and detention under mental health legislation: Systematic review and qualitative meta-synthesis. *BJPsych Open, 5*(3), e37. https://doi.org/10.1192/bjo.2019.19

Allison, R., & Flemming, K. (2019). Mental health patients' experiences of softer coercion and its effects on their interactions with practitioners: A qualitative evidence synthesis. *Journal of Advanced Nursing, 75*(11), 2274–2284. https://doi.org/10.1111/jan.14035

Aluh, D. O., Ayilara, O., Onu, J. U., Pedrosa, B., Silva, M., Grigaitė, U., et al. (2023). Use of coercion in mental healthcare services in Nigeria: Service providers' perspective. *Journal of Mental Health, 33*, 75–83. https://doi.org/10.1080/09638237.2023.2182426

Angermeyer, M. C., Matschinger, H., & Schomerus, G. (2014). Attitudes of the German public to restrictions on persons with mental illness in 1993 and 2011. *Epidemiology and Psychiatric Sciences, 23*(3), 263–270. https://doi.org/10.1017/S2045796014000183

Bak, J., Zoffmann, V., Sestoft, D. M., Almvik, R., & Brandt-Christensen, M. (2014). Mechanical restraint in psychiatry: Preventive factors in theory and practice. A Danish–Norwegian Association Study. *Perspectives in Psychiatric Care, 50*(3), 155–166. https://doi.org/10.1111/PPC.12036

Baker, J., Berzins, K., Canvin, K., Benson, I., Kellar, I., Wright, J., et al. (2021). Non-pharmacological interventions to reduce restrictive practices in adult mental health inpatient settings: The COMPARE systematic mapping review. *Health Services and Delivery Research, 9*, 5. https://doi.org/10.3310/hsdr09050

Barbui, C., Purgato, M., Abdulmalik, J., Caldas-de-Almeida, J. M., Eaton, J., Gureje, O., et al. (2020). Efficacy of interventions to reduce coercive treatment in mental health services: Umbrella review of randomised evidence. *The British Journal of Psychiatry, 218*, 185. https://doi.org/10.1192/bjp.2020.144

Barnett, P., Mackay, E., Matthews, H., Gate, R., Greenwood, H., Ariyo, K., et al. (2019). Ethnic variations in compulsory detention under the Mental Health Act: A systematic review and meta-analysis of international data. *The Lancet Psychiatry, 6*(4), 305–317. https://doi.org/10.1016/S2215-0366(19)30027-6

Basaglia, F. (2000). *Conferenze Brasiliane*. Raffaello Cortina.

BBC. (2022). *Toxic culture' of abuse at mental health hospital revealed by BBC secret filming*. https://www.bbc.com/news/uk-63045298.

Beames, L., & Onwumere, J. (2021). Risk factors associated with use of coercive practices in adult mental health inpatients: A systematic review. *Journal of Psychiatric and Mental Health Nursing, 29*, 220. https://doi.org/10.1111/JPM.12757

Beghi, M., Peroni, F., Gabola, P., Rossetti, A., & Cornaggia, C. M. (2013). Prevalence and risk factors for the use of restraint in psychiatry: A systematic review. *Rivista di Psichiatria, 48*(1), 10–22.

Belayneh, Z., Chavulak, J., Lee, D.-C. A., Petrakis, M., & Haines, T. P. (2024). Prevalence and variability of restrictive care practice use (physical restraint, seclusion and chemical restraint) in adult mental health inpatient settings: A systematic review and meta-analysis. *Journal of Clinical Nursing*. https://doi.org/10.1111/jocn.17041

Bifarin, O., Felton, A., & Prince, Z. (2022). Defensive practices in mental health nursing: Professionalism and poignant tensions. *International Journal of Mental Health Nursing, 31*(3), 743–751. https://doi.org/10.1111/INM.12936

Bilanakis, N., Kalampokis, G., Christou, K., & Peritogiannis, V. (2010). Use of coercive physical measures in a psychiatric ward of a general hospital in Greece. *The International Journal of Social Psychiatry, 56*(4), 402–411. https://doi.org/10.1177/0020764009106620

Boumans, C. E., Egger, J. I. M., Souren, P. M., Mann-Poll, P. S., & Hutschemaekers, G. J. M. (2012). Nurses' decision on seclusion: Patient characteristics, contextual factors and reflexivity in teams. *Journal of Psychiatric and Mental Health Nursing, 19*(3), 264–270. https://doi.org/10.1111/J.1365-2850.2011.01777.X

Bowers, L., James, K., Quirk, A., & Simpson, A. (2015). Reducing conflict and containment rates on acute psychiatric wards: The Safewards cluster randomised controlled trial. *International Journal of Nursing Studies, 52*, 1412.

Bregar, B., Skela-Savič, B., & Kores Plesničar, B. (2018). Cross-sectional study on nurses' attitudes regarding coercive measures: The importance of socio-demographic characteristics, job satisfaction, and strategies for coping with stress. *BMC Psychiatry, 18*(1), 1–10. https://doi.org/10.1186/S12888-018-1756-1/TABLES/5

Brooks, R. A. (2006). U.S. Psychiatrists' beliefs and wants about involuntary civil commitment grounds. *International Journal of Law and Psychiatry, 29*(1), 13–21. https://doi.org/10.1016/j.ijlp.2005.04.004

Caldas de Almeida, J. M. (2019). The CRPD Article 12, the limits of reductionist approaches to complex issues and the necessary search for compromise. *World Psychiatry, 18*(1), 46–47. https://doi.org/10.1002/wps.20602

Caldas-de-Almeida, J. M., & Horvitz-Lennon, M. (2010). Mental health care reforms in Latin America: An overview of mental health care reforms in Latin America and the Caribbean. *Psychiatric Services, 61*(3), 218–221. https://doi.org/10.1176/ps.2010.61.3.218

Chammay, R. E., Karam, E., & Ammar, W. (2016). Mental health reform in Lebanon and the Syrian crisis. *The Lancet Psychiatry, 3*(3), 202–203. https://doi.org/10.1016/S2215-0366(16)00055-9

Chieze, M., Hurst, S., Kaiser, S., & Sentissi, O. (2019). Effects of seclusion and restraint in adult psychiatry: A systematic review (systematic review). *Frontiers in Psychiatry, 10*. https://doi.org/10.3389/fpsyt.2019.00491

Clerici, M., Durbano, F., Spinogatti, F., Vita, A., De Girolamo, G., & Micciolo, R. (2020). Psychiatric hospitalization rates in Italy before and during COVID-19: Did they change? An analysis of register data. *Irish Journal of Psychological Medicine, 37*(4), 283–290. https://doi.org/10.1017/IPM.2020.29

Council of Europe. (2019). *Ending coercion in mental health: The need for a human rights-based approach*. https://pace.coe.int/en/files/28038/html

Cusack, P., Cusack, F. P., McAndrew, S., McKeown, M., & Duxbury, J. (2018). An integrative review exploring the physical and psychological harm inherent in using restraint in mental health inpatient settings. *International Journal of Mental Health Nursing, 27*(3), 1162–1176. https://doi.org/10.1111/inm.12432

Dahan, S., Levi, G., Behrbalk, P., Bronstein, I., Hirschmann, S., & Lev-Ran, S. (2018). The impact of 'Being There': Psychiatric staff attitudes on the use of restraint. *The Psychiatric Quarterly, 89*(1), 191–199. https://doi.org/10.1007/S11126-017-9524-9

Doedens, P., Vermeulen, J., Boyette, L.-L., Latour, C., & de Haan, L. (2020). Influence of nursing staff attitudes and characteristics on the use of coercive measures in acute mental health services—A systematic review. *Journal of Psychiatric and Mental Health Nursing, 27*(4), 446–459. https://doi.org/10.1111/jpm.12586

Emons, B., Haussleiter, I. S., Kalthoff, J., Schramm, A., Hoffmann, K., Jendreyschak, J., et al. (2013). Impact of social-psychiatric services and psychiatric clinics on involuntary admissions. *International Journal of Social Psychiatry, 60*(7), 672–680. https://doi.org/10.1177/0020764013511794

Erez, M. (1993). Individualism and collectivism. In M. Erez, M. Erez, & P. C. Earley (Eds.), *Culture, self-identity, and work*. Oxford University Press. https://doi.org/10.1093/acprof:oso/9780195075809.003.0004

Flammer, E., Eisele, F., Hirsch, S., & Steinert, T. (2022). Increase in coercive measures in psychiatric hospitals in Germany during the COVID-19 pandemic. *PLoS One, 17*(8), e0264046.

Fletcher, L., Bailey, C., Alfes, K., & Madden, A. (2019). Mind the context gap: A critical review of engagement within the public sector and an agenda for future research. *International Journal of Human Resource Management, 31*(1), 6–46. https://doi.org/10.1080/09585192.2019.1674358

FOSTREN. (2023). *Glossary*. www.fostren.eu

Freeman, M., Kolappa, K., Caldas de Almeida, J., Kleinman, A., Makhashvili, N., Phakathi, S., et al. (2015). Reversing hard won victories in the name of human rights: A critique of the General Comment on Article 12 of the UN Convention on the Rights of Persons with Disabilities. *The Lancet Psychiatry, 2*, 844. https://doi.org/10.1016/S2215-0366(15)00218-7

Fukasawa, M., Miyake, M., Suzuki, Y., Fukuda, Y., & Yamanouchi, Y. (2018). Relationship between the use of seclusion and mechanical restraint and the nurse-bed ratio in psychiatric wards in Japan. *International Journal of Law and Psychiatry, 60*, 57–63. https://doi.org/10.1016/J.IJLP.2018.08.001

Gagnon, M. P., Desmartis, M., Dipankui, M. T., Gagnon, J., & St-Pierre, M. (2013). Alternatives to seclusion and restraint in psychiatry and in long-term care facilities for the elderly: Perspectives of service users and family members. *Patient, 6*(4), 269–280. https://doi.org/10.1007/S40271-013-0023-2/TABLES/2

Gandré, C., Gervaix, J., Thillard, J., Macé, J. M., Roelandt, J. L., & Chevreul, K. (2017). Involuntary psychiatric admissions and development of psychiatric services as an alternative to full-time hospitalization in France. *Psychiatric Services (Washington, DC), 68*(9), 923–930. https://doi.org/10.1176/APPI.PS.201600453

German Psychiatric Association (DGPPN). (2018). *S3 Guideline: Prevention of coercion: Prevention and therapy of aggressive behaviour in adults*. https://register.awmf.org/de/leitlinien/detail/038-022

Gonzalez de Chavez, M. (1980). Historia de los cambios assistenciales y sus contextos sociales. In M. Gonzalez de Chavez (Ed.), *La transformación de la assistencia psiquiátrica* (pp. 13–106). Editorial Mayoria.

Gooding, P., McSherry, B., Roper, C., & Grey, F. (2018). *Alternatives to coercion in mental health settings: A literature review*. Melbourne Social Equity Institute. https://socialequity.unimelb.edu.au/__data/assets/pdf_file/0012/2898525/Alternatives-to-Coercion-Literature-Review-Melbourne-Social-Equity-Institute.pdf

Gowda, G. S., Lepping, P., Noorthoorn, E. O., Ali, S. F., Kumar, C. N., Raveesh, B. N., et al. (2018). Restraint prevalence and perceived coercion among psychiatric inpatients from South India: A prospective study. *Asian Journal of Psychiatry, 36*, 10–16. https://doi.org/10.1016/j.ajp.2018.05.024

Gravier, B., & Eytan, A. (2011). Ethical issues in psychiatry under coercion. *Revue Medicale Suisse*. https://europepmc.org/article/med/22016935

Guaiana, G., & Barbui, C. (2004). Trends in the use of the Italian Mental Health Act, 1979–1997. *European Psychiatry, 19*(7), 444–445. https://doi.org/10.1016/J.EURPSY.2004.07.004

Guedj, M., Sorum, P. C., & Mullet, E. (2012). French lay people's views regarding the acceptability of involuntary hospitalization of patients suffering from psychiatric illness. *International Journal of Law and Psychiatry, 35*(1), 50–56. https://doi.org/10.1016/J.IJLP.2011.11.010

Gupta, S., & Sagar, R. (2022). National Mental Health Policy, India (2014): Where have we reached? *Indian Journal of Psychological Medicine, 44*(5), 510–515. https://doi.org/10.1177/02537176211048335

Happell, B., & Koehn, S. (2010). From numbers to understanding: The impact of demographic factors on seclusion rates. *International Journal of Mental Health Nursing, 19*(3), 169–176. https://doi.org/10.1111/J.1447-0349.2010.00670.X

Hermann, R. C. (2005). *Improving mental healthcare: A guide to measurement-based quality improvement*. American Psychiatric Publishing, Inc..

Hotzy, F., & Jaeger, M. (2016). Clinical relevance of informal coercion in psychiatric treatment—A systematic review (review). *Frontiers in Psychiatry, 7*. https://doi.org/10.3389/fpsyt.2016.00197

Huckshorn, K. (2006). *Six core strategies for reducing seclusion and restraint use*. National Association of State Mental Health Program Directors. https://www.nasmhpd.org/sites/default/files/2022-08/Consolidated%2520Six%2520Core%2520Strategies%2520Document.pdf

Husum, T. L., Bjørngaard, J. H., Finset, A., & Ruud, T. (2010). A cross-sectional prospective study of seclusion, restraint and involuntary medication in acute psychiatric wards: Patient, staff and ward characteristics. *BMC Health Services Research, 10*. https://doi.org/10.1186/1472-6963-10-89

Husum, T. L., Bjørngaard, J. H., Finset, A., & Ruud, T. (2011). Staff attitudes and thoughts about the use of coercion in acute psychiatric wards. *Social Psychiatry and Psychiatric Epidemiology, 46*(9), 893–901. https://doi.org/10.1007/s00127-010-0259-2

Jalil, R., Huber, J. W., Sixsmith, J., & Dickens, G. L. (2017). Mental health nurses' emotions, exposure to patient aggression, attitudes to and use of coercive measures: Cross sectional questionnaire survey. *International Journal of Nursing Studies, 75*, 130–138. https://doi.org/10.1016/J.IJNURSTU.2017.07.018

Janssen, W., Noorthoorn, E., van Linge, R., & Lendemeijer, B. (2007). The influence of staffing levels on the use of seclusion. *International Journal of Law and Psychiatry, 30*(2), 118–126. https://doi.org/10.1016/J.IJLP.2006.04.005

Janssen, W., Noorthoorn, E. O., Nijman, H. L. I., Bowers, L., Hoogendoorn, A. W., Smit, A., et al. (2013). Differences in seclusion rates between admission wards: Does patient compilation explain? *Psychiatric Quarterly, 84*(1), 39–52. https://doi.org/10.1007/S11126-012-9225-3/TABLES/2

Joa, I., Hustoft, K., Anda, L. G., Brønnick, K., Nielssen, O., Johannessen, J. O., et al. (2017). Public attitudes towards involuntary admission and treatment by mental health services in Norway. *International Journal of Law and Psychiatry, 55*, 1–7. https://doi.org/10.1016/j.ijlp.2017.09.002

Keown, P., Weich, S., Bhui, K. S., & Scott, J. (2011). Association between provision of mental illness beds and rate of involuntary admissions in the NHS in England 1988–2008: Ecological study. *BMJ (Clinical Research Edition), 343*(7816), d3736. https://doi.org/10.1136/BMJ.D3736

Kersting, X. A. K., Hirsch, S., & Steinert, T. (2019). Physical harm and death in the context of coercive measures in psychiatric patients: A systematic review (systematic review). *Frontiers in Psychiatry, 10*. https://doi.org/10.3389/fpsyt.2019.00400

Kessell, E. R., Catalano, R. A., Christy, A., & Monahan, J. (2006). Rates of unemployment and incidence of police-initiated examinations for involuntary hospitalization in Florida. *Psychiatric Services, 57*(10), 1435–1439. https://doi.org/10.1176/PS.2006.57.10.1435/ASSET/IMAGES/LARGE/IO12T1.JPEG

Kleintjes, S., & Schneider, M. (2023). History and politics of mental health policy and care in South Africa. *SSM—Mental Health, 3*, 100206. https://doi.org/10.1016/j.ssmmh.2023.100206

Korkeila, J. A., Tuohimaki, C., Kaltiala-Heino, R., Lehtinen, V., & Joukamaa, M. (2002). Predicting use of coercive measures in Finland, *Nordic Journal of Psychiatry, 56*(5), 339–345.

Krieger, E., Moritz, S., Lincoln, T. M., Fischer, R., & Nagel, M. (2021). Coercion in psychiatry: A cross-sectional study on staff views and emotions. *Journal of Psychiatric and Mental Health Nursing, 28*(2), 149–162. https://doi.org/10.1111/jpm.12643

Laiho, T., Lindberg, N., Joffe, G., Putkonen, H., Hottinen, A., Kontio, R., et al. (2014). Psychiatric staff on the wards does not share attitudes on aggression. *International Journal of Mental Health Systems, 8*(1), 1–7. https://doi.org/10.1186/1752-4458-8-14/FIGURES/2

Lepping, P., Masood, B., Flammer, E., & Noorthoorn, E. O. (2016). Comparison of restraint data from four countries. *Social Psychiatry and Psychiatric Epidemiology, 51*(9), 1301–1309. https://doi.org/10.1007/s00127-016-1203-x

Levav, I., Kohn, R., & Schwartz, S. (1998). The psychiatric after-effects of the Holocaust on the second generation. *Psychological Medicine, 28*(4), 755–760. https://doi.org/10.1017/S0033291797005813

Looi, G. M. E., Gabrielsson, S., Sävenstedt, S., & Zingmark, K. (2014). Solving the staff's problem or meeting the patients' needs: Staff members' reasoning about choice of action in challenging situations in psychiatric inpatient care. *Issues in Mental Health Nursing, 35*(6), 470–479. https://doi.org/10.3109/01612840.2013.879629

Mann, K., Gröschel, S., Singer, S., Breitmaier, J., Claus, S., Fani, M., et al. (2021). Evaluation of coercive measures in different psychiatric hospitals: The impact of institutional characteristics. *BMC Psychiatry, 21*(1), 1–11. https://doi.org/10.1186/S12888-021-03410-Z/TABLES/3

Martin, K., Arbour, S., McGregor, C., & Rice, M. (2022). Silver linings: Observed reductions in aggression and use of restraints and seclusion in psychiatric inpatient care during COVID-19. *Journal of Psychiatric and Mental Health Nursing, 29*(2), 381–385. https://doi.org/10.1111/JPM.12752

McGarvey, E. L., Leon-Verdin, M., Wanchek, T. N., & Bonnie, R. J. (2013). Decisions to initiate involuntary commitment: The role of intensive community services and other factors. *Psychiatric Services, 64*(2), 120–126. https://doi.org/10.1176/APPI.PS.000692012

McKeown, M., Wright, K., & Mercer, D. (2017). Care planning: A neoliberal three card trick. *Journal of Psychiatric and Mental Health Nursing, 24*(6), 451–460. https://doi.org/10.1111/JPM.12356

McKeown, M., Thomson, G., Scholes, A., Jones, F., Baker, J., Downe, S., et al. (2019). "Catching your tail and firefighting": The impact of staffing levels on restraint minimization efforts. *Journal of Psychiatric and Mental Health Nursing, 26*(5–6), 131–141. https://doi.org/10.1111/JPM.12532

Modini, M., Burton, A., & Abbott, M. J. (2021). Factors influencing inpatients perception of psychiatric hospitals: A meta-review of the literature. *Journal of Psychiatric Research, 136*, 492–500. https://doi.org/10.1016/j.jpsychires.2020.10.020

Muir-Cochrane, E., & Oster, C. (2021). Chemical restraint: A qualitative synthesis review of adult service user and staff experiences in mental health settings. *Nursing & Health Sciences, 23*(2), 325–336. https://doi.org/10.1111/nhs.12822

Navarro, L. N., de Loma Osorio, V. L., Fe Bravo Ortiz, M., & Liria, A. F. (2021). Mental health and human rights: The experience of professionals in training with the use of mechanical restraints in Madrid, Spain. *Salud Colectiva, 17*, 1–26. https://doi.org/10.18294/SC.2021.3045

Newton-Howes, G., Savage, M. K., Arnold, R., Hasegawa, T., Staggs, V., & Kisely, S. (2020). The use of mechanical restraint in Pacific Rim countries: An international epidemiological study. *Epidemiology and Psychiatric Sciences, 29*, e190. https://doi.org/10.1017/S2045796020001031

NICE. (2015). *Violence and aggression. Short-term management in mental health, health and community settings.* Update Edition. NICE Guideline NG10. https://www.nice.org.uk/guidance/ng10/evidence/full-guideline-60711085

Nijman, H., Palmstierna, T., Alvmvik, R., & Stolker, J. (2005). Fifteen years of research with the Staff Observation Aggression Scale: A review. *Acta Psychiatrica Scandinavica, 111*, 12–21.

O'Brien, A. J. (2014). Community treatment orders in New Zealand: Regional variability and international comparisons. *Australasian Psychiatry, 22*(4), 352–356. https://doi.org/10.1177/1039856214531080

Pec, O. (2019). Mental health reforms in the Czech Republic. *BJPsych International, 16*(1), 4–6. https://doi.org/10.1192/bji.2017.27

Pereira, M. (2004). A Mania, o tratamento moral e os inícios da psiquiatria contemporânea. *Revista Latinoamericana de Psicopatologia Fundamenta, 7*(3), 113.

Pérez, J., Baldessarini, R. J., Undurraga, J., & Sánchez-Moreno, J. (2012). Origins of psychiatric hospitalization in medieval Spain. *Psychiatric Quarterly, 83*(4), 419–430. https://doi.org/10.1007/s11126-012-9212-8

Pescosolido, B. A., Manago, B., & Monahan, J. (2019). Evolving public views on the likelihood of violence from people with mental illness: Stigma and its consequences. *Health Affairs, 38*(10), 1735–1743. https://doi.org/10.1377/HLTHAFF.2019.00702/ASSET/IMAGES/LARGE/FIGUREEX2.JPEG

Pinel, F. (1801). *Traité Medico-Philosophique sur l'Alienation Mentale ou la Manie.* Richard, Caille et Ravier.

Porter, R. (2002). *Madness: A brief history.* Oxford University Press.

Price, O., Baker, J., Bee, P., & Lovell, K. (2018). The support-control continuum: An investigation of staff perspectives on factors influencing the success or failure of de-escalation techniques for the management of violence and aggression in mental health settings. *International Journal of Nursing Studies, 77*, 197–206. https://doi.org/10.1016/j.ijnurstu.2017.10.002

Raad, R., & Makari, G. (2010). Samuel Tuke's description of the retreat. *American Journal of Psychiatry, 167*(8), 898–898. https://doi.org/10.1176/appi.ajp.2010.10020265

Raboch, J., Kališová, L., Nawka, A., Kitzlerová, E., Onchev, G., Karastergiou, A., et al. (2010). Use of coercive measures during involuntary hospitalization: Findings from ten European countries. *Psychiatric Services, 61*(10), 1012–1017. https://doi.org/10.1176/PS.2010.61.10.1012/ASSET/IMAGES/LARGE/KL14T4.JPEG

Reid, K., & Price, O. (2022). PROD-ALERT: Psychiatric restraint open data—Analysis using logarithmic estimates on reporting trends (brief research report). *Frontiers in Digital Health, 4.* https://doi.org/10.3389/fdgth.2022.945635

Rodrigues, C. A., Rodrigues, N., Nascimento, M., & Oliveira-Silva, J. (2022). Patterns of adult and youth inpatient admissions before and after the COVID-19 pandemic in a psychiatric ward: An observational study. *BMC Health Services Research, 22*(1), 1–11. https://doi.org/10.1186/S12913-022-08374-8/TABLES/5

Rugkåsa, J. (2016). Effectiveness of community treatment orders: The international evidence. *The Canadian Journal of Psychiatry, 61*(1), 15–24. https://doi.org/10.1177/0706743715620415

Salize, H. J., & Dressing, H. (2004). Epidemiology of involuntary placement of mentally ill people across the European Union. *The British Journal of Psychiatry, 184*, 163–168. https://doi.org/10.1192/BJP.184.2.163

Sattar, S. P., Pinals, D. A., Din, A. U., & Appelbaum, P. S. (2006). To commit or not to commit: The psychiatry resident as a variable in involuntary commitment decisions. *Academic Psychiatry, 30*(3), 191–195. https://doi.org/10.1176/APPI.AP.30.3.191

Savage, M. K., Lepping, P., Newton-Howes, G., Arnold, R., Staggs, V. S., Kisely, S., et al. (2024). Comparison of coercive practices in worldwide mental healthcare: Overcoming difficulties resulting from variations in monitoring strategies. *BJPsych Open, 10*(1), e26. https://doi.org/10.1192/bjo.2023.613

Schön, U. K., Grim, K., Wallin, L., Rosenberg, D., & Svedberg, P. (2018). Psychiatric service staff perceptions of implementing a shared decision-making tool: A process evaluation study. *International Journal of Qualitative Studies on Health and Well-Being, 13*(1). https://doi.org/10.1080/17482631.2017.1421352

Sheridan Rains, L., Zenina, T., Dias, M. C., Jones, R., Jeffreys, S., Branthonne-Foster, S., et al. (2019). Variations in patterns of involuntary hospitalisation and in legal frameworks: An international comparative study. *The Lancet Psychiatry, 6*(5), 403–417. https://doi.org/10.1016/ S2215-0366(19)30090-2

Shorter, E. (1997). *A history of psychiatry: From the era of the asylum to the age of Prozac.* John Wiley & Sons.

Slemon, A., Jenkins, E., & Bungay, V. (2017). Safety in psychiatric inpatient care: The impact of risk management culture on mental health nursing practice. *Nursing Inquiry, 24*(4), e12199. https://doi.org/10.1111/NIN.12199

Smith, S., Gate, R., Ariyo, K., Saunders, R., Taylor, C., Bhui, K., et al. (2020). Reasons behind the rising rate of involuntary admissions under the Mental Health Act (1983): Service use and cost impact. *International Journal of Law and Psychiatry, 68*, 101506. https://doi.org/10.1016/J. IJLP.2019.101506

Steinberg, A. (2021). Prone restraint cardiac arrest: A comprehensive review of the scientific literature and an explanation of the physiology. *Medicine, Science and the Law, 61*(3), 215–226. https://doi.org/10.1177/0025802420988370

Steinert, T., Martin, V., Baur, M., Bohnet, U., Goebel, R., Hermelink, G., et al. (2007). Diagnosis-related frequencies of compulsory measures in ten German psychiatric hospitals and correlates with hospital characteristics. *Social Psychiatry and Psychiatric Epidemiology, 42*, 140–145.

Steinert, T., Lepping, P., Bernhardsgrütter, R., Conca, A., Hatling, T., Janssen, W., et al. (2010). Incidence of seclusion and restraint in psychiatric hospitals: A literature review and survey of international trends. *Social Psychiatry and Psychiatric Epidemiology, 45*(9), 889–897.

Strous, R. D. (2007). Psychiatry during the Nazi era: Ethical lessons for the modern professional. *Annals of General Psychiatry, 6*(1), 8. https://doi.org/10.1186/1744-859X-6-8

Sugiura, K., Pertega, E., & Holmberg, C. (2020). Experiences of involuntary psychiatric admission decision-making: A systematic review and meta-synthesis of the perspectives of service users, informal carers, and professionals. *International Journal of Law and Psychiatry, 73*, 101645. https://doi.org/10.1016/j.ijlp.2020.101645

Taylor, H. J. (2016). What are 'best interests'? A critical evaluation of 'best interest' decision-making in clinical practice. *Medical Law Review, 24*(2), 176–205. https://doi.org/10.1093/ medlaw/fww007

Thumiger, C. (2017). Ancient Greek and Roman traditions. In G. Eghigian (Ed.), *The Routledge history of madness and mental health* (pp. 42–61). Routledge.

Tingleff, E. B., Bradley, S. K., Gildberg, F. A., Munksgaard, G., & Hounsgaard, L. (2017). "Treat me with respect". A systematic review and thematic analysis of psychiatric patients' reported perceptions of the situations associated with the process of coercion. *Journal of Psychiatric and Mental Health Nursing, 24*(9–10), 681–698. https://doi.org/10.1111/jpm.12410

UN General Assembly. (1948) Universal Declaration of Human Rights. United Nations 217 A (III). https://www.refworld.org/docid/3ae6b3712c.html

United Nations. (1966). *International covenant on economic, social and cultural rights.* United Nations General Assembly. https://www.ohchr.org/sites/default/files/cescr.pdf

United Nations. (1991). *Principles for the protection of persons with mental illness and the improvement of mental health care.* United Nations General Assembly. Retrieved June 12, 2023, from https://www.ohchr.org/en/instruments-mechanisms/instruments/ principles-protection-persons-mental-illness-and-improvement

United Nations. (2008). *Convention on the rights of persons with disabilities.* United Nations General Assembly. Retrieved June 12, 2023, from https://www.ohchr.org/en/instruments-mechanisms/ instruments/convention-rights-persons-disabilities

van Bilsen, H. P. J. G. (2016). Lessons to be learned from the oldest community psychiatric service in the world: Geel in Belgium. *BJPsych Bulletin, 40*(4), 207–211. https://doi.org/10.1192/ pb.bp.115.051631

van der Post, L., Mulder, C., Bernardt, C., Schoevers, R., Beekman, A., & Dekker, J. (2009). Involuntary admission of emergency psychiatric patients: Report from the Amsterdam Study

of Acute Psychiatry. *Psychiatric Services (Washington, DC), 60*(11). https://doi.org/10.1176/
APPI.PS.60.11.1543

van der Schaaf, P. S., Dusseldorp, E., Keuning, F. M., Janssen, W. A., & Noorthoorn, E. O. (2013).
Impact of the physical environment of psychiatric wards on the use of seclusion. *British Journal
of Psychiatry, 202*(2), 142–149. https://doi.org/10.1192/bjp.bp.112.118422

Vázquez-Barquero, J. L., García, J., & Torres-González, F. (2001). Spanish psychiatric reform:
What can be learned from two decades of experience? *Acta Psychiatrica Scandinavica,
104*(s410), 89–95. https://doi.org/10.1034/j.1600-0447.2001.1040s2089.x

Walker, S., Mackay, E., Barnett, P., Sheridan Rains, L., Leverton, M., Dalton-Locke, C., et al.
(2019). Clinical and social factors associated with increased risk for involuntary psychiatric hospitalisation: A systematic review, meta-analysis, and narrative synthesis. *The Lancet
Psychiatry, 6*, 1039. https://doi.org/10.1016/S2215-0366(19)30406-7

Wierdsma, A. I., & Mulder, C. L. (2009). Does mental health service integration affect compulsory admissions? *International Journal of Integrated Care, 9*(3), e90. https://doi.org/10.5334/
IJIC.324/METRICS/

Wilson, C., Rouse, L., Rae, S., & Kar Ray, M. (2018). Mental health inpatients' and staff members'
suggestions for reducing physical restraint: A qualitative study. *Journal of Psychiatric and
Mental Health Nursing, 25*(3), 188–200. https://doi.org/10.1111/JPM.12453

World Health Organization. (2019). *Quality rights materials for training, guidance and transformation.* https://www.who.int/publications/i/item/who-qualityrights-guidance-and-training-tools

World Health Organization. (2022). *Transforming mental health for all.* World Health Organisation.

World Health Organization (WHO). (1946). *Constitution of the World Health Organization.* World
Health Organization. https://apps.who.int/gb/bd/PDF/bd47/EN/constitution-en.pdf

Zhang, J., Sun, X.-L., Yan, B.-P., Liu, J., Wu, Y.-F., & Li, K.-Q. (2016). Validity and reliability of
the Broset Violence Checklist-Extended. *Chinese Mental Health Journal, 30*(10), 752–757.

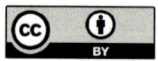

# Measurement and Prevalence of Aggression

Joanne DeSanto Iennaco, Elizabeth Molle, Christian Lauvrud, Tom Palmstierna, Henk Nijman (ID), and Roger Almvik

## 1    Introduction

Violence is a common problem in the healthcare workplace, with rate and severity differences dependent on the setting; typically psychiatric settings have the highest rates (Babiarczyk et al., 2020; United States Bureau of Labor Statistics, 2020a). This topic is complex, given that rates of patient aggression and worker aggression exposure are different, and both are important to measure. It is essential to understand the phenomenon of violence and coercive intervention, and their impact on patients, workers and the clinical environment. A multicohort study (Hanson et al., 2023) showed the seriousness of workplace violence exposure: the risk of suicide attempt or death was 1.3 times higher with workplace violence exposure, and a dose-response relationship was observed across levels of exposure, from occasional (HR 1.27) to frequent (HR 1.75) increasing suicide risk ($p < 0.0001$). Internationally, efforts are being made to reduce violence in healthcare to improve worker health, job satisfaction and patient safety and outcomes in clinical settings. The World Health Organization (WHO) identifies the inseparable interconnections between patient safety and healthcare worker safety (WHO, 2021).

Henk Nijman passed away on 24th February 2021.

J. D. Iennaco (✉) · E. Molle
Yale School of Nursing, Yale University, West Haven, CT, USA
e-mail: joanne.iennaco@yale.edu; elizabeth.molle@yale.edu

C. Lauvrud · R. Almvik
Centre for Research and Education in Forensic Psychiatry, St. Olav's University Hospital, Trondheim, Norway
e-mail: christian.lauvrud@ntnu.no; roger.almvik@ntnu.no

T. Palmstierna
Department of Clinical Neuroscience, Karolinska Institute, Huddinge, Sweden
e-mail: tom.palmstierna@ki.se

H. Nijman (Deceased)
Faculty of Social Sciences, Radboud University, Nijmegan, The Netherlands

© The Author(s) 2024
N. Hallett et al. (eds.), *Coercion and Violence in Mental Health Settings*,
https://doi.org/10.1007/978-3-031-61224-4_5

In the area of worker safety, the European Medical Organizations (European Council of Medical Orders [CEOM], 2017) have, for the first time in history, called on governments and stakeholders to 'act on the urgent need to protect medical personnel in the performance of their missions'. This includes enforcing existing laws to fight workplace violence against health professionals, establishing national reporting mechanisms across Europe and implementing violence prevention and victim assistance programmes. In the United States (US) legislature occupational health standards requiring healthcare employers to implement comprehensive violence prevention plans, with engineering and work controls to promote worker safety and security is under consideration (H.R.2663—118th Congress 2023–2024; S.1176—118th Congress 2023–2024).

The inter-relationship of worker and patient safety is important given that worker health and safety risks can lead to risks for patients, patient harm and adverse events. Physically and psychologically sound health workers are less prone to make errors, contributing to safer care. Therefore, the safety of healthcare workers directly impacts the safety of patients (WHO, 2021). One WHO strategy to mitigate workplace violence and increase patient safety is to evaluate the current patient safety incident reporting system, the Minimal Information Model for Patient Safety (MIM PS). The effort seeks to create user-friendly, confidential and effective reporting mechanisms and use the system to identify patient safety priorities to address using improvement activities (WHO, 2020).

Measuring violence in clinical settings requires approaches that address both patient events and worker exposure, as workplace violence is often met with coercive intervention by workers. This increased measurement complexity and difficulty in determining prevalence given that coercive interventions to prevent violence escalation may themselves initiate violence. An important step in understanding the complexity is to describe the incidence or prevalence of aggression or violence and coercive intervention, which require clear definitions as a starting point.

## 2    Defining Violence and Aggression

Multiple definitions of violence and aggression exist, but the most commonly used definition of aggression is based on Morrison (1990, p. 67) and is used in the Staff Observation of Aggression Scale-Revised (SOAS-R): '… any verbal, nonverbal, or physical behaviour that was threatening (to self, others, or property), or physical behaviour that actually did harm (to self, others, or property)'. Other common definitions include those by WHO and the UK's National Institute for Health and Care Excellence (NICE) Guidelines. WHO broadly defines aggression and violence as: 'the intentional use of physical force or power, threatened or actual, against oneself, another person, or against a group or community, that either results in or has a high likelihood of resulting in injury, death, psychological harm, maldevelopment, or deprivation' (Krug et al., 2002). NICE (2015, p. 20) guidelines define violence and aggression as: 'a range of behaviors or actions that can result in harm, hurt or injury to another person, regardless of whether the violence or aggression is physically or verbally expressed, physical harm is sustained, or the intention is clear'. These definitions identify the type of act, the presence of intention and harm. The WHO definition specifies the intention of the act and the potential for actual harm while being less descriptive of the type of act. The National Institute of Health and Care Excellence (NICE) definition addresses these aspects, speaking to a range of actions and outcomes. Aggressive behaviour in mental health and other healthcare settings lies on a continuum from mild, such as loud, demanding or disrespectful verbalisations, to spoken threats or gestures, to physical acts involving the body including hitting, kicking, biting, spitting, throwing things or damaging property to severe acts which regardless of intentionality have the potential to or may cause emotional and bodily injury.

Objectivity in aggression measurement is important to limit the introduction of bias, as individuals are likely to have varied perceptions regarding the nature of aggressive behaviour. However, objective aggression measurement is difficult given that it occurs as part of an interpersonal dynamic, the intention may or may not be known, and evidence shows that actual harm may be less distressing than potential harm, such as verbal threats (Gerberich et al., 2004; Whittington et al., 1996). Thus subjective perception is an important factor in understanding the impact of aggressive behaviour. Tools for measuring violence often include criteria for both subjective and objective severity regardless of the type of aggression. The subjective nature of the perception of aggression creates difficulty, for example, behaviour perceived as loud, demanding or threatening may vary based on the individual, past experiences, group norms, relationships, and unit environment and norms.

Coercion ranging from mild to severe occurs in clinical settings and may trigger agitation and aggression (i.e. restricting possessions or activity, setting limits on behaviour or activity). Coercive intervention may be a response to or result of agitated and aggressive behaviour (i.e. time out, seclusion, use of physical hold or restraint, use of mechanical or chemical restraint) and may be thought of as a negative outcome. Positive outcomes to agitation and aggression include de-escalation of behaviour to lower levels, improved therapeutic relationships and prevention of aggressive behaviour involving coercive intervention.

## 3    Principles of Aggression Measurement

From a measurement perspective, rates are the ideal way to measure and compare incidents to determine whether differences are present when comparing settings, type of patient or worker and to determine if an intervention resulted in a change. To properly determine a rate, the number of events is identified per number of people per a specific time frame. Differences between incidence and prevalence rates involve the identification of an initial or incident event versus repeated events over time. It might be of interest to measure an incidence rate (rate of first event of aggression) if determining whether differences in rates of aggression exist between persons with different diagnostic groups or treated with different types of medications. Monitoring the prevalence of aggression is useful in identifying problems with patient or worker safety and understanding whether interventions have resulted in improvement or reduction in aggressive events.

Understanding aggression and violence in the psychiatric setting involves consideration of both the patient rate of aggression, the unit rate of aggression, the staff or worker aggression exposure rate, the rate of coercion (i.e. use of coercive intervention) and the rate of successful de-escalation. Environmental and clinical practices have a significant impact on rates of aggression, more impact than psychopathology alone. These may include ward atmosphere, staff gender balance, education level, etc. (Urheim et al., 2020). Typically, settings measure rates of coercive intervention use (i.e. seclusion, physical, mechanical or chemical restraint) to determine change or improvement in aggression de-escalation and management given that it is a rate that is often required to be monitored for quality-of-care measures and to meet legal or accreditation requirements. This practice likely grossly underestimates the amount of aggressive behaviour as well as worker exposure to aggression and unfortunately may result in an inability to determine whether intervention strategies are effective due to a lack of power when coercive interventions are reduced, and outcomes are infrequent events. Measurement of the continuum of aggression from mild to severe and of successful de-escalation of aggression (i.e. near misses) offers a broader and more positive perspective on the impact of worker intervention across the continuum. While incident reporting is common in most hospital settings, reports are normally of a more generic nature (i.e. reports of falls, slippery floors) and lack information on characteristics of aggressive events, which is more useful when reducing the prevalence or monitoring effects of interventions.

## 3.1   Issues in Measurement of Aggressive Events

Measurement of aggressive events involves a variety of methods, including cross-sectional surveys of self-reported worker exposure using varied time periods (past day, week, year or career-long). Observational measures of aggression often involve form completion to report an incident. A multitude of scales exist to report incidents and include patient characteristics, events and sequelae. Some patient self-reports of aggression or hostility are used as well as staff reports of their perception of aggression. The ideal measure would provide identification of events as they occur, vs. post-event reporting which can result in under-reporting of events. A careful, evidence-based incident report should include specific information that leads to better understanding of what happened before, during and after the reported incident. This may result in improved care planning, intervention, consultation and referral. Regular reporting can identify common precipitants, effective interventions, and environmental and therapeutic 'hotspots' likely to induce conflict and coercion. Identification of a broad range of events can provide additional insight into prevention and intervention. Limitations of measures include under-reporting of events, the presence of recall bias, selection bias, impact of social desirability, and personal experiences with violence and aggression that impact measurement. A review of individual measures will highlight both the strengths and limitations of each scale.

Rates illustrate the (potential) magnitude of measurement problems. For example, nurses from the anonymous survey in East London (Nijman et al., 2005a) may have exaggerated or overestimated the prevalence of WPV. Furthermore, severely victimised caregivers may be more inclined to respond to a WPV survey. Given the low survey response rate (39%), it remains unclear whether the other 61% of nurses had similar experiences to those participating.

Such obvious limitations of survey instruments, i.e. recall and selection bias, stress the necessity for regular monitoring of aggressive occurrences in psychiatric units. Reliable and time-efficient methods of recording aggression are needed to have complete information on the magnitude of the problem. Continuous incident monitoring may be helpful in detecting typical precipitants and triggers of violent behaviour. Presumably, this information will improve intervention effectiveness in reducing aggressive behaviour. A variety of methods for measuring the aggressiveness of psychiatric patients will be reviewed. First, the use and problems with self-report questionnaires for measuring aggression, anger and hostility of psychiatric (in)patients will be briefly discussed. Following this, staff observation scales designed to observe the aggressive behaviour of patients on psychiatric wards are addressed. Finally, the prevalence of inpatient aggression in psychiatric institutions is illustrated, on the basis of the results of such aggression observation tools.

## 4    Aggression in Settings: Psychiatric vs. Other Healthcare Settings

Aggression and violence occur across healthcare clinical settings. In general, rates of aggression are higher in psychiatric settings, including inpatient psychiatry, forensic psychiatry, residential and acute or emergency services, and community-based care as compared to other healthcare settings. In the United States, psychiatric and substance use settings have the highest annual incidence rate for workplace violence injury, 124.9 per 10,000 workers compared to 12.8 per 10,000 for all hospitals and 21.1 per 10,000 for nursing and residential care facilities (US Bureau of Labor Statistics, 2023, Table 1). A recent US analysis of workplace violence (WPV) injury ($\geq$1 day lost from injury) by setting found residential workers (excluding skilled nursing) rates were higher than other healthcare workers (HCW), 44.07 vs. 6.24 per 10,000 workers in all HCWs, with rates for nursing care facilities (10.64) and hospitals (5.59) following (Hawkins & El Ghaziri, 2022). The emergency department and nursing homes are settings where aggression is more common although inpatient medical units also have aggressive events (Table 1). There seems to be a lack of similar worker injury data available for Europe but for nurses, the European Agency for Safety and Health at Work reports data from 10 European countries and 'showed that exposure to frequent violent events was highest amongst nurses from France (39%), the UK (29%) and Germany (28%). In Norway (9%) and the Netherlands (10%), nurses were less exposed to frequent violent events. The results were similar when violence from patients/their relatives was examined' (Milczarek, 2011).

**Table 1** Prevalence of HCW exposure to WPV by Clinical Setting and Region or Country

| Country or region | Psychiatric | ED | Medical | Nursing home |
|---|---|---|---|---|
| Europe | 87%[a]<br>P: 36%[a]<br>V: 94%[a]<br>47.7%[b] | 67%[a]<br>43.2%[b] | 24.4%[b] | P: 32%[a]<br>V: 83%[a]<br>30.0%[b] |
| Australia | | 70%[c]<br>87%[d]<br>P: 42.6%[e]<br>V: 88.2%[e] | | |
| Belgium | 4.3%[b] | 8.8%[b] | | |
| Canada | P: 77.2%[f] | P: 89.5%[f] | P: 86.4%[f] | P: 85%[f] |
| France | 13.2%[b] | 4.9%[b] | | 15.2%[b] |
| Germany | 5.2%[b] | 3.7%[b] | | 21.7%[b] |
| Italy | 2.7%[b] | 87%[c]<br>4.3%[b] | | 3.6%[b] |
| Jordan | | 72%[c,g]<br>14.2%[h] | 7.3%[h] | |
| Netherlands | P: 60.7%[i]<br>1.5%[b] | 2.7%[b] | | 12.6%[b] |
| Poland | 1.4%[b] | 1.1%[b] | | 5.3%[b] |
| Slovakia | 6.9%[b] | 3.4%[b] | | 18.0%[b] |
| Taiwan | 61.7%[j] | P: 30%[c]<br>V: 92%[c] | P: 27.3%[k]<br>V: 70.7%[k] | |

[a] Babiarczyk et al. (2020) (past year)
[b] Camerino et al. (2008) (nursing staff)
[c] Aljohani et al. (2021)
[d] Pich et al. (2017) (over 6m)
[e] Partridge and Affleck (2017)
[f] Havaei et al. (2020)
[g] MD/RN
[h] Ahmed (2012)
[i] van Leeuwen and Harte (2017) (past 5 years)
[j] Chen et al. (2008)
[k] Yeh et al. (2020) (nurse only)

In a meta-analysis of WPV across healthcare settings, Liu et al. (2019) estimated that 61.9% of participants reported exposure to some type of violence, with estimated rates of physical violence of 24.4% and verbal abuse of 57.6%. A recent meta-analysis of workplace violence in healthcare professionals internationally found a pooled prevalence across all studies of 19.33% and subgroups with the highest pooled prevalence in Europe and the Americas (26.38% and 23.61%, respectively, Fig. 1) and the lowest in South-East Asia (5.62%) (Li et al., 2020, pp. 9–10). A review of HCW self-reported exposure prevalence found that 10–95% of workers report WPV exposure (Fig. 2), and the kind of violence exposure varied, including verbal abuse, threats or actual physical violence. Weltens et al. (2021) reported worker exposure to any type of patient aggression on psychiatric wards ranged from 65% to 99% although prevalence decreased to 38% to 82% when measuring

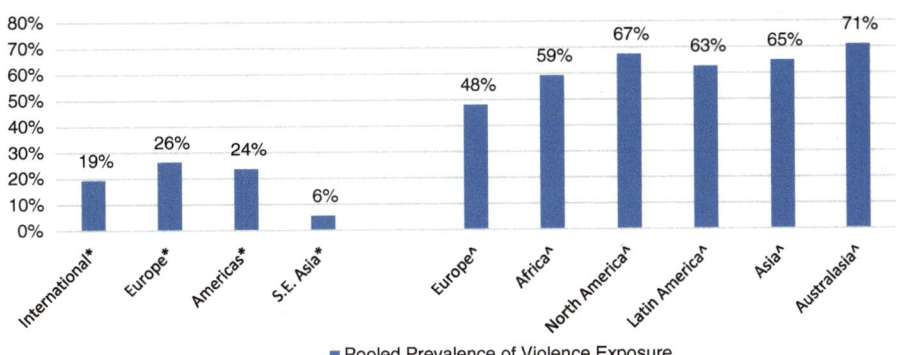

**Fig. 1** Healthcare worker (all settings) prevalence of exposure to physical aggression in the workplace by region (meta-analysis). *Li et al. (2020) 1 year prevalence of physical violence, range, individual studies: 3–88%. ^Liu et al. (2019), any type of WPV, physical violence pooled prevalence: 24.4%

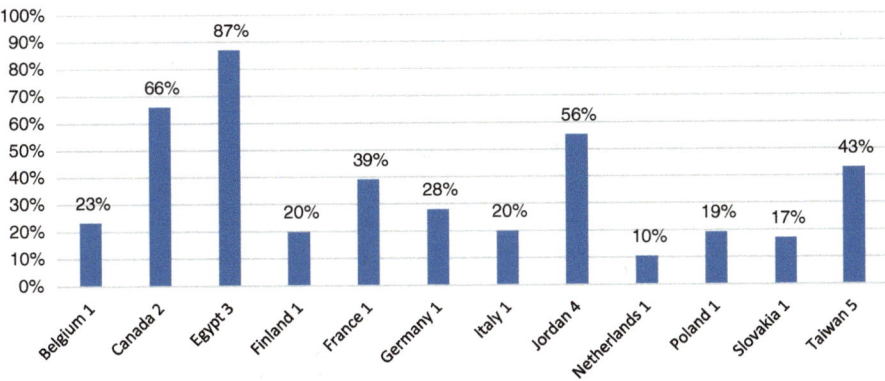

**Fig. 2** Healthcare worker (all settings) prevalence of exposure to WPV by country (self-report). [1]Camerino et al. (2008) (nursing staff), [2]Havaei et al. (2020), [3]Albadry et al. (2020) (security guards in acute care setting), [4]Ahmed (2012), [5]Chen et al. (2008)

physical aggression only (p. 6). A recent study of Dutch psychiatric settings identified that 61.9% of WPV incidents included threats (Van Leeuwen & Harte, 2017), and 47% involved actual physical violence with examples including beating, kicking, hitting, biting, spitting as well as severe acts including stabbing, taking hostage, rape or attempted strangulation (n = 130, p. 588). Babiarczyk et al.'s (2020) cross-sectional survey reports data from 1089 nurses in five European countries (Poland, the Czech Republic, the Slovak Republic, Turkey and Spain), showing that 54% had exposure to non-physical violence in the workplace, 20% experienced physical violence and 15% had suffered both forms of violence. Differences were found, with only 34% of Spanish nurses reporting non-physical violence, and significantly more Polish (34%) and Slovak (21%) nurses reporting physical violence as compared to 8% of nurses from Turkey (p < 0.001, p. 328). The nurses surveyed indicated that approximately 70% of violent incidents (both non-physical and physical) were not reported (Babiarczyk et al., 2019). Reasons for under-reporting WPV included feeling ashamed or guilty, fearing negative consequences and many felt reporting was not important or useless.

# 5 Consequences of Violence

## 5.1 Consequences of Workplace Violence: Worker Exposure and Injury

Workplace violence (WPV) can result in risks to worker safety. A critical consequence is worker injury, resulting in lost time at work. Measurement of rates of WPV in healthcare workers is a parallel area to measuring rates of patient aggression. Reporting of injury or illness due to violence at work is often reported as a rate per full-time equivalent (FTE) worker and is closely followed by occupational health and safety organisations. Studies of injury due to violence in healthcare settings indicate the most prevalent type of violence is Type II, acts by customer or client, as compared to Type I (criminal intent), Type III (worker to worker), Type IV (person known to victim) or Type V (ideological) (Adebayo et al., 2022; Center for Disease Control, 2020; Howard, 1996). Rates of injury due to WPV are gross underestimates of actual worker aggression exposure rates given that only events resulting in medical treatment are reported and only a fraction of aggressive events result in worker injury (Reilly et al., 2019). This compares to measuring toxic exposure or disease incidence vs. measuring exposure in daily work, as required in many occupations. Most aggression measurement methods omit information on worker exposure to aggressive events, focusing on patient characteristics and rates. Attention to this aspect of measurement is important. Consequences of healthcare workers' exposure to WPV include psychological distress, depression, anxiety, PTSD, decreased job satisfaction and turnover intent (Lanctôt & Guay, 2014; Pariona-Cabrera et al., 2020). A longitudinal cohort study (The Denmark Work Life Cohort) found evidence for depression as a causal effect of WPV exposure: incident depression diagnosis was significantly higher in workers with high WPV exposure, with control of depression risk factors (family history, gender, age, income) existing prior to work force entry (Madsen et al., 2021), providing compelling evidence that propensity for depression is not the source of higher rates in these workers. The most recent multicohort study, finding a dose-response relationship between increasing WPV exposure and an increased risk of suicide, highlights the importance of understanding impacts of worker exposure (Hanson et al., 2023).

## 5.2 Economic Costs of Aggression and Workplace Violence

Costs attributed to patient aggression and workplace violence include an increase in length of stay, medication use, observation levels, replacement of damaged items, costs of injury, lost time at work, job dissatisfaction and worker turnover. A recent systematic review found patient length of stay (1.5–54 days or longer), frequency of readmission (additional 1–1.8 readmissions) and medication use were significantly higher in patients with aggressive acts during inpatient psychiatric hospitalisation (Rubio-Valera et al., 2015). In addition, coercive interventions such as seclusion and restraint involve increasing the level of observation resulting in higher staffing costs (Flood et al., 2008). A recent study (Lambert et al., 2018) estimating staffing costs for aggression-related constant observation in four forensic psychiatric units in England in 2014 was €493,286.04 (converted to 2023 cost: ~€592,041.90). Costs identified from a long-term inpatient psychiatric unit in the Netherlands were €78 per aggression incident, or €7000 per patient-year based on a rate of 90 incidents per patient-year. The measure of staff time spent per incident was an average of 125 min, with a total cost of €140,000 per ward (20 patients per ward) per year (de Bles et al., 2021, p. 433). Available estimates indicate the high prevalence, costs and impact of aggressive events on workload.

Earlier studies indicated high costs associated with workplace violence, for example Lanza and Milner (1989) identified costs of $14,667 associated with staff time managing aggression annually. A much-cited study by Hunter and Carmel (1992) identified 134 serious injuries for a 973-bed forensic psychiatric hospital annually, $5719 average costs per injury were conservatively estimated, suggesting a total loss of $766,290 annually. In a survey of 148 psychiatric nurses in East London (Nijman et al., 2005a), almost one of every six nurses (16%) identified experiencing past year severe physical WPV. A little over one in five nurses (22%) revealed they have called in sick, losing an average of 5.2 workdays per nurse (range 1–23 days) in connection with WPV. Finally, a recent review found that from 13% to 60% of victims of WPV considered quitting their jobs (Lanctôt & Guay, 2014), turnover can cost employers up to three times the nurse's salary (Bae, 2022) to hire and orient new workers, and in loss of skills and knowledge, inestimable aspects of organisational human and intellectual capital (Li & Jones, 2013).

Recent rates of WPV-related injury or illness involving days away from work are highest in psychiatric settings, with rates of 18.2 per 10,000 FTE in nurses, 50.9 per 10,000 in nursing assistants, 376.7 per 10,000 in psychiatric technicians and 360.8 per 10,000 in psychiatric aides based on data from the US Bureau of Labor Statistics (USBLS, 2020a, 2020b). Healthcare and psychiatric care workers are at higher risk of WPV injury or illness compared to other workers, for example, all education and HC workers have a total rate of 13.9/10,000 FTE while the total rate for all sectors of workers is 4.0 per 10,000 FTEs (USBLS, 2020b). In summary, violence from psychiatric patients not only has considerable physical and psychological consequences but also has substantial financial implications. Estimates of medical, disability and productivity costs in 2016 were $428.5 million for US hospitals resulting from WPV (Van Den Bos et al., 2017).

## 6    Assessing the Aggression of Psychiatric Patients with Self-Report Scales

The assessment of psychiatric patients' aggression can be divided into two overarching methods: self-rated and observer-rated aggression scales (Girasek et al., 2022; Ravyts et al., 2021; Bech, 1994). A well-known self-rating scale with a long history, the Buss-Durkee Hostility Inventory (BDHI), is used for measuring hostility and anger (Buss & Durkee, 1957). Research over the years on the psycho-metric qualities of BDHI items has led to adapted versions of the BDHI, such as the Aggression Questionnaire (AQ) (Buss & Perry, 1992).

A review of the literature by Bjørkly (1995, p. 49) noted that the BDHI's 'predic-tive value for adult psychiatric patients has not been convincing so far'. A recent review of the BDHI found that few had calculated the reliability of the measure, and when available, the mean alpha estimates for the subscales were below standards, ranging from 0.55 to 0.69 (Vassar & Hale, 2009). While early research on the psy-chometric properties of aggression selfreport measures was conducted with 'nor-mal' subjects (Yudofsky et al., 1986)—for example, psychology students)—this seems to be changing rapidly (Novaco & Taylor, 2004). One of the problems with aggression self-reports may be that people with severe psychiatric disorders, for example, antisocial personality disorder or schizophrenia, lack insight into their own role in creating conflicts. However, changes in cognitive processes might lead to increased insight and change behaviour in a positive direction. This is true not only for persons with psychiatric disorders but also, for example, in staff working in mental health services (Ross et al., 2008).

Furthermore, self-reports of aggressive behaviour rely on the honesty of respon-dents about their tendency to become angry and behave aggressively. Yudofsky et al. (1986, p. 35) noted in general about aggression self-reports that: 'many patients are not angry between aggressive episodes, and do not reliably recall or admit to past violent events'.

In forensic psychiatric samples, release from custody may be based on psychiat-ric condition. The inclination to provide socially desirable answers poses problems for the validity of self-reported aggressive symptoms. A Dutch study by Hornsveld et al. (2004) found that forensic patients sentenced to Dutch 'TBS[1]' hospitals reported lower aggression and hostility scores than forensic out-patients. On the basis of the criminal, often violent histories of TBS-patients, the opposite would be expected. Out-patients' answers may be more honest given high scores would not lead to longer admission. In some countries, judges decide on the continuation or termination of a sentence. Apart from a lack of insight into one's own behaviour, one problem with aggression self-reports may be that certain subgroups have a strong interest in minimising impulse control problems.

On the other hand, several studies present evidence of the predictive validity of self-reported feelings of anger and aggressiveness, even in forensic psychiatric patient samples. For example, Novaco and Taylor (2004) measured aggressiveness and anger among 129 male forensic patients with intellectual disabilities using modified versions of the Novaco Anger Scale (NAS) (Novaco, 1994) and the Spielberger State-Trait Anger Expression Inventory (STAXI) (Spielberger, 1996). Significant correlations were found between the STAXI 'Trait Anger' and 'Anger Expression' subscales, and hospital physical assaults (correlations of 0.34 and 0.37,

---

[1] In Dutch, TBS stands for 'Ter Beschikking Stelling', which may be translated best as being 'placed at the disposal' of the government in one of the specialised maximum security institutions for forensic psychiatric care, i.e. TBS hospitals.

respectively). The correlation between hospital assaults and the NAS total score was 0.43 (Novaco & Taylor, 2004).

Further, aggression self-report scales are designed to identify tendencies to react in a hostile or angry way. Given this, aggression self-report scales are prone to social desirability bias. They rarely record discrete aggressive incidents and therefore are not designed to provide information on the prevalence of aggressive incidents. For this reason, much of the scientific literature on the prevalence and prevention of aggressive behaviour on psychiatric wards has relied on observation (observer-rated) scales. With observation scales, aggressive behaviour is recorded by staff after the aggressive incident occurrence. In contrast to self-report questionnaires, most observer-rated aggression scales measure discrete incidents. In the next section, several reliable-but easy-to-use-observer-rated scales for recording aggressive incidents of psychiatric inpatients are discussed. These instruments are aligned with the World Health Organization's (WHO) Global Patient Safety Action Plan 2021–2030 (WHO, 2021).

## 7    Assessing the Aggression of Psychiatric Patients with Observation Scales

The most widely used aggression observation scales are either completed retrospectively (e.g. over the last week) or immediately after an incident. They either identify an individual's aggressive behaviour over a specific period of time (without specific frequency information), or they are incident-based reports providing both a count and a snapshot of an incident or event.

'Period-based' aggression observation scales involve rating aggressive behaviour at predetermined times and may be less likely to be forgotten. While period-based assessment has a strength in a group coming to a consensus on severity of incidents of the past week, it also has flaws, in that individuals present for events may be absent from decision-making meetings, resulting in under-reporting. A disadvantage of 'Incident-based' scales is that they may not be easily integrated into ward routines (Sjostrom et al., 2001), particularly when the target behaviour is rare. Thus, the reliability of an incident-based method relies heavily on reporting, and staff under-reporting is problematic particularly with lower severity events, resulting in missing reports of aggressive incidents. This shows the limitations of both kinds of scales—the main issue of under-reporting of aggressive incidents. Period-based aggression observation scales may provide less information about specific circumstances leading to incidents on the ward. Therefore, researchers exploring the effects of potential aggression reducing interventions, should consider using a combination of 'incident-based' and 'period based' aggression observation scales.

A common feature of many aggression observation scales is the presence of predefined answering options, adding to time-efficiency and ease of use. The aggressive event is registered using options that apply to the observed aggressive behaviour. One could argue that easy to use time-efficient scales are more feasible, thus it is more likely that staff will record all incidents encountered regardless of severity. In recent years, some scales may be even more user-friendly due to the availability of digital versions (e.g. apps, electronic medical record integration).

## 7.1 Period-Based Aggression Observation Scales

Period-based observation scales of an individual's aggressive behaviour include:

- The Overt Aggression Scale (OAS) (Silver & Yudofsky, 1991; Yudofsky et al., 1986).
- The Modified version of the OAS (MOAS/MOAS-R) (Kay et al., 1988).
- Social Dysfunction and Aggression Scale (SDAS) (Wistedt et al., 1990).
- Ward Anger Rating Scale (WARS) (Novaco, 1994).

Due to the common use of the OAS and MOAS, these scales will be described in greater detail. The others are mentioned to provide information on available options. The SDAS was developed by Wistedt et al. (1990) to measure the full range of aggression (mild to extremely severe). The scale has nine items identifying outward aggressive behaviours (irritability, dysphoric mood, negativism, social disturbances, directed or nondirected verbal aggressiveness, and physical violence to staff, to things or to others) and two items of inward aggressive behaviour (self-mutilation, suicidal thoughts and impulses). The 11 items are rated on a scale of 0 (not present) to 4 (extremely severe) and the scale has acceptable reliability. The WARS (Novaco, 1994) was developed for staff to rate patient behaviour over the past week and includes 18 items including antagonistic behaviour, verbal and physical aggression, aggression towards self, psychotic symptoms, emotional lability and paranoid attitude. The scale has a second part rating characteristics of anger on a 5-point scale from 'not at all' to 'very often' (Novaco & Taylor, 2004, p. 45).

### 7.1.1 The Overt Aggression Scale (OAS)

Yudofsky et al. (1986) developed the OAS, a 16-item behavioural checklist that identifies four categories of aggression: verbal aggression, physical aggression against objects, physical aggression against self and physical aggression against others. Four descriptors of each behaviour are identified if present (items are ordered by severity). The scale was originally tested within a children's psychiatric service and adult intensive care units. The OAS is described as easy and adaptable for clinical use, and reliable for rating violent incidents. Limitations include a lack of definition of categories, exclusion of certain forms of aggression and the absence of a total weighted score (Jager, 2006). The OAS has, since its origin, developed into several variants including the Retrospective Overt Aggression Scale (ROAS) and Aggression Observation Short Form (AOS) (Bowers, 1999; Hvidhjelm et al., 2014).

### 7.1.2 The Modified Overt Aggression Scale (MOAS)

The MOAS is an aggression observation instrument based on a modification of the OAS using four main categories: verbal aggression, aggression against property, auto-aggression and physical aggression. With added descriptors and scoring for severity, it provides a weighted score (Kay et al., 1988). Each type of aggression is rated from zero (not present) to 4 (most severe) based on the 'most serious' aggressive act in the observation period and requires communication among team members to assure that behaviour over the entire observation period is considered. In order to calculate the overall severity, aggression against property scores are multiplied by a factor of 2, auto-aggression scores by a factor of 3 and physical aggression scores by a factor of 4, and added to the verbal aggression score. The scores of the categories are weighted so that the physical aggression score is the most important in calculating the overall severity. The total MOAS severity scores can theoretically range from zero (no aggression) to 40 (most severe aggression). The interrater reliability of MOAS, based on the total severity scores of two independent raters has been found to be good (Pearson's $r$'s of 0.85 and 0.94; Kay et al., 1988). In a subsequent validation study (Margari et al., 2005), the reliability and validity of the MOAS were found to be high, and the instrument was judged to be suitable for the assessment of aggression based on its psychometric properties.

## 7.2    Incident-Based Aggression Observation Tools

Incident-based reports of an aggressive event include:

- The Staff Observation Aggression Scale (SOAS) (Palmstierna & Wistedt, 1987).
- The revised version of the SOAS (SOAS-R) (Nijman et al., 1999).
- The Report Form for Aggressive Episodes (REFA) (Bjørkly, 1996).
- The Attempted and Actual Assault Scale (ATTACKS) (Bowers et al., 2007a).
- Patient Conflict and Containment–Shift Report (PCC-SR) (Bowers et al., 2007b).
- Patient Safety Incident Reporting Systems (PSiRS) (Kuosmanen et al., 2022).
- NDNQI Database (Press Ganey, 2023; Montalvo, 2007).
- Minimal Information Model for Patient Safety Incident Reporting and Learning Systems (MIM PS) (WHO, 2016).

### 7.2.1    The Staff Observation Aggression Scale-Revised (SOAS/SOAS-R)

The SOAS (Palmstierna & Wistedt, 1987) and a revised version, the SOAS-R (Nijman et al., 1999), aim to measure verbal and physical aggression against objects, patients or staff. The SOAS-R has five columns pertaining to specific aspects of an aggressive incident: the provocation, the means used, the target, the consequences and the measures taken to stop the aggressive incident. By reporting all aspects simultaneously, a broad context of the incident is recorded.

There are no major differences between the SOAS-R and the original SOAS. The principal structure for reporting is not changed in the SOAS-R, nor in other forms of the SOAS/SOAS-R such as the SOAS-RE and SOAS-RA. The difference in the SOAS-R as compared to the SOAS is mainly in the scoring of the reported incident. In the original SOAS design, there was no weighting of the items on the structured report form. Scoring was refined to provide validated weighting of severity, however with further study by Nijman et al., (1999), a Visual Analogue Scale (VAS) scoring of severity was added to the report form. Based on correlations between the VAS-score and the items in the report form, the revised scoring gives heavier weight to the consequences for victims and measures to stop aggression sections. A minor change was introduced in the SOAS-R report form by adding 'injury to self' to the options for the target of aggression.

Every time a staff member witnesses any form of aggression by a service user, an SOAS-R form should be completed. The first column of the SOAS-R, concerning what provoked or triggered the aggression, has been assumed to increase staff members' sensitivity to risk factors in specific patients (Nilsson et al., 1988; De Niet et al., 2005). The SOAS takes staff without training less than 90 s to fill in, compared to time-consuming communication required to complete the MOAS, suggesting an advantage in its feasibility. The adapted version, the SOAS-R,[2] has a validated severity scoring system, which may increase the ability to compare aggression rates between units. The original SOAS severity scoring system had a maximum score of 12 while the revised SOAS-R severity score ranges from 0 to 22 points with higher scores indicating greater severity. The rationale was that severity of aggressive behaviour is dependent on an array of features with some, such as the consequences for victims, more important than others, for example, means used by the aggressive patient, in calculating overall incident severity. With regression techniques, a severity scoring system was developed to weight separate features that make differential contributions to the overall aggression severity score (Nijman et al., 1999).

Studies addressing the concurrent validity of SOAS and SOAS-R severity scores with other measures of aggression severity yielded significant results, with correlations to other methods for assessing the severity of aggressive behaviour ranging from 0.38 to 0.81 (Nijman et al., 2005b). Cross-validation with clinical estimates of severity provided by staff members, who had experienced the aggressive event, indicated that the revised SOAS-R severity scores approximate the general opinion of ward staff of the severity of incidents better than those from the original SOAS (Dias Marques & Cruz Mendes, 2003; Nijman et al., 1999, 2002). A revision of the scale involved empirically testing the scoring system to make it less arbitrary. Furthermore, various studies have demonstrated that the SOAS has fair to good interrater reliability (Palmstierna & Wistedt, 1987), with similar results for the revised version, the SOAS-R (Nijman et al., 1997; Steinert et al., 1999, 2000).

The reliability of all incident-based aggression observation methods relies on the staff completing a form after each aggressive occurrence. Aggression on the SOAS-R is defined as: 'Any verbal, non-verbal, or physical behavior that was threatening (to self, others or property), or physical behavior that actually did harm (to self, others, or property)' (Morrison, 1990, p. 67). Particularly in cases of mild aggressive behaviour, inconsistency between raters could exist on whether or not the observed behaviour needs to be reported. However, none of these studies examined the reliability between raters' decisions about when, or when not, to complete

[2]For more information on the SOAS-R, contact Professor Tom Palmstierna: tom.palmstierna@ki.

an SOAS(-R) form. In addition, the instruction requires that if anyone judges an event worthy of reporting, then the SOAS(-R) should be completed. This is a precaution to prevent under-reporting and assure that no incident will be missed. Instructions for the SOAS (Palmstierna & Wistedt, 1987) direct that if more than one staff member reports the same incident, there is a strategy to handle the event as a single incident, and the highest severity score is recorded.

The SOAS-R exists in several versions adapted to an array of settings, including a geriatric version (Almvik et al., 2006). More recently, the SOAS-R was adapted for use in emergency primary health care, the Staff Observation Scale-Revised Emergency (SOAS-RE) (Morken et al., 2018) and the SOAS-R for paramedics is under development and validation in an ongoing study. Other versions of the SOAS-R include the SOAS-RI (India), the SOAS-R ER (Emergency Rooms) and SOAS-R EC (Elderly Care), they are all examples using the same five aspects of an aggressive event used in the SOAS-structure. The SOAS-R is used to report incidents that the observer defines as aggressive, which is both a strength and flaw. The strength being that defined aspects of an incident are reported on in a structured consistent manner and the flaw being that it measures just one perspective of an aggressive event, namely the observers' perception, without offering perceptions of the aggressor, or other witnesses of the event.

### 7.2.2   Report Form for Aggressive Episodes (REFA)

The REFA[3] is a scale measuring aggressive behaviour towards other persons (Bjørkly, 1996) and was designed to map situations provoking aggressive behaviour in individual patients. Compared to the SOAS-R, the focus of the REFA is on detecting situational triggers of aggression. Based on an interactional approach and situational analysis, aggression is considered a function of triggers in a situation or interaction that increase the risk of behaving aggressively towards others (Bjørkly, 2001); with similarities to behavioural analysis and cognitive therapy in analysing stimulus control factors associated with events (Foreyt & Rathjen, 1978; Marlatt & Gordon, 1985). The REFA depicts factors in the situation that increase a patient's risk for aggression. The REFA has recently been used in the Norwegian SAFE study (Bjørkly et al., 2021), a prospective study of the link between internal and external protective factors and violence prevention during treatment and after discharge from forensic facilities (Bjørkly et al., 2023).

The REFA lists 30 descriptors of aggression triggering situations or interactions grouped by type: physical contact (4 items); limit setting (6 items); problems of communication (3 items); changes/readjustments (6 items); persons (6 items); high-risk contact (2 items); drugs/stimulants (3 items); additional situations or interactions can be identified in a final row. Next to precipitants of aggression, there are columns to record characteristics by type of aggressive episode: to identify verbal or physical threat, and physical assault as well as definitions to operationalise each (Bjørkly, 2000). As with the SOAS-R, the nurse observing the event records the aggressive incident on the form for that patient as soon as possible after the

---

[3] For more information on the REFA, contact Stål Bjørkly: Stal.Bjørkly@hiMolde.no.

aggressive incident occurs; forms are used over an extended period of time to derive accurate descriptions of precipitants to aggression. A difference with the REFA is that at least one other staff member and patients are asked for relevant information on precipitants and characteristics of the actual aggressive incident. Two studies on the interrater reliability of the REFA have been conducted, one involved an acute psychiatric admission ward and a special secure ward for forensic patients (Bjørkly, 2000) and results showed that interrater agreement and reliability were high.

The REFA has been used over many years, strengths include the presence of definitions and operational criteria for aggression, the identification of situational variables and the scale is clinically useful, assisting in planning preventive interventions (Bjørkly, 2000).

## 7.3 The Attempted and Actual Assault Scale: ATTACKS

The ATTACKS was designed exclusively to measure physical violence towards a person in great detail by ward staff witnessing aggression, directly after a violent incident has taken place (Bowers et al., 2007a). One of the earliest tests of the reliability and validity of the ATTACKS (Bowers et al., 2007a) was conducted by means of video recordings of interpersonal assaults, compiled from regular television broadcasts. During a meeting of the European Violence in Psychiatry Research Group (EVIPRG), 22 members from 14 different countries were instructed to rate the assaults on both the MOAS and the ATTACKS. Interrater reliability for the ATTACKS was higher than the MOAS. The raters were also asked to provide their judgements of the severity of the assaults shown on the tape. There was a high correlation between the ATTACKS severity scores and the overall judgement of severity of the assaults. These results indicate that the ATTACKS scale may be a useful addition to scales already available for aggression research. Interestingly, despite the promising psychometric properties of the ATTACKS, no further clinical research using the ATTACKS was identified.

## 7.4 Patient-Staff Conflict Checklist–Shift Report (PCC-SR)

The Patient-staff Conflict Checklist–Shift Report (PCC-SR) is a shift report scale that identifies the rate of conflict events and containment interventions within a mental health unit (Bowers et al., 2003, 2007b). The report is completed by the nurse in charge, who records all the conflict and containment events from the shift for the entire unit. The form consists of a series of conflict events (i.e. verbal aggression, physical aggression, self-harm, refusing hygiene or meals, medication refusal) and containment interventions that may occur (i.e. use of medication, increased observation, time out, seclusion, restraint), and information on ward security (locked or open door), admissions, and number of staff on duty on one shift. The PCC-SR was developed from the Patient-staff Conflict Checklist (PCC) which is a simple checklist designed to provide count of a patient's aggressive events after inpatient admission; the events on the checklist are based on aggressive items in the OAS (Bowers et al., 2003).

Rates of aggressive events can be identified from the PCC-SR given that the report provides the frequency of each event during a particular shift. However, the measure has not been fully validated to determine its performance as a scale. While the report allows for identification of an average number of events per shift over a set period of time, it does not offer information about incidents nor event characteristics, involvement of individual patients or worker exposure. The PCC-SR was used in the City 128 Study (Bowers et al., 2007b) to provide mean daily rates of conflict and containment events for the acute psychiatric units in the study. The PCC-SR offers a way to compare event rates across units and evaluate factors associated with higher or lower levels of conflict and containment (Bowers et al., 2013).

## 8    Incident Reporting Systems (IRSs)

Incident reporting systems (IRSs) or Patient Safety Incident Reporting Systems (PSiRS) are used by healthcare organisations to report incidents, often digitally, on electronic databases within hospital systems (Arnetz et al., 2011; Kuosmanen et al., 2022; NRI, 2013a; Reilly et al., 2019; Stavropoulou et al., 2015). These tools are designed for patient safety use and to identify issues such as medical errors, close calls, and actual and potential patient harm for organisational improvement and learning. Some systems include specific workplace violence incident reporting that require employees to report all incidents, whether or not an injury is involved (Arnetz et al., 2015). PSiRS is one reporting system that consists of events such as verbal and physical assault, self-harm incidents, and can be used as a registration tool to measuring violence and aggression within healthcare settings. The National Database of Nursing Quality Indicators (NDNQI) was originally developed by the American Nurses Association (Montalvo, 2007), and now available from Press Ganey (2023); the NDNQI provides settings unit level measures to benchmark performance for comparison to competitors (Madaris & Potter, 2023).

## 8.1    The Minimal Information Model for Patient Safety Incident Reporting and Learning System (MIM PS)

A new tool, the Minimal Information Model for Patient Safety Incident Reporting and Learning System (MIM PS), was developed by the WHO to address reporting issues related to adverse events (WHO, 2020). The purpose of the MIM PS is to provide a list of information categories to include when reporting adverse events, providing a templated incident reporting system that includes important details such as contributing and mitigating factors, outcomes, and resulting actions (WHO, 2016). The MIM PS was compared to existing reporting and learning systems across the world using a stepwise approach, and the European validation of the MIM PS was part of an EU-WHO collaborative project. Further study of this reporting system is needed as it is implemented in additional settings worldwide (WHO, 2020).

## 8.2    The Prevalence of Inpatient Aggression

Identification of the prevalence of aggression by psychiatric patients is affected by aggression measurement methods, leading to identification of varying rates. Scales differ in their ability to report single versus multiple events and their characteristics. Reports of incidents combined with information about the number of patients and period of time offer the ability to provide an aggression rate or frequency (prevalence) that can be used to compare rates across settings. Aggression measurement scales are more commonly used on inpatient units, compared to outpatient or community settings. Most settings have incident reporting methods to assure patient and workplace safety. Despite this many incidents are not reported, resulting in underestimates of the prevalence of aggression (Arnetz et al., 2015; Arnetz, 2022). It is crucial to carefully consider the measurement methods when comparing rates. This section briefly summarises the evidence on the prevalence of aggression.

The prevalence of aggressive behaviour in psychiatric populations is an important issue that has been explored in numerous studies. It is worth noting that relying solely on hospitalised samples may result in an overestimation of aggressive behaviour within the overall psychiatric population (Asaoka et al., 2021). This overestimation can be attributed to the fact that violence is a significant factor considered in the selection of individuals for psychiatric hospitalisation (Weltens et al., 2021). Consequently, the frequency of aggressive acts among psychiatric inpatients is expected to be higher compared to community samples. Furthermore, empirical data has provided convincing preliminary evidence of an association between mental illness and community violence among psychiatric outpatients (Wasserman et al., 2020). Reviews on aggressive behaviour prevalence among psychiatric patients indicate hospitalised psychiatric patients have engaged in violence prior to admission (Pelto-Piri et al., 2020; Salzmann-Erikson & Yifter, 2020). Other issues that may play a role in this association include service reductions due to costs, ever increasing documentation requirements, difficulties in communication-related ineffective use of or ineffective electronic records, as well as the coercive environment present in psychiatric settings that may result in disruptive behaviour. These findings contribute to our understanding of the relationship between psychiatric populations and aggressive behaviour.

A systematic review of studies focusing on inpatient psychiatric wards, (Weltens et al., 2021) found wide ranging prevalence of aggressive behaviour, from 8% to 76%, with an average prevalence of 54%, and the highest levels occurring within the first week of admission. In addition, prior aggression predicted a 34% higher risk of subsequent aggression. A history of aggression increased aggression risk from 45% to 7.25 times higher than those without a history of aggression (Weltens et al., 2021). Similarly, Stewart and Bowers (2013) found prior history of violence predicted from 1.97 to 5.43 times the risk of various forms of verbal abuse (shouting (1.97), threats (4.20), racism (5.43), anger (3.04)) during admission, particularly during the initial weeks of admission. Chou et al. (2002) found that 77% of those who were assaultive during admission had a prior history of assault and this history significantly predicted assaultive behaviour. However, it must also be noted that some studies have not found an association between history of violence and subsequent aggression during an inpatient admission (Weltens et al., 2021, p. 9), suggesting that other factors may play a role in this result.

Using the National Database of Nursing Quality Indicators (NDNQI) database, a national US nursing database of outcome indicators, Staggs (2015) found an overall assault rate among hospitalised psychiatric patients of 9.1 per 10,000 patient days. Further injurious assault rates varied by population: adults 7.4/10,000; geriatric 13.3/10,000; and child/adolescent 17.17/10,000 patient days. Most injurious assaults resulted in minor (80.3%) compared to serious (1.9%) injuries. Staggs found prevalence of assault rates did not significantly change over the years (2007–2013) by unit or type.

In addition to rate differences by population served, rates vary internationally. Rates identified in Australia find the pooled incidence of violent patients presenting to emergency departments is 36 per 10,000 patient presentations (Lau et al., 2004). While in South Africa a rate of 3.8 patient-to-patient assaults per month and 1.3 patient-to-staff assaults per month were identified in an acute inpatient psychiatric unit (Luckhoff et al., 2013).

A study of long-term care (older adult) residents in Canada (Berry et al., 2017) found that 8.5% had at least one report of an aggressive event, and patterns show that all had impaired cognition, and most had only one ($n = 10$) or two ($n = 17$) events reported via incident report, while 7 had more than ten aggressive incidents reported ($n = 126$ incidents, p. 419). Many studies replicate the finding that a small number of individuals are often responsible for a large number of events. Chieze et al. (2021) found 16.4% of geriatric psychiatry patients in a hospital in Switzerland experienced at least one coercive measure during hospitalisation.

Rates of coercive interventions are often used as a proxy for rates of aggression with studies available from several countries internationally, offering a comparison of rates of interventions used to manage aggressive events, sometimes considered. For example, Steinert et al. (2010) reviewed the use of seclusion and restraint in different countries, finding that seclusion was used in from 0% to 15.6% of patient admissions, physical restraint was used in 2.5% to 7.3%, and mechanical restraint in 1.2% to 35.6% of admissions (pp. 893–894). This reflects that some countries rarely or never use seclusion. In Germany, a recent study of four hospitals (Mann et al., 2021) found a prevalence of 8% of patients experienced coercive measures although prevalence varied by hospital, ranging from 5.2% to 11.7% (p. 4). Välimäki et al. (2019) found the overall prevalence of use of coercive interventions was 9.8% over a 20-year period in Finland, prevalence of seclusion was 6.9% and physical restraint was 0.8% (p. 5). Miodownik et al. (2019) found that 31.3% of patients in 2014 (176 of 563 admissions) were restrained or secluded while hospitalised in an acute psychiatric unit in Israel. In the United States, from 2.16% to 2.71% of state hospital clients were secluded, while 4.62% to 6.12% were restrained over a 3.5-year period (2010–2013) (NRI, 2013a, 2013b).

Recording discrete incidents separately, immediately after they occur, has advantages for prevention of aggression in inpatient facilities. For example, the information provides the opportunity to investigate the specific circumstances and times that are connected to violent events (Nijman et al., 1997). The registration of aggressive behaviour directly after each incident may offer more insight into aggression-eliciting factors (Nilsson et al., 1988; De Niet et al., 2005). Mistler and Friedman (2022) conducted a review on observation scales, identifying 74 studies of which 74% used structured tools to measure aggression and violence on inpatient psychiatric services. It concluded that the instrument and tools identified were primarily versions of the Overt Aggression Scale (OAS), all found to be valid and reliable and easy to use in clinical practice. However, the review is limited to studies from the last 10 years (June 2008–2018) and may not offer a full picture given that many tools were developed between 1986 and 2007. Over time the SOAS-R has been used in multiple settings and offered rates of incidents over time, offering a historical perspective on rates. In addition, the use of the SOAS-R continues to evolve and be used in new settings. Reporting of SOAS or SOAS-R results (Nijman et al., 2005b) offers an opportunity to compare aggression frequencies across countries and types of units. A review of the reported SOAS-R frequencies (*n* = 54 separate observations; Nijman et al., 2005b) yielded a median value of a little under eight incidents per psychiatric patient per year. However, the reported annual number of SOAS(-R) incidents per psychiatric patient varied considerably across studies from as low as 0.4 to as high as 59.9 incidents per year, depending on the type of unit and the country involved. Rates from different settings and historical context from different time periods will be reviewed. The rate of SOAS-R incidents per patient on acute adult admission units (*n* = 38 separate observations), a mean of 9.3 incidents per bed, per year, was found (Nijman et al., 2005b). A more recent study using the SOAS-R found a rate of 13.3 incidents per bed, per year, and 7.1% of assaults required medical treatment (Iennaco et al., 2017). These rates are higher although it was found in the United States where inpatient stays range from 7 to 10 days, resulting in higher patient acuity. Several studies on aggression in psychogeriatric samples, conducted in Sweden and the UK, reported a high prevalence of aggression (more than 15 incidents per patient, per year, with a maximum of 59.9), but there is some indication that the severity of the incidents, in terms of physical consequences, on average is low on such wards. In general, the proportion of incidents leading to physical consequences, for example, pain, bruises and welts, ranges from 10% to 20% of the total number of SOAS-R assessments (Nijman et al., 2005b). Severe assaults for which victims required somatic treatment, constituted about 1–5% of all SOAS-R reports.

High SOAS-R frequencies of incidents were found on units caring for high-risk patients, for example, 29.2 and 40.2 in violent patients with schizophrenia in Finland, and 31.2 in young, high-risk, involuntary Dutch patients. With the REFA, Bjørkly (1999) found high aggression rates on specialised wards, such as a 19-bed Norwegian secure unit for dangerous psychotic patients. Rates of aggression per patient, per year, were: 25.9 (total aggressive episodes), 13.5 (verbal threats), 6.5 (physical threats) and 5.9 (physical assaults). Four patients accounted for 77% of the aggressive episodes that occurred. Interestingly, a comparison between rates of aggression in the first 5-year period and in the last 5-year period yielded a 60% reduction over the study period (Bjørkly, 1999).

Several SOAS-R studies also reported reductions in aggression reports over time that may be due to under-reporting. Nilsson et al. (1988) speculated that the 'reduction phenomenon' could be: 'Caused by a learning process from the ordinary nursing staff, who during a study of this kind are forced to systematize their observation of their patients' (p. 174). Alternatively, the 'spontaneous' decrease of the registration of incidents over time could have something to do with changes in the way aggression observation scales are completed as time progresses (De Niet et al., 2005; Shah, 1999; Sival et al., 2000).

The evidence from the SOAS-R review (Nijman et al., 2005b) carefully suggested there may be differences in the prevalence rates in various European countries and beyond. The mean number of incidents per patient, per year, from Dutch acute admission wards, for instance, was high when compared to the mean number of incidents from other countries, for example, the UK, Germany, Norway and Denmark (Nijman et al., 2005b), but the relatively low number of studies per country does not allow us to draw very firm conclusions on this finding that the availability of standardised aggression report forms is likely to improve the comparability of aggression frequencies between units, hospitals and countries. Cross-national differences may emerge when aggression frequencies are compared on a larger scale.

## 9      Innovative Measurement Methods

Aggression observation instruments may avoid many problems that arise from a lack of insight or social desirability bias. Staff themselves are also part of the interaction that leads to aggressive incidents on psychiatric wards, impacting rating objectivity (Whittington & Wykes, 1996). Models for reducing violence and coercion in mental health settings have included the key elements of the relationship between patient and staff and the environment of care as vital to improving clinical outcomes. The inclusion of these factors in measurement methods is important to fully describing the phenomenon of aggression in clinical settings (Huckshorn, 2006; Bowers et al., 2015; Duxbury et al., 2019).

One way to avoid the subjective nature of measuring aggression is to use video to record aggression-related activity as a basis for measurement of events. An early report of use of video involved review of video recordings from a mental health setting and rating of conflicts by individuals not involved in the situation (Crowner et al., 1994). Nolan and Volavka (2006) used video to better understand aggression in psychiatric patients, finding that from 20% to 40% of aggressive events (depending on level of review of tapes) were not reported. Recently use of wearable cameras has become common in some settings (law enforcement), but it has not been embraced in healthcare settings. A recent systematic review of the use of body worn cameras (Wilson et al., 2022) found only eight studies of use in healthcare, the settings included emergency medical services (5), inpatient mental health (2) and home care (1). In the emergency and home care settings, the purpose was to aid in virtual assessment and documentation. The purpose in the mental health studies was to determine the feasibility of use of body worn cameras and the studies did not involve use as an objective measure of aggression incidence, however, use in these settings was similar to the use in law enforcement: to document and deter aggressive incidents although even in law enforcement settings there is no clear evidence supporting use in reducing aggression (Wilson et al., 2022). A recent qualitative study involving mental health staff and patients on body worn cameras identified the ethical concern that wearing a camera exacerbates power dynamics and impacts therapeutic engagement and raised concerns about mistrust in mental health settings causing staff and patients to feel unsafe (Wilson et al., 2023). A difficulty in use for incident reporting is that video evaluation and interpretation is very labour intensive and may lack feasibility as well as raise concerns that surveillance adds an element of coercive control to the psychiatric environment. Due to practical and ethical problems, this approach to aggression measurement is not currently in use in clinical practice.

Other approaches to observe aggression of psychiatric patients include the use of actigraphy, handheld counters and 'wearable' technology to record incidents. For example, Lanza et al. (2009) used handheld counters to indicate an aggressive incident in real time, providing a count of verbal as well as physical aggression events, with identification of event characteristics later in the shift. A similar approach was used in a measurement study comparing multiple measures, including scales (SOAS-R, PCC-SR), restraint event reporting and incident reporting, to the use of handheld counters by staff to record 'in the moment observations' of verbal and physical aggression, with subsequent documentation of event characteristics on a counter log, providing both patient incident as well as worker exposure information (Iennaco et al., 2013). A subsequent study measuring patient aggression and worker exposure in the inpatient medical setting replicated the use of handheld counters with a log to record event characteristics (Iennaco et al., 2023). Recently, de Looff et al. (2019a) had staff use a wearable watch to 'time stamp' observation of aggressive events with later documentation of information on the nature and severity of the event using the MOAS+. One strength of noting an incident in real time is the likelihood of recording all incidents that occur in a setting, minimising the problem of under-reporting. Use of measures of skin conductance and heart rate with actigraphy or 'wearable' technology to detect changes in physiologic measures has also been investigated (Kuijpers et al., 2012; de Looff et al., 2019a), showing physiologic reactivity approximately 20 min prior to incidents of aggression. Further study of wearable technology is underway and may offer insight into physiological patterns associated with aggressive behaviour, 'just in time' preventive interventions, as well as the actual exposure and impact of workplace violence if used with workers (de Looff et al., 2019a, 2019b).

## 10  Conclusion

The measurement of aggression and violence is an important activity that can promote efforts to improve the safety and quality of patient care in a variety of settings. This chapter begins with the importance of having a common definition to study aggression and violence, discussing principles to consider in measuring aggression, as well as offering a snapshot of aggression and violence rates in psychiatric and other settings from both the perspective of worker violence exposure and later the prevalence of patient aggression. There are differences in both worker exposure and patient aggressive behaviour prevalence internationally. The chapter also provides a basis for understanding different types of measures (patient events, worker exposure, coercive intervention, preventive intervention) and highlights use of measurement tools including strengths and limitations to consider. The concept of using an incident management reporting system to track and compare aggression and violence rates is also introduced. Accurate data collection provides the foundation for predicting events and tracking the effectiveness of workplace violence interventions. Better measurement across the continuum of aggression severity provides information on preventive interventions that de-escalate aggression prior to use of coercive intervention or acts of severe consequence such as patient or worker injury.

We lack measures of worker exposure which currently range from retrospective surveys asking about past week, month, year or career-long exposure, to the use of handheld or wearable devices to immediately identify event exposure. However, most often settings identify worker exposure using injury events, which grossly underestimate individual worker exposure.

A review of a multitude of tools to measure patient aggression is offered that might be used depending on specific clinical and workplace needs, some of which have been used in multiple settings including inpatient medical units, emergency departments, as well as community-based care. There is no 'perfect' tool for use. Some of the more commonly used tools include the SOAS-R and the MOAS to record characteristics related to aggressive incidents and aggressive behaviour. The use of carefully studied and validated tools provides information to base interventions to prevent aggressive behaviour as well as reduce the use of coercive intervention in clinical settings. Some settings already collect information to monitor and prevent aggressive behaviour and worker injury as well as to inform plans of care to better understand and prevent repeated events in violent patients.

Looking to the future, technology and artificial intelligence may offer the field of aggression improved measurement methods. Current studies of measures using 'wearable' technology or in the moment recording of events may provide unique information about both patient and worker behaviour, physiologic responses and the impact of both worker exposure and preventive interventions that may benefit both patients and workers. Measurement tools, combined with predictive tools offer data-driven approaches to identify those at greatest risk of aggressive behaviour, to better intervene based on individual, staff and unit characteristics, to determine the benefit of training or other interventions implemented and plan for patient and worker safety measures to reduce aggressive events, coercive intervention, injuries and the costs and consequences associated with violence in clinical settings.

# References

Adebayo, O., Ugorji, J., Ekeh, A., Jolade, E., Odoh, N., Ikeme, A., Azoroh, N., Aloba, O., & Ogiehor-Enoma, G. (2022). The impact of workplace violence on nurses and nursing practice: A literature review. *International Journal of Science and Research Archive, 5*(1), 51–58.

Ahmed, A. S. (2012). Verbal and physical abuse against Jordanian nurses in the work environment. *Eastern Mediterranean Health Journal, 18*(4), 318–324. https://doi.org/10.26719/2012.18.4.318

Albadry, A. A., El-Gilany, A. H., & Abou-ElWafa, H. S. (2020). Workplace violence against security personnel at a university hospital in Egypt: A cross-sectional study. *F1000Research, 9*, 347. https://doi.org/10.12688/f1000research.23252.1

Aljohani, B., Burkholder, J., Tran, Q. K., Chen, C., Beisenova, K., & Pourmand, A. (2021). Workplace violence in the emergency department: A systematic review and meta-analysis. *Public Health, 196*, 186–197. https://doi.org/10.1016/j.puhe.2021.02.009

Almvik, R., Rasmussen, K., & Woods, P. (2006). Challenging behavior in the elderly—Monitoring violent incidents. *International Journal of Geriatric Psychiatry, 21*, 368–374. https://doi.org/10.1002/gps.1474

Arnetz, J. E. (2022). The Joint Commission's new and revised workplace violence prevention standards for hospitals: A major step forward toward improved quality and safety. *Joint Commission Journal on Quality and Patient Safety, 48*(4), 241–245.

Arnetz, J. E., Aranyos, D., Ager, J., & Upfal, M. J. (2011). Development and application of a population-based system for workplace violence surveillance in hospitals. *American Journal of Industrial Medicine, 54*, 925–934. https://doi.org/10.1002/ajim.20984

Arnetz, J. E., Hamblin, L., Ager, J., Luborsky, M., Upfal, M. J., Russell, J., & Essenmacher, L. (2015). Underreporting of workplace violence: Comparison of self-report and actual documentation of hospital incidents. *Workplace Health & Safety, 63*(5), 200–210. https://doi.org/10.1177/2165079915574684

Asaoka, Y., Won, M., Morita, T., Ishikawa, E., & Goto, Y. (2021). Comparable level of aggression between patients with behavioural addiction and healthy subjects. *Translational Psychiatry, 11*(1), 375.

Babiarczyk, B., Turbiarz, A., Tomagová, M., Zeleníková, R., Önler, E., & Sancho Cantus, D. (2019). Violence against nurses working in the health sector in five European countries—Pilot study. *International Journal of Nursing Practice, 25*(4), e12744. https://doi.org/10.1111/ijn.12744

Babiarczyk, B., Turbiarz, A., Tomagová, M., Zeleníková, R., Önler, E., & Cantus, D. S. (2020). Reporting of workplace violence towards nurses in 5 European countries—A cross-sectional study. *International Journal of Occupational Medicine and Environmental Health, 33*(3), 325–338. https://doi.org/10.13075/IJOMEH.1896.01475

Bae, S. H. (2022). Noneconomic and economic impacts of nurse turnover in hospitals: A systematic review. *International Nursing Review, 69*, 392–404.

Bech, P. (1994). Measurement by observations of aggressive behavior and activities in clinical situations. *Criminal Behaviour and Mental Health, 4*, 290–302.

Berry, B., Young, L., & Kim, S. C. (2017). Utility of the aggressive behavior risk assessment tool in long-term care homes. *Geriatric Nursing, 38*, 417–422.

Bjørkly, S. (1995). Prediction of aggression in psychiatric patients. A review of prospective prediction studies. *Clinical Psychology Review, 15*, 475–502.

Bjørkly, S. (1996). Report form for aggressive episodes: Preliminary report. *Perceptual and Motor Skills, 83*, 1139–1152. Retrieved from https://journals.sagepub.com/doi/epdf/10.2466/pms.1996.83.3f.1139

Bjørkly, S. (1999). A ten-year prospective study of aggression in a special secure unit for dangerous patients. *Scandinavian Journal of Psychology, 40*, 57–65.

Bjørkly, S. (2000). The inter rater reliability of the report form for aggressive episodes. *Journal of Family Violence, 15*, 269–279.

Bjørkly, S. (2001). The Report Form for Aggressive Episodes (REFA) in the treatment of violent psychotic patients. In M. Martinez (Ed.), *Prevention and control of aggression and the impact on its victims* (pp. 95–100). Springer Science + Business Media.

Bjørkly, S., Laake, P., Roaldset, J. O., & Douglas, K. S. (2021). The safe pilot study: A prospective naturalistic study with repeated measures design to test the psychosis—Violence link in and after discharge from forensic facilities. *Psychiatry Research, 298*, 113793. https://doi.org/10.1016/j.psychres.2021.113793

Bjørkly, S., Laake, P., & Douglas, K. S. (2023). The safe pilot study: A prospective naturalistic study with repeated measures design to test protective factors against violence in and after discharge from forensic facilities. *Psychiatry Research, 320*, 115017.

Bowers, L. (1999). A critical appraisal of violent incident measures. *Journal of Mental Health, 8*, 335–345.

Bowers, L., Simpson, A., & Alexander, J. (2003). Patient-staff conflict: Results of a survey on acute psychiatric wards. *Social Psychiatry and Psychiatric Epidemiology, 38*, 402–408. https://doi.org/10.1007/s00127-003-0648-x

Bowers, L., Nijman, H., & Palmstiema, T. (2007a). The Attempted and Actual Assault Scale (Attacks). *The International Journal of Methods in Psychiatric Research, 16*, 171–176. https://doi.org/10.1002/mpr.219

Bowers, L., Whittington, R., Nolan, P. Parkin, D., Curtis, S., Bhui, K., Hackney, D., Allan, T., Simpson, A., & Flood, C. (2007b). *The City 128 study of observation and outcomes on acute psychiatric wards.* Report to the NHS SDO Programme, Issue. N. S. Programme.

Bowers, L., Stewart, D., Papadopoulos, C., & Iennaco, J. D. (2013). Correlation between levels of conflict and containment on acute psychiatric wards: The City-128 study. *Psychiatric Services, 64*(5), 423–430.

Bowers, L., James, K., Quirk, A., Simpson, A., Stewart, D., & Hodsoll, J. (2015). Reducing conflict and containment rates on acute psychiatric wards: The safewards cluster randomised controlled trial. *International Journal of Nursing Studies, 52*(9), 1412–1422. https://doi.org/10.1016/j.ijnurstu.2015.05.001

Buss, A. H., & Durkee, A. (1957). An inventory for assessing different kinds of hostility. *Journal of Consulting Psychology, 21*, 343–349.

Buss, A. H., & Perry, M. (1992). The aggression questionnaire. *Journal of Personality and Social Psychology, 63*, 452–459.

Camerino, D., Estryn-Behar, M., Conway, P. M., van Der Heijden, B. I. J. M., & Hasselhorn, H.-M. (2008). Work-related factors and violence among nursing staff in the European NEXT study: A longitudinal cohort study. *International Journal of Nursing Studies, 45*(1), 35–50. https://doi.org/10.1016/j.ijnurstu.2007.01.013

Center for Disease Control. (2020). *Types of workplace violence. Unit 1: Definitions, types, and prevalence.* Retrieved March 30, 2023, from https://wwwn.cdc.gov/WPVHC/Nurses/Course/Slide/Unit1_5

Chen, W. C., Hwu, H. G., Kung, S. M., Chiu, H. J., & Wang, J. D. (2008). Prevalence and determinants of workplace violence of health care workers in a psychiatric hospital in Taiwan. *Journal of Occupational Health, 50*(3), 288–293.

Chieze, M., Kaiser, S., Courvoisier, D., Hurst, S., Sentissi, O., Fredouille, J., & Wullschleger, A. (2021). Prevalence and risk factors for seclusion and restraint in old-age psychiatry inpatient units. *BMC Psychiatry, 21*(1), 82. https://doi.org/10.1186/s12888-021-03095-4

Chou, K.-R., Lu, R.-B., & Mao, W.-C. (2002). Factors relevant to patient assaultive behavior and assault in acute inpatient psychiatric units in Taiwan. *Archives of Psychiatric Nursing, 16*(4), 187–195. https://doi.org/10.1053/apnu.2002.34394

Crowner, M. L., Stepcic, F., Perie, G., & Czobor, P. (1994). Typology of patient-patient assaults detected by video cameras. *American Journal of Psychiatry, 151*, 1669–1672.

de Bles, N. J., Hazewinkel, A. W. P., Bogers, J., van den Hout, W. B., Mouton, C., van Hemert, A. M., Ottenheim, N. R., & Giltay, E. J. (2021). The incidence and economic impact of aggression in closed long-stay psychiatric wards. *International Journal of Psychiatry in Clinical Practice, 25*(4), 430–436. https://doi.org/10.1080/13651501.2020.1821894

de Looff, P., Noordzij, M. L., Moerbeek, M., Nijman, H., Didden, R., & Embregts, P. (2019a). Changes in heart rate and skin conductance in the 30 min preceding aggressive behavior. *Psychophysiology, 56*(10), e13420. https://doi.org/10.1111/psyp.13420

de Looff, P., Didden, R., Embregts, P., & Nijman, H. (2019b). Burnout symptoms in forensic mental health nurses: Results from a longitudinal study. *International Journal of Mental Health Nursing, 28*, 306–317. https://doi.org/10.1111/inm.12536

De Niet, G. J., Hutschemaekers, G. J. M., & Lendemeijer, B. H. H. G. (2005). Is the reducing effect of the Staff Observation Aggression Scale owing to a learning effect? An explorative study. *Journal of Psychiatric and Mental Health Nursing, 12*, 687–694.

Dias Marques, M. I., & Cruz Mendes, A. (2003). Violence in psychiatry: An exploratory study in the Coimbra Psychiatric Services. In *European violence in psychiatry research group dissemination project. Report to the European Commission on behalf of the EV/PRC (EVIPACOM, QLAM-2000-00011)*. City University.

Duxbury, J., Baker, J., Downe, S., Jones, F., Greenwood, P., Thygesen, H., et al. (2019). Minimising the use of physical restraint in acute mental health services: The outcome of a restraint reduction programme ('REsTRAIN YOURSELF'). *International Journal of Nursing Studies, 95*, 40–48.

European Council of Medical Orders (CEOM) (2017) *CEOM actions: The European Observatory on Violence against Doctors*. Retrieved March 29, 2023, from https://www.ceom-ecmo.eu/en/ceom-actions-1570

Flood, C., Bowers, L., & Parkin, D. (2008). Estimating the costs of conflict and containment on adult acute inpatient psychiatric wards. *Nursing Economic, 26*, 325–330, 324.

Foreyt, J. P., & Rathjen, D. (1978). *Cognitive behavior therapy—Research and application*. Plenum Press.

Gerberich, S. G., Church, T. R., McGovern, P. M., Hansen, H. E., Nachreiner, N. M., Geisser, M. S., Ryan, A. D., Mongin, S. J., & Watt, G. D. (2004). An epidemiological study of the magnitude and consequences of work related violence: The Minnesota Nurses' Study. *Occupational and Environmental Medicine, 61*(6), 495–503. https://doi.org/10.1136/oem.2003.007294

Girasek, H., Nagy, V. A., Fekete, S., Ungvari, G. S., & Gazdag, G. (2022). Prevalence and correlates of aggressive behavior in psychiatric inpatient populations. *World Journal of Psychiatry, 12*(1), 1–23. https://doi.org/10.5498/wjp.v12.i1.1

H.R.2663—118th Congress. (April 18, 2023–2024). *Workplace Violence Prevention for Health Care and Social Service Workers Act*. Retrieved January 31, 2024, from https://www.congress.gov/bill/118th-congress/house-bill/2663

Hanson, L. L. M., Pentti, J., Nordentoft, T., Xu, T., Rugulie, R., Madsen, I. E. H., Conway, P. M., Westerlund, H., Vahtera, J., Ervasti, J., Batty, D., & Kivimäki, M. (2023). Association of workplace violence and bullying with later suicide risk: A multicohort study and meta-analysis of published data. *The Lancet Public Health, 2023*(8), e494–e503.

Havaei, F., MacPhee, M., & Ma, A. (2020). Workplace violence among British Columbia Nurses Across Different Roles and Contexts. *Healthcare (Basel, Switzerland), 8*(2), 98. https://doi.org/10.3390/healthcare8020098

Hawkins, D., & El Ghaziri, M. (2022). Violence in health care: Trends and disparities, Bureau of Labor Statistics Survey Data of Occupational Injuries and Illnesses, 2011-2017. *Workplace Health & Safety, 70*(3), 136–147. https://doi.org/10.1177/21650799221079045

Hornsveld, R. H. J., van Dam-Baggen, C. M. J., Lammers, S. M. M., Nijman, H. L. I., & Kraaimaat, F. W. (2004). Forensische patienten met geweldsdelicten: Persoonlijkheidskenmerken en gedrag. *Tijdschrift voor Psychiatrie, 46*, 133–143.

Howard, J. (1996). State and local regulatory approaches to preventing workplace violence. *Occupational Medicine, 11*(2), 293–301.

Huckshorn, K. A. (2006). Re-designing state mental health policy to prevent the use of seclusion and restraint. *Administration and Policy in Mental Health, 33*(4), 482–491.

Hunter, M., & Carmel, H. (1992). The cost of staff injuries from inpatient violence. *Hospital and Community Psychiatry, 43*, 586–588.

Hvidhjelm, J., Sestoft, D., & Bjørner, J. B. (2014). The aggression observation short form identified episodes not reported on the Staff Observation Aggression Scale-Revised. *Issues in Mental Health Nursing, 35*(6), 464–469. https://doi.org/10.3109/01612840.2013.879359

Iennaco, J., Dixon, J., Whittemore, R., & Bowers, L. (2013). Measurement and monitoring of health care worker aggression exposure. *The Online Journal of Issues in Nursing, 18*(1), Man03. https://doi.org/10.3912/OJIN.Vol18No01Man03

Iennaco, J. D., Whittemore, R., & Dixon, J. (2017). Aggressive event incidence using the Staff Observation of Aggression Scale-Revised (SOAS-R): A longitudinal study. *Psychiatric Quarterly, 88*, 485–499.

Iennaco, J. D., Molle, E., Allegra, M., Depukat, D., & Parkosewich, J. (2023). The Aggressive Incidents in Medical Settings (AIMS) study. *Joint Commission Journal on Quality and Patient Safety, 50*, 166. https://doi.org/10.1016/j.jcjq.2023.11.005

Jager, A. D. (2006). An instrument to measure violence. *CES Medicina, 20*(2), 7–18. Retrieved from https://www.redalyc.org/pdf/2611/261120979002.pdf

Kay, S. R., Wolkenfield, F., & Murril, L. (1988). Profiles of aggression among psychiatric patients. I: Nature and prevalence. *The Journal of Nervous and Mental Disease, 176*, 539–546.

Krug, E. G., Mercy, J. A., Dahlberg, L. L., & Zwi, A. B. (2002). The world report on violence and health. *Lancet, 360*(9339), 1083–1088. https://doi.org/10.1016/S0140-6736(02)11133-0

Kuijpers, E., Nijman, H., Bongers, I. M. B., Lubberding, M., & Ouwerkerk, M. (2012). Can mobile skin conductance assessments be helpful in signalling imminent inpatient aggression? *Acta Neuropsychiatrica, 24*(1), 56–59. https://doi.org/10.1111/j.1601-5215.2011.00582.x

Kuosmanen, A., Tiihonen, J., Repo-Tiihonen, E., & Turunen, H. (2022). Voluntary patient safety incidents reporting in forensic psychiatry—What do the reports tell us? *Journal of Psychiatric and Mental Health Nursing, 29*(1), 36–47.

Lambert, K., Chu, S., Duffy, C., Hartley, V., Baker, A., & Ireland, J. L. (2018). The prevalence of constant supportive observations in high, medium and low secure services. *British Journal of Psychiatry Bulletin, 42*, 54–58.

Lanctôt, N., & Guay, S. (2014). The aftermath of workplace violence among healthcare workers: A systematic literature review of the consequences. *Aggression and Violent Behavior, 19*, 492–501. https://doi.org/10.1016/j.avb.2014.07.010

Lanza, M. L., & Milner, J. (1989). The dollar cost of patient assault. *Hospital and Community Psychiatry, 40*, 1227–1229.

Lanza, M. L., Rierdan, J., Forester, L., & Zeiss, R. A. (2009). Reducing violence against nurses: The violence prevention community meeting. *Issues in Mental Health Nursing, 30*(12), 745–750. https://doi.org/10.3109/01612840903177472

Lau, J. B., Magarey, J., & McCutcheon, H. (2004). Violence in the emergency department: A literature review. *Australian Emergency Nursing Journal, 7*, 27–37.

Li, Y., & Jones, C. B. (2013). A literature review of nursing turnover costs. *Journal of Nursing Management, 21*, 405–418. https://doi.org/10.1111/j.1365-2834.2012.01411.x

Li, Y.-L., Li, R.-Q., Qiu, D., & Xiao, S.-Y. (2020). Prevalence of workplace physical violence against health care professionals by patients and visitors: A systematic review and meta-analysis. *International Journal of Environmental Research and Public Health, 17*, 299. https://doi.org/10.3390/ijerph17010299

Liu, J., Gan, Y., Jiang, H., Li, L., Dwyer, R., Lu, K., Yan, S., Sampson, O., Xu, H., Wang, C., & Zhu, Y. (2019). Prevalence of workplace violence against healthcare workers: A systematic review and meta-analysis. *Occupational and Environmental Medicine, 76*(12), 927–937.

Luckhoff, M., Jordaan, E., Swart, Y., Cloete, K. J., Koen, L., & Niehaus, D. J. (2013). Retrospective review of trends in assaults and seclusion at an acute psychiatric ward over a 5-year period. *Journal of Psychiatric and Mental Health Nursing, 20*(8), 687–695. https://doi.org/10.1111/jpm.12006

Madaris, S., & Potter, C. (2023). Your comprehensive guide to the Press Ganey National Database of Nursing Quality Indicators (NDNQI). *Healthcare experience insights*. Retrieved from https://info.pressganey.com/press-ganey-blog-healthcare-experience-insights/your-comprehensive-guide-to-the-press-ganey-national-database-of-nursing-quality-indicators-ndnqi

Madsen, I. E. H., Svane-Petersen, A. C., Holm, A., Burr, H., Framke, E., Melchior, M., Rod, N. H., Sivertsen, B., Stansfeld, S., Sorensen, J. K., Virtanen, M., & Rugulies, R. (2021). Work-related violence and depressive disorder among 955,573 employees followed for 6.99 million person-years. The Danish Work Life Course Cohort study: Work-related violence and depression. *Journal of Affective Disorders, 288*, 136–144. https://doi.org/10.1016/j.jad.2021.03.065

Mann, K., Groschel, S., Singer, S., Breitmaier, J., Claus, S., Fani, M., Rambach, S., Salize, H. J., & Lieb, K. (2021). Evaluation of coercive measures in different psychiatric hospitals: The impact of institutional characteristics. *BMC Psychiatry, 21*(1), 419. https://doi.org/10.1186/s12888-021-03410-z

Margari, F., Matarazzo, R., Casacchia, M., Roncone, R., Dieci, M., Safran, S., et al., the EPICA Study Group. (2005). Italian validation of MOAS and NOSIE: A useful package for psychiatric assessment and monitoring of aggressive behavior. *International Journal of Methods in Psychiatric Research, 14*, 109–118.

Marlatt, G. A., & Gordon, J. R. (Eds.). (1985). *Relapse prevention*. Guilford.

Milczarek, M. (2011). *European Agency for Safety and Health at Work, Workplace violence and harassment: A European picture*. Publications Office. Retrieved from https://data.europa.eu/doi/10.2802/12198

Miodownik, C., Friger, M. D., Orev, E., Gansburg, Y., Reis, N., & Lerner, V. (2019). Clinical and demographic characteristics of secluded and mechanically restrained mentally ill patients: A retrospective study. *Israel Journal of Health Policy Research, 8*(1), 9. https://doi.org/10.1186/s13584-018-0274-4

Mistler, L. A., & Friedman, M. J. (2022). Instruments for measuring violence on acute inpatient psychiatric units: Review and recommendations. *Psychiatric Services, 73*(6), 650–657. https://doi.org/10.1176/appi.ps.202000297

Montalvo, I. (2007). The National Database of Nursing Quality Indicators (NDNQI). *The Online Journal of Issues in Nursing, 12*(3), Man02. https://doi.org/10.3912/OJIN.Vol12No03Man02

Morken, T., Baste, V., Johnsen, G. E., Rypdal, K., Palmstierna, T., & Johansen, I. H. (2018). The staff observation aggression scale-revised (SOAS-R)—Adjustment and validation for emergency primary health care. *BMC Health Services Research, 18*(1), 335.

Morrison, E. F. (1990). Violent psychiatric inpatients in a public hospital. *Scholarly Inquiry for Nursing Practice, 4*, 65–82.

National Association of State Mental Health Program Directors Research Institute (NRI). (2013a). *Using data, changing practice: National public rates: Behavioral healthcare performance measurement system*. Retrieved from https://www.nri-inc.org/our-work/nri-reports/national-public-rates/

National Association of State Mental Health Program Directors Research Institute (NRI). (2013b). *National public rates 2010 to 2013 injury antipsychotic elopement seclusion restraint*. Retrieved from https://www.nri-inc.org/media/1115/2013-national-public-rates-schacht.pdf

National Institute for Health and Care Excellence (NICE). (2015). *Violence and aggression: Short-term management in mental health, health and community settings (NG10)*. Retrieved March 29, 2023, from https://www.nice.org.uk/guidance/ng10

Nijman, H. L. I., Allertz, W. W. F., Merckelbach, H., à Campo, J., & Ravelli, D. (1997). Aggressive behavior on an acute psychiatric admissions ward. *European Psychiatry, 11*, 106–114.

Nijman, H. L. I., Muris, P., Merckelbach, H. L. G. J., Palmstierna, T., Wistedt, B., Vos, A. M., et al. (1999). The Staff Observation Aggression Scale-Revised (SOAS-R). *Aggressive Behavior, 25*, 197–209. https://doi.org/10.1002/(sici)1098-2337(1999)25:3

Nijman, H., Evers, C., Merckelbach, H. L. G. J., & Palmstierna, T. (2002). Assessing aggression severity with the revised Staff Observation Aggression Scale (SOAS-R). *Journal of Nervous and Mental Disease, 190*, 198–200. https://doi.org/10.1097/00005053-200203000-00009

Nijman, H. L. I., Bowers, L., Oud, N., & Jansen, G. (2005a). Psychiatric nurses' experiences with inpatient aggression. *Aggressive Behavior, 31*, 217–227. https://doi.org/10.1002/ab.20038

Nijman, H., Palmstierna, T., Almvik, R., & Stalker, J. (2005b). Fifteen years of research with the Staff Observation Aggression Scale. A review. *Acta Psychiatrica Scandinavica, 111*, 12–21. https://doi.org/10.1111/j.1600-0447.2004.00417.x

Nilsson, K., Palmstierna, T., & Wistedt, B. (1988). Aggressive behavior in hospitalized psychogeriatric patients. *Acta Psychiatrica Scandinavica, 78*, 172–175.

Nolan, K. A., & Volavka, J. A. N. (2006). Video recording in the assessment of violent incidents in psychiatric hospitals. *Journal of Psychiatric Practice, 12*(1). Retrieved from https://journals.

lww.com/practicalpsychiatry/Fulltext/2006/01000/Video_Recording_in_the_Assessment_of_Violent.10.aspx

Novaco, R. W. (1994). Anger as a risk factor for violence among the mentally disordered. In J. Monahan & H. J. Steadman (Eds.), *Violence and mental disorder* (pp. 21–59). University of Chicago Press.

Novaco, R. W., & Taylor, J. L. (2004). Assessment of anger and aggression in male offenders with developmental disabilities. *Psychological Assessment, 16*, 42–50.

Palmstierna, T., & Wistedt, B. (1987). Staff observation aggression scale. Presentation and evaluation. *Acta Psychiatrica Scandinavica, 76*, 657–663.

Pariona-Cabrera, P., Cavanagh, J., & Bartram, T. (2020). Workplace violence against nurses in health care and the role of human resource management: A systematic review of the literature. *Journal of Advanced Nursing, 76*, 1581–1593. https://doi.org/10.1111/jan.14352

Partridge, B., & Affleck, J. (2017). Verbal abuse and physical assault in the emergency department: Rates of violence, perceptions of safety, and attitudes towards security. *Australasian Emergency Nursing Journal, 20*(3), 139–145. https://doi.org/10.1016/j.aenj.2017.05.001

Pelto-Piri, V., Warg, L. E., & Kjellin, L. (2020). Violence and aggression in psychiatric inpatient care in Sweden: A critical incident technique analysis of staff descriptions. *BMC Health Services Research, 20*, 1–11.

Pich, J. V., Kable, A., & Hazelton, M. (2017). Antecedents and precipitants of patient-related violence in the emergency department: Results from the Australian VENT Study (Violence in Emergency Nursing and Triage). *Australasian Emergency Nursing Journal, 20*(3), 107–113. https://doi.org/10.1016/j.aenj.2017.05.005

Press Ganey. (2023). *The National Database of Nursing Quality Indicators (NDNQI)*. Retrieved February 28, 2023, from https://www.pressganey.com/solutions/nursing-excellence/

Ravyts, S. G., Perez, E., Donovan, E. K., Soto, P., & Dzierzewski, J. M. (2021). Measurement of aggression in older adults. *Aggression and Violent Behavior, 57*, 101484.

Reilly, C. A., Cullen, S. W., Watts, B. V., Mills, P. D., Paull, D. E., & Marcus, S. C. (2019). How well do incident reporting systems work on inpatient psychiatric units? *The Joint Commission Journal on Quality and Patient Safety, 45*, 63–69. https://doi.org/10.1016/j.avb.2020.101484

Ross, T., Woods, P., Reed, V., Sookoo, S., Dean, A., Kettles, A., Almvik, R., Ter Horst, P., Brown, I., Collins, M., Walker, H., & Pfafflin, F. (2008). Assessing living skills in forensic mental health care with the behavioural status index: A European network study. *Psychotherapy Research, 18*(3), 334–344. https://doi.org/10.1080/10503300701508488

Rubio-Valera, M., Luciano, J. V., Ortiz, J. M., Salvador-Carulla, L., Gracia, A., & Serrano-Blanco, A. (2015). Health service use and costs associated with aggressiveness or agitation and containment in adult psychiatric care: A systematic review of the evidence. *BMC Psychiatry, 15*, 35. https://doi.org/10.1186/s12888-015-0417-x

S.1176—118th Congress (April 18, 2023–2024): *Workplace Violence Prevention for Health Care and Social Service Workers Act*. Retrieved January 31, 2024, from https://www.congress.gov/bill/118th-congress/senate-bill/1176/all-info

Salzmann-Erikson, M., & Yifter, L. (2020). Risk factors and triggers that may result in patient-initiated violence on inpatient psychiatric units: An integrative review. *Clinical Nursing Research, 29*(7), 504–520.

Shah, A. (1999). Some methodological issues in using aggression rating scales in intervention studies among institutionalized elderly. *International Psychogeriatrics, 11*, 439–444.

Silver, J. M., & Yudofsky, S. C. (1991). The Overt Aggression Scale. *Journal of Neuropsychiatry, 3*, 22–29.

Sival, R. C., Albronda, T., Haffmans, P. M. J., Saltet, M. L., & Schellekens, C. M. (2000). Is aggressive behavior influenced by the use of a behavior rating scale in patients in a psychogeriatric nursing home? *International Journal of Geriatric Psychiatry, 15*, 108–111.

Sjostrom, N., Eder, D. N., Malm, U., & Beskow, J. (2001). Violence and its prediction at a psychiatric hospital. *European Psychiatry, 16*, 459–465.

Spielberger, C. D. (1996). *State-Trait anger expression inventory professional manual*. Psychological Assessment Resources.

Staggs, V. S. (2015). Trends, victims, and injuries in injurious patient assaults on adult, geriatric, and child/adolescent pyschiatric units in US hospitals 2007-2013. *Research in Nursing and Health, 38*, 115–120. https://doi.org/10.1002/nur.21647

Stavropoulou, C., Doherty, C., & Tosey, P. (2015). How effective are incident-reporting systems for improving patient safety? A systematic literature review. *Milbank Quarterly, 93*(4), 826–866.

Steinert, T., Woefle, M., & Gebhardt, R. P. (1999). No correlation of serum cholesterol levels with measures of violence in patients with schizophrenia and non-psychotic disorders. *European Psychiatry, 14*, 80–81.

Steinert, T., Wolfie, M., & Gebhardt, R. P. (2000). Measurement of violence during in-patient treatment and association with psychopathology. *Acta Psychiatrica Scandinavica, 102*, 107–112.

Steinert, T., Lepping, P., Bernhardsgrütter, R., Conca, A., Hatling, T., Janssen, W., Keski-Valkama, A., Mayoral, F., & Whittington, R. (2010). Incidence of seclusion and restraint in psychiatric hospitals: A literature review and survey of international trends. *Social Psychiatry and Psychiatric Epidemiology, 45*(9), 889–897. https://doi.org/10.1007/s00127-009-0132-3

Stewart, D., & Bowers, L. (2013). Inpatient verbal aggression: Content targets and patient characteristics. *Journal of Psychiatric and Mental Health Nursing, 20*, 236–243. https://doi.org/10.1111/j.1365-2850.2012.01905.x

Urheim, R., Palmstierna, T., Rypdal, K., Gjestad, R., Senneseth, M., & Mykletun, A. (2020). Violence rate dropped during a shift to individualized patient-oriented care in a high security forensic psychiatric ward. *BMC Psychiatry, 20*, 200. https://doi.org/10.1186/s12888-020-02524-0

US Bureau of Labor Statistics. (2020a). *Table R100. Fact sheet: Workplace violence in healthcare, 2018*. Retrieved from https://www.bls.gov/iif/factsheets/workplace-violence-healthcare-2018.htm

US Bureau of Labor Statistics. (2020b). *Table R-75. Worker injury and illness by event or exposure and industry sector, private industry*. Retrieved from https://www.bls.gov/iif/nonfatal-injuries-and-illnesses-tables.htm

US Bureau of Labor Statistics. (2023). *Incidence rates of nonfatal occupational injuries and illnesses by industry and case types, 2020*. Retrieved from https://www.bls.gov/web/osh/sum100.htm, https://www.bls.gov/iif/nonfatal-injuries-and-illnesses-tables.htm, https://www.bls.gov/iif/nonfatal-injuries-and-illnesses-tables.htm

Välimäki, M., Yang, M., Vahlberg, T., Lantta, T., Pekurinen, V., Anttila, M., & Normand, S.-L. (2019). Trends in the use of coercive measures in Finnish psychiatric hospitals: A register analysis of the past two decades. *BMC Psychiatry, 19*(1), 230. https://doi.org/10.1186/s12888-019-2200-x

Van Den Bos, J., Creten, N., Davenport, S., & Roberts, M. (2017). *Cost of community violence to hospitals and health systems: Report for the American Hospital Association*. American Hospital Association. Retrieved from https://www.aha.org/system/files/2018-01/community-violence-report.pdf

Van Leeuwen, M. E., & Harte, J. M. (2017). Violence against mental health care professionals: Prevalence, nature and consequences. *The Journal of Forensic Psychiatry & Psychology, 28*, 581–598.

Vassar, M., & Hale, W. (2009). Reliability reporting across studies using the Buss Durkee Hostility Inventory. *Journal of Interpersonal Violence, 24*(1), 20–37.

Wasserman, D., Apter, G., Baeken, C., Bailey, S., Balazs, J., Bec, C., et al. (2020). Compulsory admissions of patients with mental disorders: State of the art on ethical and legislative aspects in 40 European countries. *European Psychiatry, 63*(1), e82.

Weltens, I., Bak, M., Verhagen, S., Vandenberk, E., Domen, P., van Amelsvoort, T., & Drukker, M. (2021). Aggression on the psychiatric ward: Prevalence and risk factors. A systematic review of the literature. *PLoS One, 16*(10), e0258346. https://doi.org/10.1371/journal.pone.0258346

Whittington, R., & Wykes, T. (1996). Aversive stimulation by staff and violence by psychiatric patients. *British Journal of Clinical Psychology, 35*, 11–20.

Whittington, R., Shuttleworth, S., & Hill, L. (1996). Violence to staff in a general hospital setting. *Journal of Advanced Nursing, 24*(2), 326–333.

Wilson, K., Eaton, J., Foye, U., Ellis, M., Thomas, E., & Simpson, A. (2022). What evidence supports the use of Body Worn Cameras in mental health inpatient wards? A systematic review and narrative synthesis of the effects of Body Worn Cameras in public sector services. *International Journal of Mental Health Nursing, 31*(2), 260–277.

Wilson, K., Foye, U., Thomas, E., Chadwick, M., Dodhia, S., Allen-Lynn, J., Brennan, G., & Simpson, A. (2023). Exploring the use of body-worn cameras in acute mental health wards: A qualitative interview study with mental health patients and staff. *International Journal of Nursing Studies, 140*, 104456.

Wistedt, B., Rasmussen, A., Pedersen, L., Malm, U., Traskman-Bendz, L., Wakelin, J., et al. (1990). The development of an observer-scale for measuring social dysfunction and aggression. *Pharmacopsychiatry, 23*, 249–252.

World Health Organization. (2016). *Minimal information model for patient safety incident reporting and learning systems—User guide*. WHO.

World Health Organization. (2020). *Patient safety incident reporting and learning systems: Technical report and guidance*. Licence: CC BY-NC-SA 3.0 IGO.

World Health Organization. (2021). *Global patient safety action plan 2021–2030: Towards eliminating avoidable harm in health care*. Licence: CC BY-NC-SA 3.0 IGO.

Yeh, T.-F., Chang, Y.-C., Feng, W.-H., Sclerosis, M., & Yang, C.-C. (2020). Effect of workplace violence on turnover intention: The mediating roles of job control, psychological demands, and social support. *INQUIRY: The Journal of Health Care Organization, Provision, and Financing, 57*, 0046958020969313.

Yudofsky, S. C., Silver, J. M., Jackson, W., Endicott, J., & Williams, D. (1986). The Overt Aggression Scale for the objective rating of verbal and physical aggression. *The American Journal of Psychiatry, 143*, 35–39.

# Violence Risk Assessment

Lisa A. Mistler, Roger Almvik, Frans Fluttert,
Øyvind Lockertsen, Angela Hassiotis, Matthew Manton,
and Jaroslav Pekara

Dr. Mistler is supported by the Health Resources and Services Administration (HRSA) of the US Department of Health and Human Services (HHS) as part of an award T32HP32520 totalling $2,496,422 (2021–2026) with 0% financed with non-governmental sources. The contents are those of the author(s) and do not necessarily represent the official views of, nor an endorsement by, HRSA, HHS or the US Government.

L. A. Mistler (✉)
Geisel School of Medicine, Dartmouth College, Hanover, NH, USA

Dartmouth & Dartmouth-Hitchcock Medical Center, Lebanon, NH, USA
e-mail: lisa.a.mistler@hitchcock.org

R. Almvik
Centre for Research and Education in Forensic Psychiatry, St. Olav's University Hospital, Trondheim, Norway
e-mail: roger.almvik@ntnu.no

F. Fluttert
Centre for Research and Education in Forensic Psychiatry, St. Olav's University Hospital, Trondheim, Norway

Department of Health and Social Sciences, Molde University College, Molde, Norway
e-mail: frans.fluttert@himolde.no

Ø. Lockertsen
Oslo University Hospital, Centre for Research and Education in Forensic Psychiatry, South-Eastern Norway Regional Health Authority, Oslo, Norway

Department of Nursing and Health Promotion, Faculty of Health Sciences, Oslo Metropolitan University, Oslo, Norway
e-mail: oylock@oslomet.no

A. Hassiotis
Epidemiology and Applied Clinical Research, Division of Psychiatry, University College London, London, UK
e-mail: a.hassiotis@ucl.ac.uk

M. Manton
Camden and Islington NHS Foundation Trust, London, UK
e-mail: matthew.manton3@nhs.net

J. Pekara
Medical College in Prague and Prague Emergency Medical Services, Prague, Czech Republic
e-mail: pekara@vszdrav.cz

# 1      Introduction

The relationship between aggression and violence and mental health is complex: compared with the general population, adults with mental illness are at higher risk for being both victims and perpetrators of violence, and this risk is heightened in the context of inpatient stays (Civilotti et al., 2021; Desmarais et al., 2012; Witt et al., 2013). A key part of psychiatric clinicians' jobs is to assess the likelihood, or risk, that an individual client with mental illness will engage in some form of violence within a particular time frame. Hart (2009) defines evidence-based assessment and management of violence risk as '…the process of gathering information about people in a way that is consistent with and guided by the best available scientific evidence and professional knowledge to understand their potential for engaging in violence in the future and to determine what should be done to prevent them from doing so'. Identifying known risk factors is only one part of thorough violence risk assessment; however, identifying protective factors within the individual or their environment that may reduce risk is equally essential. The consideration of risk and protective factors can then be used to develop a plan for managing and support that has a focus on these factors. Support services can be overly cautious when considering risk in the absence of objective risk assessment, which can lead to overly restrictive practices being used in the mistaken belief that they will be helpful (Van de Sande et al., 2013). Reliable and valid violence risk assessment allows for better use of resources to support clients. Treatment and supports can be included that are tailored approaches to address known risk factors for this person, matching treatment and support intensity to the degree of identified risk. Valid violence risk assessment should be used for ongoing monitoring to identify changes in risk. Re-assessment allows services to determine whether the support they provide is effective in reducing risk and can also help identify when they are able to reduce restrictive measures that are in place to manage risk as it decreases (Whittington et al., 2013).

The purpose of this chapter is to provide a broad introduction to the concept of risk assessment for aggression and violence directed at others by clients in mental healthcare. The scope includes information related specifically to clients involved with the criminal justice system, or forensic psychiatric populations, since much of our knowledge has been gained from studying these populations. We describe the evolution of the field of risk assessment, present a particular model called the Early Recognition Model and describe risk assessment in special populations. At the end of the chapter, we briefly review the current state of research on risk assessment and make recommendations for future research. As with other chapters in this book, we propose moving away from the oversimplified view that only clients are responsible for aggression and violence. We argue that staff members and the environment also contribute considerably. We recommend an organisational innovation to increase safety and security in clinical mental healthcare, as described by Voskes et al. (2019).

Also consistent with this book, we aim to be inclusive but remain aware that, based on the background and experience of the authors, the North-West-European point of view has possibly biased our writing. We recognise this and invite readers to consider this disclaimer whilst reading and generalising this information in their clinical practice.

## 2 Factors Associated with Aggression and Violence

Factors associated with increased risk of inpatient violence are of great interest to clinicians; hence, understanding these factors informs effective risk management and enables staff to select appropriate interventions (Szabo et al., 2015). A recent systematic review that investigated risk factors for aggression in psychiatric wards divided the factors between patients, staff and wards (Weltens et al., 2021). The 'patient risk factors' identified were diagnosis of psychotic or bipolar disorder, substance abuse, a history of aggression and younger age. 'Staff risk factors' included male gender, unqualified or temporary staff, job strain, dissatisfaction with the job or management, burnout and quality of interaction with patients. 'Staff protective factors' were a good functioning team, good leadership and involvement in treatment decisions. Significant 'ward risk factors' were higher bed occupancy, busy ward locations, an unsafe or restrictive environment, lack of structure during the day, smoking and lack of privacy.

Patient risk factors may be grouped into four categories: what a person is (e.g. age, gender), a person's prior experiences (e.g. pathological family environment, victimisation), what a person has been diagnosed with (e.g. major mental disorder, personality disorder, substance abuse disorder) and what a person has done (e.g. prior crimes, violence) (Monahan et al., 2019). Patient risk factors can also be arranged according to whether they are static (e.g. historical and unchanging), stable dynamic (modifiable but unlikely to change) or acutely dynamic (modifiable and likely to change) (Andrews & Bonta, 2010). Examples include previous violence, marital status and environmental stress, respectively. Static risk factors for violence (e.g. early onset of violence and history of violence) are historical events or variables that are not amenable to change through planned intervention over time (Chu et al., 2013; Douglas & Skeem, 2005). Dynamic risk factors for violence (e.g. active psychotic symptoms, antisocial attitudes, negative affect and present substance abuse/intoxication) are variables that are proximally associated with violence and can fluctuate with time and circumstances (Chu et al., 2013). Although most research on violence risk assessment emphasises static patient risk factors, the associations between static factors and aggression are weak (Dack et al., 2013). Research to date has been primarily on reacting to violence and patient factors contributing to it, which has limited the field in developing robust aggression prevention measures. Future studies should focus more on the earlier stages of aggression such as agitation and on factors that may be more amenable to preventing aggression, such as ward and staff factors (Weltens et al., 2021).

# 3     From Risk Prediction to Risk Assessment

The Oxford Dictionary defines risk as 'the possibility of something bad happening at some time in the future' (S.v. 'Risk (n.)', 2023). Overall, most definitions of risk focus on outcome and probability. Violence prediction is the assigning of a probability to a patient, indexing the likelihood of a patient committing harm or a violent offence (Dolan & Doyle, 2000). Violence risk assessment, however, is a clinical decision-making task that is conducted in numerous legal and clinical settings in which the possibility of a person's future violent behaviour is of concern (Douglas & Kropp, 2002).

There are three main approaches to forming opinions about violence risk: (1) unstructured professional judgement (UPJ), (2) actuarial decision-making and (3) structured professional judgement (SPJ) (Whittington et al., 2013). The different approaches refer to how information is weighted and combined to reach a final assessment, regardless of the information being considered and how it was collected (Grove, 2005; Meehl, 1954).

## 3.1     Unstructured Professional Judgement (UPJ)

Prior to the 1990s, risk assessment for violence consisted largely of UPJ. This is defined as a clinical judgement whereby the assessor, from his or her perspective of the client, gives an opinion about the expected danger. Formal or explicit rules or procedures are absent for assessing violence risk. The underlying rationale for the use of UPJ was that the complexity of risk assessment would be best approached by one expert evaluator (Hart et al., 2016). An advantage of UPJ is that it allows for flexibility and individualisation (Otto, 2000); UPJ can result in a client-centred analysis of the client's behaviour and a context-specific tailoring of risk management and violence prevention strategies. However, because the approach relies so heavily on an individual professional's expertise, it is vulnerable to biases based on the professional's training, experience, intuition and preferences, rather than on (1) well-reasoned consideration of dynamic and context-specific risk factors; and (2) intervention strategies that are either empirically valid or well accepted in the field. Within UPJ there are no constraints on the information that assessors may use to reach their decision, no guidance on what information to gather, which risk factors to consider, how to weigh them, how to define or operationalise risk factors and how to combine risk factors to reach a decision (Craig et al., 2012).

During the last half of the twentieth century, research demonstrated that violence risk predictions based on UPJ are only slightly better than chance. Additionally, it was found that predictive competence varies considerably among clinicians. These findings led to the adoption of other, more reliable and valid models (Lidz et al., 1993; Singh et al., 2011, 2016).

## 3.2     Actuarial Decision-Making

The actuarial model is the application of risk assessment instruments in which fixed items of behaviour (e.g. age, gender) are scored and the final score gives an indication of the expected risk. Actuarial methods are defined by a fixed algorithm or set of a priori decision-making rules (Meehl, 1954). Actuarial violence risk assessment instruments are designed to predict violence in a specific population within a specific time frame, with predefined rules (Bjørkly et al., 2014; Hart & Cooke, 2013). The hallmark of the actuarial approach is that, based on the information available to them, evaluators make an ultimate decision according to fixed and explicit rules (Meehl, 1954). Actuarial decision-making is based on specific risk markers, selected because they have been demonstrated empirically to be associated with violence and coded in a pre-determined manner. The combination of risk markers forms a total risk score, which represents the prognosis of future violent behaviour expressed in probabilistic terms (Douglas et al., 1999; Hart & Cooke, 2013; Nicholls et al., 2016). Several different actuarial violence risk assessment instruments for different types of violence have been developed since the 1990s with moderate to good levels of predictive accuracy (Dvoskin & Heilbrun, 2001; Yang et al., 2010). Actuarial instruments are designed not to measure anything but solely to predict the future (Douglas et al., 1999) and have the advantage of transparency and direct empirical support (Grove, 2005). However, the limited number of risk factors included and a tendency to focus on static factors limits the approach. Furthermore, crucial risk factors (e.g. individual areas of vulnerability such as physical contact with a person of the same/opposite sex, or specific sounds/smells that may evoke past trauma) may be excluded if their value has not been empirically proven, and the decisions can be non-optimal when applied in different settings (Doyle & Dolan, 2002; Norko & Baranoski, 2005).

## 3.3     Structured Professional Judgement (SPJ)

SPJ is when agreement is reached in a structured manner on the expected recurrence of relapse of violence, on the basis of scored items from risk assessment instruments merged with clinical judgement (Douglas et al., 2014). This leads to a 'risk formulation', which is the description of possible relapse scenarios (best case-, worst case-, relapse- and twist scenarios). In SPJ, the use of risk assessment instruments is linked in a structured way to risk management strategies, including development of risk interventions for relapse prevention. This is the most dynamic and recent approach to risk management.

   The primary goal of the SPJ approach to risk assessment is to prevent future violence (Douglas & Kropp, 2002; Hart & Logan, 2011). According to the SPJ approach, a comprehensive risk assessment needs to include both static and dynamic risk factors, describe scenarios in which risk may be increased or reduced and finally involve a professional clinical judgement of each factor's presence and relevance in each case (Douglas et al., 2014; Singh et al., 2016). SPJ risk assessment is guided and structured by evidence-based literature, but the overall risk decision is still based on a discretionary interpretation process (Bjørkly et al., 2014). SPJ manuals and guides have evolved to be more reflective of the complete risk assessment process, from the coding of risk factors to providing management recommendations (Douglas & Kropp, 2002). The SPJ approach has three phases: identifying facts, making meaning of those facts and then taking action (Douglas et al., 2014). The primary disadvantage of SPJ is in the process by which the evaluator intuitively combines the risk factors and arrives at a judgement about risk (Quinsey et al., 2006). In principle, this process is not different from UPJ, except the specific risk factors are outlined. Such unconstrained discretion could lead to inconsistent weighting of risk factors. Moreover, the process by which risk factors are translated into a summary of risk estimates (i.e. low, medium and high risk) is not well studied relative to studying the risk factors numerically (Douglas & Reeves, 2010).

## 3.4  Comparing the Actuarial and SPJ Models

Actuarial violence risk assessment instruments are transparent and standardised, making them a time-effective procedure that, unlike many SPJs, does not require extensive training (Nicholls et al., 2016). However, actuarial instruments tend to be comprised of static factors that do not show positive change over time, limiting their utility and relevance to risk management in healthcare settings (Douglas & Skeem 2005; Dvoskin & Heilbrun, 2001; Nicholls et al., 2016; Yang et al., 2010). SPJ models are identified through theory and empirical research, giving the assessor specific parameters to consider. SPJ models are also less rigid and mechanical than actuarial models, allowing clinical expertise and insights to inform the ultimate determination of summary risk (Nicholls et al., 2016). Neither actuarial violence risk assessment instruments nor SPJs seem to show clear superiority regarding predictive accuracy for violent outcomes (Coid et al., 2009; Guy et al., 2015; Heilbrun, 2009). Regarding predictive efficacy, SPJs and actuarial instruments seem interchangeable (Yang et al., 2010). In sum, there is virtually unanimous agreement that actuarial violence risk assessment instruments and SPJs perform equally well in predicting violence (Guy et al., 2015; Nicholls et al., 2016; Singh et al., 2011), whilst there is consensus that UPJ is not evidence-based best practice (Fazel et al., 2012; Guy et al., 2015; Heilbrun, 2009; Nicholls et al., 2016).

## 3.5  Acute Psychiatry and Violence Risk Screening

During the past several decades, the science and practice of violence risk assessment have flourished (Monahan et al., 2001). As a result, more than 400 different violence risk assessment instruments are available (Singh et al., 2016). Most instruments were developed in male-dominated populations like forensic and prison settings (Harris et al., 2004; Monahan, 1984), but many have proven to be valid in general psychiatry as well (Douglas et al., 1999).

In acute psychiatric settings, clinicians must make decisions quickly and may have less clinical and behavioural information available on admission than clinicians in long-term clinical settings (Anderson & Jenson, 2019). Often logistical constraints make it difficult to obtain much-needed information and some patients may be too ill to provide accurate information (Elbogen et al., 2003; Gardner et al., 1996). In acute psychiatric settings, a screening tool for violence may be used to identify individuals with a possible risk of violence, and the main purpose is to help identify who needs immediate measures to prevent violence and to distinguish who needs a more comprehensive risk assessment (Anderson & Jenson, 2019). The Violence Risk Screening 10 (V-RISK-10) (Roaldset et al., 2011), a brief screening checklist developed for acute and general psychiatry, is a simple screener based on risk factors with a time horizon from days to a few months (Bjørkly et al., 2009; Hartvig et al., 2006, 2011).

A literature review that examined violence risk assessment screening instruments found that the Brøset Violence Checklist (BVC), a short-term violence prediction instrument assessing confusion, irritability, boisterousness, verbal threats, physical threats and attacks on objects as either present or absent (Almvik & Woods, 1998), and the V-RISK-10 were the two instruments that provided enough statistical information to be considered for use in acute psychiatric settings (Anderson & Jenson, 2019). For the inpatient context, the retrospectively estimated net time consumption for scoring the V-RISK-10 was estimated by the assessors to be around 5 min (Hartvig et al., 2011) and for the BVC it takes about 1 min (Clarke et al., 2010), making either suitable for acute psychiatric settings.

## 4    Early Recognition Method

In any clinical situation, violence between clients or towards staff has a major impact as it can lead to stress, anger and fear in those who are involved. There are several models for risk management that attempt to account for the contributions of external and personalised factors to violent acts. The Early Recognition Method (ERM) (Fluttert et al., 2008) is a step-wise strategy that aims to identify, formulate and manage early warning signs of violence. The ERM has successfully been applied in forensic and general ambulatory psychiatry settings.

Working in a closed secure facility requires staff to keep the work environment safe. Various studies show that when staff are confronted with a high degree of stress at work, including aggression or violence, they are at higher risk of burnout (Andersen et al., 2017; Bezerra et al., 2016; Finney et al., 2013; Gadon et al., 2006). Work pressure is considerably increased under these circumstances, as staff must be constantly aware of the potential for violence (Bezerra et al., 2016). Research shows that in secured institutes, violence from clients towards staff has a major impact in that it elicits feelings of anger, fear and hopelessness (van Leeuwen & Harte, 2017).

Historically, in order to explain why violence occurs, the emphasis has often been on the personal characteristics of clients. However, research shows that situational, relational and environmental factors also contribute to the occurrence of violence (Bjørkly et al., 2019). For example, ward crowding, in which there are many people in a relatively small space, and insufficient delineation of undesirable behaviour, or boundary-setting, are associated with an increased likelihood of violence (Bezerra et al., 2016; Carlsson et al., 2006; Newbill et al., 2010; Ng et al., 2001; Nijman et al., 1997). Most studies investigate the probability and course of violence at the group level; however, for clinicians and staff, it is important to know how violence can be understood and influenced on an individual level.

In secure institutions such as forensic psychiatric clinics, risk management strategies aim to manage and prevent violence in individual patients. The emphasis has been on the risk-needs-responsivity model that treatment and care should match the patient's risk profile, the need for treatment and the patient's abilities (Bonta & Andrews, 2007). When applying the risk-needs-responsivity model in treatment, patients, in collaboration with clinicians and staff, learn to understand how violence can occur, what the consequences may be and especially how to control aggressive feelings and behaviours (Eidhammer et al., 2014; Fluttert et al., 2008; Ray & Simpson, 2019). The ERM is such a risk management strategy. Research shows that the use of ERM contributes to less frequent and less serious violence within a forensic psychiatric clinic (Fluttert et al., 2010a) and a decrease in relapse and re-admissions in ambulatory psychiatry (Johansen et al., 2021b, 2022). The ERM strategy focuses on identifying and describing early warning signs of behavioural escalation in ERM plans. The emphasis is therefore not on how violence escalates, but rather on how to develop behavioural stability and understand the warning signs which could disturb it.

## 4.1 Applying ERM

The central vision behind ERM is that disruptive behaviour, including aggression, gradually develops and that, especially in the first phase of behavioural disruption, there are opportunities for stabilising interventions (see Fig. 1). In addition, it is important to describe the context in which the early warning signs mainly occur. For example, the signal 'irritation and anger' could occur especially when too many people surround the patient.

The baseline in the figure shows the behaviour as one encounters it in stable situations. The sloping line symbolises an increasing deterioration of behaviour. In case of minor unstable behaviours patients are able to restore themselves to stable functioning. However, when stress and/or symptoms of a disorder increase, the behaviour can deteriorate further to a point where no adjustment is possible and a crisis is likely to occur. When applying ERM plans, we focus on the functional area from the start to the middle of the ascending line. In this area, the behaviour is out of balance, but not completely deteriorated. This is the area where the first early warning signs occur. This is also the area in which there are the best opportunities for influencing behaviour and prevention.

An important aspect of risk management strategies such as ERM is that care providers adopt a non-judgemental attitude and encourage the client to discuss what

**Fig. 1** Process of
deterioration (Fluttert
et al., 2021)

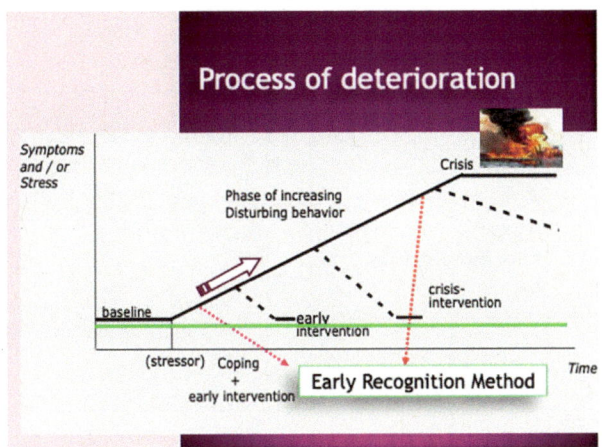

**Fig. 1** Process of deterioration (Fluttert et al., 2021)

is bothering them (Meehan et al., 2017). At the same time, a client does not have to be convinced or motivated to be able to cooperate with ERM plans. Motivation can grow over time if the client notices that working with ERM plans is not as complex or threatening as they initially thought.

The two most important factors in the process of working with ERM plans are: (1) the client learns to understand that risk management conversations are not punitive or threatening, and (2) the client learns how to work with ERM plans that support him or her. The enduring benefit of ERM is understanding, and that takes time. ERM research (Fluttert et al., 2010b) shows that the discussion between clients and staff regarding early warning signs leads to a better understanding of the client's perceptions and behaviour. Even when there is disagreement about early warning signs, these discussions may improve clients' behaviours in stable and less stable conditions.

The ERM protocol is the manual for guiding the care provider and the client in drafting and implementing an ERM plan. The protocol should be used systematically (Fluttert et al., 2011), as it is (Fluttert et al., 2010b, 2011; Van Meijel et al., 2006). Several studies show that the interaction between the care provider and client is the most important factor in influencing aggression during admission (Gildberg et al., 2021; Johansen et al., 2021a). Research into the application of ERM has also shown that weekly discussions between care providers and clients had a meaningful contribution to reducing the number and severity of aggressive incidents (Fluttert et al., 2010b).

The ERM strategy and protocol consists of four phases (Fluttert et al., 2011): (1) introduction, (2) listing early warning/identification, (3) monitoring and (4) action plan; see Fig. 2.

Phases of the protocol:

1. Introduction/preparation phase

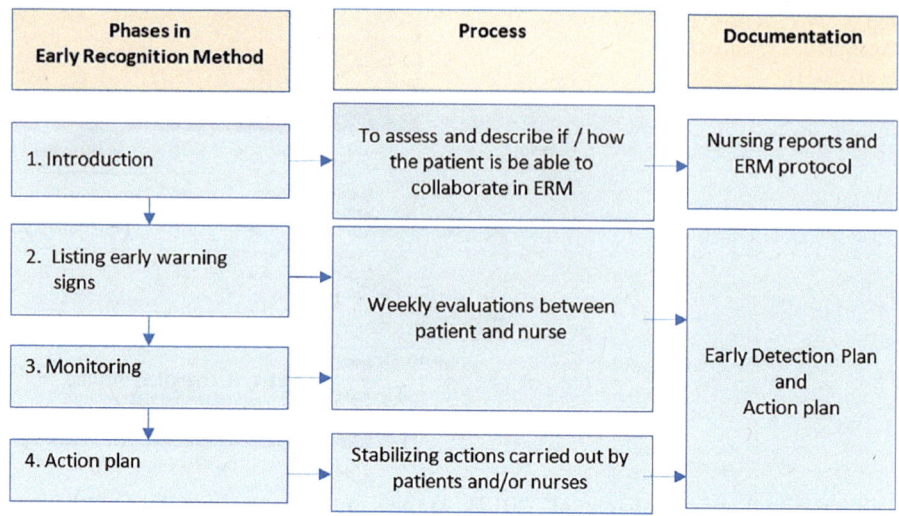

**Fig. 2** ERM framework

The client is introduced to the concept of the ERM plan and what is expected of them. At this stage, an assessment is also made as to whether and how the client will be able to work with the ERM plan. The strategy is determined and, if necessary, an ERM plan may be drawn up without the client's cooperation.

2. Listing early warning/identification phase

In this phase, it is determined in collaboration with the client which early warning signs they tend to exhibit. Each early warning sign is categorised into three levels of severity: (1) stable, (2) disrupted and (3) more disrupted. The Forensic Early Signs of Aggression Inventory (FESAI) is used to identify early warning signs (Fluttert et al., 2011). This is a list of 44 items in 15 categories, see Sect. 4.4.

3. Monitoring phase

The monitoring phase involves observing the client to recognise the occurrence of early warning signs. The dialogue between the client and the care provider about the occurrence of early warning signs occurs during this phase. As mentioned previously, the care provider remains non-judgemental, exploring with the client how he or she interprets his behaviour and creating a dialogue about the differences in perception of the behaviour.

4. Action phase

Finally, an action plan is drawn up together with the client which describes which actions can contribute to the stabilisation of behaviour.

## 4.2 Client Involvement and Shared Decision-Making in Risk Management

In recent years, there has been more recognition of the client's involvement in risk management (Gudde et al., 2015; Ray & Simpson, 2019). Shared decision-making is an approach based on the principle that there are two experts in care and treatment: the client and the care provider (Légaré et al., 2008). Care providers have expertise in the process of diagnosis, risk assessment and risk management, whilst clients are experts in their values and goals, what helps them and what gives meaning to the quality of their lives. Ideally, care providers and clients agree on the nature and purpose of the treatment and risk management. Through active participation of the client in the treatment programme, the client is more likely to follow through with the treatment plan, so that effectiveness increases (Stringer et al., 2008). Whilst the collaboration between the care provider and the client is intended to teach the client to independently control their risk (Kroner, 2012), systematic reviews show that patient involvement is rare in evidence-based risk management strategies (e.g. Eidhammer et al., 2014). In this review, only four risk management strategies were found (including ERM) where the client had an active role in its application. Client participation in risk formulation, as part of risk assessment strategies, is also described as scarce (Ray & Simpson, 2019).

## 4.3 Models of ERM Plans

Working with the ERM strategy has its origins in the treatment of patients with schizophrenia. Birchwood et al. (2000) described how early signs of psychosis could be described in a way that patients themselves learn to recognise these signs and thereby prevent psychosis. In the 1990s in the Netherlands, there was increased attention paid to relapse prevention plans based on early warning signs, which led to the development of ERM. To date four models of ERM plans can be distinguished:

1. The Basic Model. The patient is not involved in identifying and monitoring their early warning signs, due to the incapacity of the patient to actively participate.
2. The Phase Model. The patient participates in identifying their early warning signs and describes how these signs could be recognised in different phases of severity.
3. The Comprehensive Model. The patient and the social network are involved in the ERM strategy. They discuss with the caregiver not only the occurrence of the determined early warning signs but also the factors that influence their recognition.
4. The Dynamic Model (Fluttert et al., 2022). A further development of the comprehensive model is that, in addition to the early warning signs and factors in the patient and the social network, the factor context is also highlighted. These are descriptions of specific circumstances in which early warning signs could occur.

For example, a patient may notice that their increasing desire for alcohol occurs mainly when they feel more lonely and when they have less contact with family. The 'dynamic' in the dynamic model is that early warning signs and context are brought together to contribute to a more focused dialogue between the client and the care provider (Fluttert et al., 2022).

## 4.4   The 'Forensic Early Signs of Aggression Inventory' (FESAI) List of Early Warning Signs

A major obstacle in current practice is that there are few instruments available to support clients and care providers in identifying relevant early warning signs of aggression in a structured manner. For this purpose, the 'Forensic Early Signs of Aggression Inventory' (FESAI) was developed in a prison setting (Fluttert et al., 2011). In the construction of the FESAI, 167 ERM plans and 3768 descriptions of early warning signs were studied and then categorised. Validity and inter-rater reliability were tested and assessed as sufficiently adequate and reliable (Fluttert et al., 2011).

The FESAI appears to provide particularly good insight and guidance to determine the individualised early warning signs. In addition to the prison staff describing the signs in their own words, the FESAI immediately added a code corresponding to the category and the item in question in the FESAI. This provides opportunities for more systematic investigations into the ranking and classification of early warning signs in aggressive clients. It also appears that the format of the ERM plan provides sufficient guidance for adequately scoring the occurrence of signs over time. A first-ranking analysis showed that the most important early warning signs were: (1) tension, agitation and anger; (2) withdrawal from contact and fewer contacts; and (3) change in daily activities (Fluttert et al., 2013).

## 5   Summary

Working in secured mental health institutions such as with civilly committed or forensic populations requires considerable commitment and professionalism from care providers. As a consequence of daily exposure to the potential for aggression and violence, there is an increased likelihood of staff burnout, as well as physical and mental health problems. The application of risk management strategies such as ERM contributes to the timely recognition of behavioural deterioration and the ability to manage it. Research into the effects of ERM on incident management in a number of clinical environments is ongoing (Fluttert et al., 2022; Johansen et al., 2021a). This can, ultimately, contribute to both safety within the institution and the rehabilitation of detainees towards a stable existence after discharge from the institution.

The core element of ERM is to identify and adapt new behavioural strategies through the direct involvement of the client. Thus, multi-voiced collaboration is highlighted in this chapter. At present, given the evidence base for its effectiveness and its client-centred focus, the ERM strategy exemplifies the state of the art regarding violence and aggression, particularly in forensic settings. At the same time, employing ERM and, for example, the FESAI, new data could serve as input for studies that, in turn, might contribute to an even more comprehensive conceptualisation of aggression and violence, and the management and prevention of these. Current challenges are (1) the 'paradigm issue', i.e. how staff working with forensic or civilly committed clients change the culture from being more punitive to more interactive with clients, and (2) in forensic settings in particular, how to engage staff to work in a coordinated and systematic manner using knowledge, skills assessment and management instruments from mental health settings.

## 6    Assessment of Risk in Special Populations

Inpatient services work with a broad cross-section of the population and are concerned with the assessment of a variety of risks, including the risk of violence and aggression. Risk assessment can be notoriously challenging, and often involves the input of a multidisciplinary team of professionals. Risk assessment for people with neurodevelopmental disorders (NDD) and intellectual disability follow the same principles as in peers without. Whilst several risk assessment tools have been developed, no particular one is fully adapted for people with NDD and intellectual disability (Sammut et al., 2023).

### 6.1    Intellectual Disability Population vs Mainstream Population

It is estimated that 2% of the population of the UK have an intellectual disability, which is broadly in line with global estimates (2.2%) (WHO, 2011), and compared to the general population, individuals with an intellectual disability are overrepresented within the criminal justice system (Young et al., 2013). Evidence suggests that 7–10% of individuals with intellectual disability are estimated to act aggressively over a 6-month period (Cooper et al., 2009; Emerson et al., 2001; Holden & Gitlesen, 2006) and that these rates can be even greater in some subgroups. One study found that 70% of forensic inpatients with intellectual disability had been involved in at least one violent incident over a 12-month period (Malda Castillo et al., 2018), with over double the incidence compared to a non-intellectually disabled forensic population.

   Where appropriate, following a criminal act, individuals with intellectual disability may be detained under the Mental Health Act (UK, 1983) in a secure forensic inpatient unit, based on their assessed level of risk. This allows for treatment of their underlying mental health disorder, which may be done less effectively in a prison setting. Sadly, investigations into the care of inpatients with intellectual disability have highlighted suboptimal levels of care, including longer periods of compulsory detention under the Mental Health Act, representing a risk to their human rights. Violence and aggression are some of the most common barriers to discharge (Puddicombe & Lunsky, 2007), highlighting a clear benefit of accurate and validated risk assessment in forensic ID settings.

A key difference in risk assessment for those with intellectual disability compared to mainstream populations is in understanding the underlying aetiology of the risk. In mainstream populations, aggression and violence are often perceived to have antisocial intent. For those with intellectual disability, it is more likely to be interpreted as 'challenging behaviour'; a means of communicating an unmet need that the individual cannot otherwise communicate (e.g. having pain). Furthermore, those with intellectual disability can often perceive the risk and protective factors differently and can have difficulties with understanding, communication and decision-making around safety (Martí-Agustí et al., 2019). These key differences raise questions about the validity of the assessment of risk to others using standard tools and assessments.

## 6.2    Which Type of Assessment to Use?

The question for many clinicians is whether one should use a well-established tool that is not well-validated for people with intellectual disability or NDD, such as the Violence Risk Appraisal Guide related to sex offenders (VRAG) (Rice et al., 2013), or Historical Clinical Risk Management-20 (HCR-20) (Douglas & Webster, 1999), each of which was originally designed for use in correctional populations; or whether one should instead use a bespoke but less well-validated tool designed with a particular special population in mind, such as the Dynamic Risk Assessment and Management System (DRAMS) (Lindsay et al., 2004) or Current Risk of Violence (CuRV) (Lofthouse et al., 2014) tools. In the context of a paucity of good-quality research, there are potential pitfalls to both approaches. Using a 'mainstream' risk assessment tool could potentially underestimate the risk of an individual with intellectual disability, leading to less restrictive management and avoidable harm to the individual or others. Conversely, it could overestimate risk, leading to unnecessary restrictions on the rights and freedoms of the individual, extended admissions and increased cost of healthcare delivery. Overly restrictive practices have been found to increase anxious and depressive symptoms in those with intellectual disability (Tomlin et al., 2019) and extended admissions have been associated with poorer physical health outcomes (Higgins et al., 2016).

## 6.3    Evidence for the Use of Risk Assessment Tools in Intellectually Disabled Populations

A systematic review into the predictive validity of risk assessment tools for violence in those with intellectual disability concluded that several commonly used mainstream risk assessment tools (specifically VRAG and HCR-20) are valid for use in adults with intellectual disability though it also acknowledged that there is significant scope for more research in this area (Hounsome et al., 2018). The authors also noted that tools that have been designed for use specifically in intellectual disability populations—often by local services and likely lacking extensive psychometric testing—may be less valid, given their relative lack of evidence when compared with more established tools. However, Lindsay et al. (2008) demonstrated that several commonly used risk rating scales (including the HCR-20 and VRAG) had good predictive and discriminating validity in distinguishing between risks in those with intellectual disability in three separate cohorts: maximum security, medium/low security and community settings. A further meta-analysis supported the use of VRAG and HCR-20 for assessing the risk of aggression in those with intellectual disability (Lofthouse, 2016), with the caveat that novel dynamic risk assessment tools require more research before clinicians can be confident in their validity in assessing risk. Finally, most of the work on risk tools for people with intellectual disability has occurred in the area of sexual offending. Several tools have been developed and tested including the static risk assessments aided by SVR-20 (Boer et al., 1997), RM2000-V (Thornton, 2010) and the Rapid Risk Assessment for Sexual Offence Recidivism (RRASOR) (Hanson, 1997; Harris and Tough 2004) instruments and the dynamic risk instrument, Assessment of Risk Manageability for Intellectually Disabled Individuals who Offend (ARMIDILO) (Boer et al., 2004). Also see Blacker (2009) for additional information on the properties of those scales.

## 6.4    Risk Assessment in Autism Spectrum Disorder (ASD)

Those with Autism Spectrum Disorder (ASD) have 'persistent deficits in social communication and social interaction across multiple contexts' as defined by the DSM-5 (American Psychiatric Association, 2022). Autistic people can also demonstrate 'highly restricted, fixated interests that are abnormal in intensity or focus' and 'ritualized patterns of verbal and nonverbal behaviour' (American Psychiatric Association, 2022) which can increase the likelihood of offending behaviours, lead to conflicts with others and manifest in behaviours such as stalking and physical violence.

Studies on the rates of violence autistic people have suggested a wide range of estimates, from 1.5% to 67% (Del Pozzo et al., 2018). Such a broad span is hypothesised to be a consequence of the variability in ASD diagnosis of participants in the study, the types of violence included and the sample populations (e.g. forensic or community) (Del Pozzo et al., 2018). As with those with intellectual disability, studies have been designed to assess the validity of traditional risk assessment tools, such as the HCR-20, for autistic offenders. It is postulated, that given the risk profiles of autistic people are different to peers without autism, such risk assessment tools may not be valid (Westphal & Allely, 2019). However, it appears that at least the HCR-20 does have some value with people on the autistic spectrum (Girardi et al., 2019). Despite this work, there continue to be calls for further work to develop a specific risk assessment tool tailored to autistic people.

## 7    Compassionate Care

Assessment of the risk of violence requires making the difficult decision of what level of violence risk is acceptable, even when discussing the risk of violence towards others. This in itself is a significant ethical issue and triggers a fundamental debate on the concept of risk assessment in general and violence risk assessment in particular.

Whether it is possible to predict the risk of a recurrence of crime and/or violence, and with what degree of certainty is particularly salient in forensic psychiatry, in which the debate has focused on assessments by forensic psychiatry-appointed experts. It is argued, however, that being at the receiving end of criticism if something goes wrong encourages an authoritarian approach that dismisses patients' feelings for validation, leading to a further sense of erosion of physical and emotional safety (Veale et al., 2023).

This is often the case in forensic, but also general psychiatric assessments, where psychiatrists must predict who is likely to become violent even when there is a chance that the risk never manifests. Such 'false positives' can lead to multiple coercive measures, including overmedication, seclusion, refusal to leave, forced hospitalisation and forced treatment, among others. However, 'false negative' prediction can also lead to insufficient treatment and inadvertently discharging clients who are at an increased risk of violence. A more compassionate approach can lead to a positive therapeutic relationship and possibly to a full recovery in some cases. Unfortunately, we do see situations, particularly in inpatient mental healthcare, where there is a clear power imbalance and lack of patient engagement in their own care which can exacerbate the use of force and contribute to a traumatic experience (Liberati et al., 2023). Those issues apply to all inpatients with mental illness, but more so to those who are considered as lacking or having limited capacity, such as people with intellectual and developmental disorders.

This is further borne out by Skeem et al.'s (2013) findings. The researchers asked 86 inpatients with co-occurring mental illness and substance use disorders (people with schizophrenia were excluded) to complete two brief violence risk assessment tools before discharge. Two months after discharge, researchers interviewed the PWLE in the community, asking about their involvement in aggression and violence. The findings were that PWLE were very good and reliable global predictors of their own serious violence, with an area under the curve (AUC) of 0.74 and sensitivity of 50%, as compared with the predictive ability of two standard risk assessment tools they also filled out prior to discharge, which resulted in an AUC of 0.59, sensitivity 40% and AUC of 0.66, sensitivity 30%, respectively (Skeem et al., 2013). The results of this study imply that PWLE could contribute considerably to future models for risk assessment for violence.

Whilst risk assessments and their context will be an important tool that is required in clinical practice, there is currently a belief that perhaps it permits a legally enforceable removal of autonomy and is counter to respectful and empathic care for highly distressed individuals. More emphasis must be placed on the systemic reasons behind excessive application of restrictive practices; staff must be supported to avoid burnout with subsequent potential to engage in oppressive practices that will compromise their humanity and ability to provide safe care.

## 8  Conclusion

Reducing risk of aggression on psychiatric inpatient wards and forensic facilities includes not just risk assessment of the patient's potential for violence. We must also recognise that staff and ward factors contribute to the risk considerably. Some form of interaction between patient and staff precipitates aggression in 40% of the incidents (Weltens et al., 2021). These interactions include negative interactions such as poor communication, lack of empathy or respect, lack of shared decision-making, restrictions for patients, limit setting or patients being denied something and seemingly positive or neutral interactions, such as helping with activities of daily living, providing medication or discussion about medication, interaction with other patients and discussion about cigarettes. Despite our knowledge that aggression arises from a combination of patient, staff and ward factors, patient factors and treatment of aggression have been studied most often, and we are left with fewer studies on the prevention of aggression development. Future studies should focus more on the earlier stages of aggression such as agitation, and on components that are better suited for preventing aggression, such as ward and staff factors, making changes as assessed and needed. Future studies should also address patient-staff interaction and staff job strain, job dissatisfaction and overwork that influence this interaction. These factors are crucial for a safe atmosphere on wards and essential for management in guiding ward staff appropriately.

One salient example of how to approach these complex issues on inpatient psychiatric wards is the model of High Intensive Care, which has been adopted in several psychiatric institutions in Europe. This model focuses on creating an optimal healing environment, with as much autonomy and privacy as possible. Preventing unnecessary escalation is pursued through a welcoming atmosphere, frequent contact between patients and nurses that focus on the strengths of a patient, frequent contact with ambulatory carers, multidisciplinary staff, minimum use of coercive measures, and in case of agitated behaviour or aggression the possibility of one-on-one nursing (Voskes et al., 2019).

## References

Almvik, R., & Woods, P. (1998). The Broset Violence Checklist (BVC) and the prediction of inpatient violence: Some preliminary results. *Perspectives in Psychiatric Care, 5*(6), 208–211.

American Psychiatric Association. (2022). *Diagnostic and statistical manual of mental disorders* (5th ed., Text Revision). American Psychiatric Association Publishing. https://doi.org/10.1176/APPI.BOOKS.9780890425787.

Andersen, D. R., Andersen, L. P., Gadegaard, C. A., Høgh, A., Prieur, A., & Lund, T. (2017). Burnout among Danish prison personnel: A question of quantitative and emotional demands. *Scandinavian Journal of Public Health, 45*, 824–830. https://doi.org/10.1177/1403494817718644

Anderson, K. K., & Jenson, C. E. (2019). Violence risk–assessment screening tools for acute care mental health settings: Literature review. *Archive of Psychiatric Nursing, 33*(1), 112–119. https://doi.org/10.1016/j.apnu.2018.08.012

Andrews, D. A., & Bonta, J. (2010). *The psychology of criminal conduct* (5th ed.). Lexis Nexis.

Bezerra, C., Assis, S. G., & Constantino, P. (2016). Psychological distress and work stress in correctional officers: A literature review. *Ciência & Saúde Coletiva, 21*, 2135–2146.

Birchwood, M., Spencer, E., & McGovern, D. (2000). Schizophrenia: Early warning signs. *Advances in Psychiatric Treatment, 6*, 93–101. https://doi.org/10.1192/APT.6.2.93

Bjørkly, S., Hartvig, P., Heggen, F. A., Brauer, H., & Moger, T. A. (2009). Development of a brief screen for violence risk (V-RISK-10) in acute and general psychiatry: An introduction with emphasis on findings from a naturalistic test of interrater reliability. *European Psychiatry, 24*, 388–394. https://doi.org/10.1016/j.eurpsy.2009.07.004

Bjørkly, S., Hartvig, P., Roaldset, J. O., & Singh, J. P. (2014). Norwegian developments and perspectives on violence risk assessment. *Criminal Justice and Behavior, 41*(12), 1384–1397. https://doi.org/10.1177/0093854814547949

Bjørkly, S., Magnus Waerstad, J., Erik Selmer, L., Waerp, J., Bjørnstad, M., Vegard Leinslie, J., Eidhammer, G., & Douglas, K. S. (2019). Violence after discharge from forensic units in the safe pilot study: A prospective study with matched pair design. *Psychology Research and Behavior Management, 12*, 755–766. https://doi.org/10.2147/PRBM.S214270

Blacker, J. E. (2009). *The assessment of risk in intellectually disabled sexual offenders.* Unpublished master's thesis, School of Psychology, University of Birmingham.

Boer, D. P., Hart, S. D., Kropp, P. R., & Webster, C. D. (1997). *Manual for the Sexual Violence Risk-20: Professional guidelines for assessing risk of sexual violence.* British Columbia Institute Against Family Violence.

Boer, D. P., Tough, S., & Haaven, J. (2004). Assessment of risk manageability of intellectually disabled sex offenders. *Journal of Applied Research in Intellectual Disabilities, 17*, 275–283. https://doi.org/10.1111/J.1468-3148.2004.00214.X

Bonta, J., & Andrews, D. (2007). Risk-need-responsivity model for offender assessment and rehabilitation. *Rehabilitation, 6*, 1–22.

Carlsson, G., Dahlberg, K., Ekebergh, M., & Dahlberg, H. (2006). Patients longing for authentic personal care: A phenomenological study of violent encounters in psychiatric settings. *Issues in Mental Health, 27*, 287–305. https://doi.org/10.1080/01612840500502841

Chu, C. M., Thomas, S. D. M., Ogloff, J. R. P., & Daffern, M. (2013). The short- to medium-term predictive accuracy of static and dynamic risk assessment measures in a secure forensic hospital. *Assessment, 20*, 230–241. https://doi.org/10.1177/1073191111418298

Civilotti, C., Berlanda, S., & Iozzino, L. (2021). Hospital-based healthcare workers victims of workplace violence in Italy: A scoping review. *International Journal of Environmental Research and Public Health, 18*(11), 5860. https://doi.org/10.3390/IJERPH18115860

Clarke, D. E., Brown, A. M., & Griffith, P. (2010). The Brøset Violence Checklist: Clinical utility in a secure psychiatric intensive care setting. *Journal of Psychiatric and Mental Health Nursing, 17*, 614–620. https://doi.org/10.1111/j.1365-2850.2010.01558.x

Coid, J., Yang, M., Ullrich, S., Zhang, T., Sizmur, S., Roberts, C., Farrington, D. P., & Rogers, R. D. (2009). Gender differences in structured risk assessment: Comparing the accuracy of five instruments. *Journal of Consulting and Clinical Psychology, 77*(2), 337–348. https://doi.org/10.1037/a0015155

Cooper, S. A., Smiley, E., Jackson, A., Finlayson, J., Allan, L., Mantry, D., & Morrison, J. (2009). Adults with intellectual disabilities: Prevalence, incidence and remission of aggressive behaviour and related factors. *Journal of Intellectual Disability Research, 53*, 217–232. https://doi.org/10.1111/J.1365-2788.2008.01127.X

Craig, L. A., Beech, A. R., & Harkins, L. (2012). The predictive accuracy of risk factors and frameworks. In A. R. Beech, L. A. Craig, & K. D. Browne (Eds.), *Assessment and treatment of sex offenders: A handbook* (pp. 53–74). Wiley. https://doi.org/10.1002/9780470714362.CH4

Dack, C., Ross, J., Papadopoulos, C., Stewart, D., & Bowers, L. (2013). A review and meta-analysis of the patient factors associated with psychiatric in-patient aggression. *Acta Psychiatrica Scandinavica, 127*, 255–268. https://doi.org/10.1111/acps.12053

Del Pozzo, J., Roché, M. W., & Silverstein, S. M. (2018). Violent behavior in autism spectrum disorders: Who's at risk? *Aggression and Violent Behavior, 39*, 53–60. https://doi.org/10.1016/J.AVB.2018.01.007

Desmarais, S. L., Nicholls, T. L., Wilson, C. M., & Brink, J. (2012). Using dynamic risk and protective factors to predict inpatient aggression: Reliability and validity of START assessments. *Psychological Assessment, 24*, 685–700. https://doi.org/10.1037/a0026668

Dolan, M., & Doyle, M. (2000). Violence risk prediction: Clinical and actuarial measures and the role of the Psychopathy Checklist. *British Journal of Psychiatry, 177*, 303–311. https://doi.org/10.1192/bjp.177.4.303

Douglas, K. S., & Kropp, P. R. (2002). A prevention-based paradigm for violence risk assessment: Clinical and research applications. *Criminal Justice and Behavior, 29*, 617–658. https://doi.org/10.1177/009385402236735

Douglas, K. S., & Reeves, K. A. (2010). Historical-Clinical-Risk Management-20 (HCR-20) Violence Risk Assessment Scheme: Rationale, application, and empirical overview. In R. K. Otto & K. S. Douglas (Eds.), *Handbook of violence risk assessment* (pp. 147–185). Routledge/Taylor & Francis Group.

Douglas, K., & Skeem, J. L. (2005). Violence risk assessment: Getting specific about being dynamic. *Psychology, Public Policy, and the Law, 11*(3), 347–383. https://doi.org/10.1037/1076-8971.11.3.347

Douglas, K. S., & Webster, C. D. (1999). The HCR-20 violence risk assessment scheme. *Handbook of Violence Risk Assessment, 26*, 3–19. https://doi.org/10.1177/0093854899026001001

Douglas, K. S., Cox, D. N., & Webster, C. D. (1999). Violence risk assessment: Science and practice. *Legal and Criminal Psychology, 4*, 149–184. https://doi.org/10.1348/135532599167824

Douglas, K. S., Hart, S. D., Webster, C. D., Belfrage, H., Guy, L. S., & Wilson, C. M. (2014). Historical-clinical-risk management-20, version 3 (HCR-20V3). *Development and Overview, 13*, 93–108. https://doi.org/10.1080/14999013.2014.906519

Doyle, M., & Dolan, M. (2002). Violence risk assessment: Combining actuarial and clinical information to structure clinical judgements for the formulation and management of risk. *Journal of Psychiatric and Mental Health Nursing, 9*, 649–657. https://doi.org/10.1046/J.1365-2850.2002.00535.X

Dvoskin, J., & Heilbrun, K. (2001). Risk assessment and release decision-making: Toward resolving the great debate. *Journal of the American Academy of Psychiatry and the Law, 29*(1), 6–10.

Eidhammer, G., Fluttert, F. A. J., & Bjørkly, S. (2014). User involvement in structured violence risk management within forensic mental health facilities—A systematic literature review. *Journal of Clinical Nursing, 23*, 2716–2724. https://doi.org/10.1111/JOCN.12571

Elbogen, E. B., Tomkins, A. J., Pothuloori, A. P., & Scalora, M. (2003). Documentation of violence risk information in psychiatric hospital patient charts: An empirical examination. *Journal of the American Academy of Psychiatry and the Law, 31*, 58–64.

Emerson, E., Kiernan, C., Alborz, A., Reeves, D., Mason, H., Swarbrick, R., Mason, L., & Hatton, C. (2001). The prevalence of challenging behaviors: A total population study. *Research in Developmental Disabilities, 22*(1), 77–93. https://doi.org/10.1016/S0891-4222(00)00061-5

Fazel, S., Singh, J., Doll, H., & Grann, M. (2012). Use of risk assessment instruments to predict violence and antisocial behaviour in 73 samples involving 24 827 people: Systematic review and meta-analysis. *British Medical Journal (BMJ), 345*, e4692.

Finney, C., Stergiopoulos, E., Hensel, J., Bonato, S., & Dewa, C. S. (2013). Organizational stressors associated with job stress and burnout in correctional officers: A systematic. *BMC Public Health, 13*, 82. https://doi.org/10.1186/1471-2458-13-82

Fluttert, F., Van Meijel, B., Webster, C., Nijman, H., Bartels, A., & Grypdonck, M. (2008). Risk management by early recognition of warning signs in patients in forensic psychiatric care. *Archives of Psychiatric Nursing, 22*, 208–216. https://doi.org/10.1016/J.APNU.2007.06.012

Fluttert, F., van Meijel, B., Nijman, H., Bjørkly, S., & Grypdonck, M. (2010a). Detached concern of forensic mental health nurses in therapeutic relationships with patients the application of the early recognition method related to detached concern. *Archives of Psychiatric Nursing, 24,* 266–274. https://doi.org/10.1016/J.APNU.2009.09.002

Fluttert, F. A. J., van Meijel, B., Nijman, H., Bjørkly, S., & Grypdonck, M. (2010b). Preventing aggressive incidents and seclusions in forensic care by means of the "Early Recognition Method". *Journal of Clinical Nursing, 19,* 1529–1537. https://doi.org/10.1111/J.1365-2702.2009.02986.X

Fluttert, F. A. J., Van Meijel, B., Van Leeuwen, M., Bjørkly, S., Nijman, H., & Grypdonck, M. (2011). The development of the Forensic Early Warning Signs of Aggression Inventory: Preliminary findings: Toward a better management of inpatient aggression. *Archives of Psychiatric Nursing, 25,* 129–137. https://doi.org/10.1016/J.APNU.2010.07.001

Fluttert, F. A. J., Van Meijel, B., Bjørkly, S., Van Leeuwen, M., & Grypdonck, M. (2013). The investigation of early warning signs of aggression in forensic patients by means of the "Forensic Early Signs of Aggression Inventory". *Journal of Clinical Nursing, 22,* 1550–1558. https://doi.org/10.1111/J.1365-2702.2012.04318.X

Fluttert, F., Eidhammer, G., & Dale, K. Y. (2021). Early recognition method: 'Opening doors' in risk management dialogue between mental health and prison services. In S. Hean, B. Johnsen, A. Kajamaa, & L. Kloetzer (Eds.), *Improving interagency collaboration, innovation and learning in criminal justice systems.* Palgrave Macmillan. https://doi.org/10.1007/978-3-030-70661-6_11. This chapter is licensed under the terms of the Creative Commons Attribution 4.0 International License. Retrieved from http://creativecommons.org/licenses/by/4.0/

Fluttert, F. A. J., Bjørkly, S., & Dale, K. Y. (2022). The impact of a discarded diagnosis and focus on early warning signs of aggression on relations between user and municipal service providers—A narrative of a complex case. *Current Psychology, 41,* 5503–5513. https://doi.org/10.1007/S12144-020-01055-X

Gadon, L., Johnstone, L., & Cooke, D. (2006). Situational variables and institutional violence: A systematic review of the literature. *Clinical Psychology Review, 26*(5), 515–534.

Gardner, W., Lidz, C., Mulvey, E., & Shaw, E. (1996). Clinical versus actuarial predictions of violence in patients with mental illnesses. *Journal of Consulting and Clinical Psychology, 64*(3), 602–609. https://doi.org/10.1037/0022-006X.64.3.602

Gildberg, F., Fallesen, J., Vogn, D., Baker, J., & Fluttert, F. (2021). Conflict management: A qualitative study of mental health staff's perceptions of factors that may influence conflicts with forensic mental health inpatients. *Archives of Psychiatric Nursing, 35,* 407–417.

Girardi, A., Hancock-Johnson, E., Thomas, C., & Wallang, P. M. (2019). Assessing the risk of inpatient violence in autism spectrum disorder. *Journal of the American Academy of Psychiatry and the Law, 47,* 427–436. https://doi.org/10.29158/JAAPL.003864-19

Grove, W. M. (2005). Clinical versus statistical prediction: The contribution of Paul E. Meehl. *Journal of Clinical Psychology, 61,* 1233–1243. https://doi.org/10.1002/JCLP.20179

Gudde, C. B., Olsø, T. M., Whittington, R., & Vatne, S. (2015). Service users' experiences and views of aggressive situations in mental health care: A systematic review and thematic synthesis of qualitative studies. *Journal of Multidisciplinary Healthcare, 3,* 449–462. https://doi.org/10.2147/JMDH.S89486

Guy, L. S., Douglas, K. S., & Hart, S. D. (2015). Risk assessment and communication. In B. L. Cutler & P. A. Zapf (Eds.), *APA handbook of forensic psychology* (Individual and situational influences in criminal and civil contexts) (Vol. 1, pp. 35–86). American Psychological Association. https://doi.org/10.1037/14461-003

Hanson, R. K. (1997). *The development of a brief actuarial risk scale for sexual offense recidivism.* Retrieved from https://www.publicsafety.gc.ca/cnt/rsrcs/pblctns/dvlpmnt-brf-ctrl/index-en.aspx?wbdisable=true

Harris, A. J. R., & Tough, S. (2004). Should actuarial risk assessments be used with sex offenders who are intellectually disabled? *Journal of Applied Research in Intellectual Disabilities, 17,* 235–241.

Harris, G. T., Rice, M. E., & Camilleri, J. A. (2004). Applying a forensic actuarial assessment (the violence risk appraisal guide) to nonforensic patients. *Journal of Interpersonal Violence, 19*(9), 1063–1074. https://doi.org/10.1177/0886260504268004

Hart, S. D. (2009). Evidence-based assessment of risk for sexual violence. *Chapman Journal of Criminal Justice, 1*(1), 143–165.

Hart, S. D., & Cooke, D. J. (2013). Another look at the (im-)precision of individual risk estimates made using actuarial risk assessment instruments. *Behavioral Sciences & the Law, 31*, 81–102. https://doi.org/10.1002/BSL.2049

Hart, S., & Logan, C. (2011). Formulation of violence risk using evidence-based assessments: The structured professional judgment approach. In P. Sturmey & M. McMurran (Eds.), *Forensic case formulation*. John Wiley and Sons. https://doi.org/10.1002/9781119977018.ch4

Hart, S. D., Douglas, K. S., & Guy, L. S. (2016). The structured professional judgement approach to violence risk assessment. In P. Boer (Ed.), *The Wiley handbook on the theories, assessment and treatment of sexual offending* (pp. 643–666). John Wiley and Sons. https://doi.org/10.1002/9781118574003.WATTSO030

Hartvig, P., Alfarnes, S. A., Skjønberg, M., Moger, T. A., & Østberg, B. (2006). Brief checklists for assessing violence risk among patients discharged from acute psychiatric facilities: A preliminary study. *Nordic Journal of Psychiatry, 60*, 243–248. https://doi.org/10.1080/08039480600780532

Hartvig, P., Roaldset, J., Moger, T., Østberg, B., & Bjorkly, S. (2011). The first step in the validation of a new screen for violence risk in acute psychiatry: The inpatient context. *European Psychiatry, 26*, 92–99.

Heilbrun, K. (2009). *Evaluation for risk of violence in adults*. Oxford University Press.

Higgins, A., Doyle, L., Downes, C., Morrissey, J., Costello, P., Brennan, M., & Nash, M. (2016). There is more to risk and safety planning than dramatic risks: Mental health nurses' risk assessment and safety-management practice. *International Journal of Mental Health Nursing, 25*, 159–170. https://doi.org/10.1111/INM.12180

Holden, B., & Gitlesen, J. P. (2006). A total population study of challenging behaviour in the county of Hedmark, Norway: Prevalence, and risk markers. *Research in Developmental Disabilities, 27*(4), 456–465. https://doi.org/10.1016/j.ridd.2005.06.001

Hounsome, J., Whittington, R., Brown, A., Greenhill, B., & McGuire, J. (2018). The structured assessment of violence risk in adults with intellectual disability: A systematic review. *Journal of Applied Research in Intellectual Disabilities, 31*, e1–e17. https://doi.org/10.1111/JAR.12295

Johansen, K., Hounsgaard, L., Hansen, J., & Fluttert, F. (2021a). Early Recognition Method—Amplifying relapse management in community mental health care; A comprehensive study of the effects on relapse and readmission. *Archives of Psychiatric Nursing, 35*, 587–594.

Johansen, K. K., Hounsgaard, L., Frandsen, T. F., Fluttert, F. A. J., & Hansen, J. P. (2021b). Relapse prevention in ambulant mental health care tailored to patients with schizophrenia or bipolar disorder. *Journal of Psychiatric and Mental Health Nursing, 28*, 549–577. https://doi.org/10.1111/JPM.12716

Johansen, K. K., Marcussen, J., Hansen, J. P., Hounsgaard, L., & Fluttert, F. (2022). Early recognition method for patients with schizophrenia or bipolar disorder in community mental health care: Illness insight, self-management and control. *Journal of Clinical Nursing, 31*, 3535–3549. https://doi.org/10.1111/JOCN.16181

Kroner, D. G. (2012). Service user involvement in risk assessment and management: The Transition Inventory. *Criminal Behaviour and Mental Health, 22*, 136–147. https://doi.org/10.1002/CBM.1825

Légaré, F., Ratté, S., Gravel, K., & Graham, I. (2008). Barriers and facilitators to implementing shared decision-making in clinical practice: Update of a systematic review of health professionals' perceptions. *Patient Education and Counseling, 73*(3), 526–535. https://doi.org/10.1016/j.pec.2008.07.018

Liberati, E., Richards, N., Ratnayake, S., Gibson, J., & Martin, G. (2023). Tackling the erosion of compassion in acute mental health services. *British Medical Journal (BMJ), 382*, e073055. https://doi.org/10.1136/BMJ-2022-073055

Lidz, C., Mulvey, E., & Gardner, W. (1993). The accuracy of predictions of violence to others. *Journal of the American Medical Association (JAMA), 269*, 1007–1011.

Lindsay, W. R., Murphy, L., Smith, G., Murphy, D., Edwards, Z., Chittock, C., Grieve, A., & Young, S. J. (2004). The dynamic risk assessment and management system: An assessment of immediate risk of violence for individuals with offending and challenging behaviour. *Journal of Applied Research in Intellectual Disabilities, 17*, 267–274. https://doi.org/10.1111/J.1468-3148.2004.00215.X

Lindsay, W. R., Hogue, T. E., Taylor, J. L., Steptoe, L., Mooney, P., O'Brien, G., Johnston, S., & Smith, A. H. W. (2008). Risk assessment in offenders with intellectual disability: A comparison across three levels of security. *International Journal of Offender Therapy and Comparative Criminology, 52*(1), 90–111. https://doi.org/10.1177/0306624X07308111

Lofthouse, R. (2016). *Assessing and managing risk with adults with intellectual disabilities (ID).* DClinPsy thesis, Department of Clinical Psychology, University of Liverpool.

Lofthouse, R., Lindsay, W., Totsika, V., Hastings, R., & Roberts, D. (2014). Dynamic risk and violence in individuals with an intellectual disability: Tool development and initial validation. *Journal of Forensic Psychiatry & Psychology, 25*(3), 288–306. https://doi.org/10.1080/14789949.2014.911946

Malda Castillo, J., Smith, I., Morris, L., & Perez-Algorta, G. (2018). Violent incidents in a secure service for individuals with learning disabilities: Incident types, circumstances and staff responses. *Journal of Applied Research in Intellectual Disabilities, 31*, 1164–1173. https://doi.org/10.1111/JAR.12490

Martí-Agustí, G., Muñoz García-Largo, L., Martin-Fumadó, C., Martí-Amengual, G., & Gómez-Durán, E. L. (2019). Intellectual disability: Criminality, assessment and forensic issues. *Spanish Journal of Legal Medicine, 45*, 155–162. https://doi.org/10.1016/J.REMLE.2019.03.002

Meehan, T., de Alwis, A., & Stedman, T. (2017). Identifying patients at risk of inpatient aggression at the time of admission to acute mental health care. What factors should clinicians consider? *Advances in Mental Health, 15*(2), 161–171. https://doi.org/10.1080/18387357.2016.1259001

Meehl, P. (1954). *Clinical versus statistical prediction: A theoretical analysis and a review of the evidence.* University of Minnesota Press.

Monahan, J. (1984). The prediction of violent behavior: Toward a second generation of theory and policy. *American Journal of Psychiatry, 141*(1), 10–15. https://doi.org/10.1176/ajp.141.1.10

Monahan, J., Steadman, H., Silver, E., & Appelbaum, P. (2001). *Rethinking risk assessment: The MacArthur study of mental disorder and violence.* Oxford University Press.

Monahan, J., Steadman, H. J., Appelbaum, P. S., Grisso, T., Mulvey, E. P., Roth, L. H., Robbins, P. C., Banks, S., & Silver, E. (2019). The classification of violence risk. *Focus, 17*(4), 429. https://doi.org/10.1176/APPI.FOCUS.17404

Newbill, W., Marth, D., Coleman, J., Menditto, A., Carson, S., & Beck, N. (2010). Direct observational coding of staff who are the victims of assault. *Psychological Services, 7*(3), 177–189.

Ng, B., Kumar, S., Ranclaud, M., & Robinson, E. (2001). Ward crowding and incidents of violence on an acute psychiatric inpatient unit. *Psychiatric Services, 52*, 521–525. https://doi.org/10.1176/APPI.PS.52.4.521

Nicholls, T., Peterson, K. L., & Pritchard, M. M. (2016). Comparing preferences for actuarial versus structured professional judgment violence risk assessment measures across five continents: To what extent is practice keeping pace with science? In J. P. Singh, S. Bjørkly, & S. Fazel (Eds.), *International perspectives on violence risk assessment.* Oxford University Press.

Nijman, H. L. I., Allertz, W. F. F., Merckelbach, H. L. G. J., à Campo, J. M. L. G., & Ravelli, D. P. (1997). Aggressive behaviour on an acute psychiatric admissions ward. *The European Journal of Psychiatry, 11*(2), 106–114.

Norko, M. A., & Baranoski, M. V. (2005). The state of contemporary risk assessment research. *Canadian Journal of Psychiatry, 50*, 18–26. https://doi.org/10.1177/070674370505000105

Otto, R. K. (2000). Assessing and managing violence risk in outpatient settings. *Journal of Clinical Psychology, 56*, 1239–1262.

Puddicombe, J., & Lunsky, Y. (2007). Aggression and dual diagnosis: Implications for Ontario's developmental services. *Journal on Developmental Disabilities, 13*, 191–196.

Quinsey, V., Harris, G., Rice, M., & Cormier, C. (2006). *Violent offenders: Appraising and managing risk.* American Psychological Association.

Ray, I., & Simpson, A. I. F. (2019). Shared risk formulation in forensic psychiatry. *The Journal of the American Academy of Psychiatry and the Law, 1*(47), 22–28.

Rice, M. E., Harris, G. T., & Lang, C. (2013). Validation of and revision to the VRAG and SORAG: The violence risk appraisal guide-revised (VRAG-R). *Psychological Assessment, 25,* 951–965. https://doi.org/10.1037/A0032878

Roaldset, J. O., Hartvig, P., & Bjørkly, S. (2011). V-RISK-10: Validation of a screen for risk of violence after discharge from acute psychiatry. *European Psychiatry, 26,* 85–91. https://doi.org/10.1016/J.EURPSY.2010.04.002

Oxford English Dictionary, s.v. "risk (2023)," September 2024. https://doi.org/10.1093/OED/2698784569

Sammut, D., Hallett, N., Lees-Deutsch, L., & Dickens, G. L. (2023). A systematic review of violence risk assessment tools currently used in emergency care settings. *Journal of Emergency Nursing, 49,* 371–386.e5. https://doi.org/10.1016/J.JEN.2022.11.006

Singh, J., Grann, M., & Fazel, S. (2011). A comparative study of violence risk assessment tools: A systematic review and metaregression analysis of 68 studies involving 25,980 participants. *Clinical Psychology Review, 31,* 499–513.

Singh, J., Desmarais, S., Otto, R., Nicholls, T., Petersen, K., & Pritchard, M. (2016). The International Risk Survey: Use and perceived utility of structured violence risk assessment tools in 44 countries. In J. Singh, S. Bjørkly, & S. Fazel (Eds.), *International perspectives on violence risk assessment* (pp. 101–126). Oxford University Press.

Skeem, J. L., Manchak, S. M., Lidz, C. W., & Mulvey, E. P. (2013). The utility of patients' self-perceptions of violence risk: Consider asking the person who may know best. *Psychiatric Services, 64,* 410–415. https://doi.org/10.1176/APPI.PS.001312012

Stringer, B., Van Meijel, B., De Vree, W., & Van Der Bijl, J. (2008). User involvement in mental health care: The role of nurses. A literature review. *Journal of Psychiatric and Mental Health Nursing, 15,* 678–683. https://doi.org/10.1111/J.1365-2850.2008.01285.X

Szabo, K. A., White, C. L., Cummings, S. E., Wang, R. S., & Quanbeck, C. D. (2015). Inpatient aggression in community hospitals. *CNS Spectrums, 20,* 223–230. https://doi.org/10.1017/S1092852914000820

Thornton, D. (2010). *Scoring guide for risk matrix 2000.10/SVC.* Unpublished Document.

Tomlin, J., Egan, V., Bartlett, P., & Völlm, B. (2019). What do patients find restrictive about forensic mental health services? A qualitative study. *International Journal of Forensic Mental Health, 19,* 44–56. https://doi.org/10.1080/14999013.2019.1623955

Van de Sande, R., Noorthoorn, E., Wierdsma, A., Hellendoorn, E., van der Staak, C., Mulder, C. L., & Nijman, H. (2013). Association between short-term structured risk assessment outcomes and seclusion. *International Journal of Mental Health Nursing, 22,* 475. https://doi.org/10.1111/inm.12033

van Leeuwen, M. E., & Harte, J. M. (2017). Violence against mental health care professionals: Prevalence, nature and consequences. *Journal of Forensic Psychiatry and Psychology, 28,* 581–598. https://doi.org/10.1080/14789949.2015.1012533

Van Meijel, B., Kruitwagen, C., Van Der Gaag, M., Kahn, R. S., & Grypdonck, M. H. F. (2006). An intervention study to prevent relapse in patients with schizophrenia. *Journal of Nursing Scholarship, 38,* 42–49. https://doi.org/10.1111/J.1547-5069.2006.00076.X

Veale, D., Robins, E., Thomson, A. B., & Gilbert, P. (2023). No safety without emotional safety. *Lancet Psychiatry, 10,* 65–70. https://doi.org/10.1016/S2215-0366(22)00373-X

Voskes, Y., Van Melle, A. L., Widdershoven, G. A. M., Mierlo, V., Bovenberg, F. J. M., & Mulder, C. L. (2019). High and intensive care in psychiatry: A new model for acute inpatient care. *Administration and Policy in Mental Health, 46,* 34–43. https://doi.org/10.1176/APPI.PS.201800440

Weltens, I., Bak, M., Verhagen, S., Vandenberk, E., Domen, P., van Amelsvoort, T., & Drukker, M. (2021). Aggression on the psychiatric ward: Prevalence and risk factors. A systematic review of the literature. *PLoS One, 16*, e0258346. https://doi.org/10.1371/JOURNAL. PONE.0258346

Westphal, A., & Allely, C. (2019). The need for a structured approach to violence risk assessment in autism. *The Journal of the American Academy of Psychiatry and the Law, 47*, 437–439. https://doi.org/10.29158/JAAPL.003896-19

Whittington, R., Hockenhull, J. C., McGuire, J., Leitner, M., Barr, W., Cherry, M. G., Flentje, R., Quinn, B., Dundar, Y., & Dickson, R. (2013). A systematic review of risk assessment strategies for populations at high risk of engaging in violent behaviour: Update 2002-8. *Health Technology Assessment, 17*. https://doi.org/10.3310/HTA17500

WHO. (2011). *WHO: World report on disability*. World Health Organization [WWW Document]. Retrieved 2.4.24, from https://www.who.int/teams/noncommunicable-diseases/ sensory-functions-disability-and-rehabilitation/world-report-on-disability

Witt, K., van Dorn, R., & Fazel, S. (2013). Risk factors for violence in psychosis: Systematic review and meta-regression analysis of 110 studies. *PLoS One, 8*. https://doi.org/10.1371/ JOURNAL.PONE.0055942

Yang, M., Wong, S. C. P., & Coid, J. (2010). The efficacy of violence prediction: A meta-analytic comparison of nine risk assessment tools. *Psychological Bulletin, 136*, 740–767. https://doi. org/10.1037/a0020473

Young, S., Goodwin, E. J., Sedgwick, O., & Gudjonsson, G. H. (2013). The effectiveness of police custody assessments in identifying suspects with intellectual disabilities and attention deficit hyperactivity disorder. *BMC Medicine, 11*, 248. https://doi.org/10.1186/1741-7015-11-248

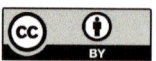

# What Is Coercion and Can Its Use Be Justified in Mental Healthcare? An Ethical Analysis

Christin Hempeler, Matthé Scholten, Anna Werning, and Jakov Gather

## 1 Introduction

The discussion about coercion has a long history in philosophy. Early theories typically understood coercion as the power of one agent to enforce certain actions of other agents. Coercion was largely discussed as an issue concerning the rights and duties held by the state, for example, the enforcement of the law, and was characterised by the use of physical force or violence, or for some, the threat thereof (Anderson, 2023).

By contrast, contemporary philosophical analyses of coercion move away from conceptualising coercion in terms of physical force. Instead, they focus on verbal proposals, mostly in the form of offers or threats, influencing their recipients' choices according to the interests of the coercer. This way of conceptualising coercion was initiated by Robert Nozick's essay 'Coercion' (1969) and has remained influential ever since (Anderson, 2023).

C. Hempeler (✉) · M. Scholten
Institute for Medical Ethics and History of Medicine, Ruhr University Bochum, Bochum, Germany
e-mail: christin.hempeler@ruhr-uni-bochum.de; matthe.Scholten@ruhr-uni-bochum.de

A. Werning
Department of Psychiatry, Psychotherapy and Preventive Medicine, LWL University Hospital, Ruhr University Bochum, Bochum, Germany
e-mail: Anna.Werning@ruhr-uni-bochum.de

J. Gather
Institute for Medical Ethics and History of Medicine, Ruhr University Bochum, Bochum, Germany

Department of Psychiatry, Psychotherapy and Preventive Medicine, LWL University Hospital, Ruhr University Bochum, Bochum, Germany
e-mail: jakov.gather@ruhr-uni-bochum.de

© The Author(s) 2024
N. Hallett et al. (eds.), *Coercion and Violence in Mental Health Settings*,
https://doi.org/10.1007/978-3-031-61224-4_7

People with a mental health condition are exposed to both coercion through physical force (formal coercion) and verbal proposals (informal coercion) in mental healthcare. The significance of the use of coercion lies in its inconsistency with voluntariness, which is a prerequisite for making autonomous choices. Autonomy is part of our self-understanding as human beings. Every individual in a liberal society has the right to live and act according to their own values (Christman, 2020). Accordingly, medical ethics places great emphasis on respecting the autonomy of patients (Beauchamp & Childress, 2019; Jennings, 2009; Pugh, 2020). Beauchamp and Childress (2019, p. 104) state that respecting a patient's autonomy means 'to acknowledge their right to hold views, to make choices and to take actions based on their values and beliefs'. In other words, patients themselves should be the ones ultimately making the decision about any medical intervention according to their values and beliefs—even if these contradict what is advised by the treatment team or relatives.

However, autonomy is not the only moral principle relevant in (mental) healthcare. Instead, it must be weighed against considerations regarding beneficence, non-maleficence and justice (Beauchamp & Childress, 2019). This is reflected in professional codes of conduct, for example, the Code of Ethics for Psychiatry of the World Psychiatric Association (2020) or the Declaration of Geneva of the World Medical Association (2017), which states that 'THE HEALTH AND WELL-BEING OF MY PATIENT will be my first consideration; I WILL RESPECT the autonomy and dignity of my patient' (emphasis adopted).

These guiding moral principles are usually compatible with each other in everyday clinical practice. However, these principles can also come into conflict, for example, when a person with anorexia nervosa refuses to eat. Under certain conditions, a patient's autonomy may be constrained in favour of their well-being, that is, with reference to the principle of beneficence, which may involve the use of coercion. Additionally, mental healthcare is often given the societal task of protecting third parties from dangers that may be posed by people with a mental health condition in both general and forensic psychiatric settings (Albrecht, 2016; Steinert, 2016; Wasserman et al., 2020). To accomplish this task, mental healthcare professionals may use coercion in particular situations.

The use of coercion in mental healthcare raises philosophically relevant questions. Wertheimer (1993, p. 239) distinguishes between two central questions: (1) the 'analytical question' of how coercion can be defined and what actions constitute coercion, and (2) the 'justification question' of whether, and if so how, the use of coercion can be morally legitimised. The aim of this chapter is to investigate these two questions.

The chapter is structured as follows. Firstly, we will consider the analytical question and expound on the distinction between formal and informal coercion. We will then turn to the justification question and differentiate between the two major argumentative strategies drawn upon to defend the use of coercion, that is, one strategy based on the harm principle, and one based on soft paternalism. We will also outline another position holding that coercion can never be justified. Finally, we will discuss self-binding directives as a specific form of psychiatric advance directives that may constitute a way to reconcile autonomy and coercion.

## 2    The Analytical Question: What Actions Amount to Coercion?

### 2.1    Formal Coercion

When speaking of coercion in mental healthcare, what is mostly referred to is formal coercion. Formal coercion, also referred to as compulsion (Szmukler, 2010), is regulated by law, which distinguishes it from so-called informal coercion (Rugkåsa et al., 2016). Formal coercion entails various involuntary interventions, such as involuntary hospital admission, coercive measures (e.g. physical or mechanical restraint, seclusion) or involuntary treatment (e.g. compulsory medication in the form of an intramuscular injection). These interventions are characterised by the fact that they are carried out using physical force and without the service user's consent (Szmukler, 2015). As Szmukler (2010, p. 322) points out, 'the patient has no choice but to accept treatment against his or her will'.

Legal regulations on formal coercion differ across European countries (Albrecht, 2016; Georgieva et al., 2019; Steinert & Lepping, 2009; Wasserman et al., 2020). There are also significant differences between countries in terms of the type and frequency of involuntary interventions (Savage et al., 2024; Sheridan Rains et al., 2019; Steinert, 2016; Steinert & Lepping, 2009). Yet, it is widely acknowledged that the use of formal coercion infringes on a person's fundamental rights, that is, their autonomy, freedom of movement and bodily integrity (Chieze et al., 2021). Furthermore, even if carried out with benevolent intentions, it is undisputed that involuntary interventions can also harm the service user in a number of ways: they may cause physical injuries, psychological traumatization or a loss of trust in the therapeutic relationship, which may lead service users to turn away from the mental healthcare system (Chieze et al., 2019; Horvath et al., 2018; Kersting et al., 2019; Soininen et al., 2016).

Therefore, the use of formal coercion in mental healthcare (and medical practice in general) needs thorough ethical and legal justification and every effort should be made to reduce its use (Herrman et al., 2022; O'Brien & Golding, 2003; Sashidharan et al., 2019).

### 2.2    Informal Coercion

Service users also regularly experience more subtle forms of coercion that, in contrast to formal coercion, are not regulated by law and are, thus, described as informal coercion (Cratsley, 2019; Hotzy & Jaeger, 2016; Yeeles, 2016). Imagine an admission interview during which a woman in a severely manic episode tells the psychiatrist that she does not want to be admitted to the mental healthcare hospital, while the psychiatrist believes she would benefit greatly from an admission. In such situations, mental healthcare professionals, relatives or friends regularly use various communicative strategies to influence the decision-making of service users with the goal of getting them to follow certain treatment recommendations or social rules (Hotzy & Jaeger, 2016; Klingemann et al., 2022; Szmukler & Appelbaum, 2008; Yeeles, 2016). Other prevalent terminologies used in the literature to describe these communicative strategies are 'treatment pressure' or 'psychological pressure' (Klingemann et al., 2022; Yeeles, 2016).[1]

In contrast to formal coercion, which is carried out against the will of service users, psychological pressure and informal coercion leave service users with a choice to make (Potthoff et al., 2022b). Since the aim is to influence service users' decision-making in a way that brings them to consent to something they previously did not want to do (e.g. to take medication or accept treatment in the hospital), the voluntariness of their consent deserves closer consideration. Table 1 shows a comparison of key features of formal and informal coercion.

While there is agreement on the definition of formal coercion, a clear understanding of psychological pressure and informal coercion is still lacking (Yeeles, 2016). One influential conceptualisation has been proposed by Szmukler and Appelbaum (2008) and describes a hierarchy with increasing pressure that includes persuasion, interpersonal leverage, inducements and threats.

According to Szmukler and Appelbaum (2008), the lowest level of pressure is exerted through *persuasion*. It involves a discussion of the arguments for and against a certain treatment option in light of the service user's beliefs and value system. Because the discussion has a preferred and intended result, persuasion goes beyond impartially listing facts, but it remains a (mainly) rational discourse. As an example, imagine a service user with schizophrenia who is reluctant to continue their antipsychotic medication. Trying to persuade them to take their medication, a psychiatrist might stress the importance of the medication for the voices not to come back: 'I

**Table 1** Comparison of formal and informal coercion

| Formal Coercion | Informal Coercion |
| --- | --- |
| Regulated by law | Not regulated by law |
| Physical | Psychological |
| No influence on decision-making | Influence on decision-making |
| Without the consent of the person affected | With the consent of the person affected (but voluntariness is compromised) |

[1] Although often used interchangeably, these terminologies have slightly different meanings (Potthoff et al., 2022b). While 'treatment pressure' was originally introduced by Szmukler and Appelbaum (2008) to describe communicative strategies used to increase treatment adherence, 'psychological pressure' is a broader term that also encompasses pressure to adhere to social rules. We will, therefore, use 'psychological pressure' in this chapter. Acknowledging that not all communicative strategies constitute coercion, we will use the term 'informal coercion' only for those communicative strategies that constitute coercion.

propose you take this medication. Last time, it helped the voices in your head to go away'.

Second in the hierarchy is *interpersonal leverage*. It is based on an emotional bond or even a certain degree of dependency that often develops between a service user and a mental healthcare professional or another care provider. The service user may feel pressured to act in a certain way to preserve that special relationship or to please rather than disappoint the other person. An example is a worried mother telling her daughter: 'I was so proud that you managed to take your medication so well on your own. It would be a pity if we were to have discussions over taking it again now'.

*Inducements* and *threats* are next. To distinguish between the two, Szmukler and Appelbaum (2008) rely on philosophical moral baseline theories of coercion, such as those proposed by Nozick (1969) and Wertheimer (1987). The moral baseline constitutes a point of reference that is based on a theory of rights, the formulation of which is left open, and describes the way that A morally ought to treat B. Regarding the context of mental healthcare, Dunn et al. (2012) suggest setting the moral baseline according to the professionals' duties of care.

According to Wertheimer (1987, 1993), a threat is made if A proposes to make B worse off compared to the moral baseline if B rejects the proposal; that is, if A proposes to make B worse off than B morally ought to be if B rejects the proposal. As an illustration, consider the following example of a mental healthcare professional telling a service user: 'If you don't take your medication, we will cancel your daughter's visit tonight' (Hempeler et al., 2023). The proposal leaves the service user with two options: (a) to take the medication and receive their daughter's visit, or (b) not to take the medication and not receive their daughter's visit. For the sake of argument, let us assume that service users have a moral right to receive visits from their relatives. This determines the moral baseline. We can see now that option (b), non-acceptance of the proposal, makes the service user worse off than they morally ought to be. The proposal, therefore, is a threat.

By contrast, an inducement (referred to as an offer by Wertheimer (1987, 1993)) is made if A proposes to make B no worse off compared to the moral baseline if they reject the proposal; that is, if A proposes to make B no worse off than they morally ought to be if they reject the proposal. Furthermore, upon acceptance of the proposal, inducements make the recipient better off compared to the moral baseline. Again, consider an example for illustration. A mental healthcare professional proposes to a service user: 'If you attend therapy, you will be given an extra cigarette'. Again, the proposal leaves the service user with a choice between two options: (a) to attend therapy and receive an extra cigarette, or (b) not to attend therapy and not receive an extra cigarette. Commonly, service users have no moral right to receive extra cigarettes from mental healthcare professionals; to come back to Dunn et al. (2012), it is not part of professional duties of care to give away cigarettes. Refusal

**Fig. 1** Hierarchy of psychological pressure based on Szmukler and Appelbaum (2008)

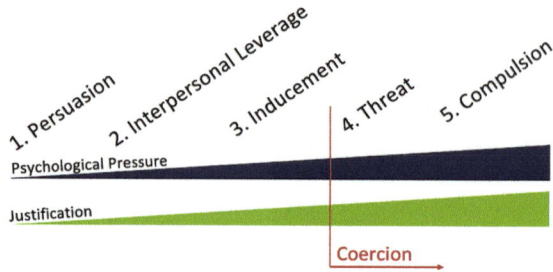

of the proposal, thus, does not leave the service user worse off than they morally ought to be. On the contrary, acceptance of the proposal makes them better off. The proposal, thus, is an inducement.

The distinction between inducements and threats is crucial because, according to baseline theories, only some types of threats—those that leave the recipient no other reasonable choice but to succumb—are coercive, while inducements are not (Wertheimer, 1987). Szmukler and Appelbaum (2008) follow baseline theories in this distinction. Acknowledging that pressure increases within their proposed hierarchy, they hold persuasion, interpersonal leverage and inducements not to be coercive, and only particular threats to constitute coercion. See Fig. 1 below for an overview.

Despite its remaining influence, there is a growing amount of research questioning Szmukler and Appelbaum's (2008) conceptualisation of psychological pressure. Particularly, both observational (Lidz et al., 1993; Sjöström, 2006, 2016) and qualitative studies with service users (Allison & Flemming, 2019; Canvin et al., 2013; Norvoll & Pedersen, 2016; Potthoff et al., 2022b; Verbeke et al., 2019) underline that the context in which an interaction takes place needs to be considered when assessing its coerciveness (Hempeler et al., 2023). For example, in an interview study conducted by our research group (Potthoff et al., 2022b), service users emphasised that contextual factors such as the style of communication, the relationship to the mental healthcare professional and the spatial surroundings play a key role in their evaluation of the coerciveness of an interaction. Similarly, Norvoll and Pedersen construe coercion as a 'relational and contextual phenomenon' (2016, p. 210) and Sjöström (2006, 2016) emphasises that a de-contextualised understanding does not do justice to the reality of coercion in clinical practice. Taking these findings into consideration, we proposed a new conception of informal coercion that incorporates both contextual factors and the service user's appreciation of the interaction (Hempeler et al., 2023). An important implication of our new conception is that not only threats but also other forms of psychological pressure, for example, persuasion, interpersonal leverage or inducements, can be coercive under certain conditions.

# 3     The Justification Question: How, If At All, Can Coercion Be Morally Justified?

There has been little elaboration of the situations and conditions under which the use of psychological pressure and informal coercion may be justified. One of Szmukler and Appelbaum's (2008) central theses is, however, that the greater the psychological pressure applied, the stronger the justification for exercising that pressure needs to be. They suggest the ethical frameworks used for the justification of formal coercion may be helpful for this evaluation.

Problematically, empirical evidence indicates that stronger justification for greater pressure may not always be given in clinical practice. A focus group study conducted by Valenti et al. (2015) showed that mental healthcare professionals often use psychological pressure without being aware of it. Additionally, other studies have found that mental healthcare professionals tend to underestimate the coerciveness of the pressures they use, especially of those higher up in Szmukler and Appelbaum's (2008) hierarchy (Elmer et al., 2018; Jaeger et al., 2014; Schori et al., 2018). Consequently, it should be imperative to increase mental healthcare professionals' understanding and awareness of psychological pressure and informal coercion in clinical practice to enable critical reflection and justification of its use. To this end, Szmukler (2015, p. 259) recommends 'clarifying practice in codes of practice or professional ethics'.

The ethical justification of the use of formal coercion in mental healthcare usually follows one of two argumentative strategies: it is defended for either (a) the protection of third parties with reference to the harm principle (situations of harm to others), or (b) the restoration of the autonomy and well-being of a person currently lacking decision-making capacity with reference to soft paternalism (situations of harm to self). Situations of harm to self and to others often occur simultaneously in clinical practice. Nevertheless, the argumentative strategy ethically justifying a specific involuntary intervention should always be made transparent.

Importantly, even if a coercive measure is considered justified in a certain situation, mental healthcare professionals are morally obliged to ensure that it is carried out appropriately. Procedural justice describes the extent to which service users believe that they were treated fairly, respectfully, and listened to, and whether mental healthcare professionals acted out of concern for them (Lidz et al., 1995). Fair treatment means that the process is transparent and service users are given the opportunity to appeal (McKenna et al., 2001). It has been shown that procedural justice influences the level of service users' perceived coercion (Katsakou et al., 2011; Lidz et al., 1995; O'Donoghue et al., 2014). Service users evaluate coercion more negatively when they experience unnecessary force, are not sufficiently informed or feel a loss of influence (Lorem et al., 2015). When carrying out a coercive measure, mental healthcare professionals should, therefore, be respectful, make their decision-making process transparent and give service users the opportunity to voice their opinions (Gather & Scholten, 2022).

We will next expound the two argumentative strategies and outline a third position that holds coercion to never be justified within mental healthcare.

## 3.1    The Harm Principle

A fundamental and widely endorsed principle in liberal societies is that everyone can do what they want as long as they do not harm others (Large et al., 2008). It follows from this inadmissibility of harming others that third parties have a right to be protected from harm caused by another person. This applies regardless of whether the harm is caused by a person with or without a mental health condition. This so-called harm principle goes back to the philosopher John Stuart Mill and is used to justify involuntary interventions in situations in which a person harms or endangers others. Mill's harm principle states that

> 'the only purpose for which power can be rightfully exercised over any member of a civilized community, against his will, is to prevent harm to others' (Mill, 2015 [1859], p. 13).

With his formulation of the harm principle, Mill states a necessary condition for involuntary interventions: they may only be used to prevent harm to others. It follows that involuntary interventions may not be applied to promote the well-being of the person concerned. Mill makes clear, however, that the harm principle applies 'only to human beings in the maturity of their faculties' (Mill, 2015 [1859], p. 13f.). We will discuss this scope limitation in the next section.

Yet, it does not follow from the harm principle that *all* involuntary interventions can be justified in *all* situations in which a person harms or endangers others: the harm principle specifies a necessary condition for restrictions of freedom, not a sufficient one. Various authors have specified criteria which must be met to justify involuntary interventions in the medical context (Gather et al., 2020; Pugh & Douglas, 2016; Scholten et al., 2022). Involuntary interventions to prevent harm or danger to others can only be justified under the additional conditions of suitability, necessity and proportionality (Gather et al., 2020; Scholten et al., 2022). Importantly, these are valid regardless of the presence of a mental health condition.

1. The intervention must be *suitable* to avert harm to others. It is considered suitable if it is effective in preventing harm to others. Involuntary admission to a psychiatric hospital, for instance, is not suitable in itself to prevent a person in a psychotic state who attacks people in a supermarket from harming others. Without further intervention, it is likely that the person will attack other people, for example, nurses or fellow service users, in the hospital.
2. The intervention must be *necessary* to avert harm to others, that is, there are no less restrictive interventions that are suitable. Mechanical restraint, for instance, is usually suitable to prevent a person from attacking others. Yet, such a drastic intervention is not necessary to protect others if the attacking person can be calmed down verbally, by providing 1:1 care or other milder means. There are a range of interventions which can prevent the use of coercion, for example, de-escalation techniques, calming methods, involvement of peer support workers or debriefing discussions and the formulation of a crisis plans after involuntary interventions have taken place (Committee on Bioethics of the Council of

Europe, 2021; Hirsch & Steinert, 2019; Steinert & Hirsch, 2020). Furthermore, considerations of necessity require that an involuntary intervention only be applied for as short a time as possible and in the least restrictive way (O'Brien & Golding, 2003). This means, for example, that the dosage of medication given for chemical restraint ought to be as low as possible or that mechanical restraint encompasses as few restraints as possible. Carrying out an intervention in the least restrictive way further urges mental healthcare professionals to consider the individual evaluation of which involuntary intervention is considered least restrictive by the service user (Georgieva et al., 2012; Hempeler et al., 2024).

3. The intervention must be *proportionate.* To assess whether an intervention is proportionate, the benefits and risks of intervening must be weighed against the harm to be averted. In other words, the risk-benefit ratio of carrying out an involuntary intervention must be weighed against the risk-benefit ratio of not carrying it out (Scholten et al., 2022). Involuntary interventions in themselves can cause significant harm to the person affected, for example, post-traumatic stress disorder after seclusion or restraint (Chieze et al., 2019) or deep vein thrombosis in conjunction with mechanical restraint (Kersting et al., 2019). Therefore, an involuntary intervention will only be proportionate if the risk averted is high, that is, of considerable impact and probability (Gather et al., 2020).

Importantly, in contrast to situations of harm to self, discussed in the next section, neither a lack of decision-making capacity nor consistency with the person's deeply held values and preferences constitute necessary conditions in situations of danger to others. This can be illustrated by means of the following example: Suppose a person attacks other people and threatens them with a knife. It should be indisputable that the individuals attacked have a right to protection even if the person attacking them has preserved decision-making capacity. No one has the right to infringe on other people's freedom. Involuntary intervention is thus justified under the criteria described.

The same applies if we imagine that the attacker lacks decision-making capacity and has previously stated in an advance directive that they never want to be restrained. Such a previous expression of preferences is irrelevant in the sense that it does not delegitimize the measure, if, and only if, a restraint measure constitutes a suitable, necessary and proportionate means to ensure the protection of third parties in a given situation. Previously expressed preferences are, however, relevant insofar as they can help to identify the least restrictive alternative in the individual case by providing information on how particular involuntary interventions are personally evaluated by a service user (Hempeler et al., 2024).

## 3.2    Soft Paternalism

The promotion of a service user's well-being is identified as the most important reason to justify the use of coercion by Hem et al. (2018) in their systematic review of ethical challenges associated with coercion in mental healthcare. The term 'paternalism' describes a person overriding the will or preferences of another person to promote the latter's well-being, which includes preventing the person from harming themselves (Beauchamp & Childress, 2019; Dworkin, 2020; Feinberg, 1989; Schöne-Seifert, 2015). The principle of respect for autonomy is, therefore, infringed upon with reference to the principle of beneficence.

A differentiation can be made between hard and soft paternalism. While hard paternalism refers to situations in which an autonomous decision is overridden, soft paternalism refers to situations in which a non-autonomous decision is overridden (Beauchamp & Childress, 2019; Dworkin, 2020; Feinberg, 1989; Schöne-Seifert, 2015). Due to the high value placed on individual autonomy, hard paternalism is not considered justified in medical practice (Schöne-Seifert, 2015). This corresponds with Mill who emphasised that involuntary intervention may only be used in cases of harm to others and clarified that

> '[h] is own good, either physical or moral, is not a sufficient warrant. He cannot rightfully be compelled to do or forbear because it will be better for him to do so, because it will make him happier, because, in the opinions of others, to do so would be wise, or even right' (Mill, 2015 [1859], p. 12).

As briefly mentioned above, Mill (2015 [1859]) makes the qualification that this statement is not valid for those who lack the capacity for autonomous choice. His allowance for soft paternalism forms the basis for the contemporary medical ethics analysis that holds soft paternalism to be justified under certain conditions that will be outlined in what follows (Schöne-Seifert, 2015; Wertheimer, 1993).

Before we proceed, let us first clarify further in which cases one can rightfully speak of soft paternalism, that is, in which cases a decision is considered non-autonomous. In the medical context, three conditions must be satisfied for a decision to be considered autonomous as captured in the concept of informed consent: the decision must be informed, voluntary and made by a person with decision-making capacity (Beauchamp & Childress, 2019; Faden & Beauchamp, 1986). Although deficits in either of the three conditions can render a decision non-autonomous, the debate about soft paternalism has largely focused on decision-making capacity.

Decision-making capacity describes 'the ability of subjects to make their own medical decisions' in the sense of ethically and legally valid informed consent (Hawkins & Charland, 2020, p. 1). According to the prominent four abilities model, a person has decision-making capacity if, and only if, they are able to clearly express their choice, understand the relevant information provided in order to make that choice, appreciate their own medical condition, apply the information given and its consequences to their own situation, and weigh the risks and benefits of the different options in light of their own values and beliefs (Appelbaum, 2007; Grisso & Appelbaum, 1998).

Adults are commonly assumed to have decision-making capacity until proven otherwise (Hawkins & Charland, 2020). Importantly, the determination of decision-making capacity must always be made regarding a specific decision at a particular time and thus is not a general judgement (Grisso & Appelbaum, 1998; Kim, 2010). Accordingly, although having a mental health condition is a risk factor for lacking decision-making capacity, it cannot be assumed that people with a mental health condition generally lack decision-making capacity (Grisso & Appelbaum, 1998; Kim, 2010).

Some legal frameworks regulating the use of coercion, for example in Germany, regard the lack of decision-making capacity as one of the preconditions for justifying the use of coercion in situations in which a person harms themselves (Henking & Scholten, 2023). This is discussed within medical ethics as the *capacity criterion* (Gather et al., 2020). The potentially far-reaching consequences of declaring that someone lacks decision-making capacity, that is, fulfilling a precondition of using coercion, underline the importance of a thorough review of decision-making capacity in clinical practice.

In accordance with the capacity criterion, soft paternalistic acts serve the purpose of compensating for a person's current lack of autonomy. The second principle of the World Psychiatric Association's Code of Ethics (2020) underlines that the objective of involuntary interventions 'is ultimately to promote and re-establish patients' autonomy and welfare'. When a person lacks decision-making capacity and capacity cannot be re-established by providing decision-making support, a substitute decision-maker must decide on their behalf (Beauchamp & Childress, 2019). To promote the person's autonomy, surrogate decisions should align with the person's autonomous preferences; this alignment is, therefore, a further necessary criterion for a soft paternalistic intervention to be justified. The surrogate decision should be guided by previously stated preferences, preferably in the form of advance directives or concrete treatment preferences expressed in the past. If there is no evidence of such concrete treatment preferences, a substitute decision should be made based on a person's deeply held values and preferences. This means that the surrogate decision-maker should make the decision the person would have made if they had decision-making capacity at the time (Buchanan & Brock, 1990; Henking & Scholten, 2023). Only if the person's preferences and values are not known, should the substitute decision be made in accordance with the objective best interests of the person (Beauchamp & Childress, 2019).

Since paternalism describes overriding a person's will or preferences for the promotion of their well-being, the justification of involuntary intervention with reference to soft paternalism further demands that the involuntary intervention promotes the service user's well-being. The aversion of serious harm to one's health may be seen as promoting one's well-being (Bester, 2020; Braun et al., 2022; Steinert, 2017; Steinert et al., 2016). In line with the World Health Organization's (1946) definition of health as 'a state of complete physical, mental and social well-being and not merely the absence of disease or infirmity', it has been proposed that not only physical harm but also subjective suffering and harm regarding daily functioning and social participation ought to be considered as potential harms to health (Steinert, 2017; Steinert et al., 2016). Importantly, a short-term harm to one's health where improvement without interference is foreseeable is insufficient to justify an involuntary intervention. Instead, the harm ought to be longer term and, without intervention, a deterioration of the condition must be foreseeable (Gather & Scholten, 2022; Steinert et al., 2016). When contemplating whether an involuntary intervention would promote a service user's well-being, it is crucial to consider the potential harms of involuntary intervention (Chieze et al., 2019; Kersting et al., 2019) as already highlighted with regard to the proportionality criterion above.

The capacity criterion and the condition that the intervention must promote the service user's well-being we have just discussed are unique to cases of harm to self. In addition, the three criteria of suitability, necessity and proportionality, discussed in Sect. 3.1 for cases of harm to others also apply (Gather et al., 2020).

## 3.3 The Use of Coercion in Mental Healthcare Is Never Justified

In their systematic review investigating ethical reasons for or against the use of involuntary interventions in mental healthcare, Chieze et al. (2021) found that most authors agree that there are exceptional situations in which the use of coercion may be justified. They also describe strong agreement that each individual case requires a thorough weighing of reasons and that efforts must be made to reduce coercion in psychiatry to an absolute minimum. However, a few articles included in the review favoured an absolute prohibition of coercion, holding that the benefits of coercion can never outweigh its violation of fundamental rights and central biomedical principles (Chieze et al., 2021). Recently, Dirk Richter (2024) has further argued that empirical research does not support the claims commonly used to ethically legitimise the use of coercive intervention. Along with others, such as Zinkler and von Peter (2019), he therefore suggests a system of psychosocial mental healthcare services without coercion, based on support offers only.

Proponents of a complete ban on the use of coercion in mental healthcare often base their views on the interpretation of the United Nations (UN) Convention on the Rights of Persons with Disabilities (CRPD) proposed by the CRPD Committee (2006). The CRPD is a human rights treaty that was adopted by the UN in 2006 and entered into force in 2008. It has been ratified by 186 States Parties to date. The CRPD Committee has the authority to write reports on States Parties' compliance with the CRPD and comment on individual articles of the convention (United Nations, Department of Economic and Social Affairs). In its General Comment No. 1 (2014, par. 42), the CRPD Committee calls for States Parties to 'abolish policies and legislative provisions that allow or perpetrate forced treatment', explaining that

'it is an ongoing violation found in mental health laws across the globe, despite empirical evidence indicating its lack of effectiveness and the views of people using mental health systems who have experienced deep pain and trauma as a result of forced treatment'.

Zinkler and von Peter (2019) highlight that, according to the CRPD Committee, involuntary hospital admission and treatment violate several articles of the CRPD, including the right to personal integrity (Art. 17), freedom from torture (Art. 15) and freedom from violence, exploitation and abuse (Art. 16).

A discussion about article 12 of the CRPD has been central to this debate (Scholten & Gather, 2018). While the second paragraph of article 12 states that 'States Parties shall recognise that persons with disabilities enjoy legal capacity on an equal basis with others in all aspects of life', the CRPD Committee (2014, par. 25) has interpreted this paragraph as saying that 'all persons, regardless of disability or decision-making skills, inherently possess legal capacity' and, hence, inherently possess the right to provide or withhold consent to hospital admission or treatment. 'At all times, including in crisis situation', the CRPD Committee (2014, par. 18) explains, 'the individual autonomy and capacity of persons with disabilities to make decisions must be respected'. It follows that 'States parties have an obligation not to permit substitute decision-makers to provide consent on behalf of persons with disabilities' (CRPD Committee, 2014, par. 41). According to the CRPD Committee (2014, par. 3), the practice of substitute decision-making should be fully replaced by the provision of supported decision-making.

This interpretation has sparked criticism from many scholars who are themselves proponents of the CRPD and who endorse its purpose and principles (Appelbaum, 2016; Dawson, 2015; Freeman et al., 2015; Scholten & Gather, 2018; Szmukler, 2019). Their criticism is not targeted at the aims and principles of the CRPD; on the contrary, their criticism is precisely that the CRPD Committee's interpretation of Article 12 has adverse effects that run counter to the CRPD's purpose and principles. The purpose of the CRPD is 'to promote, protect and ensure the full and equal enjoyment of all human rights and fundamental freedoms by all persons with disabilities' (Art. 1), and its general principles include respect for individual autonomy, non-discrimination, and full and effective participation and inclusion in society (Art. 3).

Briefly considering psychiatric advance directives will enable us to see why the critics think that the interpretation of the CRPD committee runs counter to this purpose and these principles (Scholten et al., 2019). Imagine Claire, a 23-year-old university student who has experienced several psychotic episodes in which she showed harmful behaviour and had to interrupt her studies for quite some time. Claire responds well to antipsychotic medication and believes that it helps to treat psychotic episodes. She is less convinced, however, that it helps to prevent future episodes. Since she also experiences weight gain as a side effect of the medication, she is inclined to stop taking the medication when well. After her last inpatient stay, Claire completed a psychiatric advance directive in which she documented a preference for the treatment of psychosis with second-generation antipsychotics, such as risperidone, rather than first-generation antipsychotics, such as haloperidol. Three months later, Claire is brought to the mental health hospital because she was roaming the streets without a jacket on a winter night showing self-harming behaviour. Claire agrees to stay in the hospital but refuses all treatment, believing that the staff is intent on poisoning her. Supported decision-making interventions are provided but are of no avail.

The Committee's interpretation of CRPD (2014, par. 42) Article 12 is that people's decisions must be respected 'at all times, including in crisis situations'. It, thus, implies that Claire's treatment refusal must be respected. The critics would argue that this interpretation restricts, rather than promotes Claire's autonomy, and her participation and inclusion in society. After all, in this view, Claire's psychiatric advance directive, containing her autonomous choices, is disregarded and the psychotic episode will probably be prolonged by going untreated, potentially leading to an interruption of Claire's university studies and frustration with her own life goal of attaining a university degree. Involuntary treatment with her preferred antipsychotic medication, subject to the conditions defined in Sect. 3.2 (e.g. suitability, necessity and proportionality), will in this case be more conducive to promoting Claire's autonomy and participation in society.

Another motivation for completely abandoning the practice of substitute decision-making and the use of involuntary interventions is the alleged incompatibility of mental capacity assessments with the CRPD's principle of non-discrimination. The CRPD Committee states that 'perceived or actual deficits in mental capacity must not be used as justification for denying legal capacity' (2014, para. 13) and that 'States Parties should […] [r]eform existing legislation to prohibit discriminatory denial of legal capacity, premised on status-based, functional or outcome-based models [of mental capacity]' (CRPD Committee, 2018, par. 49).

This claim might need to be nuanced. It has been argued that mental capacity assessment itself is not discriminatory, but only the restriction of legal capacity based on it (e.g. Sándor Gurbai in Craigie et al., 2019). In a broader analysis of capacity assessment and discrimination, Scholten et al. (2021a) have argued that the practice of capacity assessment can satisfy the CRPD's demand for non-discrimination only under very strict conditions. These conditions are that (i) capacity assessment is preceded by the provision of adequately supported decision-making; (ii) the diagnosis of the person concerned and the content of their decision (i.e. consent to or refusal of treatment) play no determinate role in the capacity assessment; (iii) the capacity assessment is based on functional criteria related to the person's psychological decision-making capacities which can be assessed reliably; (iv) any determination of impaired mental capacity is considered as valid only for a particular treatment decision at a given point of time; and (v) any substitute decision is based on the deeply held values and preferences of the person concerned rather than on their alleged medical best interests. Insofar as policies and practices of capacity assessment fall short of one or more of these criteria, Scholten et al. (2021a) conclude that these policies and practices discriminate against people with a mental health condition.

# 4     Self-Binding Directives: A Way to Reconcile Autonomy and Coercion?

In Sect. 3.2, we showed that the choices of people who have decision-making capacity must be respected and that people who lack such a capacity may sometimes be protected against making choices that they would not have made had they had decision-making capacity. Advance care planning can provide a way to reconcile autonomy and involuntary intervention, especially for service users with episodic disorders, such as bipolar disorders, major depression or psychotic disorders where periods in which service users have decision-making capacity are repeatedly interrupted by times in which they lack this capacity.

A good way to start thinking about advance care planning is to consider a challenge to substitute decision-making. A major issue for the practice of substitute decision-making is that there is reason to doubt that the decisions that substitute decision-makers make on behalf of people who lack decision-making capacity reliably track the decisions that these persons would have made in the situation had they had the capacity. A systematic review carried out by Shalowitz et al. (2006) showed that substitute decision-makers accurately predicted the choices of the people they represented only in about two-thirds of cases. Although the studies included in the review predominantly tested the accuracy of substitute decisions by means of hypothetical decisions related to end-of-life situations, the findings of the review give reasons not to have too great a confidence in the accuracy of substitute decisions in the context of mental healthcare.

Psychiatric advance directives provide a potential way to address this issue. Psychiatric advance directives are documents that mental healthcare service users can create when they have decision-making capacity and in which they can express their treatment preferences for future situations in which they lack decision-making capacity (Scholten et al., 2019). A service user, for example, can use their psychiatric advance directive to express a preference for second-generation antipsychotics (e.g. risperidone) over first-generation antipsychotics (e.g. haloperidol) in future situations in which they show signs of psychosis and lack decision-making capacity. Accordingly, psychiatric advance directives facilitate substitute decision-making or even make it superfluous if the content of the psychiatric advance directive is sufficiently clear and detailed. Service users strongly endorse psychiatric advance directives and see many benefits in their use, such as promoting autonomy and well-being (Braun et al., 2023). They are also the only intervention that has been shown to reduce the rates of involuntary hospital admissions (Tinland et al. 2022; de Jong et al., 2016; Molyneaux et al., 2019). Although clinicians have expressed concerns about the quality and appropriateness of the content of psychiatric advance directives, research has shown that this content is generally clear and compatible with professional standards (Gaillard et al., 2023).

Psychiatric advance directives do not achieve a full reconciliation of autonomy and coercion, however, because involuntary intervention remains subject to conditions that have been defined by statute or case law in virtually all jurisdictions. That means that service users cannot use standard psychiatric advance directives to request involuntary intervention under self-defined circumstances.

A full reconciliation of autonomy and coercion can only be achieved by means of self-binding directives (SBDs). SBDs are a specific kind of psychiatric advance directive that include a clause in which service users give advance consent to involuntary hospital admission and treatment under self-defined conditions (Gergel & Owen, 2015; Scholten et al., 2021b). They are also commonly referred to as 'Ulysses directives', contracts or arrangements. Much like Homer's Ulysses when he sailed past the isle of the Sirens, service users can use the principle of precommitment or self-binding to achieve certain life goals (e.g. returning to Ithaca or finishing a university degree) by instructing others to overrule anticipated decisions that are incompatible with these goals (e.g. jumping into the sea enchanted by the Sirens' beguiling song or refusing treatment in a manic or psychotic episode). Although service users with, for example, bipolar disorder show a high interest in SBDs (Stephenson et al., 2020), very few jurisdictions worldwide have legal provisions for SBDs, the Netherlands being a notable exception (Scholten et al., 2021b; van Melle et al., 2023).

SBDs can be a useful tool, particularly for people with fluctuating decision-making capacity who anticipate treatment refusals that they do not endorse on reflection, have experience with involuntary hospital admission and treatment, show good recovery between episodes, and have a good insight into their health condition and the possibilities of treatment (Scholten et al., 2023a). Empirical research has shown that stakeholders (e.g. service users, mental healthcare professionals and relatives) see important benefits of SBDs, such as the promotion of service user autonomy and well-being, the avoidance of self-defined harms and the possibility of early intervention (Scholten et al., 2023b). Some of these benefits have already been mentioned by academics in earlier theoretical debates about SBDs (Stephenson et al., 2023).

In these debates, academics and most prominently Rebecca Dresser (1981, 1984) also raised fundamental objections to SBDs. Some academics argued, for example, that the consent to involuntary hospital admission is invalid because it has expired by the time the involuntary interventions are initiated or the person who gave consent to the involuntary interventions is not sufficiently identical to the person who, at a later time, is subject to the involuntary interventions due to a lack of psychological continuity (Stephenson et al., 2023). Recent empirical research showed that stakeholders tend not to voice these concerns and focus more on practical implementation challenges (Potthoff et al., 2022a; Scholten et al., 2023b; van Melle et al., 2023). This suggests that the fundamental objections mentioned may have limited relevance in practice.

The practical challenges that stakeholders identify, however, suggest that SBDs can be implemented successfully only with due care and under strict safeguards. Practical challenges identified by stakeholders include a lack of awareness and knowledge among service users and mental healthcare professionals, a lack of professional support for service users in SBD completion, the presence of undue influence from mental healthcare professionals or third parties during the drafting process, the inaccessibility of SBDs in a mental health crisis, the potentially equivocal nature of SBD content and the potential restriction of therapeutic flexibility due to narrow SBD instructions (Scholten et al., 2023b).

One step in the direction of addressing these challenges is through clear legal regulation (Scholten et al., 2023a). It may, therefore, be helpful to take a brief look into the legal provisions for SBDs in the Netherlands, for which we will rely on the exposition in Scholten et al. (2021b). The formal validity criteria for SBDs in the Netherlands are as follows: the service user who drafted it was at least 16 years old and had decision-making capacity at the time of drafting; the SBD is signed by the service user, the treating mental healthcare professional and the chief psychiatrist (*geneesheer-directeur*), and the period of validity described in the SBD has not expired.

SBDs must also satisfy several content-related criteria. For an SBD to be valid, it must include a description of the circumstances in which the SBD applies, the service user's treatment preferences, the maximum duration of involuntary hospital admission and treatment, the termination criteria for these involuntary interventions, the period of validity of the SBD, and the names and contact information of designated contact people.

Involuntary hospital admission and treatment can be initiated based on SBD instructions if, and only if, the circumstances described in the SBD occur, the service user lacks decision-making capacity and shows a risk of harm to self or others, and the judge grants authorisation of involuntary hospital admission and treatment. The procedure for obtaining legal authorization for SBD activation has been subject to criticism because the time frame for this procedure is much longer than the mean time of decompensation in, for example, bipolar and psychotic disorders, as a result of which SBDs may not yield their potential benefits in practice (Scholten et al. 2021b; van Melle et al., 2023).

Other due care criteria and safeguards that have been proposed to address the challenges of SBDs mentioned above include raising awareness about SBDs through flyers and campaigns, developing training modules for mental healthcare professionals, offering professional support for SBD completion, involving a person of trust and a neutral party (e.g. a peer support worker) in the SBD drafting process, securing SBD accessibility through digital infrastructure, and regularly updating SBD content (Scholten et al., 2023a). Only if such due care criteria are fulfilled and safeguards apply, can SBDs reach their full potential of reconciling autonomy and coercion.

## 5    Self-Binding Directives: A Service User's Perspective

To close off the chapter, one of our co-authors who is an expert by experience, will share their personal view on self-binding directives:

During my first episode of bipolar disorder, I had never heard of psychiatric advance directives, let alone SBDs. Now that I have several years of experience with the disorder, I have completed a joint crisis plan. In a joint crisis plan, the treatment wishes and preferences for a future crisis are written down in a process of shared decision-making with a mental healthcare professional. In Germany, SBDs are not legally regulated or clinically implemented. However, I would strongly endorse the possibility of drafting a legally binding SBD for a tailored situation in a future crisis.

Even though I have never been admitted to the hospital against my will—one of the typical applications discussed in the context of SBDs—I went through some experiences which resulted in personal harm. Due to the mind-confusing effect of the illness, I did various inconsiderate things like excessive shopping for nonsense, for example, unusable items. Consequently, besides the loss of money, my bank account was blocked, and I got in trouble with pending important transfers. A second example is the unreflective activity on social media which led to posts and comments I regretted and found rather embarrassing in retrospect.

In these situations, I would have appreciated someone locking away my bank card and my smartphone. This is an intervention restricting personal liberty which seems less severe than keeping someone in the hospital against their will. However, it may have the potential to protect individuals in crisis from debts and social or emotional harm, which unfortunately is quite a common negative consequence of manic episodes.

SBDs, in my view, present a missing piece in the advance care planning process. After experience with crises, I would find it highly beneficial to be able to determine, for special situations, in advance: who exactly will be legitimized to do what exactly? When I am in a reflected state of mind and capable of making my own decisions, my right to make advance agreements for cases in which I'm unable to grasp the consequences of my decisions, and to take precautions by composing an SBD, should not be limited.

## References

Albrecht HJ (2016) Legal aspects of the use of coercive measures in psychiatry. In: Völlm B, Nedopil N (eds) The use of coercive measures in forensic psychiatric care. Legal, ethical and practical challenges. Springer, pp 31–48

Allison R, Flemming K (2019) Mental health patients' experiences of softer coercion and its effects on their interactions with practitioners: A qualitative evidence synthesis. J Adv Nurs 75(11):2274–2284. https://doi.org/10.1111/jan.14035

Anderson S (2023) Coercion. In: Zalta EN, Nodelman U (eds) The Stanford encyclopedia of philosophy, Summer 2021 Edition. https://plato.stanford.edu/archives/spr2023/entries/coercion/. Accessed 23 March 2023.

Appelbaum PS (2007) Clinical practice. Assessment of patients' competence to consent to treatment. N Engl J Med, 357(18):1834–1840. https://doi.org/10.1056/NEJMcp074045

Appelbaum PS (2016) Protecting the rights of persons with disabilities: An international convention and its problems. Psychiat Serv 67(4):366–368. https://doi.org/10.1176/appi.ps.201600050

Beauchamp TL, Childress JF (2019) Principles of biomedical ethics. Oxford University Press

Bester JC (2020) The two components of beneficence and wellbeing in medicine: A restatement and defense of the argument. Am J Bioethics 20(5):W4–W11. https://doi.org/10.1080/15265161.2020.1745947

Braun E, Gather J, Henking T, et al (2022) [The understanding of well-being in German guardianship law — an analysis o the ocasion of the term's removal from the reformed law]. Ethik in der Medizin 34(4):515–528. https://doi.org/10.1007/s00481-022-00697-8

Braun E, Gaillard AS, Vollmann J et al (2023) Mental health service users' perspectives on psychiatric advance directives: A systematic review. Psychiat Serv 74:381. https://doi.org/10.1176/appi.ps.202200003

Buchanan AE, Brock DW (1990) Deciding for others: The ethics of surrogate decision making. Cambridge University Press

Canvin K, Rugkåsa J, Sinclair J et al (2013) Leverage and other informal pressures in community psychiatry in England. Int J Law Psychiat 36(2):100–106. https://doi.org/10.1016/j.ijlp.2013.01.002

Chieze M, Hurst S, Kaiser S et al (2019) Effects of seclusion and restraint in adult psychiatry: A systematic review. Frontiers in Psychiatry 10:491. https://doi.org/10.3389/fpsyt.2019.00491

Chieze M, Clavien C, Kaiser S et al (2021) Coercive measures in psychiatry: A review of ethical arguments. Frontiers in Psychiatry, 12:790886. https://doi.org/10.3389/fpsyt.2021.790886

Christman J (2020) Autonomy in moral and political philosophy. In: Zalta EN The Stanford encyclopedia of philosophy, Fall 2020 Edition. https://plato.stanford.edu/archives/fall2020/entries/autonomy-moral/. Accessed 30 March 2023.

Committee on Bioethics of the Council of Europe (2021) Compendium Report: Good practices in the Council of Europe to promote voluntary measures in mental health. https://rm.coe.int/compendium-final https://rm.coe.int/compendium-final-en/1680a45740. Accessed 30 March 2023

Committee on the Rights of Persons with Disabilities (2014) General comment No. 1 Article 12: Equality before the law. CRPD/C/GC/1. United Nations. https://undocs.org/en/CRPD/C/GC/1. Accessed 4 August 2023

Committee on the Rights of Persons with Disabilities (2018) General comment No. 6 on equality and nondiscrimination. CRPD/C/GC/6. United Nations. https://undocs.org/CRPD/C/GC/6. Accessed 4 August 2023.

Craigie J, Bach M, Gurbai S et al (2019) Legal capacity, mental capacity and supported decision-making: Report from a panel event. Int J Law Psychiat 62:160–168. https://doi.org/10.1016/j.ijlp.2018.09.006

Cratsley K (2019) The ethics of coercion and other forms of influence. In: Bluhm R, Tekin S (eds) The Bloomsbury companion to philosophy of psychiatry. Bloomsbury, pp 283–304

Dawson J (2015) A realistic approach to assessing mental health laws' compliance with the UNCRPD. Int J Law Psychiat 40:70–79. https://doi.org/10.1016/j.ijlp.2015.04.003

de Jong MH, Kamperman AM, Oorschot M et al (2016) Interventions to reduce compulsory psychiatric admissions: A systematic review and meta-analysis. JAMA Psychiat 73(7):657–664. https://doi.org/10.1001/jamapsychiatry.2016.0501

Dresser RS (1981) Deception research and the HHS final regulations. IRB 3(4):3–4

Dresser R (1984) Feeding the hunger artists: Legal issues in treating anorexia nervosa. Wisc Law Rev 1984(2):297–374

Dunn M, Maughan D, Hope T et al (2012) Threats and offers in community mental healthcare. J Med Ethics 38(4):204–209. https://doi.org/10.1136/medethics-2011-100158

Dworkin G (2020) Paternalism. In: Zalta EN The Stanford encyclopedia of philosophy, Fall 2020 Edition. https://plato.stanford.edu/archives/fall2020/entries/paternalism/. Accessed 31 March 2023

Elmer T, Rabenschlag F, Schori D et al (2018) Informal coercion as a neglected form of communication in psychiatric settings in Germany and Switzerland. Psychiat Res 262:400–406. https://doi.org/10.1016/j.psychres.2017.09.014

Faden R, Beauchamp TL (1986) A history and theory of informed consent. Oxford University Press

Feinberg J (1989) Legal paternalism. In: The moral limits of the criminal law, vol 3: Harm to self. Oxford University Press. https://doi.org/10.1093/0195059239.003.0001

Freeman MC, Kolappa K, Almeida JMC et al. (2015) Reversing hard won victories in the name of human rights: A critique of the General Comment on Article 12 of the UN Convention on the Rights of Persons with Disabilities. Lancet Psychiat 2(9):844–850. https://doi.org/10.1016/S2215-0366(15)00218-7

Gaillard AS, Braun E, Vollmann J e al (2023) The content of psychiatric advance directives: A systematic review. Psychiat Serv 74(1):44–55. https://doi.org/10.1176/appi.ps.202200002

Gather J, Scholten M (2022) Ethisches Spannungsfeld—Patientenselbstbestimmung und professionelle Fürsorge. In: Ethik im Gesundheitswesen. Springer, pp 1–10. https://doi.org/10.100 7/978-3-662-58685-3_48-2

Gather J, Juckel G, Henking T et al (2020) Under which conditions are changes in the treatment of people under involuntary commitment justified during the COVID-19 pandemic? An ethical evaluation of current developments in Germany. Int J Law Psychiat 73:101615. https://doi.org/10.1016/j.ijlp.2020.101615

Georgieva I, Mulder CL, Wierdsma A (2012) Patients' preference and experiences of forced medication and seclusion. Psychiat Quart 83(1):1–13. https://doi.org/10.1007/s11126-011-9178-y

Georgieva I, Whittington R, Lauvrud C et al (2019) International variations in mental-health law regulating involuntary commitment of psychiatric patients as measured by the Mental Health Legislation Attitudes Scale. Med Sci Law 59(2):104–114. https://doi.org/10.1177/0025802419841139

Gergel T, Owen GS (2015) Fluctuating capacity and advance decision-making in Bipolar Affective Disorder—Self-binding directives and self-determination. Int J Law Psychiat 40:92–101. https://doi.org/10.1016/j.ijlp.2015.04.004

Grisso T, Appelbaum PS (1998) Assessing competence to consent to treatment. A guide for physicians and other health professionals. Oxford University Press.

Hawkins J, Charland LC (2020) Decision-making capacity. In: Zalta EN The Stanford encyclopedia of philosophy, Fall 2020 Edition. https://plato.stanford.edu/archives/fall2020/entries/decision-capacity/. Accessed 31 March 2023

Hem MH, Gjerberg E, Husum TL et al (2018) Ethical challenges when using coercion in mental healthcare: A systematic literature review. Nurs Ethics 25(1):92–110. https://doi.org/10.1177/0969733016629770

Hempeler C, Braun E, Potthoff S et al (2023) When treatment pressures become coercive: A context-sensitive model of informal coercion in mental healthcare. Am J Bioethics 1:1–13. https://doi.org/10.1080/15265161.2023.2232754

Hempeler C, Braun E, Faissner M et al (2024) Preferences of individual mental health service users are essential in determining the least restrictive type of restraint. AJOB Neuroscience 15(1):19–22. https://doi.org/10.1080/21507740.2023.2292502

Henking T, Scholten M (2023) Respect for the will and preferences of people with mental disorders in German law. In: Kong C, Coggon J, Cooper P et al (eds) Capacity, Participation, and Values in Comparative Legal Perspective. Bristol University Press. Bristol University Press, pp. 203–225. https://doi.org/10.51952/9781529224474.ch012

Herrman H, Allan J, Galderisi S et al (2022) Alternatives to coercion in mental health care: WPA position statement and call to action. World Psychiatry 21(1):159–160. https://doi.org/10.1002/wps.20950

Hirsch S, Steinert T (2019) Measures to avoid coercion in psychiatry and their efficacy. Deutsches Ärzteblatt International 116(19):336–343. https://doi.org/10.3238/arztebl.2019.0336

Horvath J, Steinert T, Jaeger S (2018) Antipsychotic treatment of psychotic disorders in forensic psychiatry: Patients' perception of coercion and its predictors. Int J Law Psychiat 57:113–121. https://doi.org/10.1016/j.ijlp.2018.02.004

Hotzy F, Jaeger M (2016) Clinical relevance of informal coercion in psychiatric treatment—A systematic review. Frontiers in Psychiatry 7:197. https://doi.org/10.3389/fpsyt.2016.00197

Jaeger M, Ketteler D, Rabenschlag F et al (2014) Informal coercion in acute inpatient setting—Knowledge and attitudes held by mental health professionals. Psychiat Res 220(3):1007–1011. https://doi.org/10.1016/j.psychres.2014.08.014

Jennings B (2009) Autonomy. In: Steinbock B (ed) The Oxford handbook of bioethics (p. 0). Oxford University Press. https://doi.org/10.1093/oxfordhb/9780199562411.003.0004

Katsakou C, Marougka S, Garabette J et al (2011) Why do some voluntary patients feel coerced into hospitalisation? A mixed-methods study. Psychiat Res 187(1–2):275–282. https://doi.org/10.1016/j.psychres.2011.01.001

Kersting XAK, Hirsch S Steinert T (2019) Physical harm and death in the context of coercive measures in psychiatric patients: A systematic review (systematic review). Frontiers in Psychiatry 10. https://doi.org/10.3389/fpsyt.2019.00400

Kim SYH (2010) Evaluation of capacity to consent to treatment and research. Oxford University Press

Klingemann J, Switaj P, Lasalvia et al (2022) Behind the screen of voluntary psychiatric hospital admissions: A qualitative exploration of treatment pressures and informal coercion in experiences of patients in Italy, Poland and the United Kingdom. Int J Soc Psychiatr 68(2):457–464. https://doi.org/10.1177/00207640211003942

Large MM, Ryan CJ, Nielssen OB et al (2008) The danger of dangerousness: Why we must remove the dangerousness criterion from our mental health acts. Journal of Medical Ethics 34(12):877. https://doi.org/10.1136/jme.2008.025098

Lidz CW, Mulvey EP, Arnold RP et al (1993) Coercive interactions in a psychiatric emergency room. Behav Sci Law 11(3):269–280. https://doi.org/10.1002/bsl.2370110305

Lidz CW, Hoge SK, Gardner W et al (1995) Perceived coercion in mental hospital admission. Pressures and process. Arch Gen Psychiat 52(12):1034–1039. https://doi.org/10.1001/archpsyc.1995.03950240052010

Lorem GF, Hem MH, Molewijk B (2015) Good coercion: Patients' moral evaluation of coercion in mental health care. Int J Ment Health Nu 24(3):231–240. https://doi.org/10.1111/inm.12106

McKenna BG, Simpson AIF, Coverdale JH et al (2001) An analysis of procedural justice during psychiatric hospital admission. Int J Law Psychiat 24(6):573–581. https://doi.org/10.1016/S0160-2527(00)00069-8

Mill JS (2015 [1859]) In: Philp M, Rosen F (eds) On liberty, utilitarianism and other essays. Oxford University Press

Molyneaux E, Turner A, Candy B et al (2019) Crisis-planning interventions for people with psychotic illness or bipolar disorder: Systematic review and meta-analyses. BJPsych Open 5(4):e53. https://doi.org/10.1192/bjo.2019.28

Norvoll R, Pedersen R (2016) Exploring the views of people with mental health problems' on the concept of coercion: Towards a broader socio-ethical perspective. Soc Sci Med 156:204–211. https://doi.org/10.1016/j.socscimed.2016.03.033

Nozick R (1969) Coercion. In: Morgenbesser S, Suppes, White M (eds) Philosophy, science, and method. Essays in Honor of Ernest Nagel. St. Martin's Press.

O'Brien AJ, Golding CG (2003) Coercion in mental healthcare: The principle of least coercive care. Journal of Psychiatric and Mental Health Nursing 10(2):167–173. https://doi.org/10.1046/j.1365-2850.2003.00571.x

O'Donoghue B, Roche E, Shannon S et al (2014) Perceived coercion in voluntary hospital admission. Psychiatry Research 215(1):120–126. https://doi.org/10.1016/j.psychres.2013.10.016

Potthoff S, Finke M, Scholten M et al (2022a) Opportunities and risks of self-binding directives: A qualitative study involving stakeholders and researchers in Germany (Original Research). Frontiers in Psychiatry 13:974132. https://doi.org/10.3389/fpsyt.2022.974132

Potthoff S, Gather J, Hempeler C et al (2022b) "Voluntary in quotation marks": A conceptual model of psychological pressure in mental healthcare based on a grounded theory analysis of interviews with service users. BMC Psychiatry 22(1):186. https://doi.org/10.1186/s12888-022-03810-9

Pugh J (2020) Autonomy, rationality, and contemporary bioethics. Oxford University Press

Pugh J, Douglas T (2016) Justifications for non-consensual medical intervention: From infectious disease control to criminal rehabilitation. Criminal Justice Ethics 35(3):205–229. https://doi.org/10.1080/0731129X.2016.1247519

Richter D (2024) Menschenrechte in der Psychiatrie—Prinzipien und Perspektiven einer psychosozialen Unterstützung ohne Zwang. Psychiatrie Verlag

Rugkåsa J, Molodynski A, Burns T (2016) Introduction. In: Rugkåsa J, Molodynski A, Burns T (eds) Coercion in community mental health care. International perspectives. Oxford University Press

Sashidharan SP, Mezzina R, Puras D (2019) Reducing coercion in mental healthcare. Epidemiol Psych Sci 28(6):605–612. https://doi.org/10.1017/S2045796019000350

Savage MK, Lepping P, Newton-Howes G et al (2024) Comparison of coercive practices in world-wide mental healthcare: Overcoming difficulties resulting from variations in monitoring strategies. BJPsych Open 10(1):e26. https://doi.org/10.1192/bjo.2023.613

Scholten M, Gather J (2018) Adverse consequences of article 12 of the UN Convention on the Rights of Persons with Disabilities for persons with mental disabilities and an alternative way forward. J Med Ethics 44(4):226–233. https://doi.org/10.1136/medethics-2017-104414

Scholten M, Gieselmann A, Gather J et al (2019) Psychiatric advance directives under the convention on the rights of persons with disabilities: Why advance instructions should be able to override current preferences. Frontiers in Psychiatry 10:631. https://doi.org/10.3389/fpsyt.2019.00631

Scholten M, Gather J, Vollmann J (2021a) Equality in the informed consent process: Competence to consent, substitute decision-making, and discrimination of persons with mental disorders. J Med Philos 46(1):108–136. https://doi.org/10.1093/jmp/jhaa030

Scholten M, van Melle L, Widdershoven G (2021b) Self-binding directives under the new Dutch Law on Compulsory Mental Health Care: An analysis of the legal framework and a proposal for reform. Int J Law Psychiat 76:101699. https://doi.org/10.1016/j.ijlp.2021.101699

Scholten M, Gather J, Vollmann J (2022) Das kombinierte Modell der Entscheidungsassistenz. Ein Mittel zur ethisch vertretbaren Umsetzung von Artikel 12 der UN-Behindertenrechtskonvention in der Psychiatrie. Der Nervenarzt 93(11/2022):1093–1103. https://doi.org/10.1007/s00115-022-01384-1

Scholten M, Efkemann SA, Faissner M et al (2023a) Implementation of self-binding directives: Recommendations based on expert consensus and input by stakeholders in three European countries. World Psychiatry: 22(2):332–333. https://doi.org/10.1002/wps.21095

Scholten M, Efkemann SA, Faissner M et al (2023b) Opportunities and challenges of self-binding directives: A comparison of empirical research with stakeholders in three European countries. Eur Psychiat 66(1):e48. https://doi.org/10.1192/j.eurpsy.2023.2421

Schöne-Seifert B (2015) Paternalism: Its ethical justification in medicine and psychiatry. In: Schramme T (ed) New perspectives on paternalism and health care. Springer, pp 145–162. https://doi.org/10.1007/978-3-319-17960-5_10

Schori D, Jaeger M, Elmer T et al (2018) Knowledge on types of treatment pressure. A cross-sectional study among mental health professionals. Arch Psychiat Nurs 32(5):662–669. https://doi.org/10.1016/j.apnu.2018.03.005

Shalowitz DI, Garrett-Mayer E, Wendler D (2006) The accuracy of surrogate decision makers: A systematic review. Arch Intern Med 166(5):493–497. https://doi.org/10.1001/archinte.166.5.493

Sheridan Rains L, Zenina T, Dias MC et al (2019) Variations in patterns of involuntary hospitalisation and in legal frameworks: An international comparative study. Lancet Psychiat 6(5):403–417. https://doi.org/10.1016/s2215-0366(19)30090-2

Sjöström S (2006) Invocation of coercion context in compliance communication—Power dynamics in psychiatric care. Int J Law Psychiat 29(1):36–47. https://doi.org/10.1016/j.ijlp.2005.06.001

Sjöström S (2016) Coercion contexts—How compliance is achieved in interaction. In: Molodynski AR, Jorun R, Burns T (eds) Coercion in community mental health care. International perspectives. Oxford University Press

Soininen P, Kontio R, Joffe G et al (2016) Patient experience of coercive measures. In: Völlm B, Nedopil N (eds) The use of coercive measures in forensic psychiatric care. Legal, ethical and practical challenges. Springer

Steinert T (2016) An international perspective on the use of coercive measures. In: Völlm B, Nedopil N (eds) The use of coercive measures in forensic psychiatric care. Legal, ethical and practical challenges. Springer, pp 87–100

Steinert T (2017) Ethics of coercive treatment and misuse of psychiatry. Psychiat Serv 68(3):291–294. https://doi.org/10.1176/appi.ps.201600066

Steinert I, Hirsch S (2020) [German S3 guidelines on avoidance of coercion: Prevention and therapy of aggressive behavior in adults]. Der Nervenarzt 91(7):611–616. https://doi.org/10.1007/s00115-019-00801-2.

Steinert T, Lepping P (2009) Legal provisions and practice in the management of violent patients. A case vignette study in 16 European countries. Eur Psychiat 24(2):135–141. https://doi.org/10.1016/j.eurpsy.2008.03.002

Steinert T, Heinz A, Hohl-Radke F et al (2016). Was ist ein "erheblicher gesundheitlicher Schaden" im Sinne des § 1906 BGB? [What is a "considerable damage to one's health" in the sense of German Guardianship Law?]. Psychiatrische Praxis 43(7):395–399. https://doi.org/10.1055/s-0042-116649

Stephenson LA, Gergel T, Gieselmann A et al (2020) Advance decision making in bipolar: A systematic review (systematic review). Frontiers in Psychiatry 11(1020). https://doi.org/10.3389/fpsyt.2020.538107

Stephenson L, Gieselmann A, Gergel T et al (2023) Self-binding directives in psychiatric practice: A systematic review of reasons. Lancet Psychiat 10(11):887–895. https://doi.org/10.1016/s2215-0366(23)00221-3

Szmukler G (2010) 'Coercive' measures. In: Helmchen H, Sartorius N (eds) Ethics in psychiatry. Springer, pp 321–340

Szmukler G (2015) Compulsion and "coercion" in mental health care. World Psychiatry 14(3):259–261. https://doi.org/10.1002/wps.20264

Szmukler G (2019) "Capacity", "best interests", "will and preferences" and the UN Convention on the Rights of Persons with Disabilities. World Psychiatry 18(1):34–41. https://doi.org/10.1002/wps.20584

Szmukler G, Appelbaum PS (2008) Treatment pressures, leverage, coercion, and compulsion in mental health care. J Ment Health 17(3):233–244. https://doi.org/10.1080/09638230802052203

Tinland A, Loubière S, Mougeot F, Jouet E, Pontier M, Baumstarck K, Loundou A, Franck N, Lançon C, Auquier P; DAiP Group (2022) Effect of psychiatric advance directives facilitated by peer workers on compulsory admission among people with mental illness: a randomized clinical trial. JAMA Psychiatry, 79(8):752–759. https://doi.org/10.1001/jamapsychiatry.2022.1627.

United Nations Treaty Collection (2006) Convention on the Rights of Persons with Disabilities. https://treaties.un.org/pages/ViewDetails.aspx?src=TREATY&mtdsg_no=IV-15&chapter=4&clang=_en. Accessed 4 August 2023

Valenti E, Banks C, Calcedo-Barba A et al (2015) Informal coercion in psychiatry: A focus group study of attitudes and experiences of mental health professionals in ten countries. Soc Psych Psych Epid 50(8):1297–1308. https://doi.org/10.1007/s00127-015-1032-3

van Melle L, van der Ham L, Voskes Y et al (2023) Opportunities and challenges of self-binding directives: An interview study with mental health service users and professionals in The Netherlands. BMC Med Ethics 24(1):38. https://doi.org/10.1186/s12910-023-00915-y

Verbeke E, Vanheule S, Cauwe J et al (2019) Coercion and power in psychiatry: A qualitative study with ex-patients. Social Science & Medicine 223:89–96. https://doi.org/10.1016/j.socscimed.2019.01.031

Wasserman D, Apter G, Baeken C et al (2020) Compulsory admissions of patients with mental disorders: State of the art on ethical and legislative aspects in 40 European countries. Eur Psychiat 63(1):e82. https://doi.org/10.1192/j.eurpsy.2020.79

Wertheimer A (1987) Coercion. Princeton University Press

Wertheimer A (1993) A philosophical examination of coercion for mental health issues. Behav Sci Law 11(3):239–258. https://doi.org/10.1002/bsl.2370110303

World Health Organization. (1946) Preamble to the Constitution of the World Health Organization as adopted by the International Health Conference. 19 January 2024. Available at: https://www.who.int/about/accountability/governance/constitution

World Medical Association. (2017) Declaration of Geneva. https://www.wma.net/policies-post/wma-declaration-of-geneva/. Accessed 30 March 30 2023

World Psychiatric Association. (2020) Code of Ethics for Psychiatry. https://www.wpanet.org/_files/ugd/842ec8_1d812c6b8a4f4d24878ee1db8a6376f6.pdf. Accessed 30 March 2023

Yeeles K (2016) Informal coercion: Current evidence. In: Molodynski AR, Jorun R, Burns T (eds) Coercion in community mental health care. International perspectives. Oxford University Press

Zinkler M, von Peter S (2019) End coercion in mental health services—Toward a system based on support only. Laws 8(3):19. https://doi.org/10.3390/laws8030019

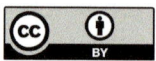

# Coercion in Psychiatry: The Human Rights Challenge

Dirk Richter

## 1 Introduction

The history of psychiatry is a history of human rights violations (Scull, 2015). Until well into the second half of the twentieth century, the rights of people with mental health problems were largely ignored, and coercion and other measures against the will were the order of the day. This changed with the psychiatric reforms of the 1960s and 1970s; now human rights were taken into account but not declared to be the yardstick for action (Zinkler & von Peter, 2019). Surprisingly, it is not only psychiatry as a whole (Hoare & Duffy, 2021), but also social psychiatry that is struggling to implement the United Nations Convention on the Rights of Persons with Disabilities (UN CRPD) (United Nations, 2006) and to completely renounce coercion and other measures against the will of the persons concerned. The following chapter provides an overview of the discussion on human rights and coercion in psychiatric care, the associated controversies and dilemmas, and the question of what significance the human rights approach could have for psychiatry. The main discussion centres on the status of the human rights approach in relation to conventional biomedical ethics and associated ideas about mental disorders.

## 2 Human Rights and Coercion in the History of Psychiatry

The history of psychiatry is part of the general history of humanity and thus also part of the history of personal and individual rights. The first codified catalogues of individual rights have been known since the twelfth century. However, these rights did not apply universally, but usually only to certain groups of people and they often

D. Richter (✉)
School of Health Professions, Division of Nursing, Bern University of Applied Sciences, Bern, Switzerland
e-mail: dirk.richter@bfh.ch

© The Author(s) 2024
N. Hallett et al. (eds.), *Coercion and Violence in Mental Health Settings*,
https://doi.org/10.1007/978-3-031-61224-4_8

excluded other groups such as women. The situation was similar to the rights of people who, according to today's understanding, had mental health problems.

The history of human rights in relation to psychiatry can be divided into three major phases. The first phase can be characterised as pre-psychiatric, as psychiatry as an institution and knowledge system did not exist having emerged only from the eighteenth century onwards. This first phase lasted in the Western world into the eighteenth and nineteenth centuries and can be described as non-medical containment of what was seen as disagreeable or problematic behaviour. Physical coercion and other measures against a person's will are therefore not only part of the present but much more so of the past. In the ancient Greek poet Aristophanes we read that 'madmen' were pelted with stones and in Plato, the 'Laws' (section 934c7) contained a passage for dealing with 'frenzy' which suggested that such persons were best kept away from the public by their own family and that violators should be fined (Thumiger, 2017). Dealing with 'madness' without coercion has never actually existed, at least in Europe, as can be assumed from this evidence.

The second phase began with the development of psychiatry as a subject. The philosopher Michel Foucault characterised the institutionalised beginning of psychiatry in the seventeenth century as a 'great confinement' (Foucault, 1961). Later historical research has confirmed the aspect of confinement in psychiatry but shifted its start to the end of the eighteenth century and the beginning of the nineteenth century and established a link with the Enlightenment. As medical historian Edward Shorter has put it: 'Thus on both sides of the Atlantic, the history of psychiatry began as the history of the custodial asylum, institutions to confine raging individuals who were dangerous to themselves and a nuisance to others'. (Shorter, 1997, p. 7). In custodial asylums, the idea of protection came before treatment. Even then, however, according to Shorter, behind the 'great confinement' was the idea that placement against one's will in the asylums could have a curative effect. This second phase can therefore be characterised as simply ignoring human rights. This phase lasted well into the 1960s and 1970s in many Western countries.

In addition to the history of psychiatry, the history of law is also of considerable importance here. In the transition to the early modern period, the notion of a benevolent state that was allowed to take decisions over its subjects in certain situations prevailed in absolutist states. In the Anglo-Saxon legal tradition, this principle from Roman law was called *parens patriae* (Custer, 1978). The ruler was identical to the state and, according to this legal doctrine, also acted as a parent. As the terminology suggests, the *parens patriae* doctrine was predominantly applied in legal matters concerning the welfare of children. However, the principle of the benevolent state was also applied to people who were considered mentally ill (Wesson, 1980). It was considered a legal principle, for example, in the United States, until well into the 1970s (Zander, 1976). On the European continent, the principle was not called this, but was handled similarly under the concept of state 'welfare' (Müller, 2012). Involuntary placements are still called 'welfare placements' in Switzerland today.

# 3  The Legitimation of Human Rights Restrictions in Contemporary Psychiatry

The pre-psychiatric phase and the human rights-ignoring phase have been followed since the 1980s by a third phase, which is still dominant today. This phase can be characterised in such a way that human rights are perceived and considered but can be restricted for medical reasons. Person-centredness and evidence-based approaches play a crucial role in this phase. The approach was to organise primarily medical psychiatry in the supposed interest of the service users, based on scientific evidence of forms of therapy.

It is one of the ambiguities of the concept of person-centredness that both recovery orientation and the perspective that professionals know what is good for service users can go hand in hand with person-centredness. It is therefore not surprising that in the relevant literature, person- or patient-centredness is seen as a concept that should contribute to the steady adherence to medication (Pyne et al., 2014). It is just another step in a dubious direction when even coercive measures are discussed as potentially person-centred (Rudnick, 2013). The fact that this abandons the notion of 'equal footing' that is inherent in shared decision-making in the context of treatment and care does not seem to matter.

Although a certain contradictoriness or even abstruseness (coercion as a person-centred intervention) must be perceived here, it should be noted that this does not necessarily have to be a contradiction to conventional medical or psychiatric ethics. Person-centredness—as just described—also has a side that is capable of being objectified, and in conventional medical ethics, decisions are generally not made from the perspective of the service user, but from an external perspective 'for the good of the person concerned'. This is also understandable insofar as many of the situations to be ethically discussed in acute somatic care assume that the persons concerned are unconscious and would consent to the measures. Legally, this is conceived as 'natural will' (Nossek et al., 2018).

This is somewhat different in psychiatric settings, as service users are usually not unconscious. Historically, the views of the responsible persons were certainly similar. Until the end of the last century, it was hardly questioned whether coercion could not be in the person's best interest, especially since, in addition to the widespread paternalistic views, there was virtually no empirical research on this question. This was to change only from the mid-1990s onwards when ethical and professional discussion became much more important (Lidz, 1998). However, as time went on, there was increasing discussion about the conditions under which it can be ethically legitimised to treat people psychiatrically against their will. Is it sufficient to establish a medical need or must the illness be accompanied by a risk to oneself and what about risks to other people? And further: what kind of therapy may be used? For example, is electroconvulsive therapy also permitted against the will, as was quite common for decades in the second half of the last century? All these things, which were practised more or less unquestioningly before, have now been ethically and empirically investigated (Tannsjo, 2004). Furthermore, ethical-practical guidelines for dealing with self-injurious or other-injurious behaviour in psychiatric settings have been developed in many countries. There have even been attempts to harmonise this within a European framework (Kallert et al., 2007).

In addition to professional and ethical aspects, legal considerations naturally play a central role in the legitimisation of coercion in psychiatric care. Both national and international courts and legal conventions have increasingly addressed this issue since the 1970s. According to a survey of the ethical and legal aspects of compulsory hospitalisation in 40 European countries, psychiatric coercion is currently legitimised by a combination of the presence of mental illness or an *unsound mind* and the risk to one's own health or the safety of others (Wasserman et al., 2020). In some countries, only the need for treatment as determined by medical professionals and a significantly impaired capacity to judge can be used as justification (Bartlett, 2012). Furthermore, it is generally accepted that the measure should be a therapeutically effective intervention, that it should be used as a *last resort* and that it should be the *least restrictive alternative*. Overall, it is assumed that the measure is in the interest or best interests of the person concerned.

These arguments are within the general framework of the ethical justification of coercion in psychiatry, as a systematic analysis of the arguments commonly used internationally has recently shown (Chieze et al., 2021). The ethical argument in favour of coercive measures in certain circumstances provides for the following aspects to be taken into account: while coercion may pose a threat to autonomy and integrity, it can also serve as a means to restore them. The same applies to human dignity. Coercion can be used for the benefit of the person concerned (benevolence) and serves to avoid harm (non-maleficence). Furthermore, coercion can be fair insofar as individual and social interests are weighed. It can ultimately serve the safety of others as well as oneself and thus also be for the good of a greater whole.

In practice, of course, these arguments also play a role. Generally speaking, in the areas that use coercion in psychiatry, the necessity and also the ultimately positive outcome of corresponding measures is assumed. It is often argued by clinicians that the measure against the person's will also have therapeutic effects, such as the promotion of 'illness insight' as well as compliance with treatment in general and the promotion of the recovery process (Paradis-Gagné et al., 2021). In addition, the use of coercion against the person's will also serves to restore social order. However, in practice, there is also a clear awareness that such measures can jeopardise the therapeutic relationship under certain circumstances (Gerace & Muir-Cochrane, 2019; Theodoridou et al., 2012). These negative consequences, which are also reflected in practice, are evidence of ambivalence in dealing with coercive measures. Nevertheless, the arguments of necessity and the ultimate benefit to the person's well-being prevail (Morandi et al., 2021).

The research literature on this topic also draws attention to a considerable societal change that has occurred in mental health care. Both in general psychiatry and especially in forensic practice, there has been a certain shift in many countries of the Western world from primarily therapeutic aspects to safety aspects as well as risk assessment and risk avoidance (Doedens et al., 2020; Oosterhuis & Loughnan, 2014). In this respect, it is not surprising that these aspects still play a strong role in the legitimisation of coercion in psychiatry.

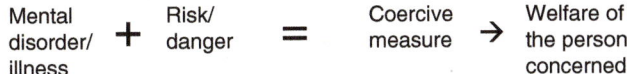

Fig. 1 Justification scheme of psychiatric coercive measures

Considering the numerous country-specific variations in the use of psychiatric coercion (Wasserman et al., 2020), the following schematic sequence for the legitimisation of coercion in psychiatric contexts emerges (Fig. 1).

The existence of a mental disorder with a perceived impaired capacity to judge, combined with a danger that has already occurred or a suspected risk to oneself or other persons, therefore justifies a coercive measure if it is used as a last resort and as the least possible restriction. The overall measure is—according to the assumption—in the interest of the person affected by the coercive measure, who would approve the measure in retrospect. It is further assumed that the compulsory measure is intended to restore the autonomy of the person affected, which is considered to be significantly impaired by the mental disorder. This all presupposes that the therapy associated with coercion is effective and produces the desired results.

## 4     The Challenge Posed by the Convention on the Rights of Persons with Disabilities

In recent years, psychiatry, which essentially takes the position outlined above in connection with coercion in treatment, has had to deal with criticism from unexpected quarters. Repeatedly, the United Nations and its sub-organisations such as the World Health Organization (WHO) have drawn attention to the aspect of violated human rights that arise, for example, through coercive measures. The starting point for this criticism is the Convention on the Rights of Persons with Disabilities (UN CRPD) adopted by the United Nations (UN) in 2006. This was developed through the participation of numerous associations representing people with disabilities. Professional and medical associations, on the other hand, have hardly participated at all in the consultations.

The first important thing to understand about the UN CRPD is that it does not only apply to people with mental or psychological problems. The Convention applies to people with any form of disability, i.e. whether physical or otherwise. The central tenet of the Convention is non-discrimination against people with disabilities. People with disabilities are to be treated in the same way as people without disabilities. They should enjoy the same rights as all other people and this also concerns their rights in health care, for example, in psychiatric treatment.

Article 1 of the UN CRPD formulates how disabilities should be understood, namely as a result of an '…interaction with various barriers may hinder their full and effective participation in society on an equal basis with others'. In other words, the concept of disability follows the so-called social model of disability (Shakespeare, 2006), in which the problem is no longer primarily located within the person, as it was in earlier medical models. Previously, the person had to adapt to an environment of whatever kind, for example, by choosing a living situation according to the person's possibilities and skills. Usually, no further development that helped the person to move out of the situation took place. Today, on the other hand, there are support services available, such as residential and occupational coaching (supported housing/supported employment), which help people cope with living situations that were previously considered impossible for them. In other words, the problem of disability arises in interaction with the social environment and the environment is adapted to the person in such a way that the person can ideally live according to his or her preferences.

Behind the entire Convention is the idea to enable affected persons 'to live independently and to participate fully in all aspects of life', as Article 9 puts it. Applied to today's mental health care, this means the full inclusion of people in society and the possibility to achieve all that people without disabilities can achieve.

Full participation consequently also means legal equality. Article 12 of the CPRD consistently calls for persons with disabilities to retain their legal capacity and to receive support, if needed, to exercise their legal capacity. In a supplementary commentary to Article 12, the responsible UN Committee has explained that—contrary to the legal traditions of many countries—the article calls for a separation of legal capacity and mental capacity (Snellgrove & Steinert, 2017). This means that people who are certified as incapable of judgement should be allowed to refuse medical treatment and thus also psychiatric coercive measures, as they retain their legal capacity in principle. The instrument of legal representation (e.g. guardianship) would thus become obsolete, at least if it were done against the will of the person concerned.

Article 15, sentence 1 of the UN CRPD reads: 'No one shall be subjected to torture or to cruel, inhuman or degrading treatment or punishment. In particular, no one shall be subjected without his or her free consent to medical or scientific experimentation'. With this sentence, involuntary confinement and treatment are defined similar to torture and degradation. It follows that any involuntary form of medical intervention related to disability should be avoided. Accordingly, treatment in psychiatric settings must be exclusively voluntary. While a negative formulation is used here, Article 25, which describes access to health services, explicitly states that 'health professionals undertake to provide care of the same quality to persons with disabilities as to others, including on the basis of free and informed consent…'.

The independent living of persons with disabilities is set out in Article 19. Among other things, it states that 'persons with disabilities must have the opportunity to choose their place of residence and where and with whom they live on an equal basis with others and are not obliged to live in a particular living arrangement' and that they should have access to support services, 'including personal assistance necessary to support living and inclusion in the community, and to prevent isolation or segregation from the community'. This is to make it clear that people with disabilities should no longer have their living arrangements dictated to them but should live as they wish and receive the necessary assistance to do so. Placement against their will in residential homes or similar settings would therefore no longer be permissible. In this context, Article 25 calls for comprehensive outpatient care, including in rural areas, regarding health services.

According to the Convention, independent living and full participation also include equal access to educational opportunities. Article 24 regulates inclusive education, which is intended to prevent the separation of services for people with and without disabilities. Building on the education article, Article 27 formulates the right regarding work and employment as 'the opportunity to gain a living by work freely chosen or accepted in a labour market and work environment that is open, inclusive and accessible to persons with disabilities' and this includes 'equal opportunities and equal remuneration for work of equal value'. Accordingly, employment in sheltered workshops is not of equal value, and persons with disabilities must first be given access to the general labour market if they wish to have it. Finally, Article 28 formulates the right to an adequate standard of living 'for themselves and their families, including adequate food, clothing and housing, and to the continuous improvement of living conditions'.

In summary, consistent implementation of the UN CRPD would not only mean the abolition of psychiatric coercion but also a fundamental prioritisation of the perspective of persons with disabilities over a professional and psychiatric perspective. The will and preferences of the persons concerned would in any case have priority over medical concerns.

---

## 5     Additional Political, Legal and Ethical Challenges in the Context of Human Rights

In connection with the UN CRPD, various UN rapporteurs have repeatedly pointed out the violation of the rights of people with mental problems and denounced coercive measures such as restraint, isolation and forced medication. Coercive measures, they claimed, should be abolished in principle. The accompanying disputes between the psychiatric professional associations and the sub-organisations of the United Nations reached a preliminary climax when the UN Human Rights Council appointed a rapporteur to deal with torture, abuse and degrading treatment in medical institutions. Psychiatric institutions were particularly affected by this report, as it argued:

> Legislation authorizing the institutionalization of persons with disabilities on the grounds of their disability without their free and informed consent must be abolished. This must include the repeal of provisions authorizing institutionalization of persons with disabilities for their care and treatment without their free and informed consent, as well as provisions authorizing the preventive detention of persons with disabilities on grounds such as the likelihood of them posing a danger to themselves or others, in all cases in which such grounds of care, treatment and public security are linked in legislation to an apparent or diagnosed mental illness (UN General Assembly, 2013)

In addition, a follow-up report established a particular link between coercion and the conventional biomedical paradigm. This report accordingly called for fundamental change:

> Coercion, medicalization and exclusion, which are vestiges of traditional psychiatric care relationships, must be replaced with a modern understanding of recovery and evidence-based services that restore dignity and return rights holders to their families and communities. People can and do recover from even the most severe mental health conditions and go on to live full and rich lives. (UN General Assembly, 2017, p. 18)

Recently, the World Health Organization (WHO) has published new guidelines for psychiatric care that focus on the avoidance of coercion and call for the respect of human rights in psychiatry. Here, too, a move away from the biomedical and primarily medication-based paradigm is called for. The guidelines explicitly expect WHO member states to ensure the right of affected people to refuse any form of psychiatric intervention. (WHO, 2021).

The reforms demanded by the UN organisations were not compatible with the traditional medical-psychiatric self-image. In addition, different ethical assessments of the importance of human rights are to be assumed. While the UN CRPD and various other UN documents ascribe a prominent position to human rights and freedoms, this is not the case according to the current mainstream position in biomedical ethics. The most cited textbook on biomedical ethics, for instance, states, '…human rights are not more basic than moral virtues in universal morality…' (Beauchamp & Childress, 2019, S. 4). In other words, human rights do not have a higher status than, for example, medical ethics.

The conflicts between the UN agencies and the medical associations culminated in an exchange of reports and letters between the World Psychiatric Association and the American Psychiatric Association on the one hand and the rapporteur on the use of torture, Juan Mendez, on the other (Grzywnowicz et al., 2013). This exchange ended in a slightly more conciliatory tone from both sides. The rapporteur, Juan Mendez, acknowledged that there may be situations that justify coercion, and the World Psychiatric Association published its own position paper a few years later, which took up many of the criticisms (Herrman et al., 2022).

# 6   'Concluding Observations': The Evaluation of the Implementation of the UN CRPD Using the Examples of Germany and Switzerland

All signatory states of the UN CRPD must regularly undergo an evaluation of their implementation by the UN's 'Committee on the Rights of Persons with Disabilities'. In Germany, at the time of writing this last occurred in 2015 (Committee on the Rights of Persons with Disabilities, 2015) and in Switzerland in 2022 (Committee on the Rights of Persons with Disabilities, 2022). These evaluations are summarised and published in the so-called 'Concluding Observations'. For the purpose of this chapter, it is relevant that the evaluations not only refer to psychiatric care but also to all areas in which people with disabilities are supported, in whatever form. In the following, I will focus on the essential aspects that are relevant for people with mental impairments in both countries.

In general, the evaluations give both states—as well as most other states—a relatively poor report card. For Germany, however, the point in time of 2015 must be considered, when the Federal Participation Act (*'Bundesteilhabegesetz'*) had not yet entered into force. This law from 2016 has the task of implementing the UN CRPD and aims to achieve greater self-determination and equal participation in social life for people with disabilities. Fundamental to both Germany and Switzerland is the criticism of the continuing systems of legal representation of persons with disabilities, i.e. 'legal guardianship' and 'assistance'. In both countries, *substituted decision-making* still takes place, which is generally not compatible with Article 12 of the UN CRPD. Instead of substituted decision-making, the Convention relies on *supported* decision-making, which is based on the separation of judgement and legal capacity (Gooding, 2017). People with any form of disability, therefore, retain their legal capacity and may need support in decision-making from a person they trust, who may, of course, be a professional. Article 12 and related documents such as WHO Quality Rights Initiative (Funk & Bold, 2020) have generated considerable controversy, which, as will be shown in a moment, has even led to suggestions that the Convention should no longer be followed.

Other measures recommended for both Switzerland and Germany concern, in particular, involuntary placement and treatment against the will of the person concerned, as is still common in psychiatric hospitals. Here, the Committee advocates without exception the abolition of placement and treatment without the person's consent. This also includes the abolition of mechanical, physical and medicinal restrictions on movement, including isolation and fixation during inpatient stays.

In the area of social rights, the Convention and subsequently also the Evaluation Committee advocate the right to independent forms of housing and living. This means that the obligation to live in a special form of housing—such as a care home—because of mental impairment, for example, should be abolished. Sheltered jobs, as they are widespread in both countries in workshops in the second labour market, should also be abolished. The general labour market should be accessible to all people with disabilities.

## 7    The Human Rights Controversy

The evaluation reports show that implementation of the UN CRPD has thus far only been successful to a certain extent. At best, in the non-medical area of accompanying persons with disabilities, there have been legal changes such as the already mentioned Federal Participation Act in Germany (Rosemann, 2018) or the so-called Bern Model in the Swiss canton of Berne (Participia, n.d.) which can certainly be seen in the sense of the UN CRPD. Both legal standards are aimed at implementing the Convention. The extent to which these initiatives have improved the situation of the persons concerned remains to be seen in future evaluations. Current data analyses from Switzerland support a relatively sceptical view of the overall development (Hess-Klein & Scheibler, 2022; Richter et al., 2023).

However, it was not only conventional biomedically oriented psychiatry that had problems with the criticism of coercion in mental health care and the accompanying demand to abolish measures against the will of the person concerned and especially the abolition of coercion in psychiatry. One could have expected professionals orientated towards social psychiatry to adopt these demands and initiatives. Although this has happened to some extent, the reactions of many professionals nevertheless look different. The general demand for the abolition of coercion in psychiatry is highly controversial even within social psychiatry. The fundamental controversy revolves around the question of whether the people affected by the care and the possible restrictions of freedom are able to decide for themselves. It is therefore a matter of judgement or mental capacity and the associated legal capacity of the person (Appelbaum, 2016).

The core issue is the relevance of the psychiatric concept of illness. Are people potentially unable to decide for themselves in particular situations due to their mental disorder, or is this an unjustified biomedical simplification of the facts and people can also be fundamentally capable of judgement and legal rights despite any difficulties? In this context, medical positions emphasise that, for example, the human rights to life and health may be jeopardised if measures cannot be taken against the person's will (Scholten & Gather, 2018). This problem is exacerbated, for example, in the context of life-threatening eating disorders.

While human rights are only one of several bases for decision-making from the point of view of conventional biomedical ethics (Beauchamp & Childress, 2019), associations of persons affected by psychiatric disorders emphasise the special relevance of human rights approaches, before which medical considerations should take a back seat (Bundesverband Psychiatrie-Erfahrener and Bundesarbeitsgemeinschaft Psychiatrie-Erfahrener, 2021). These fundamental differences in the assessment of illness and human rights have led, among others in various countries, to calls by medical professionals for their countries to withdraw from the UN CRPD (Gosney & Bartlett, 2020).

The absolute prohibition of coercion, according to this opinion, creates the opposite of rights and leads to a step backwards in humanity. It must be possible to act 'in the interest of the person' even against his or her will. However, this 'interest of the person' is ascribed too much room for interpretation by the proponents of the Convention. Instead of this construct, they seek the view expressed in a supplementary commentary to the Convention to use the 'will and preferences' of the persons. The difference is not to be able to conjecture about interest, but to actually interrogate will and preferences and to act accordingly (Szmukler, 2019).

This means that the same ethical arguments, such as human dignity and the well-being of the person, can be used to argue for the abolition of coercion as well as for its retention. Even clinical arguments can be made for both the retention and the abolition of coercion. If one side can legitimately argue that mental health problems can impair judgement, the other side can just as legitimately point out that the paternalistic approach associated with coercion does not lead to strengthening recovery.

On a political-institutional level, this stalemate has already been described as the 'Geneva impasse' (Martin & Gurbai, 2019). This refers to the fact that within the United Nations and the World Health Organization (WHO), one can find conventions that legitimise coercion (e.g. the International Covenant on Civil and Political Rights) and those that seek to abolish measures against a person's will such as the UN CRPD. This means that even at the level of human rights, both sides are equipped with good arguments. The human rights discourse from a legal perspective is not able to resolve this controversy.

## 8    Consequences of a Consistent Human Rights-Based Care

Can this fundamental contradiction in attitudes towards human rights-based mental health care be overcome? Most likely, not. The fundamental problem of human rights-based approaches such as the WHO's 'QualityRights' is that the conventional system of medical care is adhered to in principle. In various publications, the WHO, for example, has propagated a recovery-oriented approach and praised facilities and services such as Soteria and 'Open Dialogue' as positive examples of a human rights-based approach (WHO, 2021). However, it has adhered to a psychiatric concept of illness that is, in my view, incompatible with the recovery approach. If one truly takes 'will and preferences' seriously, this must also refer to the question of whether the person concerned would describe him/herself as 'ill'. A consistent human rights approach must therefore transfer the power of definition from the mental health care system to the person at stake.

What at first glance seems questionable from a professional point of view has, however, already made itself felt in various respects at present. 'Hearing voices' is no longer necessarily regarded as a symptom of psychosis but can possibly have a subjective biographical meaning. To a certain extent, voice hearing is being de-pathologised and normalised (Higgs, 2020). Something similar arises with the 'neurodiversity' approach advocated by people in the context of autism. Many people who describe themselves as autistic claim to be diverse as opposed to the so-called 'neurotypicals' (Graby, 2015). In this way, the power of definition is claimed by those affected. This is also shown by the 'Mad Pride' movement, which declares itself to be crazy but is also proud of being 'different'. (Rashed, 2019).

In contrast to the 1960s' anti-psychiatry, this is not about denying the existence of mental disorders, but about the fact that the people in question are allowed to determine for themselves whether their 'otherness' should be classified as 'disordered'. Many people would claim to be ill and this is just as unquestionable as the denial of the pathological from a person's point of view.

People who—in whatever form—would become conspicuous and would not see themselves as ill could therefore not be treated in psychiatric systems. In contrast, psychiatry would be exclusively responsible for voluntary measures for those who consider themselves as mentally disordered. Closed doors and physical and pharmacological coercion would be dispensable within the framework of psychiatric care. Individual preferences would be decisive for medical and non-medical support and accompaniment. The eternal arguments about medication would come to an end and individual discontinuation attempts could be professionally accompanied.

The same would apply to housing rehabilitation and occupational rehabilitation. Preference would be decisive for how and with whom people with mental health problems live and in what form they want to work or occupy themselves (Richter & Hoffmann, 2017). Instead of integration into forms of living and working, these would adapt to needs in the sense of inclusion. People with mental health problems could decide whether they want to be supported by trained professionals, by which professions and whether peer support should play a role in this.

Certain changes in human rights are currently visible, at least in outline. For people undergoing voluntary treatment, more freedom of choice is already visible. However, this is not yet visible for people in involuntary treatment. A consistent human rights orientation should, however, aim to fully uphold the fundamental rights and freedoms of the people who make use of the support. This would also result in a change in therapeutic practice. Instead of 'person-centredness', as it is now propagated, 'person-drivenness' should be assumed in the future (SAMHSA 2012). People affected by mental health problems should themselves control how they are treated and supported.

## 9      Dilemmas of a Consistent Human Rights Implementation in Psychiatry

The previous paragraph sounds too good to be true, given the reality of care. The positive developments described there, the avoidance of coercion and the relevance of preferences would then have massive implications for many people and institutions to consider. It is remarkable that the numerous publications of the UN, the WHO and many other advocates of a human rights-based approach to care are almost completely silent on the implications of the abolition of coercion.

At first glance, the problem becomes clear that if psychiatric care were exclusively voluntary, many people who would not classify themselves as ill would find themselves in other institutions such as police custody and prisons. However, in such institutions, as is known from numerous studies, support is hardly available (Fazel et al., 2016). A fundamental dilemma would therefore be to 'transfer' people in difficult situations to where they are likely to be met with less help than in psychiatry.

This would be particularly problematic for people in suicidal crises. A system relying exclusively on voluntariness would lead to suicides that would possibly not occur—at least in the short term—in a psychiatric system operating with coercion. Authorities—and societies as a whole—would have to be prepared to take this risk, especially if additional preventive services were not implemented.

Another problem would arise in relation to offenders. A consistent human rights approach to care would amount to exclusively voluntary forensic psychiatry. There would be a significant increase in detentions and long-term prison sentences and an increase in people with mental health problems in the conventional justice system.

A human rights-based approach to these dilemmas would amount to asking the people concerned whether they experience themselves as ill, what form of support—if any—they want to avail themselves of and whether they are prepared to bear the consequences. Of course, society also has a right to protection from people who prognostically pose a danger. Consequently, this would certainly not lead to less coercion overall, but coercion would no longer take place in psychiatry.

Beyond that, however, approaches to solutions are also conceivable. Police and judicial institutions would have to offer significantly more psychosocial services to better support people in difficult situations. For people in suicidal crises, counselling and support measures should be available that are not linked to coercive measures. This would potentially build greater trust in support services. Furthermore, greater use of advance directives should be considered. According to the existing research literature, these instruments have been shown to reduce coercive admissions (de Jong et al., 2016). Residential support services have also been shown to have a preventive effect on admission to psychiatric hospitals (Adamus et al., 2022a, b). A consistent expansion of outpatient support services, even outside of crisis situations, could make a significant contribution to reducing inpatient stays.

## 10    Conclusions

How big is the human rights challenge to the practice of psychiatric coercion? To date, psychiatry has largely been able to reject these challenges. As long as the conventional psychiatric concept of illness is not revised, psychiatry has—from its point of view and a legal perspective—good arguments against the abolition of coercion. It is difficult to convey to the general public and politicians that mental health problems should not affect legal capacity. This is made more difficult by the fact that acts of violence by people with mental problems are regularly reported in the media and courts often commit these people to forensic hospitals.

This means that the human rights argument alone is not capable of abolishing coercion in psychiatry. Nevertheless, gradual changes can already be seen today, for example, in the legal field, where the UN CRPD has been transposed into national law. However, the consistent implementation of the Convention is legally very controversial (Alexandrov & Schuck, 2021; Müller, 2018). From the legal side, the reaction to the abolition of coercion is predominantly cautious (Wilson, 2021). In contrast, service user organisations are much more positive about the convention (Minkowitz, 2012; Russo & Wooley, 2020). Therefore, it is to be expected that in the future a great impetus towards reforms in mental health care that seek to abolish coercion can be expected especially from service users' organisations.

However, there could also be movement on the issue of coercion and human rights from the medical side. A joint commission of the World Psychiatric Organisation and the journal 'Lancet Psychiatry' called for: 'Legislation (to)... be evidence-based, using evidence-based treatment outcomes informed both by patient experience as a fundamental underpinning and by research aimed at the elimination of coercion and compulsion' (Bhugra et al., 2017, p. 797). Current evidence on the outcomes of coercion in mental health care settings does not suggest that coercion can be justified. For example, the ethico-legal claim that coercion must be used in the best interests of the person is refuted by several systematic reviews (Chieze et al., 2019; Tingleff et al., 2017). From an ethical perspective, the argument of the person's best interest would mean that the person would have to consent to the coercive measure in hindsight—which is only the case for a minority of those affected.

The human rights challenge to psychiatric coercion will not diminish in the future. Psychiatric services and institutions should do their utmost to reduce coercion as much as possible and abolish it 1 day.

## References

Adamus, C., Mötteli, S., Jäger, M., & Richter, D. (2022a). Independent Supported Housing for non-homeless individuals with severe mental illness: Comparison of two effectiveness studies using a randomised controlled and an observational study design (Original Research). *Frontiers in Psychiatry, 13*, 1033328. https://doi.org/10.3389/fpsyt.2022.1033328

Adamus, C., Zürcher, S. J., & Richter, D. (2022b). A mirror-image analysis of psychiatric hospitalisations among people with severe mental illness using Independent Supported Housing. *BMC Psychiatry, 22*(1), 492. https://doi.org/10.1186/s12888-022-04133-5

Alexandrov, N. V., & Schuck, N. (2021). Coercive interventions under the new Dutch mental health law: Towards a CRPD-compliant law? *International Journal of Law and Psychiatry, 76*, 101685. https://doi.org/10.1016/j.ijlp.2021.101685

Appelbaum, P. S. (2016). Protecting the rights of persons with disabilities: An international convention and its problems. *Psychiatric Services, 67*(4), 366–368. https://doi.org/10.1176/appi.ps.201600050

Bartlett, P. (2012). A mental disorder of a kind or degree warranting confinement: Examining justifications for psychiatric detention. *The International Journal of Human Rights, 16*(6), 831–844. https://doi.org/10.1080/13642987.2012.706008

Beauchamp, T. L., & Childress, J. F. (2019). *Principles of biomedical ethics*. Oxford UP.

Bhugra, D., Tasman, A., Pathare, S., Priebe, S., Smith, S., Torous, J., et al. (2017). The WPA-Lancet Psychiatry Commission on the Future of Psychiatry. *The Lancet Psychiatry, 4*(10), 775–818. https://doi.org/10.1016/S2215-0366(17)30333-4

Bundesverband Psychiatrie-Erfahrener, & Bundesarbeitsgemeinschaft Psychiatrie-Erfahrener. (2021). Nicht in unserem Namen! Zur Kritik am Konzept einer freiwilligen Psychiatrie aus Betroffenenperspektive. *Recht und Psychiatrie, 39*, 35–38.

Chieze, M., Hurst, S., Kaiser, S., & Sentissi, O. (2019). Effects of seclusion and restraint in adult psychiatry: A systematic review. *Frontiers in Psychiatry, 10*, 491. https://doi.org/10.3389/fpsyt.2019.00491

Chieze, M., Clavien, C., Kaiser, S., & Hurst, S. (2021). Coercive measures in psychiatry: A review of ethical arguments. *Frontiers in Psychiatry, 12*, 790886. https://doi.org/10.3389/fpsyt.2021.790886

Committee on the Rights of Persons with Disabilities. (2015). *Concluding observations on the initial report of Germany; CRPD/C/DEU/CO/1*. Retrieved December 19, 2023 from https://digitallibrary.un.org/record/811105?ln=en

Committee on the Rights of Persons with Disabilities. (2022). *Concluding observations on the initial report of Switzerland; CRPD/C/CHE/CO/1*. Retrieved December 19, 2023 from https://www.edi.admin.ch/dam/edi/de/dokumente/gleichstellung/bericht/crpd_conculding_observations_2022.pdf.download.pdf/CRPD%20Concluding%20observations%20on%20the%20initial%20report%20of%20Switzerland.pdf

Custer, L. B. (1978). The origins of the doctrine of parens patriae. *Emory Law Journal, 27*, 195–208.

de Jong, M. H., Kamperman, A. M., Oorschot, M., Priebe, S., Bramer, W., van de Sande, R., et al. (2016). Interventions to reduce compulsory psychiatric admissions: A systematic review and meta-analysis. *JAMA Psychiatry, 73*(7), 657–664. https://doi.org/10.1001/jamapsychiatry.2016.0501

Doedens, P., Vermeulen, J., Boyette, L. L., Latour, C., & de Haan, L. (2020). Influence of nursing staff attitudes and characteristics on the use of coercive measures in acute mental health services-A systematic review. *Journal of Psychiatric Mental Health Nursing, 27*(4), 446–459. https://doi.org/10.1111/jpm.12586

Fazel, S., Hayes, A. J., Bartellas, K., Clerici, M., & Trestman, R. (2016). Mental health of prisoners: Prevalence, adverse outcomes, and interventions. *The Lancet Psychiatry, 3*(9), 871–881. https://doi.org/10.1016/S2215-0366(16)30142-0

Foucault, M. (1961). *Folie et Déraison: Histoire de la folie à l'âge classique*. Plon.

Funk, M., & Bold, N. D. (2020). WHO's QualityRights initiative: Transforming services and promoting rights in mental health. *Health and Human Rights, 22*(1), 69–75.

Gerace, A., & Muir-Cochrane, E. (2019). Perceptions of nurses working with psychiatric consumers regarding the elimination of seclusion and restraint in psychiatric inpatient settings and emergency departments: An Australian survey. *International Journal of Mental Health Nursing, 28*(1), 209–225. https://doi.org/10.1111/inm.12522

Gooding, P. (2017). *A new era for mental health law and policy: Supported decision-making and the UN Convention on the rights of Persons with Disabilities*. Cambridge UP.

Gosney, P., & Bartlett, P. (2020). The UK Government should withdraw from the Convention on the rights of Persons with Disabilities. *British Journal of Psychiatry, 216*(6), 296–300. https://doi.org/10.1192/bjp.2019.182

Graby, S. (2015). Neurodiversity: Bridging the gap between disabled people's movement and the mental health survivors' movement? In H. Spandler, J. Anderson, & B. Sapey (Eds.), *Madness, distress and the politics of disablement* (pp. 231–243). Policy Press.

Grzywnowicz, M., Rights, W. C. o. L. C. f. H., & Law, H. (2013). *Torture in healthcare settings: Reflections on the Special Rapporteur on Torture's 2013 Thematic Report*. Center for Human Rights and Humanitarian Law.

Herrman, H., Allan, J., Galderisi, S., Javed, A., Rodrigues, M., & The WPA Task Force on Implementing Alternatives to Coercion in Mental Health Care. (2022). Alternatives to coercion in mental health care: WPA Position Statement and Call to Action. *World Psychiatry, 21*(1), 159–160. https://doi.org/10.1002/wps.20950

Hess-Klein, C., & Scheibler, E. (2022). *Aktualisierter Schattenbericht—Bericht der Zivilgesellschaft anlässlich des ersten Staatenberichtsverfahrens vor dem UN-Ausschuss für die Rechte von Menschen mit Behinderungen*. Editions Weblaw/Inclusion Handicap. Available at: https://www.edi.admin.ch/dam/edi/de/dokumente/gleichstellung/bericht/schattenbericht_aktualisiert.pdf.download.pdf/Aktualisierter%20Schattenbericht.pdf

Higgs, R. N. (2020). Reconceptualizing psychosis: The hearing voices movement and social approaches to health. *Health and Human Rights, 22*(1), 133–144.

Hoare, F., & Duffy, R. M. (2021). The World Health Organization's QualityRights materials for training, guidance and transformation: Preventing coercion but marginalising psychiatry. *British Journal of Psychiatry, 218*(5), 240–242. https://doi.org/10.1192/bjp.2021.20

Kallert, T. W., Jurjanz, L., Schnall, K., Glöckner, M., Gerdjikov, I., Raboch, J., et al. (2007). Eine Empfehlung zur Durchführungspraxis von Fixierungen im Rahmen der stationären psychiatrischen Akutbehandlung. *Psychiatrische Praxis, 34*(Suppl 2), S233–S240. https://doi.org/10.1055/s-2006-952007

Lidz, C. W. (1998). Coercion in psychiatric care: What have we learned from research? *Journal of the American Academy of Psychiatry and Law, 26*(4), 631–637.

Martin, W., & Gurbai, S. (2019). Surveying the Geneva impasse: Coercive care and human rights. *International Journal of Law and Psychiatry, 64*, 117–128. https://doi.org/10.1016/j.ijlp.2019.03.001

Minkowitz, T. (2012). *CRPD advocacy by the World Network of Users and Survivors of Psychiatry: The emergence of an user/survivor perspective in human rights.* Retrieved December 19, 2023 from https://papers.ssrn.com/sol3/papers.cfm?abstract_id=2326668

Morandi, S., Silva, B., Mendez Rubio, M., Bonsack, C., & Golay, P. (2021). Mental health professionals' feelings and attitudes towards coercion. *International Journal of Law and Psychiatry, 74*, 101665. https://doi.org/10.1016/j.ijlp.2020.101665

Müller, M. (2012). Individuelle Selbstbestimmung und staatliche Fürsorge. *Zeitschrift für Schweizerisches Recht, 131*, 63–86.

Müller, S. (2018). Einfluss der UN-Behindertenrechtskonvention auf die deutsche Rechtsprechung und Gesetzgebung zu Zwangsmaßnahmen. *Fortschritte der Neurologie und Psychiatrie, 86*(08), 485–492. https://doi.org/10.1055/a-0597-2031

Nossek, A., Gather, J., & Vollmann, J. (2018). Natürlicher Wille, Zwang und Anerkennung—Medizinethische Überlegungen zum Umgang mit nicht selbstbestimmungsfähigen Patienten in der Psychiatrie. *Ethik in der Medizin, 30*(2), 107–122. https://doi.org/10.1007/s00481-018-0478-8

Oosterhuis, H., & Loughnan, A. (2014). Madness and crime: Historical perspectives on forensic psychiatry. *International Journal of Law and Psychiatry, 37*(1), 1–16. https://doi.org/10.1016/j.ijlp.2013.09.004

Paradis-Gagné, E., Pariseau-Legault, P., Goulet, M. H., Jacob, J. D., & Lessard-Deschênes, C. (2021). Coercion in psychiatric and mental health nursing: A conceptual analysis. *International Journal of Mental Health Nursing, 30*(3), 590–609. https://doi.org/10.1111/inm.12855

Participia. (n.d.). *Berner Behindertenkonzept.* Retrieved August 02, 2022 from https://www.participa.ch/berner-modell/berner-modell/

Pyne, J. M., Fischer, E. P., Gilmore, L., McSweeney, J. C., Stewart, K. E., Mittal, D., et al. (2014). Development of a patient-centered antipsychotic medication adherence intervention. *Health Education and Behavior, 41*(3), 315–324. https://doi.org/10.1177/1090198113515241

Rashed, M. A. (2019). *Madness and the demand for recognition: A philosophical inquiry into identity and mental health activism.* Oxford UP.

Richter, D., & Hoffmann, H. (2017). Preference for independent housing of persons with mental disorders: Systematic review and meta-analysis. *Administration and Policy in Mental Health, 44*(6), 817–823. https://doi.org/10.1007/s10488-017-0791-4

Richter, D., Rühle Andersson, S., Burr, C., Domonell, K., Melina, H., Hegedüs, A., et al. (2023). Menschenrechte in der schweizerischen Psychiatrie—Zum Stand der Umsetzung der UN-BRK. *Psychiatrische Pflege, 8*(2), 9–12. https://doi.org/10.1024/2297-6965/a000479

Rosemann, M. (2018). *BTHG: Die wichtigsten Neuerungen für die psychiatrische Arbeit.* Psychiatrie-Verlag.

Rudnick, A. (2013). Commentary: Can seclusion and restraint be person-centered? *The Israel Journal of Psychiatry and Related Sciences, 50*(1), 11–12.

Russo, J., & Wooley, S. (2020). The implementation of the convention on the rights of persons with disabilities: More than just another reform of psychiatry. *Health and Human Rights, 22*(1), 151–161.

SAMHSA (2012). SAMHSA's Working Definition of Recovery. https://store.samhsa.gov/sites/default/files/pep12-recdef.pdf. Retrieved October 14, 2024.

Scholten, M., & Gather, J. (2018). Adverse consequences of article 12 of the UN Convention on the rights of Persons with Disabilities for persons with mental disabilities and an alternative way forward. *Journal of Medical Ethics, 44*(4), 226–233. https://doi.org/10.1136/medethics-2017-104414

Scull, A. (2015). *Madness in civilization: A cultural history of insanity from the Bible to Freud, from the madhouse to modern medicine.* Princeton UP.

Shakespeare, T. (2006). The social model of disability. In L. J. Davis (Ed.), *The disability studies reader* (pp. 197–204). Routledge.

Shorter, E. (1997). *A history of psychiatry: From the era of the asylum to the age of Prozac*. Wiley.

Snellgrove, B. J., & Steinert, T. (2017). Einwilligungsfähigkeit vor dem Hintergrund der UN-Behindertenrechtskonvention. *Forensische Psychiatrie, Psychologie, Kriminologie, 11*(3), 234–243. https://doi.org/10.1007/s11757-017-0427-2

Szmukler, G. (2019). "Capacity", "best interests", "will and preferences" and the UN Convention on the rights of Persons with Disabilities. *World Psychiatry, 18*(1), 34–41. https://doi.org/10.1002/wps.20584

Tannsjo, T. (2004). The convention on human rights and biomedicine and the use of coercion in psychiatry. *Journal of Medical Ethics, 30*(5), 430–434. https://doi.org/10.1136/jme.2002.000703

Theodoridou, A., Schlatter, F., Ajdacic, V., Rössler, W., & Jäger, M. (2012). Therapeutic relationship in the context of perceived coercion in a psychiatric population. *Psychiatry Research, 200*(2), 939–944. https://doi.org/10.1016/j.psychres.2012.04.012

Thumiger, C. (2017). Ancient Greek and Roman traditions. In G. Eghigian (Ed.), *The Routledge history of madness and mental health* (pp. 42–61). Routledge.

Tingleff, E. B., Bradley, S. K., Gildberg, F. A., Munksgaard, G., & Hounsgaard, L. (2017). "Treat me with respect". A systematic review and thematic analysis of psychiatric patients' reported perceptions of the situations associated with the process of coercion. *Journal of Psychiatric and Mental Health Nursing, 24*(9–10), 681–698. https://doi.org/10.1111/jpm.12410

UN General Assembly. (2013). *Report of the Special Rapporteur on Torture and Other Cruel, Inhuman or Degrading Treatment or Punishment, Juan E. Méndez*. A/HRC/22/53.

UN General Assembly. (2017). *Report of the Special Rapporteur on the Right of Everyone to the Enjoyment of the Highest Attainable Standard of Physical and Mental Health*. A/HRC/35/21.

United Nations. (2006). *UN Convention on the Rights of Persons with Disabilities*. Retrieved December 19, 2023 from https://www.un.org/development/desa/disabilities/convention-on-the-rights-of-persons-with-disabilities/convention-on-the-rights-of-persons-with-disabilities-2.html

Wasserman, D., Apter, G., Baeken, C., Bailey, S., Balazs, J., Bec, C., et al. (2020). Compulsory admissions of patients with mental disorders: State of the art on ethical and legislative aspects in 40 European countries. *European Psychiatry, 63*(1), e82. https://doi.org/10.1192/j.eurpsy.2020.79

Wesson, M. (1980). Substituted judgment: The parens patriae justification for involuntary treatment of the mentally ill. *Journal of Psychiatry & Law, 8*, 147–165.

WHO. (2021). *Guidance on community mental health services: Promoting person-centred and rights-based approaches*. World Health Organisation. Available at: https://www.who.int/publications/i/item/9789240025707

Wilson, K. (2021). *Mental health law: Abolish or reform?* Oxford University Press.

Zander, T. K. (1976). Civil commitment in Wisconsin: The impact of Lessard v. Schmidt. *Wisconsin Law Review, 1976*, 503–562.

Zinkler, M., & von Peter, S. (2019). End coercion in mental health services—Toward a system based on support only. *Laws, 8*(3), 19. https://www.mdpi.com/2075-471X/8/3/19

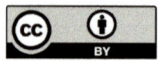

# Reducing Involuntary Admissions

Jim Maguire, Trond Hatling, and Solveig Kjus

## 1 Introduction

Modern psychiatry was once described as being 'uncomfortably wedged between the territories of law and medicine, between coercion and care' (Welsh & Deahl, 2002) as cited in Feiring and Ugstad (2014, p. 10). One of the areas where this tension is most evident is that of involuntary admission[1] and treatment, both controversial practices within mental health services worldwide. This chapter will focus on involuntary admission only, with other non-consensual practices being addressed elsewhere within the book. The controversy is multidimensional, encompassing effects on therapeutic relationships (Balducci et al., 2017) and the principles of recovery (Courtney & Moulding, 2014), psychological consequences, substituted and supported decision-making, possibilities for misuse or abuse, lack of standardisation (Fistein et al., 2016), public safety (Balducci et al., 2017) and denial of human rights (Pūras, 2017). It is no surprise then that a push for reform of related legislation and policy, and even for the abolition of involuntary admission, has gained considerable momentum in recent decades.

---

[1] Also known as involuntary/forced detention/commitment, compulsory admission/detention/commitment, civil commitment (US), formal admission (UK), sectioning (UK, IRL), certification (IRL). In this text, *admission* and *detention* are used interchangeably.

---

J. Maguire (✉)
Department of Health Sciences, Technological University of the Shannon,
Athlone, Westmeath, Ireland
e-mail: jim.maguire@tus.ie

T. Hatling · S. Kjus
Norwegian Resource Center for Community Mental Health (NAPHA), NTNU Social
Research, Trondheim, Norway
e-mail: trond.hatling@samforsk.no; solveig.kjus@samforsk.no

© The Author(s) 2024                                                        191
N. Hallett et al. (eds.), *Coercion and Violence in Mental Health Settings*,
https://doi.org/10.1007/978-3-031-61224-4_9

## 2    Involuntary Admission as a Concept

Defining exactly what involuntary admission is can be problematic. Put simply, it is the detention of a person, against their will, within a mental health facility. However, criteria for its use, and how it is initiated, arranged, monitored and reviewed vary considerably in Europe, depending on socio-cultural and legislative contexts (Johnson et al., 2016; Kallert et al., 2005), as do rates of admissions and processes involved. Even the concept of voluntariness is not straightforward, with many purportedly voluntary patients reporting they felt their admission was coerced (Gerle et al., 2019; Silva et al., 2023). Feeling compelled to voluntarily accept treatment because of fear that refusal may result in the use of coercion was labelled the 'coercive shadow' by Szmukler (2015), indicating that the binary legal concept of voluntary or involuntary status is insufficient to describe the phenomenon. The concept is commonly divided into three: formal coercion (regulated by law), informal status (different measures not regulated by the law) and perceived coercion (whether the patient feels coerced or not). This chapter primarily deals with involuntary admission as formal coercion.

The usual justifications in legislation for the use of involuntary admission are dangerousness/risk to self or others, need for treatment and diminished decision-making capacity (mental capacity or competence) (Gooding, 2017). These are clinically important concepts but notoriously difficult ones to define in legislation and all have been eruditely challenged and defended within the literature (Akther et al., 2019; Callaghan & Grundy, 2018). It is still useful to consider each of these in turn, keeping in mind that these concepts are not uniformly defined across countries.

## 2.1    Dangerousness

Dangerousness is the propensity to engage in self-harming, suicidal, impulsive or reckless behaviours, intolerable harassment and threats or actual violence towards others. Justification for detaining someone under this criterion incorporates the utilitarian position of protecting the greater good, i.e. society (Lepping et al., 2004). Clinicians make determinations of dangerousness or risk to self or others mainly based on their intuition and experience, combined with known client history. Though the use of actuarial or structured risk assessment is increasing, nurses have been noted to still defer to their clinical intuition over scores from a structured risk assessment instrument, when making clinical judgements (Conlon et al., 2019).

However, risk assessment by any means is fraught with difficulties. It may do little to reduce harm and increase people's safety and it has been reported as being individual-centric, ignoring wider environmental, societal and behavioural influences that foment violence and has been described as stigmatising and discriminatory (Callaghan & Grundy, 2018). Citing dangerousness as grounds for the admission of an individual is controversial. Experienced clinicians contend that they know when there is a risk of harm posed by a patient. Sometimes this multifactorial, complex 'reading' of a situation has been referred to as 'situation awareness'

(Endsley, 2015; Patterson et al., 2016). However, preventative detention has often been applied unequally to people with a diagnosis of mental illness. An example, given by Gooding and Flynn (2015), is where other groups who are credibly more likely to be violent to others (such as young men consuming alcohol or known perpetrators of domestic violence) do not face similar curtailments of liberty and autonomy.

The attribution by the public of dangerousness to people with mental illness has been shown to be increasing over the past three decades (Pescosolido et al., 2019). Dangerousness and calls for the protection of others are common criteria for involuntary detention and treatment. The potential for mental health teams to expand activities directed at social control in response to community fears must be recognised (Szmukler & Appelbaum, 2008). A dialogue between those advocating on behalf of patients with mental illness and a community increasingly preoccupied with risk is essential if abuses are to be avoided.

Using dangerousness as a criterion for involuntary admission has been declared a breach of Article 12 of the United Nations Convention on the Rights of People with Disabilities (CRPD), which requires people with disabilities to be recognised equally before the law. In general society, predictions of dangerousness have little legal standing and a person is innocent until they are proven to have committed a criminal act. The CRPD committee argues that people with mental health problems have no more right to pose danger to others than people without disabilities but where they do pose such risks, criminal or other legislation is in place to deal with those matters. However, when the danger to others is associated with mental illness, the person is derogated to a separate track of law, i.e. mental health legislation (Skoric & Gagro, 2020). The CRPD contends these laws have a lower standard of human rights protection, and this is inequality before the law.

## 2.2     Need for Treatment

The mental health legislation of many countries uses the need for treatment as a prerequisite for involuntary detention, either as the sole criterion or in addition to the danger criterion (Salize et al., 2002). While in some countries involuntary detention also includes the right to treat the patient with medication without consent, in other countries this requires a separate decision (Kallert et al., 2006). The need for treatment is founded on the ethical principle of responsibility of care; the right to necessary help and the health professional's duty to give help. The contention is that society thus has an obligation to give such help if the individual is not able to take self-care and, if necessary, to do so by coercion. The clinical argument points to the purported benefits of early interventions, but the evidence for such benefits is often unclear (Malhi et al., 2021).

Treating someone against their will requires that there is an effective treatment for the mental illness and that this treatment also works if it is given compulsorily. A further requirement is that the positive effect of the treatment outweighs the negative effects. Evidencing effectiveness and weighing the positive and negative effects of interventions are difficult to do due to non-standardisation of measures subjectivity, and multiple variables.

## 2.3    Mental Capacity for Decision-Making

Lack of mental capacity, competence or decision-making capacity, herein referred to as capacity, is a criterion for involuntary admission and treatment in many jurisdictions. However, the assessment of capacity is a controversial and inexact practice (Berens & Kim, 2022). Grisso and Appelbaum (1998) classically identified four abilities as evidence of capacity — understanding, appreciation, reasoning and expressing a choice, and these abilities have formed the basis of capacity assessment tools such as the much-used MacArthur Competence Assessment Tool (MacCAT-T). Concerns have been expressed that capacity tests are ill-suited to the distinctive features of psychiatric illness that may undermine capacity, which may be more related to values and less related to cognitive processes (Owen et al., 2013).

There are three approaches for determining mental capacity: the status approach, the outcome approach and the functional approach. Respectively, these refer to determining capacity based on diagnosis (status), the reasonableness or correctness of the decisions made by the person (outcome) or the person's ability to make a specific decision at a specific time and in a particular context (functional). All are problematic. Even though the latter, functional approach may seem the most reasonable, the CRPD committee rejects all three, saying the functional approach is discriminatorily applied to people with disabilities and denies them a core human right — the right to equal recognition before the law (CRPD, 2014). Flynn and Astein-Kerslake (2014, p. 87) concur, stating that the functional approach, when showing an impairment, quickly 'circle(s) back to the status-based approach'. The CRPD considers mental capacity determinations as discriminatory denial of legal capacity, the ability of a person to make decisions about their own life, including decisions related to medical treatment and care, and holds that legal capacity persists during mental illness. Others disagree, in particular in relation to the functional approach. Scholten et al. (2021b) contend their model for determining competence, which combines supported decision-making with a functional assessment of competence, does not discriminate against persons with mental disorders and so, is not contrary to Article 12 of the CRPD.

One well-debated proposal for addressing what the CRPD calls unequal treatment before the law is known as 'Fusion Law', defined as a generic law applying to all persons lacking the ability to make a treatment decision, whether resulting from a 'mental' or 'physical' illness (Szmukler, 2020). Under this type of law, the main criterion for involuntary admission (and treatment) would be diminished decision-making capacity, regardless of what is causing that diminishment. Put more clearly, involuntary admission or treatment is not based on diagnosis or disability but rather on the inability to make a decision even with the help of others. Sometimes, this approach is referred to as being disability-neutral. However, the CRPD, with logic that is difficult to dispute, regards impaired decision-making ability as another type of disability (Szmukler & Kelly, 2016), so Fusion Law is still deemed as contrary to Article 14 which states 'the existence of a disability shall in no case justify a deprivation of liberty'. (Flynn, 2016).

## 3    Variations and Changes in Involuntary Admission

Data on rates of involuntary detention, like those for all non-consensual interventions, are difficult to measure, compare and analyse (Hofstad et al., 2021b; Kallert et al., 2006). The reporting unit is generally the number of involuntary detentions per 100,000 population, but some reports are based on involuntary detention as a percentage of all admissions.

Much has been written about the variability of involuntary admission rates both within and between countries. Rains et al. (2019), comparing involuntary admission rates in 22 countries, show the incidence ranging from 14.5 per 100,000 population for Italy to 282 per 100,000 for Austria (median rate 106.4 and IQR 58.5 to 150.9). Hofstad et al. (2022) found rates vary even from one hospital to another within the same region, something referred to by Lay et al. (2015) as a 'centre effect', i.e. local factors and tradition. Many hypotheses are put forward to explain these differences, so far without solid evidence to support most of them. The difficulty in comparing figures is illustrated by Kelly (2019) who points out that, for example, in the case of the Italian data, many people in that country are treated in community facilities, which are commonly excluded from bed counts. He contends that if they were included, the Italian data on involuntary admission rates would be similar to those in the UK and elsewhere. Hofstad et al. (2021b, p. 2) state 'such large differences indicate that some areas might use more compulsion than necessary'. This would constitute 'unwanted variation' which Wennburg (2010, p. 4) defined as 'variation that cannot be explained on the basis of illness, medical evidence or patient preference'.

With increased awareness of the contentiousness of the practice, mental health acts in many countries underwent a period of widespread reform during the 1990s, with mixed impacts on detention rates. Sometimes there was a marked drop in the number of persons detained, and occasionally this change was sustained, but often the rates returned to previous levels after a year or so, hence Appelbaum's book title at the time, *Almost a Revolution: Mental Health Law and the Limits of Change* (Appelbaum, 1997 p. 145). He wrote, 'not everything that comes advertised as a revolution turns out to be one', that mental health professionals tend to find practical ways of operating at the fringes of the law, and that one should never underestimate the power of the *'ancien regime'*.

Rates can increase even after greater restrictions on the use of involuntary admission have been legislated for. This paradoxical situation has multifactorial explanations; increasing shortages of acute services, increasingly risk-averse clinicians, patients' increased reluctance to go into crowded, unpleasant facilities, increased social isolation/exclusion, rising substance misuse, and a decline in deference of patients to clinicians' instructions (Johnson, 2013).

## 4    The Multifactorial Process of Involuntary Admission

A complex constellation of factors may influence the decision to detain someone involuntarily (Fistein et al., 2016). Factors correlated with higher rates include gender (male) (Hustoft et al., 2013), age (<30 years) (Singh et al., 2014), being single (Chang et al., 2013), foreignness (Ng & Kelly, 2012), being Black, Asian or Minority Ethnic (BAME) (Gajwani et al., 2016), and socioeconomic deprivation (Karasch et al., 2020). Rössler (2019) categorised the numerous factors into three levels: a macro-level, including the wider societal perspective and the national legislation; a meso-level, including the organisation of mental health care and in particular the implementation of intervention strategies aimed to reduce those admissions; and a micro-level, including the sociodemographic and clinical features of the affected persons as well as the attitudes of their caregivers.

The pathway to hospital, where an admission is against the person's wishes, is relatively under-examined in the literature (Svindseth et al., 2013), despite it being of major significance to patients and their families (Røtvold & Wynn, 2016). Once a decision is made to initiate an involuntary detention process, many formalities need to be completed and many factors need to be considered. The approaches used depend on governing legislation, clinical traditions and the multiple personnel involved, so they vary substantially between services and countries. Factors include who makes the application, who approves it, which personnel are involved in bringing the person into the hospital (hospital staff, other branches of the health service, appointed officers, police, taxi drivers, assisted admission teams, general practitioners, paramedics, community nurses, family members or friends), how discretely or publicly it is done, the right of the person to know who has applied for them to be detained, the level of information-giving to the person and family during the process, and many others.

Wormdahl et al. (2021) investigated the contextual characteristics surrounding individuals' paths to referral and involuntary psychiatric admission. They found that initial deterioration of mental health, together with the presence of other risk factors such as inadequate housing, unemployment and loneliness, were often not detected, partly due to complex and unclear referral channels and insufficient collaboration between services. When symptoms become acute, restrictive or coercive interventions are often the likely outcome. A year later, Wormdahl et al. (2022) identified and detailed six strategy areas to collectively reduce the need for involuntary admissions: (1) management, (2) involving persons with lived experience and family carers, (3) competence development, (4) collaboration across primary and specialist care levels, (5) collaboration within the primary care level, and (6) tailoring individual services.

Georgieva et al. (2017) looked at admission processes in an Irish context, interviewing the various stakeholders involved in bringing persons to hospital against their will. Respondents in the study expressed general dissatisfaction with the usual pathways to involuntary admission, saying significant delays occur, the process is undignified and that more use should be made of staff with whom the patient is acquainted. Police respondents said they did not like being involved and that they had insufficient training for those situations. Family members were concerned about the impact on relationships after being involved in the process (Georgieva et al., 2017). Wyder et al. (2018) concluded that information, reassurance and greater partnership with families are needed in involuntary admission processes.

## 5    The Experience of Involuntary Admission

Of course, pathways to involuntary admission and the experiences of travelling those paths are inextricably linked. The experiences of people who have been subjected to involuntary admission, as well as those of carers and staff, are now presented.

## 5.1    Personal Experiences of Being Involuntarily Detained

People with lived experiences (PLE) of involuntary admission have variously reported positively and negatively about the intervention. Positive comments are associated with some time having passed since the episode and an improvement in the patient's mental health, and with positive engagement and meaningful information-giving throughout the process. Many PLEs state that if trust is present, the experience feels less coercive and several have said the admission kept them safe, something Seed et al. (2016) themed as 'sanctuary', but that was often something they could not recognise at the time (Akther et al., 2019). Some saw involuntary admission as a necessary form of protection or stated they recognised their need for treatment, but these respondents tend to be those patients described as having higher levels of insight into their condition at, or shortly after the detention (Bainbridge et al., 2018).

Negative reports are more usual. These can be subdivided into feelings and consequences. Feelings include loss of dignity, humiliation, powerlessness and distrust, and fear of being arrested, imprisoned, stigmatised or alienated (Raboch et al., 2010). Negative consequences of involuntary admission include a longer length of stay (Balducci et al., 2017), service avoidance due to loss of trust (Katsakou et al., 2012), and physical injury and damage to the staff–patient relationship. De Brito et al. (2019, p. 201)[2] write 'deprivation of the right to liberty leads to deprivation of all other rights, in particular, the maximum preservation of legal capacity; the right to be treated in the least restrictive environment; the right to live and be included in the community; and the right to privacy and integrity'. However, such experiences are greatly ameliorated by certain factors such as being familiar with the personnel involved and being given information about what is happening and why, what is likely to happen, and how to access legal information about their rights and entitlements (Akther et al., 2019; de Brito et al., 2019). A synthesis of the qualitative evidence of patients who experienced coercion during voluntary and involuntary

---

[2] De Brito and colleagues elaborate on each right within their article.

psychiatric hospitalisation by Silva et al. (2023) summarises such experiences as being mainly negative but includes several personal accounts of involuntary admission, describing feelings of being cared for, being safe, and feeling relieved because they were exhausted.

The way in which the admission is carried out is of decisive importance for the experience. For example, being taken away from home by force by the police can be very frightening. It might also cause neighbours to become afraid and hamper reintegration into the community after the detention. In addition, patients may feel betrayed if they perceive family members have been involved in initiating the admission (McGuinness et al., 2018). Two of the informants in that study describe the experience of being taken by force in order to be involuntarily admitted:

> I was taken from my place of work against my will... I was very annoyed and furious... I was taken out of my surroundings... without being explained to me why and... that a GP [general practitioner] could turn around and do something like that and then go off about his business as if nothing happened ...
> ... they [assisted admission team] just dragged me... They put me against the floor, used violence... they handcuffed me and they put me in this plastic yellow blanket and put me in a van or something... I didn't know where I was going. (McGuinness et al., 2018, p. 503)

Giving patients information about what is happening, in an individualised and repeated format, using understandable language can lead to empowerment and increased confidence. Patients want a trusting relationship with staff, based on human connection. It is important that staff are friendly and respectful and take the time to talk to them (Akther et al., 2019).

Involuntary admission should not be the first-line strategy. In many cases, former patients believe that their problems could have been dealt with by less coercive community interventions or a shorter voluntary hospitalisation (Katsakou et al., 2012). When patients feel coerced, and restrictions are perceived as unfair, they might resort to various coping strategies like resignation and pretending acceptance. This in turn amplifies their loss of self-esteem and can result in service disengagement after discharge (Silva et al., 2023).

## 5.2 Staff Attitudes and Experiences of Involuntary Admission Processes

The issue of staff attitudes and experiences of being involved *specifically* in involuntary admission appears to be less well studied than those of PLEs and carers. A review by Sugiura et al. (2020) found that staff generally view involuntary admission as justified when dangerousness is perceived as a risk, even if family members are opposed to admission. Regarding admission decision-making, professional groups experienced a lack of communication and demarcation disputes. Two decades ago, Lepping et al. (2004) compared the attitudes of mental health professionals and lay people in Germany and England. They found that the views of staff and the general public about involuntary admission appear to differ little and that the professionals most likely to be critical of involuntary admission were those least involved in the process, i.e. that direct involvement in the detention process seems to increase, rather than diminish, support for its use. This ties in with the theory that individuals strive to decrease the discomfort generated by conflicting cognitions, by modifying their cognitions, something defined in Leon Festinger's seminal paper as 'cognitive dissonance reduction' (Festinger, 1962, p. 94), i.e. 'I have compelled somebody but I am a good person, so compulsion must be good'.

### 5.3    Carers' Experiences of Involuntary Admission Processes

Carers also refer to conflicting feelings in relation to the involuntary admission of people they care for. There can be positive feelings such as relief, hope and gratitude because their concerns are being taken seriously and the person is in a safe place. In addition, they get respite from care provision, and in some cases a diagnosis is finally made, leading to more information about the illness. Carers are generally eager to receive information about prognosis, treatments and the person's needs, as well as plans for assessment, admission, care and discharge. They also want information about hospital and community care processes, the legal rights of those in their care and their own legal rights concerning involuntary admission processes (Akther et al., 2019). Carers state that they struggle to be recognised by healthcare professionals and often feel that they are undervalued (Sugiura et al., 2020).

Other feelings described by carers are anger, disappointment and frustration. In some cases, they may feel responsible that an intervention ended with involuntary admission and that they should have done more to prevent it (Finlay-Carruthers et al., 2018). Others perceive that healthcare professionals blame them for the illness. In some cases, both the patient and carer experience involuntary admission as humiliating. Carers also become particularly vulnerable and isolated if, for the sake of the PLE, they feel they cannot talk to friends and family about the person's mental illness. In some cases, admission was described by carers as humiliating both for the patient and themselves (Stuart et al., 2020).

### 6    CRPD and Involuntary Admission

Although it has been controversial for many decades now, involuntary admission has been particularly debated since 2006 when the UN adopted the Convention on the Rights of People with Disabilities (CRPD) (UN General Assembly, 2006). The articles of this Convention amount to a paradigm shift in how people with disabilities are to be viewed and treated. The shift is from a medico-legal basis for mental health care to a human rights-based framework. Article 1 of the CRPD includes mental and intellectual impairment in its definition of disabilities. This is an important basis for all that follows within the Convention's text.

The CRPD Committee contends that criteria offered to justify involuntary admission are often based on the person's diagnosis and include assumptions of diminished decision-making capacity, of risk of harm to self or others and/or that in-patient treatment is needed. Under the terms of the CRPD, making such determinations, largely unilaterally and based on disability (in this case, a mental health diagnosis or psychosocial disability), is discriminatory and amounts to arbitrary deprivation of liberty, breaching Article 12 (Equal recognition before the law), Article 14 (Liberty and security of the person) and several other CRPD Articles (e.g. 15, 16, 17, 19, 20, 21, 25).

Looking specifically at involuntary admission, the Convention stresses that such detention (and treatment) is a violation of the right to equal recognition before the law (Article 12), freedom from torture and ill-treatment (Article 15), freedom from violence, exploitation and abuse (Article 16), and personal integrity (Article 17). Furthermore, in one of its General Comments (GC1, 2014), the CRPD committee declares that states parties have an obligation to replace substitute decision-making with supported decision-making (Committee on the Rights of Persons with Disabilities, 2014). The Committee contends that substitute decision-making means that people are deprived of the right to make decisions and, instead, decisions are made for them by others. Substitute decision-makers may be members of the family, mental health and other practitioners or people appointed by a court. Sometimes substitute decision-making is a formal process (e.g. someone is appointed to be a 'guardian' by law). At other times, substitute decision-making happens informally, with family members or practitioners automatically and systematically taking over all decisions for the person concerned. In yet other circumstances, laws allow others (e.g. a court, or the director or manager of a mental health or social service) to make decisions for people, even when a guardian has not been appointed (World Health Organisation, 2019a). The WHO (ibid) states that supported decision-making entails a support person never making decisions for/on behalf of/instead of another person. With supported decision-making, all forms of support, including the most intensive, are based on the will and preferences of the person concerned. Today, most mental health laws continue to restrict the aforementioned rights in favour of substitute decision-making. In some countries, people with mental health problems lose nearly all of their civil rights, sometimes termed 'civil death' (Szmukler, 2019).

The CRPD Committee took the view that it would not be enough to simply consolidate existing legislation; what was needed was a completely new approach, i.e. a paradigm shift (Bartlett, 2014; Pūras, 2017). Both conventional mental health law and capacity-based law are deemed to violate the Convention. The Convention says the involuntary detention of persons with disabilities based on risk, dangerousness, alleged need for care or treatment, or other reasons tied to an impairment or health diagnosis amounts to arbitrary deprivation of liberty. Essentially, it states that 'the existence of a disability shall in no case justify a deprivation of liberty' *(14(1)(b))*.

An impasse arises from the fact that the CRPD appears to state involuntary admission is unacceptable, but no country's mental health legislation has followed suit. Most mental health professionals, legal personnel and even society as a whole consider involuntary admission to be justified in certain circumstances (Angermeyer et al., 2017; Joa et al., 2017). The fact that almost all nations of the world have ratified the Convention, but continue to detain involuntarily, exemplifies the procedural stalemate.

Still, no modern mental health or capacity legislation is drafted without taking cognisance of CRPD stipulations (Gooding, 2017). The problem is in understanding the stipulations; are they absolute or merely strong guidance? Can involuntary admission ever comply with UN human rights standards? An authoritative interpretation of the CRPD would be that, in stating '... the existence of a disability shall in no case justify a deprivation of liberty' (Art. 14(1)(b)), it takes an absolutist stance, condemning involuntary admission as a violation of the Convention, but others (Scholten et al., 2021a; Szmukler et al., 2010) see room for manoeuvre within sections of the CRPD, such as Article 12.4, which states that

> ... safeguards shall ensure that measures relating to the exercise of legal capacity respect the rights, will and preferences of the person, are free of conflict of interest and undue influence, are proportional and tailored to the person's circumstances, apply for the shortest time possible and are subject to regular review by a competent, independent and impartial authority or judicial body.

The CRPD objections to involuntary admission are (a) the use of involuntary admission based on one's disability and (b) the use of 'substituted decision-making' rather than 'supported decision-making'. A 'substitute decision' is one made by another person, one who can be appointed against the will of the person with a disability, and not based on the will and preferences of the person with the disability, but typically on what is believed to be in their 'best interests' (Szmukler, 2020). The CRPD states a 'supported decision' is one where the person is assisted to identify and give effect to their will and preferences. On occasions where, despite significant efforts being made, it is not possible to ascertain these, then a 'best interpretation' (Skowron, 2019) of such will and preferences can be made. Stavert (2021) states the Committee's reasoning here is that diagnosis and mental capacity assessments are often used to justify substitute decisions, but that these are influenced by subjective assessments of what is in the individual's best interests, which results in discrimination.

However, potential problems have been identified even for supported decision-making (Scholten et al., 2021b). Supported decision-making (or decision-making assistance) arrangements may still involve undue influence. Support persons may unduly influence decision-making because they pursue their own interests rather than the best interest of the person concerned. Undue influence is not necessarily exerted in bad faith and can happen even when intentions are honourable. Also, given that responsibility for treatment decisions generally rests with those supported to make the decisions, there may be reduced accountability for clinicians in supported decision-making scenarios; the beneficiaries bear responsibility for treatment decisions no matter how much support they receive (Scholten et al., 2021b).

The CRPD sees respect for a person's will and preferences as vital. It does not, however, define the terms, or how to deal with changes of will or preference over time and the meaning of these terms is much debated within the literature (Skowron, 2019; Szmukler, 2019).

## 6.1    Criticisms of the CRPD Stipulations on Deprivation of Liberty

The fact that involuntary admission is seen to be necessary and continues in all jurisdictions despite the widespread ratification of the CRPD, indicates there is a fundamental problem with an absolutist interpretation of Article 14(1)(b) of the Convention. Another UN organisation, the Human Rights Committee (UNHRC),[3] is less absolutist when it comments that the deprivation of liberty of persons with disabilities could be

> … necessary and proportionate for the purpose of protecting the individual… from serious harm or preventing injury to others (and) must be applied only as a measure of last resort and for the shortest appropriate period of time, and must be accompanied by adequate procedural and substantive safeguards, including initial and periodic judicial reviews. (UN Human Rights Committee, 2014) Art.14

Article 5(1)(e) of the European Convention on Human Rights (ECHR) states that a person may be lawfully detained for, among other things, being of unsound mind (European Court of Human Rights, 2022). The UK Law Commission document, *Mental Capacity and Deprivation of Liberty* declares 'it is not on its face possible to comply with both Article 5(1)(e) of the ECHR and (certain) interpretations of Article 14 of the CRPD' (UK Law Commission, 2017).

What is important to note here is that these stances and statements are not necessarily contradictory. The UNHRC statement above is a paraphrasing of Article 14(2) of the Convention, which states that where deprivation of liberty is necessary, human rights protections must be guaranteed, and Article 14(1)(b) of the Convention elaborates on the protection of the right to liberty and security of the person when it states that no one shall be

> … deprived of their liberty unlawfully or arbitrarily, and that any deprivation of liberty [showing it does foresee such situations] is in conformity with the law, and that the existence of a disability shall in no case justify a deprivation of liberty.

Martin and Gurbai (2019), who called this procedural stalemate 'the Geneva Impasse', note that there is a lack of consensus even among the UN and other international human rights organisations about how to rectify the Convention's abolitionist ideals with everyday clinical practices. The CRPD has been criticised for being ambivalent in creating an unrealistic ideal but failing to suggest how it can be achieved in practice (Szmukler, 2019). Some contend that, in drafting the Convention, the Committee 'was captured by some of the most radical elements of

---

[3] Though both the Committee for the Rights of People with Disabilities and the UNHRC are UN entities, the former is an elected committee, independent of the UN. The relationship between these two entities lies in their common goal of upholding and promoting human rights. The CRPD Committee focuses specifically on the rights of persons with disabilities, while the UNHRC deals with a broader spectrum of human rights concerns. Both entities work to ensure that member states adhere to international human rights standards and commitments.

the patients' rights movement, which are willing to sacrifice the well-being of persons with disabilities to achieve what they see as their long-term political goals' (Appelbaum, 2019, p. 1). Appelbaum also suggests that many governments thoughtlessly ratified the CRPD without considering its implications.

Fundamentally, the CRPD stipulations leave states parties with a stark choice; either they abolish involuntary admissions and treatments, or they operate in breach of the Convention. Anna Nilsson (2021) proposes a solution in her 2021 book, claiming it is possible to identify a line between lawful and unlawful uses of compulsion using 'proportionality reasoning'. She says that by applying four criteria, originally described by Robert Alexy (2010), one can assess the proportionality or reasonableness of an involuntary intervention. The criteria or questions are: (i) Does the practice under scrutiny have a legitimate aim? (ii) Does the practice contribute to that aim? (iii) Is the practice necessary? and (iv) Are the reasons in favour of the practice 'on balance with' the reasons against it? She claims that meeting these criteria, in particular the fourth one, which is of a higher order, constitutes a justifiable use of an involuntary intervention that wouldn't be in breach of the Convention. Fanning (2022) disagrees, stating that CRPD Article 14(1)(b) is indeed absolutist when it states '… the existence of a disability shall *in no case* justify a deprivation of liberty'. He adds that the language used by the CRPD 'seems much more definitive than Nilsson suggests' (Fanning, 2022, p. 561).

## 7    Justifying Involuntary Admission

The literature is replete with examples of situations where involuntary admission has been justified; the manic person who, untreated, poses catastrophic financial or interpersonal relationship risks to family or friends (Appelbaum, 2019); the psychotic person who believes self-harm or other aggression will serve a higher cause (Gooding & Flynn, 2015) or the person with dementia who insists on being discharged when it seems unsafe to do so (Craigie et al., 2019). Substituted decision-making in these situations had rarely been challenged prior to the CRPD. The paradoxical argument is often made that involuntary admission is necessary for restoring, rather than removing, patients' autonomy and capacity, and that failure to admit and treat can leave a person's actions being dictated by illness and put them and others at risk (Hegarty & Brusasco, 2021). Freeman et al. (2015, p. 4) state that prohibiting involuntary admission or treatment 'close(s) viable options for saving lives and is especially tragic where the suicidal ideation is directly linked with impaired decision-making capacity and could have been changed through admission or treatment'. They add 'when there is conflict between different rights, the right to life should trump the other rights'. Appelbaum (2019, p. 1) writes, 'In the name of protecting all these people (suicidal, psychotic, manic-reckless) from discrimination, they would be free to destroy their own lives and ruin the lives of their loved ones'.

Scholten et al. (2021b) argue that adhering to CRPD directives could adversely affect persons with mental health disabilities; when a person's decision-making competency is substantially impaired, the practice of informed consent loses its point. Failure to provide appropriate interventions when necessary can create a cycle in which a patient's actions are dictated by illness, and they are denied opportunities to regain their right to liberty (Hegarty & Brusasco, 2021).

## 8 How to Move Away from Involuntary Admission

While the CRPD has been ratified by a majority of countries, many have reservations about its interpretation, and the laws and standard practices in many countries still allow for the use of involuntary admission and other coercive practices. For several reasons 'mental health reform remains extremely challenging in all countries' (Funk & Drew-Bold, 2020, p. 71). Some of the main initiatives/strategies to reduce involuntary admissions are subsumed within coercion-reduction efforts, which makes sense as the solutions, when they work, tend to have effects across-the-board rather than changing any one type of coercive intervention. The following sections consider some such strategies.

### 8.1 Advance Treatment Directives

Advance treatment directives are a much-lauded development towards respecting human rights and reducing involuntary admissions. Whatever the precise meanings, one way of giving voice to one's will and preferences concerning future detention and treatment is via advance directives. Also known as Psychiatric Advance Directives (PADs), advance instructions, or advance refusals, the concept has almost universal acceptance as a progressive development in mental health care. PADs are designed to prevent involuntary interventions by enabling people with serious mental illnesses to plan for their own treatment during a future incapacitating crisis, to put their preferences in writing while they are competent, and to authorise a trusted family member or friend to make decisions on their behalf (Easter et al., 2021). The advance instruction can include a description of desired support, recovery options, treatments and place of care. People may make an advance refusal of certain support, care or treatment options. Some of the excitement about PADs has been based on the likelihood that they would reduce involuntary admission rates. Evidence is mixed on this, perhaps because the implementation of these legal documents in psychiatric emergency settings is far from perfect (de Jong et al., 2016).

Regardless of the inherent difficulties, it appears that the use of advance directives is a step in the right direction, allowing greater autonomy, with supported decision-making if acceptable to the person. PADs are usually written with the support of health professionals, but there is increasing evidence that involving peer workers enhances the benefits associated with PAD use. In a large randomised controlled trial (RCT), where a majority of the intervention group completed PADs with the support of peer workers, there was a 32% decrease in involuntary admissions compared with the control group, while the overall rate of admissions barely changed (Tinland et al., 2022). The authors speculate that the process of making the PAD, and the inherent interactions with support persons, may make participants more willing to consider a voluntary admission when a crisis occurs.

Szmukler (2020, p. 223) defines 'will' as possibly being 'a resolute or determined intention based on a person's relatively stable … beliefs, values or commitments', whereas a 'preference' is a more 'in the moment' belief, value or desire'. Through a PAD, and ideally with the support of relatives/friends/clinicians/peer workers, a person expresses their will for future management of their mental health condition.

However, problems arise with PADs too. It is not always clear what to do when a person refuses to follow their own advance directive. A patient cannot always accurately anticipate contexts and potential situations and make appropriate advance choices (Philip et al., 2019). There is also a type of PAD, permissible in some jurisdictions, called a 'self-binding' advance directive. The person inserts a clause(s) authorising mental health services to act over their objections/refusals during a crisis. This is known as a 'Ulysses' clause. Another problem hindering more widespread use of PADs/advance refusals is that services are slow to put in place the resources necessary to support the person making the directive (Henderson et al., 2017).

## 8.2 Joint Crisis Plans

Joint Crisis Plans (JCPs) often incorporate PADs and the two are easily confused. While JCPs are based on a contractual-like agreement between patients and physicians, PADs can be composed without the consultation of a medical expert. JCPs are in more widespread use than PADs (Radenbach et al., 2014). A JCP is broader than a PAD, often being formulated and agreed upon by the service user and a full mental health team. Like a PAD, it contains the patient's treatment preferences for any future psychiatric emergency, when they may be too unwell to express clear views. A JCP aims to empower mental health patients, facilitating early detection and treatment, and mitigating some of the negative consequences of relapse, including involuntary admission to hospital and use of coercion (Barrett et al., 2013).

Molyneaux et al. (2019) conducted a meta-analysis of five randomised control trials studying the effect of crisis plans on compulsory admissions. They found that using crisis planning reduced involuntary admissions by 25%. This reduction was not followed by an overall reduction in admissions, indicating that it is possible to turn some of the compulsory admissions into voluntary ones. The trials had common elements regarding crisis planning, but varied in content and intensity, making it difficult to define the optimal model of crisis planning for reducing involuntary admissions.

## 8.3    Patient-Controlled Admissions

Patient-controlled admission (PCA) is a concept that invites patients with long-term mental illness to decide for themselves when in-patient treatment is necessary without a clinician serving as gatekeeper (Strand & von Hausswolff-Juhlin, 2015). So far, it is mainly used in Scandinavian mental health services, to see if patient satisfaction and access to services can be improved. One study, which assessed whether implementing patient-controlled admission can reduce coercion and improve other clinical outcomes for psychiatric in-patients, included involuntary admission rates. No significant coercion-reduction effects were found. However, research in this area is still very limited and, given reports that patients are very satisfied with opportunities to easily self-refer when they feel they need help (Nyttingnes et al., 2021), PCAs have the potential to ease the admission process and perhaps reduce the incidence of involuntary admission.

## 8.4    'QualityRights' Training

In 2019, the WHO developed practical solutions to bring laws and practices in line with the CRPD, in three areas:

- building capacity among all stakeholders to improve attitudes and practices to address stigma and discrimination and promote human rights and recovery,
- supporting countries in the creation of community-based services and supports that respect and promote human rights,
- supporting national policy and law reform in line with the CRPD and other international human rights standards.

Based on this work, the WHO launched its QualityRights Initiative (World Health Organization, 2019b). Training, guidance materials and tools were designed to address topics like recovery, human rights and freedom from coercion, violence and abuse as well as courses directed at reducing specific restrictive practices. The WHO has also developed an extensive e-training package in many languages. The courses and the e-training package are meant for politicians, leaders of services, professionals, service users, their families and the public in general. In order for this global initiative to have any impact on rates of involuntary admission, it needs to be adopted and implemented on a national level, supported by stakeholders like national health authorities, service leadership and professional bodies.

## 8.5    Integrated Treatment

The integration of all aspects of care, primary, secondary and tertiary, community organisations, neighbours, support groups and so on constitutes a holistic integrated approach to care. It seems logical that linking all helpful elements of care and community will promote early detection and treatment of mental health problems, but would it reduce involuntary admissions? In a meta-analysis of studies of interventions to reduce involuntary admissions, De Jong et al. (2016) included four RCTs on integrated treatment as one of four subgroups[4]. Integrated treatment was understood as an augmentation of standard care and included such varied practices as crisis resolution teams and integrated services. Although there was no statistically significant risk reduction in the subgroup of integrated treatment, it showed a potentially clinically-relevant risk reduction of 29% for involuntary admission. The authors commented that this subgroup of interventions might be most promising for further research and development.

Wormdahl et al. (2021) wrote that most efforts to reduce levels of involuntary admissions have traditionally been directed towards secondary health care services. They concluded from interviews with staff and patients (where one respondent stated 'it was like there was nothing between no help and coercion') that a gap existed at primary care levels and any policy to reduce involuntary admissions needs to include primary mental health care service development. Such policies need to include measures like housing, employment and activities for people with severe mental illness and collaboration between services. This would enable and simplify timely access to services, which should consequently reduce the incidence of detentions.

The most extensive recent review of strategies and methods to promote voluntary measures is the scoping review by Gooding et al. (2020). Although the review found little on reducing involuntary admissions specifically, it is a much-needed compilation of integrative care initiatives across the Council of Europe member states. Following the logic of the opening sentences of this subsection, such initiatives have the potential to enhance mental health care and empower PLEs, which may in turn reduce involuntary measures. However, none of the studies had an RCT design so scientific evidence for these interventions is weak. Gooding et al. (2020, p. 27) state that 'no jurisdiction seems to have combined the full suite of laws, policies and practices that are available, and which taken together might further the goal of eliminating coercion'.

## 8.6   Other Initiatives

Mental health services, policymakers and legislators around the world have developed programmes or initiatives to reduce coercive practices in mental health care. These programmes generally, and by necessity, have a broad anti-coercion or even a recovery-focused remit and are not usually specifically targeted at one intervention such as involuntary admission reduction. The hope is that if they are well planned and carefully implemented, involuntary admission rates will improve, together with many other aspects of the services. This rising-tide-lifts-all-boats

---

[4] The other subgroups were advance statements, community treatment orders, and compliance enhancement.

**Table 1** Examples of programmes or initiatives to reduce coercive practices in mental health care

| Programme/initiative | References |
|---|---|
| Peer delivered care | Acri et al. (2017), Puschner (2018) |
| Staff training (better listening and viewing patient as expert) | Van den Hooff and Goossensen (2014) |
| Shared, assisted or supported decision-making | Wied et al. (2021), Scholten et al. (2021b) |
| More integrated care, for example, crisis response teams | WHO (2019c) |
| More resources in the community/primary care services | Hofstad et al. (2021a) |
| Domiciliary interventions | Gomis et al. (2017) |
| Open dialogue | Galbusera and Kyselo (2018) |
| Online social media technology – Novel user-led interventions | Alvarez-Jimenez et al. (2014) |
| Clubhouses | Battin et al. (2016) |
| Personal ombudsman systems | Council of Europe (2023) |
| Circle of care models/circles of support | Cavoukian (2009) |
| Improving social and environmental factors | Curley et al. (2016) |
| Using local rather than unfamiliar personnel for assisted admission teams and officers | Georgieva et al. (2017) |
| CBT strategies and family education | Georgieva et al. (2017) |
| Carer support workers (the triangle of care) | Hannan (2013) |

effect is quite a practical approach where staff training, environmental enhancements, improved communication, organisational change, service user inputs and research, when properly implemented, should reduce all coercion in mental health services. Some of these are listed in Table 1.

# 9 Conclusion

Reduction of the use of involuntary admission is a complex issue, made increasingly so by the authoritative declarations of the CRPD concerning the rights of persons with disabilities. Interpretation of the CRPD articles has proven difficult and generated almost two decades of discourse with often extremely different views being expressed and conclusions drawn. The ethical issues surrounding will and preferences, rights, safety, paternalism and autonomy will continue to spark debate and that is no bad thing. In fact, many positives have come from this heightened focus on traditional coercive practices. There is consensus on a few important priorities: that involuntary admission rates are rising but need to reduce (Rains et al., 2019), that the viewpoints of all those availing of mental health services need to be more valued and better understood, that their will and preferences should be sought and respected, and that supported decision-making processes should be implemented or better utilised wherever possible.

By their very nature, interventions to reduce involuntary admission rates do not lend themselves easily to empirical measurement or analysis. It should be clear from this chapter that the key elements likely to lower rates are paradoxically both simple and complex. The simple elements that patients are repeatedly saying they need, via the literature and through advocacy groups, include better communication of what is happening, what is expected of them and more dignified treatment in the form of privacy, listening to them and expressions of kindness and concern so that they feel safe and respected. The complex elements identified in this chapter include improved communication between staff and agencies, availability of early intervention and monitoring services, better training of personnel involved with symptom control, stigma reduction, changing public expectations, risk assessment, pathways to care and admissions to services. At a macro level, the picture is even more complex. International and national organisations and health services can state and recommend what seem to be best practices but experience to date has shown that interpretation, implementation and ensuring compliance with such policies/laws is fraught with difficulties.

Much remains to be done to redefine practices, policy and law, across European countries regarding involuntary admissions. Cases where decision-making capacity is deemed to be absent, and claims that substituted decision-making is sometimes necessary, will continue to pose ethical and clinical dilemmas for all stakeholders but at least the era of discussion and genuine willingness to improve is well underway. Many of the initiatives to reduce involuntary admission rates have been outlined in this chapter. Inevitably, those trying to implement them will experience varying degrees of success, and measurement of success will continue to be an inexact science due to the multiple confounding factors that exist in any mental health service and the people and communities it serves.

Though there is conceptual and political, as well as scientific agreement for the need to protect the civil rights of patients, there is still quite some way to go in order to establish an agreement between the legal perspective focusing on protecting human rights, and the clinical perspective focusing on treating the patient for their illness.

## References

Acri, M., Hooley, C. D., Richardson, N., & Moaba, L. B. (2017). Peer models in mental health for caregivers and families. *Community Mental Health Journal, 53*, 241–249.

Akther, S. F., Molyneaux, E., Stuart, R., Johnson, S., Simpson, A., & Oram, S. (2019). Patients' experiences of assessment and detention under mental health legislation: Systematic review and qualitative meta-synthesis. *BJPsych Open, 5*(3), e37.

Alexy, R. (2010). *A theory of constitutional rights*. Oxford University Press.

Alvarez-Jimenez, M., Alcazar-Corcoles, M. A., Gonzalez-Blanch, C., Bendall, S., McGorry, P. D., & Gleeson, J. F. (2014). Online, social media and mobile technologies for psychosis treatment: A systematic review on novel user-led interventions. *Schizophrenia Research, 156*(1), 96–106.

Angermeyer, M. C., Van Der Auwera, S., Carta, M. G., & Schomerus, G. (2017). Public attitudes towards psychiatry and psychiatric treatment at the beginning of the 21st century: A systematic review and meta-analysis of population surveys. *World Psychiatry, 16*(1), 50–61.

Appelbaum, P. S. (1997). Almost a revolution: an international perspective on the law of involuntary commitment. *Journal of the American Academy of Psychiatry and the Law Online*, 25(2), pp.135–147.

Appelbaum, P. S. (2019). Saving the UN Convention on the Rights of Persons with Disabilities– from itself. *World Psychiatry*, *18*(1), 1.

Bainbridge, E., Hallahan, B., McGuinness, D., Gunning, P., Newell, J., Higgins, A., Murphy, K., & McDonald, C. (2018). Predictors of involuntary patients' satisfaction with care: Prospective study. *BJPsych Open, 4*(6), 492–500.

Balducci, P. M., Bernardini, F., Pauselli, L., Tortorella, A., & Compton, M. T. (2017). Correlates of involuntary admission: Findings from an Italian inpatient psychiatric unit. *Psychiatria Danubina, 29*(4), 490–496.

Barrett, B., Waheed, W., Farrelly, S., Birchwood, M., Dunn, G., Flach, C., Henderson, C., Leese, M., Lester, H., & Marshall, M. (2013). Randomised controlled trial of joint crisis plans to reduce compulsory treatment for people with psychosis: Economic outcomes. *PLoS One, 8*(11), e74210.

Bartlett, P. (2014). *Implementing a paradigm shift: Implementing the Convention on the Rights of Persons with Disabilities in the context of mental disability law*. http://antitorture.org/wp-content/uploads/2014/03/PDF_Torture_in_Healthcare_Publication.pdf

Battin, C., Bouvet, C., & Hatala, C. (2016). A systematic review of the effectiveness of the clubhouse model. *Psychiatric Rehabilitation Journal, 39*(4), 305.

Berens, N. C., & Kim, S. Y. (2022). Should assessments of decision-making capacity be risk-sensitive? A systematic review. *Frontiers in Psychology, 13*, 897144. https://doi.org/10.3389/fpsyg.2022.897144

Callaghan, P., & Grundy, A. (2018). Violence risk assessment and management in mental health: A conceptual, empirical and practice critique. *The Journal of Mental Health Training, Education and Practice, 13*(1), 3–13.

Cavoukian, A. (2009). Circle of care: Sharing personal health information for health-care purposes. *Office of the Information and Privacy Commissioner of Ontario*.

Chang, T. M. M., Ferreira, L. K., Ferreira, M. P., & Hirata, E. S. (2013). Clincal and demographic differences between voluntary and involuntary psychiatric admissions in a university hospital in Brazil. *Cadernos De Saude Publica, 29*, 2347–2352.

Committee on the Rights of Persons with Disabilities. (2014). *General Comment No. 1. Article 12: Equal Recognition before the Law*. https://www.ohchr.org/en/documents/general-comments-and-recommendations/general-comment-no-1-article-12-equal-recognition-1

Conlon, D., Raeburn, T., & Wand, T. (2019). Disclosure of confidential information by mental health nurses, of patients they assess to be a risk of harm to self or others: An integrative review. *International Journal of Mental Health Nursing, 28*(6), 1235–1247.

Council of Europe. (2023). *Community-based initiatives—Personal Ombud Service, Sweden*. https://www.coe.int/en/web/bioethics/-/personal-ombud-programme-sweden

Courtney, M., & Moulding, N. T. (2014). Beyond balancing competing needs: Embedding involuntary treatment within a recovery approach to mental health social work. *Australian Social Work, 67*(2), 214–226.

Craigie, J., Bach, M., Gurbai, S., Kanter, A., Kim, S. Y., Lewis, O., & Morgan, G. (2019). Legal capacity, mental capacity and supported decision-making: Report from a panel event. *International Journal of Law and Psychiatry, 62*, 160–168.

Curley, A., Agada, E., Emechebe, A., Anamdi, C., Ng, X. T., Duffy, R., & Kelly, B. D. (2016). Exploring and explaining involuntary care: The relationship between psychiatric admission status, gender and other demographic and clinical variables. *International Journal of Law and Psychiatry, 47*, 53–59.

de Brito, E. S., Gallagher, A., Jago, R., Victorino, J. P., & Arena Ventura, C. A. (2019). Mental health and involuntary admission as a means to restricting rights. *Medicine and Law, 38*, 193.

de Jong, M. H., Kamperman, A. M., Oorschot, M., Priebe, S., Bramer, W., van de Sande, R., Van Gool, A. R., & Mulder, C. L. (2016). Interventions to reduce compulsory psychiatric admissions: A systematic review and meta-analysis. *JAMA Psychiatry, 73*(7), 657–664.

Easter, M. M., Swanson, J. W., Robertson, A. G., Moser, L. L., & Swartz, M. S. (2021). Impact of psychiatric advance directive facilitation on mental health consumers: Empowerment, treatment attitudes and the role of peer support specialists. *Journal of Mental Health, 30*(5), 585–593.

Endsley, M. R. (2015). Situation awareness: Operationally necessary and scientifically grounded. *Cognition, Technology & Work, 17*(2), 163–167.

European Court of Human Rights. (2022). *Guide on Article 5 of the European Convention on Human Rights; Right to liberty and security.* European Court of Human Rights. https://www.echr.coe.int/documents/guide_art_5_eng.pdf

Fanning, J. (2022). Anna Nilsson—Compulsory mental health interventions and the CRPD—Minding equality. Book review. *Medical Law Review, 30*(3), 555–562.

Feiring, E., & Ugstad, K. N. (2014). Interpretations of legal criteria for involuntary psychiatric admission: A qualitative analysis. *BMC Health Services Research, 14*, 500. (2014). https://doi.org/10.1186/s12913-014-0500-x

Festinger, L. (1962). Cognitive dissonance. *Scientific American, 207*(4), 93–106.

Finlay-Carruthers, G., Davies, J., Ferguson, J., & Browne, K. (2018). Taking parents seriously: The experiences of parents with a son or daughter in adult medium secure forensic mental health care. *International Journal of Mental Health Nursing, 27*(5), 1535–1545.

Fistein, E. C., Clare, I. C., Redley, M., & Holland, A. J. (2016). Tensions between policy and practice: A qualitative analysis of decisions regarding compulsory admission to psychiatric hospital. *International Journal of Law and Psychiatry, 46*, 50–57.

Flynn, E. (2016). Disability, deprivation of liberty and human rights norms: Reconciling European and International Approaches. *International Journal of Mental Health and Capacity Law, 22*, 75–101.

Flynn, E., & Arstein-Kerslake, A. (2014). Legislating personhood: Realising the right to support in exercising legal capacity. *International Journal of Law in Context, 10*(1), 81–104.

Freeman, M. C., Kolappa, K., de Almeida, J., Kleinman, A., Makhashvili, N., Phakathi, S., Saraceno, B., & Thornicroft, G. (2015). Reversing hard won victories in the name of human rights: A critique of the General Comment on Article 12 of the UN Convention on the Rights of Persons with Disabilities. *The Lancet Psychiatry, 2*, 844–850.

Funk, M., & Drew-Bold, N. D. (2020). WHO's QualityRights initiative: Transforming services and promoting rights in mental health. *Health and Human Rights, 22*(1), 69.

Gajwani, R., Parsons, H., Birchwood, M., & Singh, S. P. (2016). Ethnicity and detention: Are Black and minority ethnic (BME) groups disproportionately detained under the Mental Health Act 2007? *Social Psychiatry and Psychiatric Epidemiology, 51*(5), 703–711.

Galbusera, L., & Kyselo, M. (2018). The difference that makes the difference: A conceptual analysis of the open dialogue approach. *Psychosis, 10*(1), 47–54.

Georgieva, I., Bainbridge, E., McGuinness, D., Keys, M., Brosnan, L., Felzmann, H., Maguire, J., Murphy, K., Higgins, A., & McDonald, C. (2017). Opinions of key stakeholders concerning involuntary admission of patients under the Mental Health Act 2001. *Irish Journal of Psychological Medicine, 34*(4), 223–232.

Gerle, E., Fischer, A., & Lundh, L. (2019). "Voluntarily admitted against my will": Patient perspectives on effects of, and alternatives to, coercion in psychiatric care for self-injury. *Journal of Patient Experience, 6*(4), 265–270.

Gomis, O., Palma, C., & Farriols, N. (2017). Domiciliary intervention in psychosis: A systematic review. *Actas Españolas de Psiquiatría, 45*(6), 290–302.

Gooding, P. (2017). *A new era for mental health law and policy: Supported decision-making and the UN Convention on the Rights of Persons with Disabilities.* Cambridge University Press.

Gooding, P., & Flynn, E. (2015). Querying the call to introduce mental capacity testing to mental health law: Does the doctrine of necessity provide an alternative? *Laws, 4*(2), 245–271.

Gooding, P., McSherry, B., & Roper, C. (2020). Preventing and reducing 'coercion' in mental health services: An international scoping review of English-language studies. *Acta Psychiatrica Scandinavica, 142*(1), 27–39.

Grisso, T., & Appelbaum, P. S. (1998). *Assessing competence to consent to treatment: A guide for physicians and other health professionals*. Oxford University Press.

Hannan, R. (2013). The triangle of care: Carers included. *Journal of Public Mental Health, 12*(13), 171–172.

Hegarty, L., & Brusasco, M. (2021). Life, liberty and the therapeutic relationship: Examining the place of compulsory treatment in modern psychiatry. *Australasian Psychiatry, 29*(1), 66–68.

Henderson, C., Farrelly, S., Flach, C., Borschmann, R., Birchwood, M., Thornicroft, G., Waheed, W., & Szmukler, G. (2017). Informed, advance refusals of treatment by people with severe mental illness in a randomised controlled trial of joint crisis plans: Demand, content and correlates. *BMC Psychiatry, 17*(1), 1–8.

Hofstad, T., Rugkåsa, J., Ose, S. O., Nyttingnes, O., Kjus, S. H. H., & Husum, T. L. (2021a). Service characteristics and geographical variation in compulsory hospitalisation: An exploratory random effects within–between analysis of Norwegian municipalities, 2015–2018. *Frontiers in Psychiatry, 12*, 2099.

Hofstad, T., Rugkåsa, J., Ose, S. O., Nyttingnes, O., & Husum, T. L. (2021b). Measuring the level of compulsory hospitalisation in mental health care: The performance of different measures across areas and over time. *International Journal of Methods in Psychiatric Research, 30*(3), e1881.

Hofstad, T., Husum, T. L., Rugkåsa, J., & Hofmann, B. M. (2022). Geographical variation in compulsory hospitalisation–ethical challenges. *BMC Health Services Research, 22*(1), 1–12.

Hustoft, K., Larsen, T. K., Auestad, B., Joa, I., Johannessen, J. O., & Ruud, T. (2013). Predictors of involuntary hospitalizations to acute psychiatry. *International Journal of Law and Psychiatry, 36*(2), 136–143.

Joa, I., Hustoft, K., Anda, L. G., Brønnick, K., Nielssen, O., Johannessen, J. O., & Langeveld, J. H. (2017). Public attitudes towards involuntary admission and treatment by mental health services in Norway. *International Journal of Law and Psychiatry, 55*, 1–7.

Johnson, S. (2013). Can we reverse the rising tide of compulsory admissions? *Lancet, 381*(9878), 1603–1604.

Johnson, S. B., De Rosa, C., Musalek, M., Fiorillo, A., Volpe, U., & Bhugra, D. (2016). Involuntary hospitalizations in psychiatry: What to do and what to avoid. In *Psychiatry in practice: Education, experience, and expertise*. Oxford University Press.

Kallert, T. W., Glöckner, M., Onchev, G., Raboch, J., Karastergiou, A., Solomon, Z., Magliano, L., Dembinskas, A., Kiejna, A., & Nawka, P. (2005). The EUNOMIA project on coercion in psychiatry: Study design and preliminary data. *World Psychiatry, 4*(3), 168.

Kallert, T. W., Rymaszewska, J., & Torres-Gonzáles, F. (2006). The clinical point of view: Comparing differences of legal regulations related to involuntary admission and hospital stay in twelve European countries. In *Legislation on coercive mental health care in Europe. Legal documents and comparative assessment of twelve European countries* (pp. 375–400). Peter Lang.

Karasch, O., Schmitz-Buhl, M., Mennicken, R., Zielasek, J., & Gouzoulis-Mayfrank, E. (2020). Identification of risk factors for involuntary psychiatric hospitalization: Using environmental socioeconomic data and methods of machine learning to improve prediction. *BMC Psychiatry, 20*(1), 1–14.

Katsakou, C., Rose, D., Amos, T., Bowers, L., McCabe, R., Oliver, D., Wykes, T., & Priebe, S. (2012). Psychiatric patients' views on why their involuntary hospitalisation was right or wrong: A qualitative study. *Social Psychiatry and Psychiatric Epidemiology, 47*(7), 1169–1179.

Kelly, B. D. (2019). Variations in involuntary hospitalisation across countries. *The Lancet Psychiatry, 6*(5), 361–362.

Lay, B., Blank, C., Lengler, S., Drack, T., Bleiker, M., & Rössler, W. (2015). Preventing compulsory admission to psychiatric inpatient care using psycho-education and monitoring: Feasibility and outcomes after 12 months. *European Archives of Psychiatry and Clinical Neuroscience, 265*(3), 209–217.

Lepping, P., Steinert, T., Gebhardt, R., & Röttgers, H. R. (2004). Attitudes of mental health professionals and lay-people towards involuntary admission and treatment in England and Germany—A questionnaire analysis. *European Psychiatry, 19*(2), 91–95.

Malhi, G. S., Bell, E., Hamilton, A., & Morris, G. (2021). Early intervention for risk syndromes: What are the real risks?. Schizophrenia Research. 227, 4–9.

Martin, W., & Gurbai, S. (2019). Surveying the Geneva impasse: Coercive care and human rights. *International Journal of Law and Psychiatry, 64*, 117–128.

McGuinness, D., Murphy, K., Bainbridge, E., Brosnan, L., Keys, M., Felzmann, H., Hallahan, B., McDonald, C., & Higgins, A. (2018). Individuals' experiences of involuntary admissions and preserving control: Qualitative study. *BJPsych Open, 4*(6), 501–509.

Molyneaux, E., Turner, A., Candy, B., Landau, S., Johnson, S., & Lloyd-Evans, B. (2019). Crisis-planning interventions for people with psychotic illness or bipolar disorder: Systematic review and meta-analyses. *BJPsych Open, 5*(4), e53.

Ng, X. T., & Kelly, B. D. (2012). Voluntary and involuntary care: Three-year study of demographic and diagnostic admission statistics at an inner-city adult psychiatry unit. *International Journal of Law and Psychiatry, 35*(4), 317–326.

Nilsson, A. (2021). *Compulsory mental health interventions and the CRPD: Minding equality.* Bloomsbury Publishing.

Nyttingnes, O., Šaltytė Benth, J., & Ruud, T. (2021). Patient-controlled admission contracts: A longitudinal study of patient evaluations. *BMC Health Services Research, 21*(1), 1–13.

Owen, G. S., Szmukler, G., Richardson, G., David, A. S., Raymont, V., Freyenhagen, F., Martin, W., & Hotopf, M. (2013). Decision-making capacity for treatment in psychiatric and medical in-patients: Cross-sectional, comparative study. *The British Journal of Psychiatry, 203*(6), 461–467.

Patterson, C., Procter, N., & Toffoli, L. (2016). Situation awareness: When nurses decide to admit or not admit a person with mental illness as an involuntary patient. *Journal of Advanced Nursing, 72*(9), 2042–2053.

Pescosolido, B. A., Manago, B., & Monahan, J. (2019). Evolving public views on the likelihood of violence from people with mental illness: Stigma and its consequences. *Health Affairs, 38*(10), 1735–1743.

Philip, S., Rangarajan, S. K., Moirangthem, S., Kumar, C. N., Gowda, M. R., Gowda, G. S., & Math, S. B. (2019). Advance directives and nominated representatives: A critique. *Indian Journal of Psychiatry, 61*(Suppl. 4), S680.

Pūras, D. (2017). *Report of the special rapporteur on the right of everyone to the enjoyment of the highest attainable standard of physical and mental health.* United Nations Office of the High Commissioner for Human Rights, Available Online. https://daccess-ods.un.org/TMP/6425942.77858734.html

Puschner, B. (2018). Peer support and global mental health. *Epidemiology and Psychiatric Sciences, 27*(5), 413–414.

Raboch, J., Kališová, L., Nawka, A., Kitzlerová, E., Onchev, G., Karastergiou, A., Magliano, L., Dembinskas, A., Kiejna, A., & Torres-Gonzales, F. (2010). Use of coercive measures during involuntary hospitalization: Findings from ten European countries. *Psychiatric Services, 61*(10), 1012–1017.

Radenbach, K., Falkai, P., Weber-Reich, T., & Simon, A. (2014). Joint crisis plans and psychiatric advance directives in German psychiatric practice. *Journal of Medical Ethics, 40*(5), 343–345.

Rains, L. S., Zenina, T., Dias, M. C., Jones, R., Jeffreys, S., Branthonne-Foster, S., Lloyd-Evans, B., & Johnson, S. (2019). Variations in patterns of involuntary hospitalisation and in legal frameworks: An international comparative study. *The Lancet Psychiatry, 6*(5), 403–417.

Rössler, W. (2019). Factors facilitating or preventing compulsory admission in psychiatry. *World Psychiatry, 18*(3), 355.

Røtvold, K., & Wynn, R. (2016). Involuntary psychiatric admission: How the patients are detected and the general practitioners' expectations for hospitalization. An interview-based study. *International Journal of Mental Health Systems, 10*(1), 1–8.

Salize, H. J., Dreßing, H., & Peitz, M. (2002). Compulsory admission and involuntary treatment of mentally ill patients-legislation and practice in EU-member states. *Central Institute of Mental Health Research Project Final Report, Mannheim, Germany, 15*, 3–4.

Scholten, M., Gather, J., & Vollmann, J. (2021a). Equality in the informed consent process: Competence to consent, substitute decision-making, and discrimination of persons with mental disorders. *The Journal of Medicine and Philosophy: A Forum for Bioethics and Philosophy of Medicine, 46*(1), 108–136.

Scholten, M., Braun, E., Gather, J., & Vollmann, J. (2021b). Combining supported decision-making with competence assessment: A way to protect persons with impaired decision-making capacity against undue influence. *The American Journal of Bioethics, 21*(11), 45–47.

Seed, T., Fox, J. R., & Berry, K. (2016). The experience of involuntary detention in acute psychiatric care. A review and synthesis of qualitative studies. *International Journal of Nursing Studies, 61*, 82–94.

Silva, B., Bachelard, M., Amoussou, J. R., Martinez, D., Bonalumi, C., Bonsack, C., Golay, P., & Morandi, S. (2023). Feeling coerced during voluntary and involuntary psychiatric hospitalisation: A review and meta-aggregation of qualitative studies. *Heliyon, 9*(2), e13420.

Singh, S. P., Burns, T., Tyrer, P., Islam, Z., Parsons, H., & Crawford, M. J. (2014). Ethnicity as a predictor of detention under the Mental Health Act. *Psychological Medicine, 44*(5), 997–1004.

Skoric, M., & Gagro, S. F. (2020). Mental health legislation through history and challenges in implementing Article 14 of the Convention on the rights of persons with disabilities. *Anali Pravnog fakulteta u Beogradu, 68*, 56–79.

Skowron, P. (2019). Giving substance to 'the best interpretation of will and preferences'. *International Journal of Law and Psychiatry, 62*, 125–134.

Stavert, J. (2021). Supported decision-making and paradigm shifts: Word play or real change? *Frontiers in Psychiatry, 11*, 571005.

Strand, M., & von Hausswolff-Juhlin, Y. (2015). Patient-controlled hospital admission in psychiatry: A systematic review. *Nordic Journal of Psychiatry, 69*(8), 574–586.

Stuart, R., Akther, S. F., Machin, K., Persaud, K., Simpson, A., Johnson, S., & Oram, S. (2020). Carers' experiences of involuntary admission under mental health legislation: Systematic review and qualitative meta-synthesis. *BJPsych Open, 6*(2), e19.

Sugiura, K., Pertega, E., & Holmberg, C. (2020). Experiences of involuntary psychiatric admission decision-making: A systematic review and meta-synthesis of the perspectives of service users, informal carers, and professionals. *International Journal of Law and Psychiatry, 73*, 101645.

Svindseth, M. F., Nøttestad, J. A., & Dahl, A. A. (2013). Perceived humiliation during admission to a psychiatric emergency service and its relation to socio-demography and psychopathology. *BMC Psychiatry, 13*(1), 1–8.

Szmukler, G. (2015). Compulsion and "coercion" in mental health care. *World Psychiatry, 14*(3), 259.

Szmukler, G. (2019). "Capacity", "best interests", "will and preferences" and the UN Convention on the Rights of Persons with Disabilities. *World Psychiatry, 18*(1), 34–41.

Szmukler, G. (2020). Involuntary detention and treatment: Are we edging toward a "Paradigm Shift"? *Schizophrenia Bulletin, 46*(2), 231–235.

Szmukler, G., & Appelbaum, P. S. (2008). Treatment pressures, leverage, coercion, and compulsion in mental health care. *Journal of Mental Health, 17*(3), 233–244.

Szmukler, G., & Kelly, B. D. (2016). We should replace conventional mental health law with capacity-based law. *The British Journal of Psychiatry, 209*(6), 449–453.

Szmukler, G., Daw, R., & Dawson, J. (2010). A model law fusing incapacity and mental health legislation. *International Journal of Mental Health and Capacity Law. Special Ed. No. 20.*

Tinland, A., Loubière, S., Mougeot, F., Jouet, E., Pontier, M., Baumstarck, K., Loundou, A., Franck, N., Lançon, C., & Auquier, P. (2022). Effect of psychiatric advance directives facilitated by peer workers on compulsory admission among people with mental illness: A randomized clinical trial. *JAMA Psychiatry, 79*(8), 752–759.

UK Law Commission. (2017). *Mental Capacity and Deprivation of Liberty (Law Com No. 372).*

UN General Assembly. (2006). Convention on the Rights of Persons with Disabilities. *General Assembly Resolutions, 61*, 106.

UN Human Rights Committee. (2014). *General comment no. 35, article 9 (Liberty and security of person) (GC35).* https://documents-dds-ny.un.org/doc/UNDOC/GEN/G14/244/51/PDF/ G1424451.PDF?OpenElement

Van den Hooff, S., & Goossensen, A. (2014). How to increase quality of care during coercive admission? A review of literature. *Scandinavian Journal of Caring Sciences, 28*(3), 425–434.

Welsh, S., & Deahl, M. P. (2002). Modern psychiatric ethics. *The Lancet, 359*(9302), 253–255.

Wennberg, J. E. (2010). Tracking medicine: a researcher's quest to understand health care. Oxford University Press.

Wied, T. S., Haberstroh, J., Gather, J., Karakaya, T., Oswald, F., Qubad, M., Scholten, M., Vollmann, J., Pantel, J., & ENSURE Consortium. (2021). Supported decision-making in persons with dementia: Development of an enhanced consent procedure for lumbar puncture. *Frontiers in Psychiatry, 12*, 780276.

World Health Organization. (2019a). *Supported decision-making and advance planning— Substitute versus supported decision-making.* WHO QualityRights Specialized Training Report. https://www.jstor.org/stable/resrep27901.14

World Health Organization. (2019b). *Advocacy for mental health, disability and human rights: WHO QualityRights guidance module.*

World Health Organization. (2019c). *Strategies to end seclusion and restraint: WHO QualityRights specialized training.* https://apps.who.int/iris/bitstream/handle/10665/329605/9 789241516754-eng.pdf.

Wormdahl, I., Husum, T. L., Kjus, S. H. H., Rugkåsa, J., Hatling, T., & Rise, M. B. (2021). Between no help and coercion: Toward referral to involuntary psychiatric admission. A qualitative interview study of stakeholders' perspectives. *Frontiers in Psychiatry, 6*(12), 708175. https://doi.org/10.3389/fpsyt.2021.708175

Wormdahl, I., Hatling, T., Husum, T. L., Kjus, S. H. H., Rugkåsa, J., Brodersen, D., Christensen, S. D., Nyborg, P. S., Skolseng, T. B., Ødegård, E. I., & Andersen, A. M. (2022). The ReCoN intervention: A co-created comprehensive intervention for primary mental health care aiming to prevent involuntary admissions. *BMC Health Services Research, 22*(1), 1–17.

Wyder, M., Bland, R., McCann, K., & Crompton, D. (2018). The family experience of the crisis of involuntary treatment in mental health. *Australian Social Work, 71*(3), 319–331.

# Part III

# Human and Physical Context

# Ward Design, Coercion and Aggression in Psychiatric (Intensive) Care

Eric Noorthoorn van der Kruijff, Petra van der Schaaf, Paul Doedens, Bas Lamers, and Bart Thomas

## 1    Introduction

In psychiatry, discussions about the ward environment have often focused on Psychiatric Intensive Care Units (PICUs) (Baker et al., 1959; Crain & Jordan, 1979; Goldney et al., 1985; Gove & Lubach, 1969; Higgs, 1970; Mounsey, 1979). In general medicine, literature has demonstrated an association between the ward environment and (mental) health (Gross et al., 1998; Wilson et al., 1983). Studies in this area, including those by Dijkstra et al. (2006) and Watts and Wilson (2009), have connected factors such as hygiene, logistics, design, lighting, colour, accessibility, atmosphere and ambience to the concept of a healing environment.

Evidence of the association between ward design and mental health is, however, limited. This chapter provides a historical overview of research and practical experience into the impact of the ward environment on mental health, aggression, and

E. N. van der Kruijff (✉)
Human Resources—Section Research and Development, Ggnet Mental Health Centre, Warnsveld, The Netherlands
e-mail: e.noorthoorn@ggnet.nl

P. van der Schaaf
Oazis, Onderzoek & Advies, Gouda, The Netherlands
e-mail: info@oazis.nl

P. Doedens
Department of Psychiatrie, Amsterdam University Medical Center, Amsterdam, The Netherlands
e-mail: p.doedens@amsterdamumc.nl

B. Lamers
Interior Design Care Environments, Burobas Interior Architecture, Waalre, The Netherlands
e-mail: b.lamers@burobas.com

B. Thomas
NMRC-SBRC-CEMA-Down, UZ Gent, Ghent, Belgium
e-mail: bart.thomas@uzgent.be

© The Author(s) 2024                                                                                   219
N. Hallett et al. (eds.), *Coercion and Violence in Mental Health Settings*,
https://doi.org/10.1007/978-3-031-61224-4_10

coercive measures in psychiatry. After describing the main developments of Psychiatric Intensive Care Units within mental health, we present some general findings of studies into healing environments, both outside and within psychiatry. In many countries, PICU guidelines first concern a methodical approach to applying evidence-based nursing and team interventions and second, more recently, evidence-based ward design.

In several countries, building guidelines have been developed over the last 20 years. When we look at the development of PICUs, we observe several developments. The first descriptions of PICUs cover initiatives in the United States (Baker et al., 1959; Crain & Jordan, 1979; Gove & Lubach, 1969), England (Basson & Woodside, 1981; Dix & Williams, 1996; Mounsey, 1979), Ireland (Patton, 2013; Raaj et al., 2023), Canada (Musisi et al., 1989), New Zealand (Corey et al., 1986) and Australia (Goldney et al., 1985). In more recent years, PICUs have been established in Norway, Sweden (Faerden et al., 2023), Denmark (Simonsen & Duff, 2020a, 2020b) and the Netherlands (van der Schaaf et al., 2013; Voskes et al., 2021; Vruwink et al., 2012). Most of these countries have or are currently developing PICU guidelines. Many recent guidelines are based on a similar body of evidence. A report for the European Commission (Pincus, 2019) identified PICUs in 14 countries—Australia, Canada, the Czech Republic, Ireland, Wales, Japan, the Netherlands, New Zealand, Switzerland, Sweden, the UK and the USA. As well as these countries, we recently identified PICUs in Denmark (Berring et al., 2023) and Belgium (Zorgnet-Icuro, 2023).

## 2     History of Psychiatric Intensive Care

One of the first publications covering the concept of a Psychiatric Intensive Care Unit (PICU) concerns a working group document of the World Health Organization (WHO) expert committee on mental health (Baker et al., 1959), which defined several design criteria for psychiatric wards and facilities. This report describes one of the earliest conceptual designs for intensive care units in psychiatry. The criteria were based on expert opinion and included suggestions for single rooms, ward overview, ward design, lighting, colour, location of team rooms and ward accessibility. Ward design varied depending on its function and target population, whether for outpatients, youth, adults, acute admissions or the elderly. Important suggestions of the working group were to organise team rooms and ward management offices near the ward and to divide wards into smaller units with different treatment intensities. However, even though these suggestions were made in the late 1950s, many of the suggestions took decades to be carried out in mental health care.

Gove and Lubach (1969) provided the first evaluation of treatment in a Psychiatric Intensive Care Unit (PICU). This study described the establishment of a stepped-care intensive treatment program for acutely admitted service users of a single county in the west of the USA. The pilot program included all 258 consecutive admitted service users between December 1962 and December 1964. All 171 service users admitted to the same ward a year before were treated as the control group.

The hospital stay for the control group was two and a half times longer than for those in the program, yet no differences in patient characteristics were observed.

Historically, the development of PICUs can be observed to progress in three phases. During the 1960s, 1970s and 1980s, psychiatric intensive care was a methodical approach detailed in various publications, including those mentioned previously. Most of the publications were policy evaluation documents providing limited underlying evidence. Apart from ward size, no other ward-level variables were yet included in any of these reports. This approach mirrored that of intensive care in general hospitals, focusing on specialised care delivered by highly trained professionals, guided by various protocols. However, evidence for this approach was limited because its integration into a rigorous randomised-controlled trial design would have been challenging. Findings were at best based on prospective observational data as in the study by Musisi et al. (1989), but mostly concerned retrospective findings with many shortcomings (Bowers et al., 2008).

Crain and Jordan (1979) published an empirical evaluation of an initiative concerning a new ward environment of eight beds, combined with a stepped-care treatment approach. Tied into each step was a specific nursing care plan, which defined the extent of supervision, privacy, limit-setting techniques and privileges, as well as a set of activities deemed safe for the assessed risk. As many features of the ward milieu were incorporated into the steps, this system began to resemble a contingency hierarchy that progressively reinforced service users' behaviour in the direction of non-destructiveness. In practice, the service user would gain increasing token economy benefits as they advanced from lower to higher steps. The ward was equipped with ample space and also had a high staff-to-patient ratio of above one staff member per patient. The study showed that this separate unit led to fewer violent incidents and shorter hospital stays. It was also associated with fewer staff injuries. The main conclusion of the study was that the PICU did not completely prevent violent incidents. It did, however, 'provide a more humane treatment setting for [violent] individuals whose behavior ordinarily would provoke angry, punitive responses from the environment' (Crain & Jordan, 1979, p. 197).

A later study was conducted in Glenside Hospital, Adelaide, Australia, involving a 3-year observational study in an eight-bed PICU, with six beds located in single rooms (Goldney et al., 1985). Stay at the ward was short at a mean of 5 to 6 days. Approximately 60% of the service users were admitted with psychosis and received haloperidol as treatment. Contrary to previous research by Crain and Jordan (1979), Mounsey (1979), and Basson and Woodside (1981), the hospital stay in the Australian ward was much shorter and only provided the function of crisis intervention and stabilisation through a high-dosage medication protocol.

A study by Musisi et al. (1989) described a PICU in a rural psychiatric hospital. This was a six-bed ward, with a large central room, a television and a conference room. The ward had a nursing desk near the entrance with an overview of all single rooms. The introduction of the ward in 1984 led to a decrease in staff and service users' accidents, a decrease in constant observation and seclusion hours, and a decrease in the number of nursing hours lost to injuries at work. The PICU was appreciated by nursing staff who preferred to work in its more consistent and controlled environment. In addition, it was felt that the ward environment in other parts of the hospital became more therapeutic. The authors, therefore, concluded that PICUs along such a design were a useful addition to psychiatric settings with important cost and care implications. In effect, this study was the first one to show some empirical benefits of PICUs.

In the 1990s, many of the protocols described by the earlier studies were included in the development of PICU guidelines. From this time onwards, the PICU approach was increasingly confined to small wards, which were partitioned out of larger admission wards and accompanied by building criteria as depicted in the publication by Dix and Williams (1996). They suggested the ward should be positioned at a central location on the ground floor and suggested several security measures including electronic keys, lockable doors and monitoring devices. A clear view of staff over the ward is essential and, therefore, small corridors and dark corners should be avoided in the design. The patient–staff ratio on these wards should be higher, while the nurses should be trained in de-escalation, handling aggression and other techniques to prevent the use of coercive measures.

Moreover, the ward should have practical and recreational facilities, such as sports facilities and a ward telephone. Plants and accessories can be added to create a homely environment. The ward should be designed in a way that facilitates one-to-one guidance and close observation and has between four and eight single bedrooms, aligned along several central rooms.

Subsequently, an evidence-based body of knowledge developed, accompanied by guidelines in several countries between 2002 and the present day. The guidelines include evidence-based nursing and team interventions alongside adjustments to building facilities informed by architectural and social psychological studies of the healing environment. The healing environment, as developed in general hospital care, identifies elements such as space, overview, ward structure, lighting, colour and ward design. The application of healing environment principles in the design of many PICUs varied depending on the ward's location within the hospital design.

## 3    Healing Environment: A General Hospital Concept Adjusted for Psychiatry

A healing environment refers to a physical setting as well as the organisational culture that supports patients or service users in their recovery (DuBose et al., 2018). As stated, much work has been undertaken examining the effects of the healing environment on patient outcomes in general hospital settings. A study by Stichler (2001) showed that patients in critical care wards of general hospitals have a shorter length of stay, take less pain medication and have fewer notations of disordered behaviour (such as violence) in nursing reports, than those in a less welcoming environment. The following domains were identified by Stichler (2001) as being associated with better outcomes:

1. Ward design.

2. Light, colour, furnishing, sound and privacy.
3. Room design and furbishing as well as an optimal number of rooms.
4. Visibility of all parts of the ward.
5. Family space.
6. Nursing station design and staff support areas.
7. Unit support areas.
8. A circular, triangular or rectangular design.

Dijkstra et al. (2006) published a systematic review of the healing environment in the general healthcare setting. Outcomes predominately concerned clinical recovery and social and psychological well-being. Predominantly positive effects were found for sunlight, windows, odour and seating arrangements. Inconsistent effects were found for sound, nature, spatial layout, television and multiple stimuli interventions. The authors identified important architectural factors: ward layout and placing, and ambient features such as sunlight, sound, odour, window size and spatial design. In addition to these immutable characteristics, interior design features such as plants, seating provisions, television facilities, music facilities and ward colouring were also evaluated. Predominantly positive effects were found for sunlight, windows, odour and seating arrangements. Inconsistent effects were found for sound, nature, spatial layout, presence of a television and multiple stimuli interventions. In general, both the size and direction of effects seem highly dependent on the characteristics of service user populations and healthcare settings.

Similarly, Watts and Wilson (2009) published a review on evidence-based design in paediatric hospitals, examining the impact of physical elements on clinical, psychological and patient/family perceptions. They identified eight studies, published between 1980 and 2008, which found that private space, small ward size, single-room design for intensive care units, specially designed gardens, play centres and nature art were associated with benefits including reducing infections, promoting engagement and supporting coping with illness, particularly for adolescents and their parents.

The concept of a healing environment in psychiatry was first identified and conceptualised from both an architectural and a psychosocial viewpoint within a psychiatric context by Gross et al. (1998). In a large psychiatric hospital in Israel, ward design (along with healing environment principles) was developed by a multidisciplinary team of architects, psychiatrists, other mental health professionals, administrators and service users. The design of inpatient wards in this centre followed several principles of healing environment guidelines for ward design. Service users were not overcrowded or confined to overly small spaces, thereby avoiding forced interaction with too many people. Service users had the opportunity to retreat to their own, single rooms when feeling threatened, and to form beneficial relationships with staff or other patients of their own choice as the ward provided enough space to do so. This was achieved by providing a variety of spaces that supported social interaction, such as a large living room, a dining room with adequate lighting and ventilation, and a spacious lobby and corridors, with residential furniture rather than commonly used institutional pieces. The open porches of this one-story building showed a gradual transition from the ward to the garden, thus providing further spaces for social interaction, and creating a free and unthreatening atmosphere while at the same time helping to define the environment.

For the design of the ward by Gross et al. (1998), several findings from previous studies were included in the design. In previous years, empirical studies evaluating the impact of ward design revealed various effects of the physical environment on behaviour. Higgs (1970), for example, found a decrease in pathological behaviour after moving service users with schizophrenia to a newly rebuilt, larger unit that featured a comprehensive ward overview and single rooms. Another architectural change that reportedly might bring clinical benefits is the structural division of the ward into smaller units. Wilson et al. (1983) showed the division of wards into small units increased the risk of aggression and coercion, due to less overview and diminished opportunity of keeping enough eye on the patients. Corey et al. (1986) showed even simple redecorations in psychiatric wards, such as changes in furniture style, floor covering and colour scheme, could have a favourable impact on staff and service user perceptions of their physical environment.

These experiences contributed to the concept of a healing environment, which suggests that the ward environment can make a difference in the recovery of the service user. An important body of literature from the 1970s to the 1990s demonstrated that service users have a better outcome in an environment with natural light, elements of nature, soothing colours, meaningful and varying stimuli, peaceful sounds, pleasant views and a sense of beauty (Berring et al., 2023).

Lundin (2021) published a discussion paper presenting a theoretical framework identifying why a healing environment could contribute to increased safety at psychiatric wards. Ulrich et al. (2018) developed this idea into a theoretical model, describing the association between psychiatric disorder, ward design and service user outcome (Fig. 1). The main theoretical point presented in this model is that reduced stress will reduce the risk of negative emotions and thereby reduce aggressive behaviour (Ulrich, 1991; Ulrich et al., 2018).

This stress-reducing theory is possibly the most widely used and accepted theory when it comes to explaining the mechanism between physical interventions, ward environment and health outcomes in general. Ulrich et al. (2018) suggest that when a ward has more stress-reducing factors, coercive measures such as forced medication and physical restraints occur less. The impact of the building environment on ward interaction is complex (van der Schaaf et al., 2013). Collaboration among staff, service users, experts and architects is crucial to address various concerns. Balancing the preferences of all stakeholders can create a healing and secure environment. However, conflicting needs may arise between safety and a healing environment, potentially affecting feelings of safety. While some environments may enhance physical safety, they may compromise the sense of safety for either staff or service users. Staff safety encompasses measures to prevent physical or mental harm during interactions. Improvements in the environment aimed at enhancing staff safety may not simultaneously benefit user safety. For instance, creating command areas can make staff feel more secure by establishing control zones, yet this might reduce patients' sense of safety by introducing a perceived barrier or distance

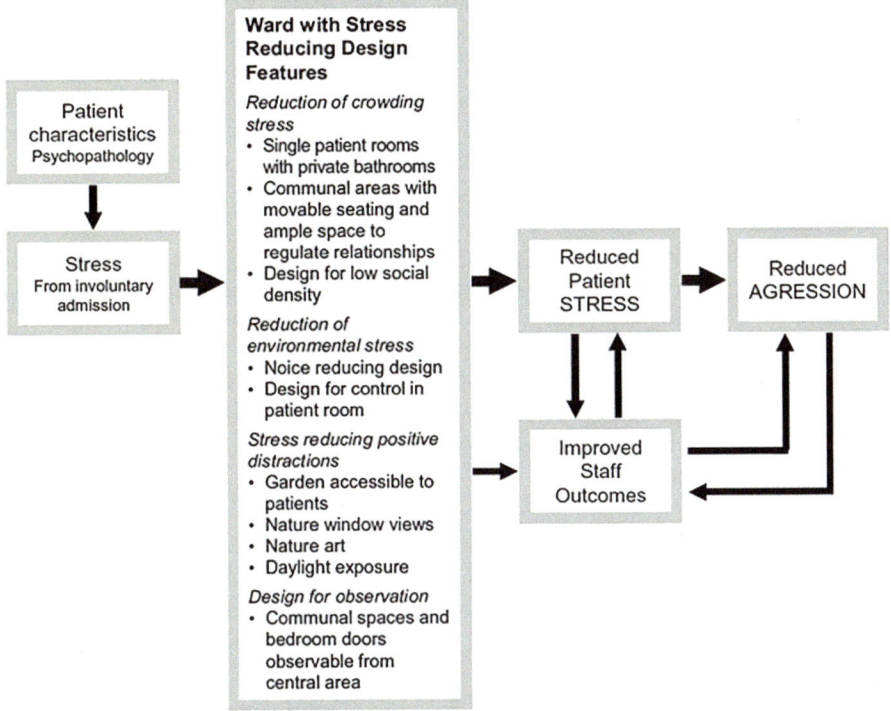

**Fig. 1** Theoretical model of ward design (Ulrich et al., 2018). 'Reprinted from Journal of Environmental Psychology, Vol. 57, Author(s), Psychiatric ward design can reduce aggressive behavior, page 14, 2018, with permission from Elsevier'

between them and the staff. Effective communication and spatial planning are essential for mitigating safety threats within the ward (Ulrich et al., 2018).

The threat of aggression is associated with the way nurses deal with service users, but also how the ward environment supports nurses in maintaining safety. Service user safety aims to prevent suicide, self-harm and harm against others (Svensson, 2022; Ulrich et al., 2018). It implies close observation of staff. It implies stepped care of increasing intensive treatment and close observation in different phases of dealing with the service user (Svensson, 2022). Service users should not have the opportunity to plan or act impulsively, resulting in suicide or self-harm. Civil protection aims to prevent service users, who are considered a danger to themselves and others, escape and becoming a threat to society (Svensson, 2022).

The service user's desire for a healing perspective could contradict the safety concerns of the staff or the service user's family (Svensson, 2022). One of the recurring issues concerns the placement of the bed in the services user's room (van der Schaaf et al., 2013). Staff may prefer to see the service user immediately when opening the door; it gives them a feeling of safety to know where the service user is. Additionally, staff want to avoid having to go further into the room, which might disturb the service user. However, from the service user's perspective, it is not certain that they want to be directly observed. A bed placement by staff requests could imply that the service user's head usually ends towards the façade wall but hinders looking out the window.

Karlin and Zeiss (2006) reviewed publications identifying environmental and therapeutic issues in psychiatric hospital design at a single-ward level. They identified five categories: ambient features, architectural features, interior design features, social features and specific issues related to the service users in care. Ambient features concern lighting, air quality, space and noise. Architectural features are about the constant characteristics of the building. The layout, size and shape of wards, and single or shared rooms promote or hinder participation in treatment activities. Interior design features are about the non-permanent features of a ward. This concerns features as placing of the reception area, the nursing office, the dining room and other common facilities. These features, together with the design and furnishing of service users' rooms, constitute a certain atmosphere which can contribute to a feeling of being at home.

The concept of a healing environment was a major issue in a large nationwide observational Dutch study into the association of psychiatric ward characteristics to the use of seclusion, which may be seen as a proxy for aggressive outbursts (van der Schaaf et al., 2013). It examined seclusion incidents and ward design in 199 wards over 12 months, gathering data from 77 hospitals and a benchmark study. Analysis showed certain design features increased seclusion risk, like limited outdoor space and high service user density, while others, like more private space and comfort, reduced it. The study emphasised the importance of a healing environment, suggesting that intrusive safety measures should be balanced with creating a homelike atmosphere to improve service user well-being and reduce seclusion and restraint needs. Several of the findings of the study were included in the Dutch national guidelines for the High and Intensive Care (HIC) model (Voskes et al., 2021). The guideline included items such as individual rooms and personal bathrooms, comfort rooms, diversity of shared spaces, outside space, a family room, a time-out room, an open nursing front desk, and the use of single intensive care units and a high-security room for emergency interventions. At a national level, these items are seen as contributing to the quality of care. Therefore, they are also considered in the inspections of the Dutch Mental Health Inspectorate.

Variations in ward features within a ward are important for a healing environment in psychiatry (van der Schaaf et al., 2013). Consideration of colours may be important with some authors suggesting incorporating neutral colours in the interior; different colour combinations can have varying effects on mood (Dalke et al., 2006). Brighter colours may be necessary for service users with depression or cognitive disorders (Dalke et al., 2006). Warm blue tones are known to have a soothing or sedating effect (Dalke et al., 2006). Also, closely related colours of the same value and intensity have been reported to have a calming effect. Blue-green colours can harm the mood of service users with depression and less energy. Seclusion room walls should be a calm, but definitive colour, not white or grey (Dalke et al., 2006).

In short, while many publications discuss environment as important in (mental) health care, few studies present real evidence of the effect of ward design on service user outcomes, including symptoms, well-being or recovery, or disordered behaviour, violence or coercion (van der Schaaf et al., 2013; van Melle et al., 2020; Voskes et al., 2021; Vruwink et al., 2012). Most of the studies about healing environments described in this chapter have been small, covering single wards. The studies within the reviews that we have identified in general and psychiatric settings (Dijkstra et al., 2006; Karlin & Zeiss, 2006; Watts & Wilson, 2009), combined many ward features. However, none covered more than one hospital. Evidence was obtained from the combination of data from the different review articles, but not confirmed by studies, combining or pooling any data.

## 4    Ward Design and Aggression

Around the turn of the twenty-first century, Henk Nijman, a leading researcher in aggression and psychiatry, published two small studies on the association between aggression and ward environment. The first investigated the incidence of aggressive incidents at an acute psychiatric admissions ward in the Netherlands (Nijman et al., 1997). It tested the reliability of the Staff Observation and Aggression Scale–revised (SOAS-r). Importantly, this was the first study looking into the location of incidents within the ward. They found that 48.6% of the incidents took place in day rooms, 19.5% near the staff offices, 14.6% near the outside door of the ward, 7.3% in service users' bedrooms and 6.1% outside the ward, while in 3.9% of incident reports that the location was not specified. The study also identified that the incidents at the ward's main entrance were less severe than those in service user's rooms. In a second study performed in a ward undergoing reconstruction, a modest association between crowding, aggression and ward occupation ratio was identified (Nijman & Rector, 1999). No association, however, between ward design and aggression was found.

Sato et al. (2017) investigated the association between ward characteristics and aggression in 30 wards across 20 Japanese psychiatric hospitals. Over 6 months, they collected violence data using the Japanese version of the Staff Observation Aggression Scale—revised (SOAS-r), during which 443 incidents were reported. The study differentiated between three types of psychiatric wards: emergency wards for severely ill patients for short stays, featuring spacious environments, higher patient-staff ratios and better-trained staff, probably comparable to a PICU; acute wards for less severely ill patients, also for short stays; and standard wards for longer-term treatment aimed at full recovery. Aggression was mostly directed at staff in acute and emergency wards, with medication enforcement being a leading provocation in acute wards and verbal aggression the most common method. Conversely, in standard wards, aggression typically involved other service users, with physical means used, leading to reported pain and the application of seclusion. The findings underline the ward environment's significant role in influencing aggressive behaviour, with acute wards experiencing the highest aggression rates, followed by emergency and standard wards, respectively. They did not find any difference in the time of day that incidents occurred but did find that the characteristics of aggressive incidents are shaped by the clinical condition of patients, their interactive relationships with staff and the ward environment, which includes staff assignments.

Similarly, Vaaler et al. (2006) compared the number of aggressive incidents in a PICU to those in a regular admission ward. The PICU was a small unit of four single rooms, a sitting room, a dining room and a staff room providing a full ward overview through one-way screens at the centre of the ward. This study showed that in the PICU, there was a lower risk of aggression, as assessed by the Brøset Violence Checklist (BVC), and fewer actual aggression incidents, as measured with the SOAS-r. Even after adjusting for service user characteristics and the severity of psychosis, the difference remained significant.

Weltens et al. (2021) conducted a systematic review of the association between aggression and service user, staff and ward factors. The prevalence of aggressive behaviour in psychiatric wards varied substantially (8–76%). Service user risk factors were diagnosis of psychotic disorder or bipolar disorder, substance abuse, a history of aggression and younger age. Staff risk factors included male gender, unqualified or temporary staff, job strain, dissatisfaction with the job or management, burn-out and quality of the interaction between service users and staff. Staff protective factors were a good functioning team, good leadership and being involved in treatment decisions. Significant ward risk factors were higher bed occupancy, busy places on the ward, walking rounds, an unsafe environment, a restrictive environment, lack of structure during the day, smoking and lack of privacy.

In short, the studies of Nijman (Nijman et al., 1997; Nijman & Rector, 1999) suggest that aggression is often determined by interactions between staff and users. Most of the aggression occurred at the locations where staff and users come together, such as day rooms and staff offices. This is supported by many studies that have shown that staff–patient interaction is the most frequent precursor of patient violence, as identified in a large literature review by Bowers et al. (2011). Crowding and ward occupation rates have shown some association with aggression, while ward design has shown none. Sato et al. (2017) found that ward type was a predictor of the frequency and severity of aggression, with acute psychiatry wards showing the highest rates, followed by emergency wards—like PICUs—and the lowest in standard wards. In acute and emergency wards, staff were primarily the targets of aggression, whereas in standard wards, other patients were more often targeted. Similarly, Vaaler et al. (2006) found that a PICU experienced less aggression compared to a regular admission ward, even after accounting for patient characteristics. The review by Weltens et al. (2021) supported these findings indicating that factors such as high bed occupancy, crowded areas, an unsafe and restricted environment with limited overview, lack of structure and privacy issues were linked to increased aggression.

## 5    Ward Design Processes in Clinical Practice

To illustrate the process of redesigning an acute admission ward following the guiding principles of a healing environment and current knowledge about ward design, we give an example of the renovation of the High Intensive Care ward at Amsterdam University Medical Center in the Netherlands. The ward of interest is a 12-bed closed psychiatric admission ward in a university hospital. Service users admitted to the ward are adults with various psychiatric diagnoses, with potential somatic co-morbidity. Most admissions are acute and involuntary. Approximately one-quarter of admissions are tertiary referral admissions, the majority are general psychiatric admissions from the municipal psychiatric crisis facilities. The original (pre-renovation) ward consisted of two separate units with six single-service user rooms with private bathrooms. Both units had a multifunctional room for (primarily) private conversations or activities, a living room, kitchen, dining room and smoking room. Both units had access to an enclosed garden and to a large nursing station. Next to (but outside), the ward was a laundry room, four seclusion rooms, offices of the ward manager and secretary, a meeting room and a room designed for occupational therapy.

This ward was renovated in 2019 after years of preparation. Part of the preparation was the implementation of the High Intensive Care model (Voskes et al., 2021) and changing (nursing) staff's attitudes towards ward safety and the use of coercive measures using regular training and supervision. The mission of the future ward design was to support and facilitate the wards' ambition to improve the recovery-oriented environment, intensify close contact between service users and staff members and reduce coercive measures. Specifically, the ward required more facilities for intensive (one-to-one) nursing care without using coercive measures and more space to prevent overcrowding. Coincidentally, the hospital would become smoking-free (inside and outside) during the renovation, so the smoking rooms would not return afterwards.

To create a more spatial ward design, the concept of two separate units was abandoned, and a larger, 12-bed ward was created. Furthermore, the corridor where the seclusion rooms, offices and occupational therapy room were situated was included in the ward. As a result, the size of the ward increased by (approximately) 30%, and we substantially improved the possibilities of service users to, e.g., do their laundry or go to the therapy room without needing staff members to unlock doors for them. The ward consisted of three different areas. These areas were not separated by walls or doors but became recognisable by different colours on the wall. Two of these areas were considered 'living areas'. The service user's rooms, comfort rooms, living rooms, dining rooms, kitchens and sports rooms were situated here. The third is the 'working area'. The conversation rooms, therapy rooms, laundry room, front desk and intensive care units were situated here. By dividing living areas and working areas, we aimed to create a safe space for service users where no intense therapy, meetings or interventions were performed. Although exceptions were possible, this remains a guiding principle for care planning at the ward.

The environment was designed to encourage interaction and engagement but to prevent moments of potential conflict between service users. Rooms and corridors were designed so that service users could always avoid a confrontation with another service user. This meant a minimum of corners and more than one entrance/exit in common areas. Rooms were divided with large closets that do not reach the ceiling, also to establish a feeling of openness for those present in the ward. When designing the ward, we used lots of wood and warm, natural colours. When choosing materials and furniture, we maintained a delicate balance between hospitality and aesthetics on the one hand and molest-proof and hygiene on the other. Materials and furniture needed to be strong and easy to clean, but not have a molest-proof, institutional look. When making choices about floors, ceilings and curtains, we chose materials that could improve the acoustics of the ward. The ward implemented several acoustic panels on the wall with a comforting print to improve the sound even more. Lights had warm colours and could be switched off during the night (contrary to the old situation). Furthermore, lighting in the ward was evenly divided in the room by large ceiling lamps. The old situation with small, bright lights resulted in 'light stains' on the ceiling, resulting in a disharmonious picture of the environment.

The nursing station was transformed into an open front desk, which is the heart of the work area and basically, the heart of the ward. The front desk contained a workstation and telephone, but nurses usually work throughout the ward with mobile phones and computers on wheels (COWs). Behind the front desk, locked closets contained all systems that were previously situated in the nursing station, such as telephones, walkie-talkies, light buttons and fire extinguishers. A large round table was placed in the space in front of the front desk to create a hospitable reception area. This has proven to be a popular meeting area for service users and staff members. Also, for hospitality purposes, this area contained a panel with names, professions and pictures of the wards' medical, nursing, therapeutic and supporting staff members. Care workers created a book with personal information for service users to get to know them to improve the feeling of equality between service users and staff members (based on Safewards 'Know each other' intervention) and a guestbook for service to leave hopeful messages at discharge for current or future service users (based on Safewards 'Goodbye messages' intervention).

The corridor next to the work area contained three small conversation rooms, one large meeting room, a laundry room for service users and a room for occupational therapy. Furthermore, two intensive care units (ICUs) were situated in this area. The ICUs were designed to provide intensive nursing care to individual service users in a private area when interaction with other service users counteracts their recovery process. The ICUs contained a bedroom, a small living room with a television and a bathroom. Both units also had access to a private garden. One of the ICUs had room for a next-of-kin to stay overnight if necessary. One of the ICUs was equipped with a high-security room (HSR) in which seclusion is possible in case of an emergency. The HSR had a large window, so the secluded service user could always see the staff member on duty. Furthermore, the HSR contained a toilet, sink, bed and multimedia system. The service user secluded in the HSR could use the multimedia system to operate several aspects of the room, such as light, colours, music, curtains and the window that can be opened for fresh air. This system is important to give a service user in seclusion a minimum amount of autonomy. The personal belongings of a service user in seclusion can be stored in a closet with a transparent front, which is visible from the window of the HSR. This can prevent conflict about the security of personal belongings between service users and staff members. Other than the HSR, none of the doors inside the ward can be closed from the outside. Not every room is accessible for all, but once inside, one can freely exit any room.

In the living areas, service users can use the living room with a television and a decently equipped kitchen. The cooker and stove can be switched off by staff members when specific service users may cause dangerous situations using them. The comfort rooms also had a television and an electric fireplace to induce a warm atmosphere, together with a couch and relax-seat. Every service user had a single bedroom with an en suite bathroom. The rooms had a bed that could be moved, a closet and a table and chair. The rooms and bathrooms were built to prevent the opportunity for hanging, such as acclivous doorknobs, shower heads and flexible coat racks. The floor had two different colours as a natural boundary for staff members to wait by the door until they were invited to come in. Every service user had a patient badge to enter their room whenever they wanted.

With these and many other design features, we aimed to combine a healing environment with the environmental safety precautions that are needed at a closed ward for acute psychiatric admissions. Some staff members were sceptical towards not having a nursing station and the abandonment of closed rooms (in the old situations, the ward had access to 4 seclusion rooms, and 4 of our 12 service user's rooms could be used to seclude a service user in its room). However, the warm and hospitable environment had an effect not only on service users but also on staff members. Service users responded on numerous occasions that they felt like they checked into a hotel, despite their mostly coerced situation. While psychiatric wards tend to deteriorate faster than other professional environments and vandalism does still occur occasionally, warm surroundings stimulate staff members and service users to keep the environment clean and intact. We believe that the ward design now supports and stimulates our perspective on high-quality, intensive psychiatric care, which could only be accomplished by a long and intense collaboration between service users, staff members, administrators, architects and contractors to achieve such goals.

## 6    Summary

This chapter has offered an overview of the knowledge regarding the impact of the ward environment on service users, including the incidence of aggression and the application of seclusion and restraint. Since the 1970s, the physical ward environment has been incorporated into mental health policy. Especially over the last two decades, studies have provided evidence of the association between ward environment, safety and the risk of aggression or the use of coercive measures. Several concepts are important in this respect: the healing environment, the establishment of PICUs and the identification of the ward environment as a risk factor for aggression.

For each specific situation, tailor-made advice is needed on how to ensure a safe ward through adjustments to the ward environment and, potentially, its location.

The healing environment relates to many aspects including the ward overview, colour, lighting, the use of plants at the ward and the proximity of a garden or outdoor space. Regarding PICUs, there is a broad consensus that small wards, staffed by highly trained nurses and maintaining a high patient-to-staff ratio are important during the acute phase of the psychiatric illness. The findings of studies investigating the relationship between ward environment and aggression, as well as the use of seclusion and restraint, align with many of the recommendations made in the healing literature. Overall, replacing the classic nursing station with an open front desk and preventing overcrowding are considered key factors in enhancing safety. Additionally, room design and bed placement contribute to increased safety. In designing wards, it is advised to engage service users and experiential experts along with staff in creating a safe environment for the care of those in the acute phase of their illness.

Concerning the direct association between ward environment and aggression, only a few quite small studies could be found covering an investigation of ward design and aggression. The findings of these studies are corroborated by a large study about coercion, which may be seen as a reasonably good proxy for aggression. The first investigated the association between ward design and seclusion and identified 14 design features of wards that had a significant effect on the risk of being secluded (van der Schaaf et al., 2013).

## 7    Recommendations

From all these studies as well as from practical experience, we can identify several building environment recommendations associated with improving well-being and reducing aggression or coercive measures. Reasoning from outwards inside the first is the placing of the ward within its environment. Preferably a psychiatric (intensive care) ward should be on the ground or on the first floor. It should be not completely incorporated into a general hospital but placed in a separate building with a limited number of beds. It should be in an environment providing direct access to nature. The ward itself should preferably have enough common space to allow a good overview of each of the service users' rooms. The rooms should be for one service user. The interior of the rooms should be adjusted to the service user's preference, except when the service user's behaviour cannot be relied upon. In that case, the placing of the bed needs to be done in a way the space around the bed is enough to move around, both for the professional and the service user. For all these spaces, factors such as light, colour, furnishing and size all contribute to less aggression, less coercion inversely and more safety. Preferably ward redesigning should occur in close collaboration with service users. Whenever psychiatric intensive care wards are meant to move or be refurbished or even rebuilt these recommendations could be considered. Supervision by an expert in the domain of healing environment is crucial, to avoid making errors in the building environment, as these errors can be very expensive and may consume an important portion of a hospital's operational capacity.

## References

Baker, A., Davies, R. L., & Sivandon, P. (1959). *Psychiatric Services and Architecture*. World Health Organization.

Basson, J. V., & Woodside, M. (1981). Assessment of a secure intensive care-forensic ward. *Acta Psychiatrica Scandinavica, 64*, 132–141.

Berring, L. L., Bak, J., & Hvidhjelm, J. C. (2023). National strategies to reduce the use of coercive measures in psychiatry in Denmark—A review of two decades of initiatives. *Issues in Mental Health Nursing, 44*(1), 35–47.

Bowers, L., Jeffery, D., Bilgin, H., Jarrett, M., Simpson, A., & Jones, J. (2008). Psychiatric intensive care units: a literature review. *International Journal of Social Psychiatry, 54*(1), 56–68.

Bowers, L., Stewart, D., Papadopoulos, C., Dack, C., Ross, J., Khanom, H., et al. (2011). *Inpatient violence and aggression: A literature review*. King's College. http://www.kcl.ac.uk/iop/depts/hspr/research/ciemh/mhn/projects/litreview/LitRevAgg.pdf

Corey, L. J., Wallace, M. A., Harris, S. H., & Casey, B. (1986). Psychiatric ward atmosphere. *Journal of Psychosocial Nursing and Mental Health Services, 24*(10), 10–16.

Crain, P. M., & Jordan, E. G. (1979). The psychiatric intensive care—an inhospital treatment of violent adult patients. *Bulletin of AAPL, 2*, 192–198.

Dalke, H., Little, J., Niemann, E., Camgoz, N., Steadman, G., Hill, S., & Stott, L. (2006). Colour and lighting in hospital design. *Optics and Laser Technology, 38*, 343–365.

Dijkstra, K., Pieterse, M., & Pruyn, A. (2006). Physical environmental stimuli that turn healthcare facilities into healing. *Journal of Advanced Nursing, 56*(2), 166–181.

Dix, R., & Williams, K. (1996). Psychiatric intensive care units a design for living. *Psychiatric Bulletin, 20*, 527–529.

DuBose, J., MacAllister, L., Hadi, K., & Sakallaris, B. (2018). Exploring the concept of healing spaces. *HERD, 11*(1), 43–56.

Faerden, A., Rosenqvist, C., Håkansson, M., Strøm-Gundersen, E., Stav, A., Svartsund, J., Røssæg, T., Davik, N., Kvarstein, E., Pedersen, G., Dieset, I., Nyrud, A. Q., Weedon-Fekjær, H., & Misvær, K. K. (2023). Environmental transformations enhancing dignity in an acute psychiatric ward: outcome of a user-driven service design project. *Health Environments Research and Design Journal, 16*(2), 55–72.

Goldney, R., Bowes, J., Spence, N., Czechowicz, A., & Hurley, R. (1985). The psychiatric intensive care unit. *British Journal of Psychiatry, 146*, 50–54.

Gove, W., & Lubach, J. E. (1969). An intensive treatment program for psychiatric inpatients: A description and evaluation. *Journal of Health and Social Behavior, 10*(3), 225–236.

Gross, R., Sasson, Y., Zarhy, M., & Zohar, J. (1998). Healing environment in psychiatric hospital design. *General Hospital Psychiatry, 20*(2), 108–114.

Higgs, W. (1970). Effects of gross environmental change upon behavior of schizophrenics: a cautionary note. *Journal of Abnormal Psychology, 26*, 421–422.

Karlin, B. E., & Zeiss, R. A. (2006). Best practices: Environmental and therapeutic issues in psychiatric hospital design: Toward best practices. *Psychiatric Services, 57*, 1376–1378.

Lundin, S. (2021). Can Healing architecture increase safety in the design of psychiatric wards? *Health Environments Research and Design Journal, 14*(1), 106–117.

Mounsey, N. (1979). Psychiatric intensive care. *Nursing Times, 75*, 1811–1813.

Musisi, S. M., Wasylenki, D. A., & Rapp, M. S. (1989). A psychiatric intensive care unit in a psychiatric hospital. *Canadian Journal of Psychiatry, 34*(3), 200–204.

Nijman, H. L. I., Allertz, W., Merckelbach, H. L. G. J., Campo, J. J., & Ravelli, D. P. (1997). Aggressive behaviour on an acute psychiatric admissions ward. *European Journal of Psychiatry, 11*(2), 106–114.

Nijman, H. L. I., & Rector, G. (1999). Crowding and aggression on inpatient psychiatric wards. *Psychiatric Services, 50*, 830–831.

Patton, D. (2013). Strategic direction or operational confusion: Level of service user involvement in Irish acute admission unit care. *Journal of Psychiatric and Mental Health Nursing, 20*(5), 387–395. https://doi.org/10.1111/j.1365-2850

Pincus, J. (2019). *International Mental Health Comparison in fourteen countries: Child and adolescent, adult, older adult services.* https://s3.eu-west-2.amazonaws.com/nhsbn-static/Other/2019/International-MH-report-31-October-2019.pdf

Raaj, S., Navanathan, S., Matti, B., Bhagawan, A., Twomey, P., Lally, J., & Browne, R. (2023). Admission patterns in a psychiatric intensive care unit in Ireland: a longitudinal follow-up. *Irish Journal Psychological of Medicine, 40*(3), 361–368.

Sato, M., Noda, T., Sugiyama, N., Yoshihama, F., Miyake, M., & Ito, H. (2017). Characteristics of aggression among psychiatric inpatients by ward type in Japan: Using the Staff Observation Aggression Scale—Revised (SOAS-R). *International Journal of Mental Health Nursing, 26*(6), 602–611.

Simonsen, T., & Duff, C. (2020a). Healing architecture and psychiatric practice (re)ordering work and space in an in-patient ward in Denmark. *Sociology of Health & Illness, 42*(2), 379–392.

Simonsen, T. P., & Duff, C. (2020b). Mutual visibility and interaction staff reactions to the 'healing architecture' in Denmark. *BioSocieties, 89*, 1–21.

Stichler, J. F. (2001). Creating healing environments in critical care units. *Critical Care Quarterly, 24*(3), 1–20.

Svensson, J. (2022). Patient safety strategies in psychiatry and how they construct the notion of preventable harm: A scoping review. *Journal of Patient Safety, 18*(3), 245–252.

Ulrich, R. S. (1991). Effects of health facility interior design on wellness: Theory and recent scientific research. *Journal of Health Care Design, 3*, 97–109.

Ulrich, R. S., Bogren, L., Gardiner, S. K., & Lundin, S. (2018). Psychiatric ward design can reduce aggressive behaviour. *Journal of Environmental Psychology, 57*, 53–66.

Vaaler, A. E., Morken, G., Fløvig, J. C., Iversen, V. C., & Linaker, O. M. (2006). Effects of a psychiatric intensive care unit in an acute psychiatric department. *Nordic Journal of Psychiatry, 60*(2), 144–149.

van der Schaaf, P. S., Dusseldorp, E., Keuning, F. M., Janssen, W. A., & Noorthoorn, E. O. (2013). Impact of the physical environment of psychiatric wards on the use of seclusion. *British Journal of Psychiatry, 202*, 142–149.

van Melle, A. L., Noorthoorn, E. O., Widdershoven, G. A. M., Mulder, C. L., & Voskes, Y. (2020). Does high and intensive care reduce coercion? Association of HIC model fidelity to seclusion use in the Netherlands. *BMC Psychiatry, 20*, 469. https://doi.org/10.1186/s12888-020-02855-y

Voskes, Y., van Melle, A. L., Widdershoven, G. A. M., van Mierlo, A. F. M. M., Bovenberg, F. J. M., & Mulder, C. L. (2021). High and intensive care in psychiatry: A new model for acute inpatient care. *Psychiatric Services, 72*(4), 475–477.

Vruwink, F. J., Noorthoorn, E. O., Nijman, H. L., Vandernagel, J. E., Hox, J. J., & Mulder, C. L. (2012). Determinants of seclusion after aggression in psychiatric inpatients. *Archives Psychiatric Nursing, 4*, 307–315.

Watts, R., & Wilson, S. (2009). Impact of the physical environment in paediatric hospitals on health outcomes a systematic review. *JBI Library of Systematic Reviews, 7*(20), 908–941.

Weltens, I., Bak, M., Verhagen, S., Vandenberk, E., Domen, P., van Amelsvoort, T., & Drukker, M. (2021). Aggression on the psychiatric ward: Prevalence and risk factors. A systematic review of the literature. *PLoS One, 16*(10), e0258346.

Wilson, M. R., Soth, N., & Robak, R. (1983). Managing disturbed behaviour by architectural changes: making space fit the program. *Milieu Therapy, 3*(2), 15–24.

Zorgnet-Icuro. (2023). *15 Miljoen extra voor High and Intensive care* [15 million extra for High and intensive care]. https://www.zorgneticuro.be/nieuws/15-miljoen-euro-extra-voor-high-intensive-care-afdelingen-het-hele-land

## *Further Reading*

Gutheil, T. G., & Daly, M. (1980). Clinical considerations in seclusion room design. *Hospital and Community Psychiatry, 31*(4), 268–270. https://doi.org/10.1176/ps.31.4.268

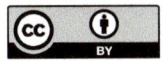

# Safety and Security: A Delicate Balance

Paul Doedens, Sofia Wikman, Hadassah Kuper,
and Hülya Bilgin

## 1 Introduction

Safety and security are broad concepts of a complex nature. Everyone involved in mental health wards (e.g. service users, staff members, visitors or family members) can experience an event that compromises their (feeling of) safety and security. However, everyone involved in mental health wards can also contribute to these events. Traditionally, scientific literature in mental health care focuses on the safety and security of staff members and the deterioration of safety and security due to aggressive and violent behaviour by service users. By embracing a broader perspective in recent years, the importance of a clear understanding of the concepts of safety and security for all increases. Although we aim to write an inclusive chapter, we are aware that (based on the background and experience of most of the authors), the North-West-European point of view possibly biased our writing. We recognise this and invite readers to consider this disclaimer while reading and generalising this information in their clinical practice.

P. Doedens (✉)
Department of Psychiatry, Amsterdam University Medical Center,
Amsterdam, The Netherlands
e-mail: p.doedens@amsterdamumc.nl

S. Wikman
Department of Social Work, Criminology and Public Health Sciences, The Academy for
Health and Occupational Studies, Gavle, Sweden
e-mail: Sofia.Wikman@hig.se

H. Kuper
Hadassah Faciliteert Herstel, Wolvega, The Netherlands
e-mail: h.kuper89@gmail.com

H. Bilgin
Mental Health and Psychiatric Nursing, Istanbul University-Cerrahpaşa, Istanbul, Turkey
e-mail: hulya.bilgin@iuc.edu.tr

© The Author(s) 2024
N. Hallett et al. (eds.), *Coercion and Violence in Mental Health Settings*,
https://doi.org/10.1007/978-3-031-61224-4_11

Aggressive and violent behaviour are still important risks for safety and security in clinical mental health care. When the victims of aggressive and violent behaviour are staff members, the literature defines this as workplace violence. Several studies identify mental health care as a high-risk sector for workplace violence (Li et al., 2020; Liu et al., 2019). Perpetrators of workplace violence can be service users, visitors or even co-workers (Civilotti et al., 2021). However, service users are also at high risk of being the victim of aggressive and violent behaviour by other service users or staff members (Frueh et al., 2005; Jenkin et al., 2022).

Furthermore, service users are at risk of numerous adverse events, such as suicide, self-harm, falls, medication errors or erroneous clinical judgement by staff members (Marcus et al., 2018; Nilsson et al., 2020; Vermeulen et al., 2018). An important safety risk for service users is the use of coercive measures, such as seclusion, restraint and forced medication. Although these measures are (ideally) solely used to prevent service users from harm, coercive measures have a substantial risk in themselves to harm psychological and physical health, due to violated personal dignity, anxiety and post-traumatic stress disorder (Kersting et al., 2019). The fact that staff members tend to use coercive measures in response to behaviour that staff members find difficult to understand and (possibly) perceive as dangerous (regardless of the service users' intention), such as violence, suicidal behaviour or absconding, complicates the mutual interest of service users and staff members concerning safety and security.

This chapter reviews the current knowledge on safety and security in clinical mental health services. The scope of this chapter is to focus on the safety and security of service users and staff members concerning aggressive and violent behaviour and the use of coercive measures. Besides a review of current knowledge, we postulate societal dilemmas that complicate the therapeutic partnership of service users and staff members to increase safety and security. Furthermore, we suggest some organisational innovations to increase safety and security in clinical mental healthcare. We end this chapter with a case report to illustrate the impact of such innovations and our thoughts on necessary developments to increase safety and security in the future.

## 2　Definitions

Safety and security were always subjects of interest in mental health services. Traditionally, the primary objective of large asylums and psychiatric hospitals was to use security to keep the mentally ill away from society. Safety and security were the primary reasons for large walls around institutions, barred windows, locked doors and restrictive institutional routines. These conditions provided an internal structure and environment, which was safe and secure for staff members and society.

Wide recognition of challenges and serious problems around safety and security dates around the 1980s. At the same time, mental health policy in many European countries began to move from a predominant model of institutional care to a more open and integrated model of community care. Back then, safety already had an accepted set of methods and solutions, such as local safety procedures, checklists and medication distribution protocols. Policymakers considered the 'new' problem of security initially as a variant of safety and treated it analogously, with secure ward design, prevention of, and protection against security hazards as the predominant strategies. Security, however, differs significantly from safety, both because security breaches are intentional rather than accidental, and because the secondary effects (i.e. postponed or long-term consequences) are more serious than the primary (i.e. immediate hazards or harm) (Hollnagel, 2021).

One of the differences between the two terms is their definition. Safety means the absence of potential harm, whether the cause of harm is deliberate or not. Security refers to the protection of individuals, organisations and properties against deliberate, external threats that are likely to cause harm. Security generally focuses on ensuring that external factors do not cause trouble or unwelcome situations to the organisation, individuals and the properties within the premises, while on the other hand, safety is the feeling of protection from factors that cause harm.

Another difference between safety and security in practice is that security is the protection against deliberate threats while safety is the aspect of being secure against unintended threats. It is common to protect people and properties against deliberate threats caused by criminals that have the intention to harm individuals, sabotage the operations of the organisation or steal the resources of the organisation. This means that security targets the protection against unlawful activities, caused by criminal behaviour. On the other hand, safety targets the protection of a person against unintended accidents.

However, in the context of mental health settings, both concepts are relevant. Some languages translate safety and security into one word, e.g. *veiligheid* (Dutch) and *säkerhet* (Swedish). Of equal importance as the meaning of the concepts is for whom they are applicable. In addition to the objective, both concepts have a subjective element as well. Organisational procedures can increase the safety and security of service users but might not increase their feeling of safety and security. Several mental traits and states of service users influence their feelings of safety, such as their current psychiatric state of the service users (e.g. anxiety disorders, paranoid delusions) and understandable emotions following (involuntary) admission due to a psychiatric crisis (e.g. despair, inequity, grief). Additionally, the attitude of staff members can influence the subjective feeling of safety and security.

## 3    Historical Perspective

Over recent decades, workplace violence has emerged as one of the principal occupational health hazards for many people at work. Workplace violence has become an increasingly high-profile societal problem. The increased attention and sensitivity to workplace violence may even increase the impact of officially registered violence in human services. Research indicates that there has been a shift from viewing workplace violence as a problem that should be resolved at the workplace as a health-and-safety issue, to increasingly viewing it as a problem that should be resolved externally with the help of the justice system (Wikman, 2016). This shift might reflect a societal move from safety to security.

Around 2000, Kennedy (2002) and Kinsley (1998) defined safety and security in three main contexts: (1) environmental; (2) relational; and (3) procedural. Environmental safety and security refer to construction and hardware issues, relational safety and security refer to interactional variables between service users and staff members and procedural safety and security focus on protocols, systems and risk management policy around this topic.

Since then, the concept of safety management has evolved from Safety-I to Safety-II (Hollnagel, 2014). Safety has traditionally been defined as a condition where the number of adverse outcomes is as low as possible (Safety-I). From a Safety-I perspective, the purpose of safety management is to make sure that the number of accidents and incidents is kept as low as possible, or as low as is reasonably possible. This means that safety management must start from the manifestations of the absence of safety and that—paradoxically—counting the number of cases where it fails rather than by the number of cases where it succeeds gives information on the 'magnitude' of safety. This unavoidably leads to a reactive approach based on responding to what goes wrong or what is a risk of harm. Focusing on and learning from what goes right, rather than on what goes wrong, change the definition of safety from 'avoiding that something goes wrong' (Safety-I) to 'ensuring that everything goes right' (Safety-II). More precisely, Safety-II is the ability to succeed under varying conditions so that the number of intended and acceptable outcomes is as high as possible. From a Safety-II perspective, the purpose of safety management is to ensure that as much as possible goes right, in the sense that everyday work achieves its objectives. This means that the achievement of safety (successes, things that go right) defines it, supported by counting the number of cases where things go right. To do this, safety management cannot only be reactive; it must also be proactive. Nevertheless, its proactive nature must be focussed on successful practice and everyday acceptable performance, rather than on prevention of failure, as traditional risk analysis does (Hollnagel, 2014). Safety-II has its influence on safety management policy at national and institutional levels. However, this philosophy also influences direct patient care. For instance, a proactive attitude of staff members (in partnership with service users) to learn from successful approaches in achieving commitment with service users, instead of the focus on failed approaches, increases the quality and safety of care.

There are several ways available to measure safety climate and safety culture, depending on the needs and capacity of an organisation. To measure these phenomena, organisations can use survey tools designed to assess an individual's response to key areas of the safety climate. These results can help to improve practice across an organisation. Several free tools are available that measure safety climate, most of them developed in the aviation and industrial sectors. The open-access publication 'Occupational Safety and Health culture assessment - A Review of main approaches and selected tools' summarises several free tools (EU-OSHA, 2011). Such tools can enable comparisons between different 'risks' or 'dangers' of workplaces, organisations, and industries. Furthermore, these tools can contribute to the exchange of experience and further theory development about how to prevent complex social problems, such as violence on an organisational level. The point of introducing these concepts is that they can broaden the theoretical understanding of and increase the spread of knowledge about complex phenomena, to which violence belongs. For an overview of diagnostic tools to measure safety climate and safety culture, see HSE (2005) or EU-OSHA (2011).

These tools are primarily to measure safety and safety climate from an (assumed) professional point of view. Service user experiences, such as satisfaction, empowerment and recovery, also give valuable information on the safety and safety climate of mental health organisations. Numerous scales for service user-reported experiences are available for mental care, although with very limited standardisation of the topics concerning service users' experiences (Fernandes et al., 2020).

## 4    Societal Dilemmas—Safety and Security for Whom?

Service users, staff members and others involved in clinical mental health care find common ground in the wish for safety and security for themselves and each other. However, there are circumstances in which interests are (or seem) contradictory. Those cases result in trade-off dilemmas; actions to improve safety and security on one side can compromise safety and security on another side. In this section, we provide some examples of such dilemmas.

### 4.1    Perpetration Versus Victimisation

An important negative stereotype about mental health service users is the perceived risk of being the perpetrator of violent crimes. Excessive media attention to tragic violent incidents serves as an accelerator of this belief. Several authors report an increased risk of violent offences perpetrated by persons with certain psychiatric illnesses, although these incidents are only a very small proportion of total violent crimes on the national level (Arseneault et al., 2000; Fazel et al., 2014; Guo et al., 2022; Kim, 2019). However, persons with psychiatric illness, in general, are at high risk of victimisation by (violent) crimes (Dean et al., 2018; Kamperman et al., 2014; Khalifeh et al., 2015; Meijwaard et al., 2015; Teplin et al., 2005). Choe et al. (2008) suggest that this victimisation is a more important societal concern than violent crimes committed by persons with psychiatric illnesses. In short, there is a wide (probably exaggerated) belief in society about the dangers of mental health service users, while protection of this group against criminal behaviour receives (too) little attention.

### 4.2    Involuntary Admission

Involuntary admission of service users has strict regulations and boundaries in most countries, including an obligation of care providers to provide service users with sufficient possibilities for person-centred voluntary care to prevent involuntary admission and treatment as much as possible. A typical part of the legal framework is the presence of danger for the service user or others due to severe mental illness (Carballedo & Doyle, 2011; de Stefano & Ducci, 2008). In case of an uncontrolled situation, involuntary admission serves as a protective measure for service users and their surroundings. The use of involuntary admissions differs substantially among European countries (de Stefano & Ducci, 2008). Literature shows ambivalent views towards involuntary admission; it is associated with positive outcomes in case of a psychiatric crisis in terms of clinical outcomes (e.g. symptoms or access to hospital care), but many service users hold negative feelings afterwards (Hofmann et al., 2022; Jones et al., 2021). Contrary to service users, informal caregivers view involuntary admission in a more positive light (Giacco et al., 2012), presumably due to concerns about the well-being of their loved ones. In a systematic review by Kallert et al. (2008), there seems to be some evidence that involuntary admission is associated with negative outcomes, such as longer admissions and a higher risk of suicide, but most studies that report such an effect do not control for the severity of psychiatric symptoms.

However, despite possible positive outcomes, involuntary admission is, without a doubt, a violation of the autonomy of service users. Every individual has the right to liberty and security, according to Article 5 of the European Convention on Human Rights (Council of Europe, 1950). Detention to protect 'persons of unsound minds' is one of the exceptions mentioned in section 1e of this article, though the European Court of Human Rights ruled that article 5 was violated with several persons with schizophrenia, among others, by involuntary admission (Wigand et al., 2021). However, it remains important to realise that the main interpretation of the term 'unsound mind' is from the perspective of others, rather than the service user. The Convention on the Rights of Persons with Disabilities (CRPD) by the United Nations describes 'respect for inherent dignity, autonomy including the freedom to make one's own choices, and independence of persons' as one of its leading principles, which makes involuntary admission at least a questionable practice (UN General Assembly, 2006). Involuntary admission hence is a delicate balance between respect for the service users' liberty and autonomy on the one hand and providing safety and security for the service users and their surroundings on the other. Furthermore, involuntary admission may expose service users to harmful events, such as violence by other service users and coercive treatment (Frueh et al., 2005; Hodgins et al., 2007; Jina-Pettersen, 2022). Thereby, involuntary admission may serve as a protective measure for society but can both benefit and violate the safety and security of service users.

## 4.3    Use of Coercive Measures in the Context of Safety and Security

The use of coercive measures in clinical mental health services is controversial and has been since the asylums of the nineteenth century (Hill, 1839; Topp, 2018). Besides the violation of service users' autonomy and human rights, there is no evidence of any therapeutic advantages of the use of coercive measures, such as seclusion and restraint (Sailas & Fenton, 2000). Seclusion and restraint qualify as interventions of last resort in case of dangerous situations when other interventions have failed (Doedens et al., 2020); they are associated with physical and psychological harm for service users (Frueh et al., 2005; Nath & Marcus, 2006; Rakhmatullina et al., 2013; Steinert et al., 2013). Although the use of coercive measures in clinical mental health differs substantially around Europe, in most countries mental health institutions still use coercive intervention (Duxbury & Whittington, 2005; Salzmann-Erikson et al., 2008). Imminent danger is the only legitimate reason for using coercive measures. However, other (informal) reasons to use coercive measures still occur in clinical practice, such as punishment, erroneous clinical judgement and neglect. In many countries, the use of coercive measures has led to public controversy after media reports of service users who have faced severe (sometimes even lethal) physical injuries after the use of coercive measures. This has led to the ambition to abandon the use of coercive measures entirely in several regions, e.g. the Dolhuys-manifest in the Netherlands (Dolhuys, 2016).

Due to these risks, service users and society commonly label seclusion and restraint as acts of abuse or violence, from staff members towards service users. Subsequently, service users, staff members and outsiders often agree that coercive interventions such as seclusion and restraint should not have a place in modern mental health care. However, some coercive measures, such as compulsory medication, at least have some intended therapeutic purposes. The purpose of such compulsory treatment is to deal with symptoms that cause a psychiatric crisis, although service users may experience serious side effects of psychiatric treatment and, above all, a major violation of their right to refuse treatment. Other measures, such as seclusion and restraint, can only serve as a crisis intervention in case of (perceived) dangerous behaviour of service users. Considering safety and security, the use of seclusion and restraint as a last resort in case of danger results in a catch-22 situation. The use of these coercive measures introduces a high risk of harm to the service user and violates their safety.

Furthermore, the use of seclusion and restraint potentially increases the risk of violent encounters with service users, as service users can easily experience these interventions as aggression from staff members. However, violence and other harmful behaviours impose a risk to the safety and security of other service users, staff members and visitors on the ward. Coercive measures, especially seclusion and restraint, should improve safety and security in clinical mental health care, but simultaneously introduce a threat to the safety of the service user undergoing the intervention and the staff delivering it.

## 4.4    Zero-Tolerance Towards Violence

Violence in clinical mental health care poses a major threat to service users, staff members and others involved. Service users and staff members in clinical mental health wards have a relatively high risk of being victimised and traumatised by violence (Flood et al., 2008; Hilton et al., 2022; Itzhaki et al., 2018). It seems obviously that professionals, institutions, governments and society reject the use of violence and stand strongly for the security of those involved in clinical mental health care. This could lead to the wish for a firm, zero-tolerance policy against service users and others who use violence. It is important to maintain awareness that violence is not by definition part of working in or using the services of clinical mental health care, as long-term exposure to (high risk of) workplace violence can impose the belief that it is a common feature of the job. However, recent insights argue against the efficacy of a zero-tolerance policy.

Research suggests that zero-tolerance might not be a helpful attitude for staff members in clinical mental health care to improve staff's understanding and resilience towards violence (Beattie et al., 2020; Fan et al., 2022). Whittington (2002) responded to the zero-tolerance movement in the United Kingdom to argue that the 'tolerance' of staff members towards aggressive behaviour is a complex phenomenon and that a strict zero-tolerance policy might not help staff members further. In other studies, Whittington and Higgins (2002) and Secker et al. (2004) viewed the zero-tolerance campaign in the UK as infeasible without attention to interactional and environmental factors that can influence the occurrence and course of events of aggressive behaviour of service users. A zero-tolerance policy can result in a rigid attitude of staff members towards service users that does not contribute to the safety, security and (especially) recovery of service users (Middleby-Clements & Grenyer, 2007).

Society should never accept a violation of service users' and staff members' safety and security by violence. However, to prevent violence, strict intolerance towards service users who act out due to frustration, desperation or anxiety does not seem helpful. An outreaching approach to support service users in a psychiatric crisis, with clear boundaries, with a focus on building a supportive relationship seems more feasible to contribute to safety and security in clinical mental health care than a strict zero-tolerance policy. One of the key features of building a supportive relationship is staff members being present and available for service users. This involves active and attentive listening, without judgement or rushing to conclusions. Policymakers need to address the delicate balance between the rejection of violent behaviour and a supportive culture and environment for service users and staff members.

Whilst we go through the process of identifying violent behaviour, we must not lose sight of the fact that some violence is a reaction to the culture of the organisation itself. Dysfunctional behaviour in a healthy and functional organisational climate might look the same as an understandable coping mechanism in an unhealthy, dysfunctional environment. It is not just 'bad apples' that must concern us, we must also focus on the possibility of a 'bad barrel' (Bowie, 2011). When focusing on individuals (service users or staff in the health care system), such an approach operates on a 'bad apple' response to managing and preventing violence in the workplace. However, there has been growing awareness of the role organisations may play in creating oppressive and violent climates within their workplace, which may in turn trigger violence by staff, service users or others. This latter 'bad barrel' approach to managing violence is a continuous and ongoing process (Bowie, 2011).

Mullen and Kelloway (2011) studied major factors of leadership that contributed to organisational health claims and found that almost every outcome measure in health psychology is associated with organisational leadership. Oppressive organisational cultures may come in many forms such as autocratic management, unreasonable workloads, takeovers, downsizing and retrenchments, reduced benefits and conditions or individual work contracts. These factors might relate to an oppressive culture and might justify a zero-tolerance policy, while this probably would not increase safety and security for service users and staff members.

## 4.5    Prosecution of Violence

Despite the negative consequences of zero-tolerance policies, in case of severe violent behaviour with (high risk of) physical harm to other service users or staff members, mental health institutions need to respond appropriately. Whether or not victims of violence in clinical mental health care should report the perpetrator to the police is a subject of ongoing debate. After several publications in the 1980s and 1990s, the subject did not receive a lot of attention in literature after 2000. Appelbaum and Appelbaum (1991) and Norko et al. (1992) suggested guidelines to determine whether mental health institutions should seek prosecution of a violent incident. According to these authors, mental health institutions should have a clear policy on the decision-making processes around reporting to the police. In addition, the wishes and needs of the victim must have a central place in the process. Hospital administrators should consider the treatment context (e.g. coerced treatment or involuntary admission) and the current medical condition of the service user who acted violently before reporting to the police. However, this can (but should not) lead to a climate in which psychiatric symptoms and involuntary admission serve as a multifunctional excuse for violence. Studies from the Netherlands and New Zealand showed that staff members in clinical mental health care are reluctant to report violent incidents to the police and that conviction of aggressors is highly uncommon (Harte et al., 2013; Kumar et al., 2006). Judges also seem reluctant to convict service users to avoid interference with their treatment process (Visscher et al., 2019).

Some studies problematise how legislation works as governance to regulate workplace violence (Almond, 2015; Almond & Gray, 2017; Haines & Almond, 2014; Schindeler & Ransley, 2016; Schuilenburg, 2015). Whether or not prosecution is (sometimes) appropriate in cases of violence in clinical mental health care is debatable and will benefit from more attention in the scientific literature. However, to support the safety and security of service users and staff members, healthcare administrators, and governments should work on clear guidelines on this matter. These guidelines should address the balance between recognising the circumstances of the incident but should also acknowledge that service users are (or should be) capable of being accountable for their (criminal) actions. At least the perception of safety and security of service users and staff members could benefit from knowing what to do and when, and what to expect from law enforcement, lawyers and judges.

## 5        Safety and Security for Everyone

To obtain a safe and secure environment for service users, staff members, visitors and others involved in clinical mental health services, a multifactorial perspective is necessary. Previously, safety and security in mental health wards primarily focused on the safety and security of staff members. Service users' behaviour potentially threatened safety and security, and staff members tried to protect themselves from harm. This type of discrimination is erroneous and toxic, and, fortunately, increasingly rare in clinical practice. Moreover, the rise of the Safety-II framework makes it irrelevant to divide those involved into service users and staff members. The focus on maximisation of positive outcomes (Safety-II) instead of minimising negative outcomes (Safety-I) nudges staff members to ally with service users to work on mutual safety and security.

As mentioned earlier, Kennedy (2002) and Kinsley (1998) state that safety and security have environmental, relational and procedural properties. Environmental safety and security refer to the hardware of clinical wards (e.g. architecture, accessibility and materialisation) and technical solutions to support safety and security (e.g. closed-circuit television [CCTV], alarm buttons and mobile phones). This chapter focuses on relational and procedural safety and security, as Chapter 10 discusses environmental safety and security in detail. Relational safety and security refer to the quality of care, service user/staff ratios, treatment, recreational regimes and therapeutic rapport. Procedural safety and security are the focus of much attention at an operational level. At the service user level, it means systems and routines for checking and searching for risks of harm. On a system level, it means arrangements for risk management, professional governance and audit. Management of violent incidents, control and restraint, de-escalation training, breakaway techniques, risk assessment and coercive measures are also features of procedural safety and security. When reviewing the concepts of relational and procedural safety, we argue that relational characteristics of safety and security have the most influence on the subjective part of safety and security, but so do objective markers, such as incidents of violence or absconding. Environmental and procedural aspects of safety and security, as well as organisational aspects of relational safety and security, serve as a supportive framework for service users and staff members to engage in meaningful relationships to establish safety and security on both an objective and subjective level. Therefore, we describe procedural safety and security as a necessary condition to facilitate service users and staff members to work on relational safety and security.

### 5.1     Procedural Safety and Security

Procedural safety and security represent policy and procedures on various levels that contribute to the safety and security of individuals. When viewed on a macro-level, healthcare authorities and non-profit organisations, such as the Joint Commission, audit the procedural safety and security of healthcare institutions.

National and international laws, quality standards and risk management programs form the basis of its supervision. On a meso-level, healthcare institutions translate these systems into institutional policy, procedures and protocols, also based on the institutions' general mission and identity. These institutional regulations form the framework for staff members in clinical mental health wards to do their job. At the micro- (ward) level, staff members formulate written and unwritten daily routines to achieve safety and security. Procedures around medication administration, prevention of falls, food safety, hygiene and prevention of infectious diseases are key topics in most parts of the healthcare system. In clinical mental health wards, prevention of violence, drug use, suicide, absconding and other major adverse events, but also patients' satisfaction and recovery-oriented care are major subjects. A traditional response to such threats is controlling practices, such as searching a service user's personal belongings for drugs and sharp objects, routine checks by staff members during the night and regulations around visits of family and friends. These controlling practices likely result in strict ward rules, which apply to the majority (or all) service users who stay on the ward (with all the negative consequences these entail for service users). In addition, staff members receive training in risk assessment, verbal de-escalation, personal safety and physical techniques for responding to aggressive behaviour.

The focus on the prevention of adverse events and training to cope with potentially dangerous behaviour is a typical Safety-I response. Although prevention of adverse events is feasible, controlling and restrictive policies might also impose an increased risk of dangerous behaviour in itself (Price et al., 2018). Environmental and procedural safety and security provide tools to contribute to a safe and secure ward that may be highly effective in preventing medication errors and transmission of infectious diseases. However, if applied to behavioural risks, these aspects of safety and security can also interfere with achieving safety and security from a relational perspective.

## 5.2    Relational Safety and Security

Kennedy (2002) and Kinsley (1998) described relational safety in terms of quality of care, service user/staff ratios, treatment, recreational regimes and therapeutic rapport. We argue that this is a narrow view of relational aspects of safety and security. Furthermore, one might consider the quality of care and service user/staff ratios as elements of procedural safety. We, however, consider every interaction between service users, staff members and others involved in clinical mental health care as an influential factor in relational safety and security.

Interaction between service users and staff members plays a vital role in achieving safety and security. Aggressive behaviour in clinical mental health wards occurs mostly during these interactions (Bowers et al., 2011). However, interaction is also a vital part of the de-escalation of (emerging) aggression. Other risk behaviours, such as self-harm, attempted suicide or absconding happen mostly during moments without interaction between service users and staff members. Interpersonal interaction at least has two actors; these actors have (approximately) equal influence on the course of their interaction. From this point of view, service users and staff members can both influence their interactions and share a certain responsibility for the quality of that interaction.

The definition of safety and security suggests some objectivity. However, safety especially has a major subjective component. When a person receives adequate protection against harm due to intended or unintended external threats, the person does not necessarily feel safe and secure as well. Service users stay in clinical mental health wards because of a (psychiatric) crisis or their recovery from a crisis. These crises can influence feelings of safety and security, for example, due to paranoid delusions, anxiety or trauma. The disparity between objective and subjective safety and security components can negatively influence the ability to interact with others. This is one of the complicating factors of interaction between service users and staff members in clinical mental health wards. When the ability of service users to interact effectively with others decreases, staff members need more effort to create adequate interactions. However, factors such as work stress, fear or trauma can reduce the interactional skills of staff members. Because both actors might not be capable of optimal interaction, we argue that improving social interaction and mutual feelings of being capable and empowered is a key contribution to relational safety and security.

## 5.3 Social Interaction and the Actor, Partner, Relation, Activities, Context and Evaluation (APRACE) Framework

When viewing communication from an interactional point of view, it is a process in which participants interchange roles as sender and receiver of a message and give meaning to the interaction by sending messages and responding to the messages of the other (i.e. feedback) within physical, psychological and environmental contexts (Schramm, 1997). Publications about social interaction go back to Aristotle and other ancient Greek and Roman philosophers. Several frameworks are available to describe necessary and optional components of social interaction. Hoppler et al. (2021) suggested that social interaction consists of six components: Actor, Partner, Relation, Activities, Context, and Evaluation (APRACE). The Actor and Partner describe the persons engaged in social interaction, and the Relation represents their bond. During the interaction, the behaviour and actions of the Actor and Partner are Activities, and the interaction takes place in a certain Context. Evaluation resembles the constant (and commonly subconscious) evaluation of social interaction by the Actor and Partner (Hoppler et al., 2021).

The APRACE framework, when applied to clinical mental health care exposes challenges in social interaction in this specific setting. The service user and staff member take the role of Actor and Partner in the framework. Given that the Actor initiates the interaction, the role of the service user and staff member, as Actor or Partner, is interchangeable. The relationship between service users and staff members can be essential in establishing effective and equal interaction. However, establishing a meaningful relationship between service users and staff members takes time and, especially in acute and emergency settings, such time is not always sufficiently available.

Furthermore, due to several circumstances (e.g. holidays, sick leave, temporary staff, etc.), service users typically need to deal with a constantly changing treatment team, which does not contribute to their recovery. This lack of continuity in the interaction between service users and staff members needs constant awareness of staff. In short, Relation is an essential, though challenging component of social interaction in clinical mental health care.

The behaviour of the Actor and Partner plays a major role in the Activities component of social interaction. Their behaviour can be helpful to the interaction but can also be detrimental to the point that the interaction ends (e.g. the service user or staff member ends the conversation due to unwanted behaviour from the other). However, the interpretation of the behaviour of the other, especially in the light of safety and security, also has a major influence on the social interaction between service users and staff members. For example, if staff members assess the service users' behaviour as a threat to staff or ward safety and security, staff members can set boundaries or even apply coercive measures. From a social interaction point of view, these actions can result in a vicious cycle towards the escalation of the interactional problem. Thereby, adequate assessment of the behaviour and (especially) the underlying problem, frustration, stressor or other reason for the behaviour is a requirement for maintaining helpful social interaction. This might be challenging while interacting with a service user in crisis, especially since both the Actor and Partner are (equally) responsible for the quality of the social interaction. However, staff members can (and should) feel responsible for initiating helpful Activities to make social interaction with the service user, who may be in a psychiatric or psychological crisis, successful. The aim is not to free the service user from responsibility regarding the interaction but to support the service user in sharing this responsibility with the staff member.

Every aspect of our lives contains some sort of social interaction with others. Each Context leads to a different role, style or behaviour. Clinical mental health care consists of a series of specific contexts with some challenges and peculiarities when engaging in social interaction. First, many service users do not choose to be there, due to involuntary admission. This results in an (unwanted) hierarchical difference of power between service users and staff members. These power differences complicate social interaction in many ways. For instance, the service user can feel the need to please the staff member or to resist their involuntary admission. Staff members can feel uncomfortable with the difference in power or abuse these differences. In addition, environmental and procedural interventions to increase safety and security (such as CCTV, ward rules and other physical or procedural boundaries) are examples of contextual factors that can limit social interaction between service users and staff members. The key to overcoming these limitations is to recognise and acknowledge these as limitations to social interaction and to express the will to engage in effective social interaction, nevertheless. Staff members should show in their attitude that effective social interaction is their top priority. This message, and its underlying attitude, is the first step in constant Evaluation of the interaction. Service users in crisis and staff members under high pressure might not be able to give adequate feedback to each other during social interaction. However, it is a form of empowerment to stimulate service users and staff members to exchange feedback on social interaction and to open up to the feedback of their interactional counterparts. Besides attitude, a learning ward culture and relational safety are required to create space to give and receive feedback between Actors and Partners. Evaluation (and social interaction as a whole) is, thereby, essential for relational safety and security to create a safe and secure environment.

## 5.4    Safety and Security for All?

In this section, we discuss the importance of social interaction as a requirement for environmental, relational and procedural safety and security as conditional to establishing relational safety and security. We argue that rooms, locks, guards, cameras, rules, procedures, legislation and all the other procedural measures can increase safety and security for staff members, but to establish safety and security for all involved in clinical mental health care, relational safety and security are keys. Focus on relational safety and security needs implementation within ward culture, staff attitude and institutional policy. The UK government Department of 'An organization with a memory' (2000) summarised features of an organisation's culture that promoted safety. Such features included:

- People are prepared to report problems, errors and 'near misses'.
- There is an atmosphere of trust.
- There is respect for the skills and abilities of frontline staff.
- There is an ability and willingness to learn and to implement improvements.

In the next section, we describe how three models assist institutions, wards, staff members and service users to obtain or sustain focus on relational safety and security: High Intensive Care (Voskes et al., 2021), Six Core Strategies (Huckshorn, 2006) and Safewards (Bowers, 2014).

## 6    Organisational Innovations to Improve Safety and Security

In this section, we describe three models (High Intensive Care, Six Core Strategies and Safewards) for improving safety and security in clinical mental health wards with special emphasis on relational safety and security. Furthermore, we present a case report about a (fictional) service user to illustrate the use of these models in clinical mental health wards.

## 6.1    High Intensive Care

The High Intensive Care (HIC) model is an organisational approach to improve care for service users with (severe) mental illness (Van Mierlo et al., 2013; Voskes et al., 2021). The HIC model centralises the recovery-oriented approach (Lorien et al., 2020) and combines this with the medical model. The HIC model prioritises the recovery of service users in the roles that they find important, so mental health treatment is more than treating symptoms of psychiatric illness. Besides recovery-oriented care, the HIC model aims to minimise the use of involuntary treatment or coercive interventions and to include next-of-kin in every aspect of treatment, if the service user chooses to do so.

Outpatient treatment is the basis of the HIC model. The aim is to allow service users to recover in their (home) environment, with appropriate care from mental health institutions, next-of-kin and other potential sources of support. If a service user experiences a (psychiatric) crisis, the care in the outpatient situation is intensified using the intensive home treatment (IHT) model (Barakat et al., 2021). If the crisis escalates, the service user can choose for admission to the High Care Unit (HCU). If the service user does not agree with psychiatric admission, involuntary admission is an option according to the appropriate legislation if staff members and next-of-kin argue that admission is necessary to maintain safety and security for the service user and others involved.

The HCU is a closed admission ward of a hospital or mental health institution. The HCU has an open culture, with special concern for recovery, hospitality and feelings of safety. Staff members are present at the unit for service users to engage with, in a physical sense, but also due to their supportive attitude towards service users. The HCU has single rooms, shared areas where staff is present, sports facilities and comfort rooms for relaxation. A multidisciplinary treatment team (psychiatrist, nurse, psychologist, occupational therapist, expert-by-experience, etc.) invites the service users and their next-of-kin to a care-planning meeting to establish treatment goals and the interventions to reach those goals. The care-planning meeting is preferably due within 24 h after the service user enters the unit. Before the care-planning meeting, the treatment team is acquainted with the service user and performs structured risk assessment and psychiatric, neurological and physical examinations to collect information for the treatment plan. In addition, rooming-in of next-of-kin is also an option to support service users during every step of their recovery process. The overall objective of admission to the HCU is crisis intervention and stabilisation to help service users regain control and return to their home environment for further recovery from the crisis. The goal is to end the admission at the HCU within 3 weeks.

The HIC model uses a stepped-care approach to intensify care if the crisis deteriorates further. The first step is to intensify home treatment, followed by admission to the HCU when no other intervention is suitable to prevent serious harm to the service user or others. When admission to the HCU is not enough to ensure safety and security due to the risk of aggressive behaviour, self-harm or other harmful situations, one-on-one care is the next step in the stepped-care approach to maintaining safety and security. When a service user receives one-on-one care, a nurse is constantly present, nearby the service user and committed to the recovery process of the service user. One-on-one care in the HCU is possible, but if the HCU is too crowded, stimulating or provocative for the service user, the service user and staff member can transfer to the intensive care unit (ICU). The ICU is a private area close to the HCU with a living room, bedroom and bathroom that is fully equipped to perform one-on-one care. Staff members of the HCU join the service user in the ICU, which is unlocked and therefore no form of seclusion. If the crisis deteriorates further to the extent that safety and security for staff members who perform one-on-one care are at stake, a time-out in the high-security room (HSR) is possible. The HSR is a seclusion area with facilities for the service user to maintain some control over their environment, such as lights, privacy screens and room temperature.

Furthermore, the HSR has some form of entertainment system to prevent boredom and to facilitate external stimuli for service users. One-on-one care does not end when the service user is in the HSR; staff members stay present next to the windows to maintain interaction with the service user. The HSR is only an emergency facility for a short period (more like hours than days). When the risk of harm for staff members decreases, seclusion in the HSR ends and the service users return to the ICU with one-on-one care.

## 6.2 Six Core Strategies

The first publication of Six Core Strategies emerged around 2002, because of a national effort in the United States to prevent conflict, violence, and the use of seclusion and restraint (Azeem et al., 2011; Duxbury et al., 2019; Huckshorn, 2006; LeBel et al., 2014). It originates from a prevention-oriented, trauma-informed care framework, which considers restrictive procedures problematic from a quality improvement perspective. These are the Six Core Strategies, described below:

1. Leadership towards organisational change
2. Use of data to inform practice
3. Workforce development
4. Use of seclusion and restraint prevention tools
5. Service user roles in inpatient settings
6. Debriefing techniques

### 6.2.1 Leadership Towards Organisational Change

The first strategy includes direction, guidance, participation and ongoing review by executive leadership throughout all projects, plans and services to reduce or eliminate seclusion and restraint. This includes daily involvement of the executive director in all seclusion and restraint to investigate causality (antecedents), review and revise facility policies and procedures that may lead to conflict, monitor and improve staff development issues, and involve administration with direct care staff in these activities (Gaynes et al., 2017; Huckshorn, 2006). The action plan needs a firm foundation in a public health approach and continuous quality improvement principles. This strategy also suggests the use of a multidisciplinary performance improvement team or task force. The public health approach allows the prevention of coercive measures and their associated consequences.

Furthermore, it supports the prevention of violent behaviour in clinical mental health wards by eliminating risk factors as much as possible through universal precautions and selected interventions. Based on indicated interventions, extensive analysis and subsequent policy changes lead to secondary and tertiary prevention after the use of coercive measures. In this way, safe and secure mental health facilities should be possible for both users and staff.

### 6.2.2   Use of Data to Inform Practice

The second strategy includes the use of data based on baseline and after with ongoing monitoring over time. Possible data sources are characteristics of service provision in terms of unit, shift/day, employee, etc. (Gaynes et al., 2017; Huckshorn, 2006). Routine collection and analysis of data facilitate finding in the current conditions and can lead to proactive interventions to prevent adverse events. In addition, the use of data encourages the workforce to set goals, e.g. to reduce seclusion and restraint and monitor the success of these goals over time.

### 6.2.3   Workforce Development

The third strategy includes staff training programs focused on primary and secondary strategies, risk assessment and consequences of seclusion and restraint as well as multi-dimensional modelling of conflict (Gaynes et al., 2017; Huckshorn, 2006). The goals of this strategy are to improve workforce quality, especially around their de-escalation skills and their ability to perform person-centred care in a highly complex environment.

### 6.2.4   Use of Seclusion and Restraint Prevention Tools

The fourth strategy includes the integration of several tools aimed at preventing seclusion and restraint into clinical practice, such as risk assessment (e.g. Brøset Violence Checklist), the conflict escalation model, early warning signs, coping methods and environmental changes, to create individualised care plans (Gaynes et al., 2017; Huckshorn, 2006).

### 6.2.5   Service User Roles in Inpatient Settings

The fifth strategy includes the full and formal inclusion of consumers or people personally experienced in recovery, carers and families, in a variety of roles in the service to assist in the reduction of seclusion and restraint (Huckshorn, 2006). The role of service users in the care process can vary, but the service user perspective is necessary for the level of direct care, management and policy. In addition, extensive support of service users in their role as staff members is part of this strategy.

### 6.2.6    Debriefing Techniques

The sixth strategy includes analysing reasons for seclusion and restraint after the event and examining the impacts of these practices on individuals with lived experience. The goal of this strategy is not only to learn from an event for prevention in the future but also to mitigate any adverse consequences that the service users experience after seclusion and restraint. This strategy explicitly defines and implements tertiary prevention within the public health approach (Gooding, 2021).

The fundamental principles of Six Core Strategies are leadership strategies for effective change, public health prevention approach, recovery/resiliency strategies, valuing persons served and staff, sticking to continuous quality improvement (CQI) strategies and trauma knowledge operationalised (LeBel et al., 2014). The National Association of State Mental Health Program Directors' Six Core Strategies strongly influenced the alternatives to reduce and/or remove seclusion and restraint interventions. Several countries adopted Six Core Strategies including the UK, Australia, Finland, New Zealand, Germany, Canada and Japan (Duxbury et al., 2019).

## 6.3    Safewards

Safewards is a model of interventions to keep wards safe and secure by prevention of conflict (i.e. aggressive behaviour, self-harm, absconding, etc.) and containment (i.e. seclusion, restraint and other formal and informal coercive measures) (Bowers, 2014). The Safewards framework argues that service user characteristics, regulatory framework (e.g. local legislation), staff team variables, physical environment, stressors from outside the hospital and patient community are variables that influence conflict and containment. Due to service user- and staff modifiers, so-called flash points (such as denial of requests, bad news or on-ward stressors) can emerge that lead to conflict and containment. By breaking conflict and containment into several categories of influential factors, Safewards aims to intervene in the process to prevent flashpoints or to mitigate the effect of flashpoints to prevent conflict and containment.

From the Safewards framework, several interventions emerged with a focus on maintaining relational safety and security. In a clinical intervention study, Safewards was effective in reducing conflict and containment in clinical mental health care (Bowers et al., 2015). Safewards is an open-source model, with materials published on its website (www.safewards.net) and is available in ten languages. The Safewards website describes the interventions in detail and gives recommendations on the implementation of the Safewards framework. Therefore, we discuss some examples of Safewards interventions that we believe directly influence relational safety and security.

One of the interventions is 'Know Each Other'. Earlier in this chapter, we discussed the importance of establishing a therapeutic relationship between service users and staff members to facilitate effective social interaction. We also pointed out the challenges within the context of clinical mental health care in establishing a therapeutic relationship. This intervention stimulates staff members to provide personal (though not sensitive) information about themselves to allow service users to get to know them. This could be information about their favourite meal, book or movie, music preferences or hobbies. Service users might use this information to start a conversation and it invites service users to open up on these subjects themselves. It serves as a starting point for forming a therapeutic relationship. Many units implemented this intervention by forming profiles of staff members in public areas of the unit, alongside names and pictures of staff members. In addition, the intervention could imply that service users also share such personal (non-medical) information to enhance social interaction.

Another example of an intervention is 'Clear Mutual Expectations'. Every service user and staff member have certain expectations about the behaviour or attitude of the people surrounding him or her. Differences in expectations can lead to frustration, despair and agitation. When establishing a therapeutic relationship, staff members need to investigate the expectations of the service user about, for example, the admission process, staff's behaviour or the care they can receive. Furthermore, their expectations and possibilities must be clear and explicit. When service users and staff members communicate about their expectations and try to synchronise their expectations, concerning each other's boundaries and possibilities, they are likely to prevent conflicts around this subject. Safewards suggests some templates to assist units to be clear on their expectations and invite service users to communicate their expectations as well.

The final example we discuss is 'Positive words'. The choice of words is a vital part of social interaction. People in clinical mental health wards interact constantly with one another, whether service users interact with staff members, other service users or visitors or staff members interact with their colleagues, other disciplines, service users or next-of-kin. Especially during the interaction between staff members, the focus can be on the challenging behaviour of service users on the ward. Challenging behaviour can trigger emotional responses in staff members. This can lead to a negative discourse about specific service users between staff members which influence their attitude towards the service user. Safewards encourages staff members to use positive language about service users during the interaction between staff members. This does not imply ignoring challenging behaviour, but it means that staff members also share moments where the service users interacted in a positive way or interventions with a positive outcome. In addition, using positive language in the interaction between service users and staff members is helpful in their social interaction. It encourages staff members to promote helpful behaviour, instead of setting boundaries on behaviour that is not helpful.

## 7    Case Report as an Example of Clinical Practice

To illustrate the impact of organisational innovations in clinical practice, we present a case report about a service user in a mental health crisis.

Our case report is about Jill. She is a 24-year-old female from Curaçao, living in Amsterdam, the Netherlands. She lives together with her boyfriend. She originated from a warm and safe family and has close contact with her parents and two older brothers. She finished nursing vocational school 2 years ago and works part-time in a nursing home. When she was 19, Jill had her first manic episode due to bipolar disorder. She recovered from this episode through intensive home treatment, intensive care from her relatives and the use of quetiapine. Several months after her symptoms were in remission, she stopped taking her medication due to side effects.

Lately, Jill has encountered high work stress due to a staff shortage. She works extra shifts, especially night shifts and weekends. Jill is fine with that; she has lots of energy and does not feel the urge to sleep. To relax, she buys many clothes on the Internet. She sees this as an investment; she wants to prepare a career switch to the fashion industry by setting up her own brand. Her boyfriend and parents are worried about her increased spending and sleeping less than usual. When they confront her, her response is agitated, and she threatens to break up with her boyfriend. After a violent incident in a fashion store, where she planned to present her brand without permission of the store manager and slapped this manager in the face, the police arrested her, and she received an order for involuntary admission.

When Jill arrived at the ward, the nurse welcomed her to the ward with a cup of tea. She can use a single room, where she found information about involuntary admission and a welcoming package with toiletries. The nurses gave her time and space to settle on the ward and to get to know the ward, staff and other service users. A warm welcome to a service user in crisis at the ward is part of the 'First Five Minutes', which is a key feature of the HIC model. Jill feels angry and helpless due to the admission, but the welcome has a calming effect. The following day, she engaged in a meeting with the psychiatrist, her boyfriend and mother, one of the nurses from the ward and her outpatient psychiatrist from her previous manic episode. The HIC model refers to such a meeting as the care-planning meeting, aimed at not losing any recovery time by waiting for a mutually supported treatment plan. Together, they plan to start medication again but choose one with fewer sedative side effects as quetiapine. Despite the closed door, she can go outside the ward with the nurses, her parents and her boyfriend for walks. However, on the second night, Jill is very emotional and desperately wants to go home. She feels alone and wants to be with her family. She sets off the fire alarm, hoping that the door will unlock so she can escape the ward. Due to the alarm and her screams, other patients are waking up. The night nurse sits down with her and invites her to go to the Intensive Care Unit. The nurse does not set boundaries to her loud voice but talks to her calmly and tries to comfort her by talking about her hobbies and dreams for the future, using de-escalation techniques as described in Safewards. The nurse stays with her until she finally falls asleep. In the next few days, Jill relaxes more and starts to have better nights of sleep. The social worker helped her to call in sick with her employer because this also gave her a lot of stress. The expert-by-experience offers Jill to talk about her experiences in the Intensive Care Unit. This might not be seclusion, but it can have an impact. Therefore, debriefing (as described in Six Core Strategies) is appropriate. The manic symptoms decrease after about a week. After 10 days of admission, another meeting takes place with Jill and her family, the clinical and outpatient teams. Together they decide that Jill can go home with care from her family and the outpatient treatment team, who visit her every other day for the first 2 weeks.

## 8    Keep on Dreaming—Future Developments for a Safe and Secure Environment

Safety and security in clinical mental health care remain subjects of high interest and importance. Although primarily defined as objective traits, safety and security both have a subjective component, i.e. people not only need to *be* safe and secure but also must *feel* safe and secure. The context of clinical mental health care introduces several dilemmas around safety and security, which can distract from the fact that every person involved is an actor and has a certain responsibility for establishing safety and security. Recent innovation in safety management encourages staff members and institutions to focus on learning from what goes right (Safety-II), instead of only responding to what goes wrong (Safety-I). The presence of adequate procedures around safety and security, and an environment that supports safety and security are important conditions to allow service users and staff members to create safety and security in clinical mental health wards. However, we argue that 'true' safety and security are only achievable when service users and staff members establish a meaningful therapeutic relationship.

High Intensive Care, Six Core Strategies and Safewards aim to improve the quality of care, and the well-being of service users, and minimise conflict and containment, ultimately leading to the improvement of safety and security for all involved in clinical mental health wards. High Intensive Care is an organisational model, with a clear mission towards recovery-oriented care and prevention of coercive measures. Six Core Strategies provides a framework to improve the quality of care, aimed to sustainably improve quality and reduce seclusion and restraint. Safewards is a conceptual model to prevent conflict and containment with several hands-on interventions to do so. Although conclusive evidence on the direct influence of these towards relational safety and security is absent, these models centralise the therapeutic relationship and social interaction between service users and staff members from a recovery-oriented point of view. The key attributes of recovery-supporting staff members are (Dröes & Plooy, 2010):

- Having an attitude of hope and optimism
- Being present and available
- Being mindful of the limitations of their professional frameworks
- Being able to stimulate, support, recognise and empower the personal recovery of the service user
- Acknowledging the expertise of the service user
- Acknowledging and facilitating the support of the service user's significant others

To achieve this, staff members are encouraged to have a proactive attitude towards interaction and de-escalation. Furthermore, staff members should invite service users explicitly to interact and influence their recovery process.

High Intensive Care, Six Core Strategies and Safewards have similarities but are complementary in their approach towards safety and security. However, due to general or specific challenges (e.g. shortages of staff or funding, unhelpful legislation, etc.), healthcare institutions and mental health systems still struggle with safety and security issues. These challenges also complicate the implementation of organisational changes. It would be a dream to expect that these challenges would disappear soon. However, institutions around the world prove that full implementation of innovative interventions and explicit focus on social interaction between service users and staff members do decrease (or even eliminate in some cases) conflict and containment and thereby improve safety and security. Future developments should focus on improving preconditions for staff members to focus primarily on interaction with service users and the implementation of models that stimulate therapeutic relationships and social interaction. Thereby, all actors can collaborate to provide safety and security in clinical mental health services for everyone involved.

# References

Almond, P. (2015). Revolution blues: The reconstruction of health and safety law as 'common-sense' regulation. *Journal of Law and Society, 42*(2), 202–229. https://doi.org/10.1111/j.1467-6478.2015.00705.x

Almond, P., & Gray, G. C. (2017). Frontline safety: Understanding the workplace as a site of regulatory engagement. *Law & Policy, 39*(1), 5–26. https://doi.org/10.1111/lapo.12070

Appelbaum, K. L., & Appelbaum, P. S. (1991). A model hospital policy on prosecuting patients for presumptively criminal acts. *Hospital & Community Psychiatry, 42*(12), 1233–1237. https://doi.org/10.1176/ps.42.12.1233

Arseneault, L., Moffitt, T. E., Caspi, A., Taylor, P. J., & Silva, P. A. (2000). Mental disorders and violence in a total birth cohort: Results from the Dunedin study. *Archives of General Psychiatry, 57*(10), 979–986. https://doi.org/10.1001/archpsyc.57.10.979

Azeem, M. W., Aujla, A., Rammerth, M., Binsfeld, G., & Jones, R. B. (2011). Effectiveness of six core strategies based on trauma informed care in reducing seclusions and restraints at a child and adolescent psychiatric hospital. *Journal of Child and Adolescent Psychiatric Nursing, 24*(1), 11–15. https://doi.org/10.1111/j.1744-6171.2010.00262.x

Barakat, A., Blankers, M., Cornelis, J. E., Lommerse, N. M., Beekman, A. T. F., & Dekker, J. J. M. (2021). The effects of intensive home treatment on self-efficacy in patients recovering from a psychiatric crisis. *International Journal Mental Health Systems, 15*(1), 1. https://doi.org/10.1186/s13033-020-00426-y

Beattie, J., Innes, K., Griffiths, D., & Morphet, J. (2020). Workplace violence: Examination of the tensions between duty of care, worker safety, and zero tolerance. *Health Care Management Review, 45*(3), E13–E22. https://doi.org/10.1097/hmr.0000000000000286

Bowers, L. (2014). Safewards: A new model of conflict and containment on psychiatric wards. *Journal of Psychiatric Mental Health Nursing, 21*(6), 499–508. https://doi.org/10.1111/jpm.12129

Bowers, L., Stewart, D., Papadopoulos, C., Dack, C., Ross, J., & Khanom, H. (2011). *Inpatient violence and aggression: A literature review.* Kings College.

Bowers, L., James, K., Quirk, A., Simpson, A., Stewart, D., & Hodsoll, J. (2015). Reducing conflict and containment rates on acute psychiatric wards: The Safewards cluster randomised controlled trial. *International Journal of Nursing Studies, 52*(9), 1412–1422. https://doi. org/10.1016/j.ijnurstu.2015.05.001

Bowie, V. (2011). An emerging awareness of the role organizational culture and management style can play in triggering workplace violence. In M. Privitera (Ed.), *Workplace violence in general health settings* (pp. 43–58). Jones and Bartlett.

Carballedo, A., & Doyle, M. (2011). Criteria for compulsory admission in some European countries. *Psychiatry International, 8*(3), 68–71.

Choe, J. Y., Teplin, L. A., & Abram, K. M. (2008). Perpetration of violence, violent victimization, and severe mental illness: Balancing public health concerns. *Psychiatric Services, 59*(2), 153–164. https://doi.org/10.1176/ps.2008.59.2.153

Civilotti, C., Berlanda, S., & Iozzino, L. (2021). Hospital-based healthcare workers victims of workplace violence in Italy: A scoping review. *International Journal of Environmental Research and Public Health, 18*(11), 5860. https://doi.org/10.3390/ijerph18115860

Council of Europe. (1950). *European Convention on Human Rights*. Council of Europe. https:// www.echr.coe.int/Documents/Convention_ENG.pdf

de Stefano, A., & Ducci, G. (2008). Involuntary admission and compulsory treatment in Europe: An overview. *International Journal of Mental Health, 37*(3), 10–21. https://doi.org/10.2753/ IMH0020-7411370301

Dean, K., Laursen, T. M., Pedersen, C. B., Webb, R. T., Mortensen, P. B., & Agerbo, E. (2018). Risk of being subjected to crime, including violent crime, after onset of mental illness: A Danish National Registry Study Using Police Data. *JAMA Psychiatry, 75*(7), 689–696. https:// doi.org/10.1001/jamapsychiatry.2018.0534

Department of Health. (2000). *An organization with a memory*. Department of Health.

Doedens, P., Vermeulen, J., Boyette, L. L., Latour, C., & de Haan, L. (2020). Influence of nursing staff attitudes and characteristics on the use of coercive measures in acute mental health services—A systematic review. *Journal of Psychiatric and Mental Health Nursing, 27*(4), 446–459. https://doi.org/10.1111/jpm.12586

Dolhuys. (2016). *Dolhuys-manifest*. https://www.hetdolhuys.nl/wp-content/uploads/2017/06/ Dolhuys-Manifest-separeervrij-juni-2016.pdf

Dröes, J., & Plooy, A. (2010). Herstelondersteunende zorg in Nederland: vergelijking met Engelstalige literatuur. *Tijdschrift voor Rehabilitatie, 19*(2), 6–17.

Duxbury, J., & Whittington, R. (2005). Causes and management of patient aggression and violence: Staff and patient perspectives. *Journal of Advanced Nursing, 50*(5), 469–478. https://doi. org/10.1111/j.1365-2648.2005.03426.x

Duxbury, J., Thomson, G., Scholes, A., Jones, F., Baker, J., Downe, S., et al. (2019). Staff experiences and understandings of the REsTRAIN Yourself initiative to minimize the use of physical restraint on mental health wards. *International Journal of Mental Health Nursing, 28*(4), 845–856. https://doi.org/10.1111/inm.12577

EU-OSHA. (2011). *Occupational safety and health culture assessment—a review of main approaches and selected tools*. Publication Office of the European Union.

Fan, S., An, W., Zeng, L., Liu, J., Tang, S., Chen, J., & Huang, H. (2022). Rethinking "zero tolerance": A moderated mediation model of mental resilience and coping strategies in workplace violence and nurses' mental health. *Journal of Nursing Scholarship, 54*(4), 501–512. https:// doi.org/10.1111/jnu.12753

Fazel, S., Wolf, A., Palm, C., & Lichtenstein, P. (2014). Violent crime, suicide, and premature mortality in patients with schizophrenia and related disorders: A 38-year total population study in Sweden. *Lancet Psychiatry, 1*(1), 44–54. https://doi.org/10.1016/s2215-0366(14)70223-8

Fernandes, S., Fond, G., Zendjidjian, X. Y., Baumstarck, K., Lançon, C., Berna, F., et al. (2020). Measuring the patient experience of mental health care: A systematic and critical review of patient-reported experience measures. *Patient Preference and Adherence, 14*, 2147–2161. https://doi.org/10.2147/ppa.S255264

Flood, C., Bowers, L., & Parkin, D. (2008). Estimating the costs of conflict and containment on adult acute inpatient psychiatric wards. *Nursing Economic$, 26*(5), 325–330. 324.

Frueh, B. C., Knapp, R. G., Cusack, K. J., Grubaugh, A. L., Sauvageot, J. A., Cousins, V. C., et al. (2005). Patients' reports of traumatic or harmful experiences within the psychiatric setting. *Psychiatric Services, 56*(9), 1123–1133. https://doi.org/10.1176/appi.ps.56.9.1123

Gaynes, B. N., Brown, C. L., Lux, L. J., Brownley, K. A., Van Dorn, R. A., Edlund, M. J., et al. (2017). Preventing and de-escalating aggressive behavior among adult psychiatric patients: A systematic review of the evidence. *Psychiatric Services, 68*(8), 819–831. https://doi.org/10.1176/appi.ps.201600314

Giacco, D., Fiorillo, A., Del Vecchio, V., Kallert, T., Onchev, G., Raboch, J., et al. (2012). Caregivers' appraisals of patients' involuntary hospital treatment: European multicentre study. *British Journal of Psychiatry, 201*(6), 486–491. https://doi.org/10.1192/bjp.bp.112.112813

Gooding, P. (2021). *Compendium report: Good practices in the Council of Europe to promote Voluntary Measures in Mental Health Services.* Council of Europe. https://www.coe.int/en/web/bioethics/compendium-report-good-practices-in-the-council-of-europe-to-promote-voluntary-measures-in-mental-health-

Guo, Y., Yang, X., Wang, D., Fan, R., Liang, Y., Wang, R., et al. (2022). Prevalence of violence to others among individuals with schizophrenia in China: A systematic review and meta-analysis. *Frontiers in Psychiatry, 13*, 939329. https://doi.org/10.3389/fpsyt.2022.939329

Haines, F., & Almond, P. (2014). Criminalization and occupational health and safety. In G. Bruinsma & D. Weisburd (Eds.), *Encyclopedia of criminology and criminal justice* (pp. 838–847). Springer.

Harte, J. M., van Leeuwen, M. E., & Theuws, R. (2013). [The nature, extent and judicial response to aggression and violence directed against care workers in psychiatry]. *Tijdschrift voor Psychiatrie, 55*(5), 325–335.

Health and Safety Executive. (2005). *A review of safety culture and safety climate literature for the development of the safety culture inspection toolkit—Research report 367.* https://www.hse.gov.uk/research/rrpdf/rr367.pdf

Hill, R. G. (1839). Lincoln lunatic asylum. *The Lancet, 32*(827), 554–555. https://doi.org/10.1016/S0140-6736(02)80065-4

Hilton, N. Z., Addison, S., Ham, E., Rodrigues, N. C., & Seto, M. C. (2022). Workplace violence and risk factors for PTSD among psychiatric nurses: Systematic review and directions for future research and practice. *Journal of Psychiatric and Mental Health Nursing, 29*(2), 186–203. https://doi.org/10.1111/jpm.12781

Hodgins, S., Alderton, J., Cree, A., Aboud, A., & Mak, T. (2007). Aggressive behaviour, victimization and crime among severely mentally ill patients requiring hospitalisation. *British Journal of Psychiatry, 191*, 343–350. https://doi.org/10.1192/bjp.bp.106.06.029587

Hofmann, A. B., Schmid, H. M., Hofmann, L. A., Noboa, V., Seifritz, E., Vetter, S., & Egger, S. T. (2022). Impact of compulsory admission on treatment and outcome: A propensity score matched analysis. *European Psychiatry, 65*(1), e6. https://doi.org/10.1192/j.eurpsy.2022.4

Hollnagel, E. (2014). *Safety-I and safety-II – The past and future of safety management.* Ashgate.

Hollnagel, E. (2021). Managing for security. In G. Jacobs, I. Suojanen, K. E. Horton, & P. S. Bayerl (Eds.), *International security management: New solutions to complexity* (pp. 43–53). Springer Nature.

Hoppler, S. S., Segerer, R., & Nikitin, J. (2021). The six components of social interactions: Actor, partner, relation, activities, context, and evaluation. *Frontiers in Psychology, 12*, 743074. https://doi.org/10.3389/fpsyg.2021.743074

Huckshorn, K. A. (2006). *Six core Strategies for reducing seclusion and restraint use.* National Association of State Mental Health Program Directors. https://www.nasmhpd.org/sites/default/files/Consolidated%20Six%20Core%20Strategies%20Document.pdf

Itzhaki, M., Bluvstein, I., Peles Bortz, A., Kostistky, H., Bar Noy, D., Filshtinsky, V., & Theilla, M. (2018). Mental health Nurse's exposure to workplace violence leads to job stress, which leads to reduced professional quality of life. *Frontiers in Psychiatry, 9*, 59. https://doi.org/10.3389/fpsyt.2018.00059

Jenkin, G., Quigg, S., Paap, H., Cooney, E., Peterson, D., & Every-Palmer, S. (2022). Places of safety? Fear and violence in acute mental health facilities: A large qualitative study of staff and service user perspectives. *PLoS One, 17*(5), e0266935. https://doi.org/10.1371/journal.pone.0266935

Jina-Pettersen, N. (2022). Fear, neglect, coercion, and dehumanization: Is inpatient psychiatric trauma contributing to a public health crisis? *Journal of Patient Experience, 9*, 23743735221079138. https://doi.org/10.1177/23743735221079138

Jones, N., Gius, B. K., Shields, M., Collings, S., Rosen, C., & Munson, M. (2021). Investigating the impact of involuntary psychiatric hospitalization on youth and young adult trust and help-seeking in pathways to care. *Social Psychiatry and Psychiatric Epidemiology, 56*(11), 2017–2027. https://doi.org/10.1007/s00127-021-02048-2

Kallert, T. W., Glöckner, M., & Schützwohl, M. (2008). Involuntary vs. voluntary hospital admission. A systematic literature review on outcome diversity. *European Archives of Psychiatry and Clinical Neuroscience, 258*(4), 195–209. https://doi.org/10.1007/s00406-007-0777-4

Kamperman, A. M., Henrichs, J., Bogaerts, S., Lesaffre, E. M., Wierdsma, A. I., Ghauharali, R. R., et al. (2014). Criminal victimisation in people with severe mental illness: A multi-site prevalence and incidence survey in The Netherlands. *PLoS One, 9*(3), e91029. https://doi.org/10.1371/journal.pone.0091029

Kennedy, H. G. (2002). Therapeutic uses of security: Mapping forensic mental health services by stratifying risk. *Advances in Psychiatric Treatment, 8*(6), 433–443. https://doi.org/10.1192/apt.8.6.433

Kersting, X. A. K., Hirsch, S., & Steinert, T. (2019). Physical harm and death in the context of coercive measures in psychiatric patients: A systematic review. *Frontiers in Psychiatry, 10*, 400. https://doi.org/10.3389/fpsyt.2019.00400

Khalifeh, H., Johnson, S., Howard, L. M., Borschmann, R., Osborn, D., Dean, K., et al. (2015). Violent and non-violent crime against adults with severe mental illness. *British Journal of Psychiatry, 206*(4), 275–282. https://doi.org/10.1192/bjp.bp.114.147843

Kim, A. M. (2019). Crimes by people with schizophrenia in Korea: Comparison with the general population. *BMC Psychiatry, 19*(1), 377. https://doi.org/10.1186/s12888-019-2355-5

Kinsley, J. (1998). Security and therapy. In C. Kaye & A. Franey (Eds.), *Managing high security psychiatric care*. Jessica Kingsley Publishers.

Kumar, S., Fischer, J., Ng, B., Clarke, S., & Robinson, E. (2006). Prosecuting psychiatric patients who assault staff: A New Zealand perspective. *Australasian Psychiatry, 14*(3), 251–255. https://doi.org/10.1080/j.1440-1665.2006.02296.x

LeBel, J. L., Duxbury, J. A., Putkonen, A., Sprague, T., Rae, C., & Sharpe, J. (2014). Multinational experiences in reducing and preventing the use of restraint and seclusion. *Journal of Psychosocial Nursing and Mental Health Services, 52*(11), 22–29. https://doi.org/10.3928/02793695-20140915-01

Li, Y. L., Li, R. Q., Qiu, D., & Xiao, S. Y. (2020). Prevalence of workplace physical violence against health care professionals by patients and visitors: A systematic review and meta-analysis. *International Journal of Environmental Research and Public Health, 17*(1), 299. https://doi.org/10.3390/ijerph17010299

Liu, J., Gan, Y., Jiang, H., Li, L., Dwyer, R., Lu, K., et al. (2019). Prevalence of workplace violence against healthcare workers: A systematic review and meta-analysis. *Occupational and Environmental Medicine, 76*(12), 927–937. https://doi.org/10.1136/oemed-2019-105849

Lorien, L., Blunden, S., & Madsen, W. (2020). Implementation of recovery-oriented practice in hospital-based mental health services: A systematic review. *International Journal of Mental Health Nursing, 29*(6), 1035–1048. https://doi.org/10.1111/inm.12794

Marcus, S. C., Hermann, R. C., Frankel, M. R., & Cullen, S. W. (2018). Safety of psychiatric inpatients at the Veterans Health Administration. *Psychiatric Services, 69*(2), 204–210. https://doi.org/10.1176/appi.ps.201700224

Meijwaard, S. C., Kikkert, M., de Mooij, L. D., Lommerse, N. M., Peen, J., Schoevers, R. A., et al. (2015). Risk of criminal victimisation in outpatients with common mental health disorders. *PLoS One, 10*(7), e0128508. https://doi.org/10.1371/journal.pone.0128508

Middleby-Clements, J. L., & Grenyer, B. F. (2007). Zero tolerance approach to aggression and its impact upon mental health staff attitudes. *Australian and New Zealand Journal of Psychiatry, 41*(2), 187–191. https://doi.org/10.1080/00048670601109972

Mullen, J. E., & Kelloway, E. K. (2011). Occupational health and safety leadership. In J. C. Quick & L. E. Tetrick (Eds.), *Handbook of occupational health psychology* (pp. 357–372). American Psychological Association. https://doi.org/10.1037/10474-000

Nath, S. B., & Marcus, S. C. (2006). Medical errors in psychiatry. *Harvard Review of Psychiatry, 14*(4), 204–211. https://doi.org/10.1080/10673220600889272

Nilsson, L., Borgstedt-Risberg, M., Brunner, C., Nyberg, U., Nylén, U., Ålenius, C., & Rutberg, H. (2020). Adverse events in psychiatry: A national cohort study in Sweden with a unique psychiatric trigger tool. *BMC Psychiatry, 20*(1), 44. https://doi.org/10.1186/s12888-020-2447-2

Norko, M. A., Zonana, H. V., & Phillips, R. T. (1992). Prosecuting assaultive psychiatric patients. *Journal of Forensic Sciences, 37*(3), 923–931.

Price, O., Baker, J., Bee, P., & Lovell, K. (2018). The support-control continuum: An investigation of staff perspectives on factors influencing the success or failure of de-escalation techniques for the management of violence and aggression in mental health settings. *International Journal of Nursing Studies, 77*, 197–206. https://doi.org/10.1016/j.ijnurstu.2017.10.002

Rakhmatullina, M., Taub, A., & Jacob, T. (2013). Morbidity and mortality associated with the utilization of restraints: A review of literature. *Psychiatric Quarterly, 84*(4), 499–512. https://doi.org/10.1007/s11126-013-9262-6

Sailas, E. E. S., & Fenton, M. (2000). Seclusion and restraint for people with serious mental illnesses. *Cochrane Database of Systematic Reviews, 2000*, CD001163. https://doi.org/10.1002/14651858.CD001163

Salzmann-Erikson, M., Lutzen, K., Ivarsson, A. B., & Eriksson, H. (2008). The core characteristics and nursing care activities in psychiatric intensive care units in Sweden. *International Journal of Mental Health Nursing, 17*(2), 98–107. https://doi.org/10.1111/j.1447-0349.2008.00517.x

Schindeler, E., & Ransley, J. (2016). *Prosecuting workplace violence: The utility and policy implications of criminalization.* Criminology Research Advisory Council. https://www.aic.gov.au/sites/default/files/2020-05/31-1213-FinalReport.pdf

Schramm, W. (1997). *The beginnings of communication study in America.* Sage.

Schuilenburg, M. (2015). *The securitization of society. Crime, risk, and social order.* New York University Press.

Secker, J., Benson, A., Balfe, E., Lipsedge, M., Robinson, S., & Walker, J. (2004). Understanding the social context of violent and aggressive incidents on an inpatient unit. *Journal of Psychiatric and Mental Health Nursing, 11*(2), 172–178. https://doi.org/10.1111/j.1365-2850.2003.00703.x

Steinert, T., Birk, M., Flammer, E., & Bergk, J. (2013). Subjective distress after seclusion or mechanical restraint: One-year follow-up of a randomized controlled study. *Psychiatric Services, 64*(10), 1012–1017. https://doi.org/10.1176/appi.ps.201200315

Teplin, L. A., McClelland, G. M., Abram, K. M., & Weiner, D. A. (2005). Crime victimization in adults with severe mental illness: Comparison with the National Crime Victimization Survey. *Archives of General Psychiatry, 62*(8), 911–921. https://doi.org/10.1001/archpsyc.62.8.911

Topp, L. (2018). Single rooms, seclusion and the non-restraint movement in British asylums, 1838–1844. *Social History of Medicine, 31*(4), 754–773. https://doi.org/10.1093/shm/hky015

UN General Assembly. (2006). *Convention on the Rights of Persons with Disabilities.* A/RES/61/106, Annex. U. G. Assembly. 13 Dec 2006. https://www.refworld.org/docid/4680cd212.html

Van Mierlo, T., Bovenberg, F., Voskes, Y., & Mulder, C. L. (2013). *Werkboek HIC. High en Intensive Care in de psychiatrie.* Uitgeverij de Tijdstroom.

Vermeulen, J. M., Doedens, P., Cullen, S. W., van Tricht, M. J., Hermann, R., Frankel, M., et al. (2018). Predictors of adverse events and medical errors among adult inpatients of psychiatric units of acute care general hospitals. *Psychiatric Services, 69*(10), 1087–1094. https://doi.org/10.1176/appi.ps.201800110

Visscher, A. J. E., Tonkens, E., & Braam, A. W. (2019). Reflecting on intramural incidents: How do judges think about intramural crimes in mental health care? *Tijdschrift voor Psychiatrie, 61*(8), 536–543.

Voskes, Y., van Melle, A. L., Widdershoven, G. A. M., van Mierlo, A., Bovenberg, F. J. M., & Mulder, C. L. (2021). High and intensive care in psychiatry: A new model for acute inpatient care. *Psychiatric Services, 72*(4), 475–477. https://doi.org/10.1176/appi.ps.201800440

Whittington, R. (2002). Attitudes toward patient aggression amongst mental health nurses in the 'zero tolerance' era: Associations with burnout and length of experience. *Journal of Clinical Nursing, 11*(6), 819–825. https://doi.org/10.1046/j.1365-2702.2002.00659.x

Whittington, R., & Higgins, L. (2002). More than zero tolerance? Burnout and tolerance for patient aggression amongst mental health nurses in China and the UK. *Acta Psychiatrica Scandinavica Supplement, 412*, 37–40. https://doi.org/10.1034/j.1600-0447.106.s412.8.x

Wigand, M. E., Orzechowski, M., Nowak, M., Becker, T., & Steger, F. (2021). Schizophrenia, human rights and access to health care: A systematic search and review of judgements by the European Court of Human Rights. *International Journal of Social Psychiatry, 67*(2), 168–174. https://doi.org/10.1177/0020764020942797

Wikman, S. (2016). Varför ökar det arbetsrelaterade våldet. *Arbetsmarknad & Arbetsliv, 22*(2), 49–66.

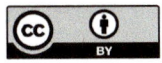

# Ward Culture and Atmosphere

Nutmeg Hallett, Joy A. Duxbury, Anna Björkdahl, and Sheena Johnson

## 1    Introduction

In mental health inpatient settings, the significance of ward climate as a crucial factor in the efficacy of inpatient care has been acknowledged for decades. Indeed as early as the 1950s, the World Health Organization (1953, p. 17) stated that 'the single most important factor in the efficacy of treatment given in a mental hospital appears to the committee to be an intangible element which can only be described as its atmosphere'. This chapter explores the multifaceted nature of ward culture and atmosphere, where these elements actively shape the therapeutic journey.

The functions of a ward, as summarised by Gunderson (1978)—containment, support, structure, involvement and validation—play a critical role in understanding the ward atmosphere and its impact on patient care. These functions highlight the dynamic nature of the ward environment, responsive to each patient's needs (Norton, 2004). Additionally, the work of Rudolf Moos since the 1960s has been instrumental in this field. Moos' conceptualisation of psychiatric hospital environments as having 'unique personalities' (Insel & Moos, 1974) comprises three dimensions: relationship, personal development and system maintenance and change. His research

N. Hallett (✉)
School of Nursing and Midwifery, University of Birmingham, Birmingham, UK
e-mail: n.n.hallett@bham.ac.uk

J. A. Duxbury
Institute of Health, University of Cumbria, Lancaster, UK
e-mail: Joy.duxbury@cumbria.ac.uk

A. Björkdahl
Centre for Psychiatric Research, Karolinska Institutet, Stockholm, Sweden
e-mail: anna.bjorkdahl@ki.se

S. Johnson
Alliance Manchester Business School, University of Manchester, Manchester, UK
e-mail: Sheena.johnson@manchester.ac.uk

© The Author(s) 2024                                                                                    265
N. Hallett et al. (eds.), *Coercion and Violence in Mental Health Settings*,
https://doi.org/10.1007/978-3-031-61224-4_12

underscores the influence of an individual's perception of their environment on their behaviour, challenging the notion of personality as a predictor of behaviour irrespective of environmental context (Insel & Moos, 1974; Moos, 1973).

This chapter examines organisational culture within healthcare settings, particularly psychiatric wards, and its impact on patient outcomes and staff well-being. Staff attitudes and training significantly affect the ward's climate—a concept distinct yet related to culture. This climate, more temporal and malleable than culture, reflects current psychological conditions within the ward, playing a crucial role in patient and staff experiences. Also discussed is the role of the ward's physical environment in patient care. Research indicates that design elements like ward layout, safety measures and access to outdoor spaces significantly influence the use of seclusion and other coercive measures. The physical space is not just a setting but an active component in the therapeutic process. Central to the dynamics of a psychiatric ward are the rules that govern patient and staff behaviour. The manner in which rules are constructed, understood and enforced can either facilitate a therapeutic environment or contribute to a culture of control and coercion.

This chapter aims to provide a comprehensive understanding of the intricate aspects of ward culture and atmosphere. By examining the interdependencies between organisational culture, staff attitudes and training, the physical environment, and the rules and power dynamics, we seek to offer insights into creating more effective, compassionate and therapeutic psychiatric ward environments. The goal is to enhance both patient care and staff well-sbeing, fostering a culture of understanding, respect and collaboration within these critical healthcare settings.

## 2    Organisational Culture

Harrison (1972) defined organisational culture in terms of the beliefs and values of the organisation, which act as prescriptions for the way in which organisational members should work. Similarly, Smircich (1983, p. 346) stated that 'culture serves as a sense-making device that can guide and shape behavior'. The study of organisational culture is, therefore, about understanding people's perceptions of the organisations in which they work, and how these perceptions influence their attitudes and behaviour towards, and within, their work environment.

The general concept of culture has been around for many years with intellectual influences from both anthropology and sociology (Ouchi & Wilkins, 1985). However, the study and application of culture within an organisational context predominantly date from the 1970s and, in a reflection of its utility as a tool with which to gain insight into organisations, remain a large and growing area of organisational research. An influential theorist, Schein (2004), believed that culture existed across three main levels: artefacts, e.g. organisational rules, procedures and observable behaviours of employees; espoused values (which serve to determine employee beliefs about how things ought to be and what is important in the organisation); and basic assumptions (unconscious assumptions about appropriate behaviour and reactions in any given situation). Schein (2004, p. 17) defined culture as:

A pattern of shared basic assumptions that the group learned as it solved its problems of external adaptation and internal integration that has worked well enough to be considered valid and, therefore, to be taught to new members as the correct way to perceive, think, and feel in relation to those problems.

A similar concept to culture, primarily based on social and organisational contexts, is evident in 'climate' literature and research. In brief, culture is typically viewed as a deeper, more stable phenomenon than climate, which is temporal and less resistant to change. The study of organisational climate preceded that of organisational culture; climate has been conceptualised as a 'snapshot' of organisational culture (Mearns et al., 1998). Although there is some disagreement between researchers as to the definitions and appropriate measurement methods of culture and climate, indeed the terms are often used interchangeably, e.g. Glisson and James (2002), Rousseau's (1988) description of climate demonstrates the close relationship the concepts of climate and culture have in practice. She, along with others, considered climate as consisting of shared perceptions and beliefs. Having acknowledged the confusion that often exists between the two terms, the term culture is used throughout this section in an effort to ease comprehension for the reader.

It is widely accepted that organisations do not operate in one overall culture, rather they are composed of subcultures. Martin et al. (1985) detailed how it is more realistic to study organisational culture as an umbrella under which multiple subcultures exist, for example, corporate, departmental, divisional, geographical location, issue-related and professional (Jansen, 1994). The attention to culture at the ward level, as opposed to the broader organisational, e.g. hospital, level is therefore appropriate.

Culture is widely promoted as a tool for gaining insight into the workings of an organisation. Researchers have discussed culture as the key to understanding what makes some organisations more successful than others (Martin, 1992; Peters & Waterman, 1982). Others have looked at the impact that culture has on the well-being and performance of organisations (Denison, 1996; Wilkins, 1983). Specific elements of culture have also been examined, for example a positive safety culture is recognised as important in terms of reducing the risk of accident or error occurrence. Enquiries following safety incidents repeatedly identify cultural factors which significantly contributed to the chain of events preceding an incident, for example the Piper Alpha oil rig fire (Cullen, 1990), the Ladbroke Grove rail crash (Cullen, 2001) and the Deepwater Horizon explosion (Reader & O'Connor, 2014). While there is little agreement as to a definition of safety culture, commonly cited dimensions are leadership commitment to safety; open, trusting communication; organisational learning; a non-punitive approach to adverse event reporting; teamwork; and a shared belief in the importance of safety (Halligan & Zecevic, 2011). Much of this is captured in the concept of a 'just culture', which is gaining traction in healthcare and is a framework for addressing patient safety incidents and near-misses that moves away from blaming individuals to looking at systems (Paradiso & Sweeney, 2019). Similar non-blaming error reporting systems have been utilised in other industries, such as aviation, since the 1970s to improve safety and reliability (Gerstle, 2018) with blame cultures believed to impede reporting and restrict learning from incidents (Swuste et al., 2020). A just culture is underpinned by openness with the intention to repair harm and to learn from incidents rather than to assign individual blame. A just culture has been attributed to significantly reducing air traffic incidents since the 1970s (Gerstle, 2018) and is beginning to deliver improvements in healthcare. In an examination of initiatives to foster a just culture in five healthcare organisations in the Netherlands, healthcare professionals highlighted the importance of open communication in incident analysis yet noted potential tension between openness and accountability (van Baarle et al., 2022). However, a study assessing the implementation of a just culture in a UK mental health trust observed positive outcomes, including reduced staff suspensions, dismissals and illness-related absences, alongside increased adverse event reporting (Kaur et al., 2019). Moreover, the total economic benefit of the introduction of a just culture was estimated to be about £2.5 million, which was approximately 1% of total costs and 2% of labour costs.

The role that organisational culture plays in violence is being increasingly recognised. Historically, patient violence was viewed as an individual issue, with most research, globally, focused on individual demographic factors related to violence such as age, gender and marital status (Bowers et al., 2011). Where staff were seen as causative they would be viewed as a 'bad apple', and whilst this can be the case, of more concern is the 'bad barrel', i.e. organisations that create oppressive and violent workplace environments (Bowen et al., 2011). Behaviours do not occur in isolation but rather within social and organisational contexts, and so improving the organisational culture, particularly where the culture has become toxic, can lead to a reduction of violence perpetrated by all the individuals within that culture. Toxic cultures have been demonstrated in numerous exposés of patient abuse in mental health settings in the UK, as seen recently on the BBC's *Panorama* (BBC, 2022). The relevance of culture within a ward environment and its influence on employee and patient attitudes and behaviour in relation to violent incidents is therefore clearly indicated.

Several researchers have looked at culture in a healthcare context; Braithwaite et al. (2017) identified 62 articles that explored the association between organisational and workplace cultures and patient outcomes, and they found that positive cultures were consistently associated with improved patient outcomes. In relation to violence and the way it is managed by staff, there is clear evidence that management practices are culturally local. There are national differences—data suggests that the Netherlands has higher rates of seclusion and restraint than three other European countries (Ireland, Germany and Wales) (Lepping et al., 2016)—and also regional differences—rates of restraint vary significantly across the UK (Care Quality Commission, 2020).

## 3    Ward Culture

Staff–patient interaction and the rules of the ward are of particular importance in the healthcare setting, and the ward culture is significantly shaped by the organisation of and the philosophy and nursing style adopted. According to Cortis (2003, p. 55), it is 'within this reality, or world view, an individual's purpose in life is defined, and appropriate, sanctioned behavior within the social group is prescribed'. Kagawa-Singer and Chung (1994) argue that culture serves an integrative function, with beliefs and values providing an individual's sense of identity, and is also functional, in that the rules for behaviour allow a group to survive.

This is important in a potentially dangerous environment. Bowers (2002) endeavoured to establish what underpins a good ward culture, suggesting six underlying mechanisms: (1) a psychiatric philosophy, (2) a belief in the importance of psycho-social factors, (3) moral commitments and choices such as bravery, honesty and equality, (4) cognitive-emotional self- management, (5) technical mastery using interpersonal skills such as solving conflicts, teamwork skills to share the burden of care and maintain consistency in relation to rules and (6) organisational support.

Anna Björkdahl, one of this chapter's authors, argues that 'the only way to achieve a long-standing reduction in violence and aggression on acute [mental health] wards is to make fundamental changes to their culture' (cited in Parish, 2013). Promoting a recovery-based approach has been used successfully to overcome a risk-averse ward culture by supporting patient autonomy and independence to reduce incidents of deliberate self-harm, attempted suicide, absconding, and verbal and physical aggression (Henderson, 2013). Similarly, implementation of Safewards—the programme of interventions designed to promote a collaborative approach to creating safer and calmer mental health wards—has been shown to create a positive ward culture; two interventions, 'Know Each Other' and 'Clear Mutual Expectations' specifically facilitate culture change by increasing the sense of community (Fletcher et al., 2019).

## 4    Ward Atmosphere: Definitions and Measurement

Definitions of what constitutes ward atmosphere are difficult to find. This is hardly surprising given the complexity of factors involved. A lack of distinction between a plethora of terms such as 'ward and social atmosphere' (Jansson & Eklund, 2002), social ecology (Moos, 1974), social climate (Dickens et al., 2022), ward culture, ward milieu, ward environment and ward climate further complicates the issue. Edvardsson (2005, p. 8) uses the term 'atmosphere' to 'include the understanding and description of a tone or mood in care settings or…of what is contained 'within the walls' of that setting'. He sees the concepts of atmosphere and climate as interchangeable metaphors describing the psychological conditions of a social region. Schalast and Redies (2005), in a similar fashion, suggest that 'the interaction of aspects of the material, social and emotional conditions of a ward, which may—over time—influence the mood, behavior and self concept of the persons involved' are indicative of a 'ward atmosphere'.

The term 'ward atmosphere' in particular seems to be most commonly adopted in studies that focus on psychiatric settings. Moos (1974) may have been influential in this trend, devising what soon became known as the Ward Atmosphere Scale (WAS). This was developed in the 1960s in an attempt to describe and measure the therapeutic atmosphere in psychiatric and drug treatment settings.

The WAS consists of a 100-item questionnaire that measures views about the actual real ward, preferences about the ideal ward and individual expectations about the ward in general. It comprises three dimensions that highlight relationships, personal growth and system maintenance, each of which is reflected in ten subscales.

The WAS is still widely used to measure ward atmosphere in inpatient settings (Banks & Priebe, 2020), despite criticisms that it is dated, lacking content validity, its extensive size and limited psychometric properties. Partly to address these criticisms, Schalast et al. (2008) developed the Essen Climate Evaluation Schema (EssenCES), a 15-item scale measuring three dimensions of the social climate: therapeutic hold, patients' cohesion and mutual support and experienced safety. A review of scales to assess the social climate of prisons and forensic units found that the EssenCES was the second most used scale after the WAS (Tonkin, 2015). While the WAS and the EssenCES aim to assess the ward atmosphere as a whole, other scales have been developed to address specific aspects of the ward atmosphere, for example, the violence prevention climate, which can be described as the primary and secondary actions of staff and patients on a ward that prevent violence, as measured by the E13 (Björkdahl et al., 2013) and the VPC-14 (Hallett et al., 2018). All these measures, and more, have been used in studies assessing the impact of interventions to improve the social climate of acute mental health wards but most seem to lack robustness and sensitivity to change over time (Dickens et al., 2022). Dickens et al. (2022) in their review of just this identified that the interventions most likely to facilitate change in the social climate were Safewards and a ward-based psychological intervention described by Berry et al. (2016).

Ward atmosphere is a complex phenomenon because it describes the way a ward feels, which becomes difficult to define in concrete terms. A welcoming atmosphere may be created by (Weltens et al., 2021):

- Frequent strengths-based contact between patients and staff
- A multidisciplinary staff team
- Minimal use of coercive measures
- One-to-one nursing for agitated patients

While it may be difficult to explain the elements of ward atmosphere, it has been suggested that one gets a sense of the atmosphere as soon as one enters a ward; in the words of one mother, 'I can tell what kind of care my daughter is going to get within 15 steps of walking on to every new ward' (NHS England, 2017, p. 5). To this end, assessment of the ward atmosphere should be integral to approaches aimed at improving care. One method to do just this is the Fifteen Steps Challenge, which is a suite of toolkits that are used to explore healthcare settings through the eyes of patients and their carers (NHS England, 2017). This involves coordinating a 'walkaround team' who briefly visits wards to explore the quality of care under the headings of welcoming, safe, caring and involved, and well organised and calm. These are assessed by a series of prompts and questions.

**The Fifteen Steps Challenge (https://www.england.nhs.uk/wp-content/uploads/2017/11/15-steps-mental-health.pdf)**

**Welcoming**

- How does this ward make me feel?
- What interactions are taking place between staff and service users?
- Is there visible information that is useful and re-assuring? What is it?

Things to look out for

- Staff introducing themselves.
- Service users able to approach staff
- Staff photo boards with names.
- Body language of staff

**Safe**

- Can I identify staff? How are they identifiable?
- What tells me that staff take safety seriously?
- What did I experience that made me feel safe?

Things to look out for

- Information boards with transparent safety information e.g. safety crosses, graphs and charts.
- No clutter or overflowing bins.
- Staff in communal areas.
- Equipment and environment well maintained.

**Caring and involving**

- What can I understand about the service user experience on this ward?
- Is there evidence that service users and carers are involved in their own care?
- How do staff interact with service users?

Things to look out for

- Staff and service users positively interacting.
- Meaningful activities taking place.
- Service users speaking positively about staff and the care being received.
- Staff acknowledging service users and visitors with warmth and kindness.

**Well organised and calm**

- Does the ward feel calm even though it may be busy?
- Are resources/equipment stored in designated places?
- Does it feel like a therapeutic environment?

Things to look out for

- Staff not looking like they are under pressure.
- Organised and tidy communal areas.
- Service users and visitors looking relaxed.

## 5    The Relationship Between Ward Culture, Restrictive Interventions and Violence

Ward culture and restrictive interventions are intimately linked. Secker et al. (2004) suggest that the organisation of care can be hugely influential in levels of aggression and violence within the ward environment; this then forms the basis of a well-defined ward atmosphere. The ward culture, which includes the attitudes and beliefs of the staff and patients, can significantly impact the use of restrictive interventions such as seclusion and restraint. Staff attitudes towards coercive measures have seen a paradigm shift from a therapeutic paradigm to a safety paradigm (Doedens et al., 2020). The therapeutic paradigm viewed coercive measures as 'harsh, but helpful', extolling the calming nature of seclusion as an example. It is important to note that this view was not shared by patients. There are numerous qualitative accounts of patients' negative experiences with coercive measures at the time when the therapeutic paradigm was at its zenith. Restraint could leave people feeling afraid, powerless and helpless (Sequeira & Halstead, 2002; Smith, 1995; Wynn, 2004) while seclusion was described as punitive and could also leave people feeling afraid and helpless (Holmes et al., 2004; Lendemeijer & Shortridge-Baggett, 1997). More recently, the therapeutic paradigm has increasingly been viewed by staff as anathema, with attitudes shifting to the safety paradigm, where staff members view coercive measures as a last resort (Doedens et al., 2020). This can create feelings of conflict in staff who view coercive measures as a necessary evil.

A positive ward culture that prioritises collaboration, communication and person-centred care can help reduce the use of restrictive interventions (Department of Health, 2014). Staff members who work in such a culture recognise the importance of primary prevention interventions, i.e. interventions that prevent known reasons behind conflicts, as part of their everyday work. They are trained in de-escalation techniques and are more likely to recognise and respond to patients' needs before they escalate to the point of requiring restraint or seclusion. Additionally, staff members who feel empowered and supported in their work are less likely to resort to restrictive interventions as a means of managing challenging behaviours.

Conversely, a negative ward culture that prioritises control and coercion can lead to an increase in the use of restrictive interventions. This can create a culture of 'us versus them', where patients and staff are in conflict, rather than working towards a shared vision (Butterworth et al., 2022). Staff members who feel disempowered or unsupported in their work are more likely to resort to restrictive interventions as a way of exerting control over patients. Moreover, these interventions can create a negative feedback loop by eroding trust between staff and patients and contributing to a hostile and coercive ward culture.

## 6      Interplay Between Ward Atmosphere and External Factors

In mental health inpatient settings, the atmosphere and culture of the ward are influenced by, and affect, various interconnected factors. This section explores the elements relevant to the environment where patients and healthcare professionals interact. The quality of care, and the safety and well-being of individuals receiving treatment are significantly affected by many factors (Care Quality Commission, 2023; Pelto-Piri et al., 2019). Elements such as staff attitudes and training, the physical ward layout and the governing policies all contribute to these aspects. While other chapters in the book provide in-depth information on training, the physical environment and organisational policies, this section specifically focuses on their impact on the ward's atmosphere and culture.

## 6.1    Staff Attitudes and Training

While various studies have examined staff attitudes and characteristics, and their association with ward atmosphere and culture (e.g. Tuvesson & Eklund, 2017), few, if any, have demonstrated the impact of staff attitudes on ward atmosphere. Despite the lack of causal research, there is some evidence of a relationship between staff attitudes and ward atmosphere. In a cross-sectional study with staff working in a medium secure unit in the UK, Berry and Robertson (2019) found that a positive ward atmosphere was associated with lower levels of burnout. Furthermore, staff perceptions of ward climate may be a predictor of perceived barriers to change (Laker et al., 2020), meaning that implementing service-level changes may be more successful in wards with a positively perceived climate. This supports an earlier realist review of achieving lasting change when undertaking recovery-oriented training, which found that a challenging organisational climate could be a barrier to change (Gee et al., 2017).

The evidence for staff training is similarly scarce, although the available evidence does suggest that training can positively affect perceptions of ward atmosphere. A 3-week training programme aimed at raising awareness of the therapeutic environment, for nursing staff in a regional forensic hospital in Norway, improved patients' perceptions of the ward atmosphere as well as patient satisfaction (Nesset et al., 2009). Moreover, staff and patients on wards that received training based on the Bergen model (a violence prevention training programme based on the positive appreciation of patients, emotional regulation and effective structure) had significantly higher perceptions of ward atmosphere than wards without that training (Björkdahl et al., 2013). Staff mindfulness training has also demonstrated an improvement in perceptions of ward atmosphere (Eliassen et al., 2016).

## 6.2 Physical Environment

The physical environment of a ward can have a significant impact on patient violence in mental health settings. Inpatient aggression and conflict result from a complex interaction of the individual characteristics of patients, staff characteristics and contextual characteristics, such as the physical environment of the ward. A study exploring the effect of design features on the risk of being secluded found that certain physical design features of psychiatric wards, such as outdoor spaces, special safety measures and the number of patients in a building, can affect the likelihood of using seclusion as an intervention (van der Schaaf et al., 2013). Specifically, a higher number of patients and special safety measures increased the risk, while more private space per patient, a higher level of comfort and better visibility within the ward were associated with a decreased risk. These findings highlight the importance of considering the physical ward environment in efforts to reduce the use of seclusion.

The Care Quality Commission (CQC), the independent regulator of health and social care in England, found that the physical environment and condition of mental health inpatient wards are 'not good enough', with many wards in need of urgent updates and repair (CQC, 2023). Issues that were observed included broken windows, holes in walls, dirty wards, and fixtures and fittings in need of repair. In many cases, the condition of wards has been made worse by the additional wear and tear created during lockdowns in the COVID-19 pandemic years. Many inpatient wards are in old and outdated buildings that lack the space and ventilation of newer buildings. This can lead to issues around privacy and dignity for patients, as well as compromise the safety of patients and staff. The relationship between a dignity-promoting culture and the preservation of dignity underscores the importance of both physical and interpersonal elements in healthcare environments. A study in a surgical ward found that a lack of privacy and staff behaviours that seem dismissive, too controlling or intrusive can threaten patient dignity (Baillie, 2009). Conversely, a physical space that respects privacy, coupled with a culture that values dignity and support from fellow patients, enhances it.

The field of 'health geography' explores how 'space, place, environment and landscape' can impact health professionals and patients (Philo, 1997). Philo (1997) offers a multifaceted examination of the geographical studies of asylums, emphasising the importance of understanding the complex interplay between societal perceptions, policy decisions and the physical environment in shaping mental health facilities. One study explored ward atmosphere and its relationship to the physical environment, through the relocation of a ward to a purpose-built acute facility (Nicholls et al., 2015). While significant improvements were observed in some of the subscales of the WAS (order and organisation, and programme clarity), other indicators did not show improvement. This suggests that ward atmosphere encompasses more than just the physical environment; it also involves social interactions and occupation within that environment.

## 6.3 Organisational Policies and Procedures

Organisational frameworks and protocols are integral to ward atmosphere and can impact rates of incidents in mental health inpatient settings. Factors contributing to workplace violence include the unpredictable behaviours of emotionally stressed patients and relatives, alongside systemic issues such as stressful working conditions, staffing deficits, inadequate policies and training and operational inefficiencies like overcrowding and extended waiting periods (Jones et al., 2023). A supportive culture can reduce the impact of these factors. Evidence from other workplace settings, in this case social enterprises, suggests that a supportive management structure, clear role definitions and robust organisational processes are essential for sustaining staff morale (Joyce et al., 2022). Evidence from mental health settings underlines the critical role of leadership in fostering a supportive culture (Weltens et al., 2021). It suggests that while factors such as job strain, dissatisfaction with management and staff burnout can increase the risk of aggression, protective factors include effective teamwork and strong leadership.

An inflexible organisational culture can have unintentional consequences for patient dignity, as highlighted in a review of dignity as perceived by patients in hospital environments, including mental health settings (Ekpenyong et al., 2021). Patients highlighted situations where their choices were limited and their preferences overlooked, all in the effort to adhere to the organisational policies or frameworks; this was deemed to be 'undignified care'.

One policy example that could be attributed to create an inflexible organisational culture is the 'zero-tolerance' approach to violence. While the aims of such an approach—to protect the workforce against violence from patients, their families and the public—are laudable, zero-tolerance approaches overlook the multifaceted nature of violence, attributing it merely to individual failings rather than organisational or systemic issues (Patterson et al., 2005). Zero-tolerance policies have been implemented across health services globally, yet the incidence of workplace violence remains high (Fan et al., 2022), suggesting that despite their popularity, they may be unsuccessful. Perhaps their popularity can be attributed to the fact that implementing such policies is a way for organisations to show support to their workforce. For example, despite being dropped by NHS Security Management in the early 2000s, the UK Government recently announced a 'new, zero-tolerance approach … to protect he NHS workforce against deliberate violence' (Department of Health and Social Care, 2018).

While zero-tolerance policies can create an inflexible ward culture, open door policies—maintaining open doors in hospital settings that would otherwise be locked (Gooding, 2021)—can have a positive effect on ward atmosphere. Staff and patients, according to an early review of locked doors in acute inpatient settings, identified that locked doors in psychiatric wards offer benefits, such as preventing the entry of illegal substances and reducing absconding and potential harm, and drawbacks, including negative psychological impacts on patients, increased feelings of confinement and additional workload for staff (van der Merwe et al., 2009). Furthermore, the practice of locking wards was linked to higher levels of patient aggression, decreased satisfaction with treatment and worsened symptomatology. Since that review there has been a proliferation of research examining the benefits of open door policies, much of which has found that such policies may actually decrease absconding and potential harm from, e.g. suicide, aggression and coercive interventions (Cibis et al., 2017; Huber et al., 2016; Lang et al., 2010; Schneeberger et al., 2017; Schreiber et al., 2022). Some authors postulate that the reduction in absconding behaviours may be due to improvements in the ward atmosphere (Lang et al., 2010). This supposition is supported by various studies that have examined the relationship between open doors and ward atmosphere, which indicate that open door policies in mental health hospitals are associated with improved ward atmosphere, including enhanced feelings of safety and patient coherence, without negatively impacting the therapeutic climate of existing open wards (Blaesi et al., 2015; Efkemann et al., 2019; Lo et al., 2018). Open settings are preferred over locked ones by involuntarily committed patients, showing higher ratings in safety and therapeutic hold, as measured by the EssenCES (Efkemann et al., 2019). The transition from locked to open wards may not compromise care quality or safety (Blaesi et al., 2015; Lo et al., 2018), suggesting that open door policies may foster a more positive therapeutic environment conducive to patient well-being.

Patient safety is intertwined with culture, policies and procedures, indeed, the World Health Organization (2021, p. vii) describes patient safety as:

A framework of organized activities that creates cultures, processes, procedures, behaviours, technologies and environments in health care that consistently and sustainably lower risks, reduce the occurrence of avoidable harm, make errors less likely and reduce the impact of harm when it does occur.

Many of the policies and procedures of healthcare organisations in the UK are overseen by the CQC. To improve patient safety, the CQC (2024) promotes a learning culture, expecting that providers, commissioners and leaders adhere to the following statement:

We have a proactive and positive culture of safety based on openness and honesty, in which concerns about safety are listened to, safety events are investigated and reported thoroughly, and lessons are learned to continually identify and embed good practices.

Furthermore, the NHS has created the just and learning culture charter, in a bid to embed the value of a person-centred workplace that is compassionate, safe and fair when care goes wrong (NHS Resolution, 2023). According to the charter, to have a learning culture, organisations must address accountability, leadership, patient and staff well-being, compassion, inclusivity, respect, candour, learning, best practice and evaluation. Adhering to the charter will include developing policies and procedures that align with a learning culture. The efforts of the CQC and NHS illustrate the UK's commitment to enhance patient safety by fostering learning cultures. Globally, the trend towards improving patient safety through the cultivation of various supportive cultures is gaining momentum. For instance, in the USA, changing from a blame culture to a learning culture has been used to improve patient safety (Hewitt et al., 2017). Furthermore, a patient safety institute in Singapore has demonstrated that enhancing patient safety involves cultivating various cultures, including 'speak up', 'reporting', 'learning', 'patient-centric' and 'just' (Tan et al., 2019). These cultures collectively contribute to a more open, informed and equitable healthcare environment.

While some may view restrictive interventions as necessary and unavoidable, aligning them with patient safety events is contentious. According to the World Health Organization (2021), such interventions could be seen as 'avoidable harm' rather than unavoidable measures. Furthermore, the World Health Organization (2019) categorises restrictive interventions as indicative of service and system failures, or sometimes failures on the part of individual staff members, suggesting that each instance should be regarded as an adverse event. This perspective shifts the view of restrictive interventions from being necessary and unavoidable to potentially being considered as adverse events, highlighting a need for change in organisational culture. This change, according to the World Health Organization's stance, would necessitate revisions in organisational policies and procedures to prevent what is deemed 'avoidable harm', thus challenging the notion that such interventions are a standard and acceptable part of patient care.

## 7 Rules and Power

From a more social perspective, the use of ward rules can be instrumental in the development and maintenance of the positive, or negative, culture of a ward. Indeed, the way rules are created and applied can be instrumental in setting the 'tone' or 'mood' of the ward; tone being one of the key features of Edvardsson's (2005, p. 8) definition of ward atmosphere. Rules in mental health settings are designed to maintain safety and order. They can include guidelines for patient behaviour, protocols for staff response to certain situations and procedures for managing crises (National Institute for Health and Care Excellence, 2015). Ward rules are necessary for maintaining order and safety but enforcement of rules can exacerbate the power imbalance that is inherent between staff and patients.

In their early review of ward rules, Alexander and Bowers (2004) found ambiguity in the literature. Many studies supported the use of highly structured approaches to reduce aggressive behaviour. However, a similar number found that strict settings can actually provoke violence in patients. Alexander (2005), in her subsequent PhD, found that clarity and consistency of rules, and also flexibility, contributed to a calm ward atmosphere. Patients have identified that staff taking a flexible approach to rules is an important aspect of staff de-escalation (Price et al., 2018). Since de-escalation is the key secondary prevention tactic that staff can use to prevent imminent violence, this suggests that taking a pragmatic approach to rules may reduce violence.

Bowers et al. (2011) conducted a comprehensive literature review of nearly 1000 studies on inpatient violence and aggression. They found that limit setting was a precursor to violence in about half of the studies that identified antecedents. This is not surprising given the literature reviewed by Doyle and Clark (2020), which examined how ward rules and limit setting impact challenging behaviour. They found that enforcing hospital ward rules with a therapeutic intent, such as involving patients in rulemaking and understanding their behaviour, leads to positive outcomes like increased patient responsibility and reduced aggression. However, when rules were applied non-therapeutically, such as when staff made moral judgments about patient behaviour, it could negatively impact patients and exacerbate challenging behaviour.

Doyle and Clark (2020) found that understanding the reasoning behind rules may be important in reducing the negative impact of rules and limit setting. When patients do not understand the rules, they experience negative emotions. For example, Alexander (2006) found that patients felt claustrophobic and resentful when the ward was locked without explanation. Similarly, Gros et al. (2017) found that patients felt frustrated and disrespected when rules did not make sense to them. In a qualitative study by Price et al. (2018) about effective de-escalators, most patient participants felt that numerous arbitrary rules impacted challenging behaviour. For instance, patients were required to turn off the television at set times and had restricted access to water coolers at night. Enforcement of these rules was perceived as petty and negatively affected patients' relationships with staff. As a result, when the need for de-escalation arose, patients were less receptive to it. However, rules that promote safety, such as no hitting, may be seen as sensible and valued by patients (Gros et al., 2017; Johnson & Delaney, 2006). A solution to this issue is provided within the Safewards suite of interventions. 'Mutual Expectations' involves clarifying the expectations that staff and patients have of each other, which allows the staff to be consistent and the patients to understand their obligations and those of staff (Safewards, 2024). By implementing the 'Mutual Expectations' intervention, patients can have a better understanding of the rules and expectations, which can reduce negative emotions and improve their relationship with the staff. This can lead to a more positive and therapeutic environment.

It is useful to explore patients' motivations for following rules (Doyle & Clark, 2020). Patients who understand and agree with the rationale behind rules, seeing their connection to treatment, are more likely to follow them (Gros et al., 2017). On the other hand, patients adhering to rules without true agreement may show signs of withdrawal or disengage from the therapeutic process (Alexander, 2006; Gros et al., 2017). Such behaviour is often overlooked by medical staff, potentially leading to unmet patient needs or an unacknowledged risk of institutionalisation. Furthermore, patients often adhere to rules to gain privileges, avoid penalties or secure other advantages (Bos et al., 2012; Gros et al., 2017). Some staff suggest that this adherence might mask underlying feelings of anger or thoughts of aggression and absconding (Alexander, 2006).

Finally, a section on rules would not be complete without consideration of blanket restrictions. Blanket restrictions are measures uniformly applied to all patients, such as fixed activity times, locked doors and limited facility access. They are sometimes mistakenly seen as general rules, as highlighted in the study by Price et al. (2018), where participants described them as rules that could be arbitrary and trivial. However, unlike ward rules, which are fixed and less frequently assessed because they are less likely to infringe on personal liberties (e.g. banning weapons and illegal substances), blanket restrictions require regular evaluation and adjustment based on fluctuating risk levels (Hinchcliffe, 2020). These measures aim to find a balance between safeguarding safety and minimising infringements on liberty and dignity, ensuring they are justified and proportional to the evaluated risk. Yet, an excessive focus on safety can foster a culture averse to any risk, which, as identified in a review of restrictiveness in forensic psychiatric care, can inadvertently legitimise the implementation of blanket restrictions (Tomlin et al., 2018). In CQC inspection reports of three high-secure hospitals in England, inspectors and patients highlighted the application of excessive restrictions, often viewed as unnecessary or illegal (Rabab et al., 2020). Issues were notably found with blanket restrictions affecting privacy, as well as access to food and kitchen areas. A specific instance highlighted was the denial of garden access to patients due to a lack of supervisory staff.

# 8    Implications and Hopes for the Future

In this chapter, a range of literature has been explored, some of which directly relates to ward atmosphere and coercion, but much of which has been applied given the limited research available. Implications for policy, particularly in terms of standardising procedures are evident. With regard to organisational culture, Scott et al. (2003) suggest that there should be an increase in the use of theoretical culture knowledge in empirical work, in addition to longitudinal and cross-sectional studies. Ultimately, the immediate and primary function of social science research should be to direct the process of change in mental healthcare and examine indiscriminate phenomena such as the ward culture and atmosphere. The need to examine this at different levels and from different perspectives cannot, therefore, be underestimated, and larger-scale studies are warranted.

In concluding this chapter, it is useful to consider what the implications are for practice, research and education. Practices within mental health settings should evolve towards a patient-centred approach, echoing the early insights about the significance of ward atmosphere highlighted by the World Health Organization (1953). This approach involves developing staff capabilities in nurturing a therapeutic ward environment where patients are integral to their treatment process. It also suggests reevaluating the physical ward space to ensure it supports therapeutic goals and respects the dignity and individuality of each patient. Research in this field would benefit from a deeper exploration into the complex relationship between ward culture and patient outcomes, including staff well-being. This exploration should seek to understand the long-term effects of ward atmosphere on patient recovery. It could be beneficial to study the subtleties of rule enforcement and its psychological impact on patients, potentially leading to significant improvements in care. The education of mental health professionals could include an in-depth understanding of ward culture. This involves training future healthcare professionals in skills to positively influence the ward atmosphere, creating an environment conducive to healing. Such education should also emphasise empathy and respect for the complexities of the psychiatric ward, preparing practitioners to contribute effectively in these settings.

The ideal ward atmosphere in a mental health hospital setting, drawing from the historical insights and discussions within this chapter, should be a harmonious blend of various critical elements. It would embody a space where containment is balanced with compassion, ensuring patients' physical well-being while preventing violence in a manner that respects their dignity. Support should be a cornerstone, with an environment that makes patients feel comfortable and secure and reduces stress and anxiety. A structured approach to organising the ward, in terms of time, place and person, is crucial for providing predictability and stability. Involvement is another key aspect, where patients are encouraged and supported to engage with their social environment, facilitating a sense of community and belonging. Lastly, validation is paramount, where processes affirm each patient's individuality, acknowledging and respecting their unique experiences and perspectives. Such an atmosphere, responsive to each patient's needs, would not only enhance the efficacy of treatment but also promote a sense of well-being and empowerment among patients and staff. This environment would be underpinned by a culture of empathy, understanding and continuous learning, ensuring that the ward remains a dynamic space that adapts to the evolving needs of all.

## References

Alexander, J. (2005). *Ward rules for patient conduct*, PhD, City University.

Alexander, J. (2006). Patients' feelings about ward nursing regimes and involvement in rule construction. *Journal of Psychiatric and Mental Health Nursing, 13*(5), 543–553.

Alexander, J., & Bowers, L. (2004). Acute psychiatric ward rules: A review of the literature. *Journal of Psychiatric and Mental Health Nursing, 11*(5), 623–631. https://doi.org/10.1111/j.1365-2850.2004.00770.x

Baillie, L. (2009). Patient dignity in an acute hospital setting: A case study. *International Journal of Nursing Studies, 46*(1), 23–37. https://doi.org/10.1016/j.ijnurstu.2008.08.003

Banks, C., & Priebe, S. (2020). Scales for assessing the therapeutic milieu in psychiatric inpatient settings: A systematic review. *General Hospital Psychiatry, 66*, 44–50. https://doi.org/10.1016/j.genhosppsych.2020.06.014

BBC. (2022). 'Panorama' *undercover hospital: Patients at risk*. https://www.bbc.co.uk/iplayer/episode/m001ckxr/panorama-undercover-hospital-patients-at-risk

Berry, S., & Robertson, N. (2019). Burnout within forensic psychiatric nursing: Its relationship with ward environment and effective clinical supervision? *Journal of Psychiatric and Mental Health Nursing, 26*(7), 212–222.

Berry, K., Haddock, G., Kellett, S., Roberts, C., Drake, R., & Barrowclough, C. (2016). Feasibility of a ward-based psychological intervention to improve staff and patient relationships in psychiatric rehabilitation settings. *British Journal of Clinical Psychology, 55*(3), 236–252. https://doi.org/10.1111/bjc.12082

Björkdahl, A., Hansebo, G., & Palmstierna, T. (2013). The influence of staff training on the violence prevention and management climate in psychiatric inpatient units. *Journal of Psychiatric and Mental Health Nursing, 20*(5), 396–404. https://doi.org/10.1111/j.1365-2850.2012.01930.x

Blaesi, S., Gairing, S. K., Walter, M., Lang, U. E., & Huber, C. G. (2015). [Safety, therapeutic hold, and patient's cohesion on closed, recently opened, and open psychiatric wards]. *Psychiatrische Praxis, 42*(02), 76–81. https://doi.org/10.1055/s-0033-1359871.

Bos, M., Kool-Goudzwaard, N., Gamel, C. J., Koekkoek, B., & Van Meijel, B. (2012). The treatment of 'difficult' patients in a secure unit of a specialized psychiatric hospital: The patient's perspective. *Journal of Psychiatric and Mental Health Nursing, 19*(6), 528–535. https://doi.org/10.1111/j.1365-2850.2011.01827.x

Bowen, B., Privitera, M. R., & Bowie, V. (2011). Reducing workplace violence by creating healthy workplace environments. *Journal of Aggression, Conflict and Peace Research, 3*(4), 185–198. https://doi.org/10.1108/17596591111187710

Bowers, L. (2002). *Dangerous and severe personality disorder: Reaction and role of the psychiatric team.* Routledge.

Bowers, L., Stewart, D., Papadopoulos, C., Dack, C., Ross, J., Khanom, H., et al. (2011). *Inpatient violence and aggression: A literature review.* King's College. http://www.kcl.ac.uk/iop/depts/hspr/research/ciemh/mhn/projects/litreview/LitRevAgg.pdf

Braithwaite, J., Herkes, J., Ludlow, K., Testa, L., & Lamprell, G. (2017). Association between organisational and workplace cultures, and patient outcomes: Systematic review. *BMJ Open, 7*(11), e017708. https://doi.org/10.1136/bmjopen-2017-017708

Butterworth, H., Wood, L., & Rowe, S. (2022). Patients' and staff members' experiences of restrictive practices in acute mental health in-patient settings: Systematic review and thematic synthesis. *BJPsych Open, 8*(6), e178. https://doi.org/10.1192/bjo.2022.574

Care Quality Commission. (2020). *Out of sight—Who cares?: Restraint, segregation and seclusion review.* https://www.cqc.org.uk/sites/default/files/20201218_rssreview_report.pdf

Care Quality Commission. (2023). *Monitoring the Mental Health Act in 2021 to 2022: Ward environments.* https://www.cqc.org.uk/publications/monitoring-mental-health-act/2021-2022/ward-environments

Care Quality Commission. (2024). *Learning culture.* https://www.cqc.org.uk/assessment/quality-statements/safe/learning-culture

Cibis, M.-L., Wackerhagen, C., Müller, S., Lang, U. E., Schmidt, Y., & Heinz, A. (2017). Comparison of aggressive behavior, compulsory medication and absconding behavior between open and closed door policy in an acute psychiatric ward. *Psychiatrische Praxis, 44*(3), 141–147. https://doi.org/10.1055/s-0042-105181

Cortis, J. D. (2003). Culture, values and racism: Application to nursing. *International Nursing Review, 50*(1), 55–64. https://doi.org/10.1046/j.1466-7657.2003.00152.x

Cullen, W. D. (1990). *The public inquiry into the Piper Alpha disaster* (Vol. 1 & 2). HMSO.

Cullen, W. D. (2001). *The Ladbroke Grove rail inquiry.* HSE Books.

Denison, D. R. (1996). What is the difference between organizational culture and organizational climate? A native's point of view on a decade of paradigm wars. *The Academy of Management Review, 21*(3), 619–654. https://doi.org/10.2307/258997

Department of Health. (2014). *Positive and proactive care: Reducing the need for restrictive interventions.* Department of Health.

Department of Health and Social Care. (2018). *Stronger protection from violence for NHS staff.* https://www.gov.uk/government/news/stronger-protection-from-violence-for-nhs-staff

Dickens, G. L., Johnson, A., Steel, K., Everett, B., & Tonkin, M. (2022). Interventions to improve social climate in acute mental health inpatient settings: Systematic review of content and outcomes. *SAGE Open Nursing, 8,* 23779608221124291. https://doi.org/10.1177/23779608221124291

Doedens, P., Vermeulen, J., Boyette, L.-L., Latour, C., & de Haan, L. (2020). Influence of nursing staff attitudes and characteristics on the use of coercive measures in acute mental health services—A systematic review. *Journal of Psychiatric and Mental Health Nursing, 27*(4), 446–459. https://doi.org/10.1111/jpm.12586

Doyle, A., & Clark, L. L. (2020). How ward rules and limit setting contribute towards restrictive practices and presentations of challenging behaviour in patients on mental health wards. *British Journal of Mental Health Nursing, 9*(2), 1–9. https://doi.org/10.12968/bjmh.2019.0008

Edvardsson, D. (2005) *Atmosphere in care settings: Towards a broader understanding of the phenomenon.* PhD, Omvårdnad.

Efkemann, S. A., Bernard, J., Kalagi, J., Otte, I., Ueberberg, B., Assion, H.-J., et al. (2019). Ward atmosphere and patient satisfaction in psychiatric hospitals with different ward settings and door policies. Results from a mixed methods study (Original Research). *Frontiers in Psychiatry, 10,* 576. https://doi.org/10.3389/fpsyt.2019.00576

Ekpenyong, M. S., Nyashanu, M., Ossey-Nweze, C., & Serrant, L. (2021). Exploring the perceptions of dignity among patients and nurses in hospital and community settings: An integrative review. *Journal of Research in Nursing, 26*(6), 517–537. https://doi.org/10.1177/1744987121997890

Eliassen, B. K., Sørlie, T., Sexton, J., & Høifødt, T. S. (2016). The effect of training in mindfulness and affect consciousness on the therapeutic environment for patients with psychoses: An explorative intervention study. *Scandinavian Journal of Caring Sciences, 30*(2), 391–402. https://doi.org/10.1111/scs.12261

Fan, S., An, W., Zeng, L., Liu, J., Tang, S., Chen, J., et al. (2022). Rethinking "zero tolerance": A moderated mediation model of mental resilience and coping strategies in workplace violence and nurses' mental health. *Journal of Nursing Scholarship, 54*(4), 501–512. https://doi.org/10.1111/jnu.12753

Fletcher, J., Hamilton, B., Kinner, S. A., & Brophy, L. (2019). Safewards impact in inpatient mental health units in Victoria, Australia: Staff perspectives (Original Research). *Frontiers in Psychiatry, 10,* 462. https://doi.org/10.3389/fpsyt.2019.00462

Gee, M., Bhanbhro, S., Cook, S., & Killaspy, H. (2017). Rapid realist review of the evidence: Achieving lasting change when mental health rehabilitation staff undertake recovery-oriented training. *Journal of Advanced Nursing, 73*(8), 1775–1791. https://doi.org/10.1111/jan.13232

Gerstle, C. R. (2018). Parallels in safety between aviation and healthcare. *Journal of Pediatric Surgery, 53*(5), 875–878. https://doi.org/10.1016/j.jpedsurg.2018.02.002

Glisson, C., & James, L. R. (2002). The cross-level effects of culture and climate in human service teams. *Journal of Organizational Behavior, 23*(6), 767–794. https://doi.org/10.1002/job.162

Gooding, P. (2021). *Compendium report: Good practices in the Council of Europe to promote voluntary measures in mental health services.* Council of Europe.

Gros, C. P., Parr, C., Wright, D. K., Montreuil, M., & Frechette, J. (2017). Hospital rules and regulations: The perspectives of youth receiving psychiatric care. *Journal of Child and Adolescent Psychiatric Nursing, 30*(1), 18–24. https://doi.org/10.1111/jcap.12166

Gunderson, J. G. (1978). Defining the therapeutic processes in psychiatric milieus. *Psychiatry, 41*(4), 327–335.

Hallett, N., Huber, J., Sixsmith, J., & Dickens, G. L. (2018). Measuring the violence prevention climate: Development and evaluation of the VPC-14. *International Journal of Nursing Studies, 88,* 97–103. https://doi.org/10.1016/j.ijnurstu.2018.09.002

Halligan, M., & Zecevic, A. (2011). Safety culture in healthcare: A review of concepts, dimensions, measures and progress. *BMJ Quality and Safety, 20*(4), 338. https://doi.org/10.1136/bmjqs.2010.040964

Harrison, R. (1972). Understanding your organization's character. *Harvard Business Review, 50,* 119–128.

Henderson, J. (2013). How the tidal model was used to overcome a risk-averse ward culture. *Mental Health Practice, 17*(1), 34–37.

Hewitt, D. B., Godlstein, S. D., Isenberg, G. A., Phillips, B. R., & Cowan, S. W. (2017). Patient safety culture: The key to sustained quality improvement. *Journal of Perioperative & Critical Intensive Care Nursing, 3*(1), 1000135. https://doi.org/10.4172/2471-9870.1000135

Hinchcliffe, G. (2020). *Justifying blanket restrictions: Resource pack.* https://q.health.org.uk/document/justifying-blanket-restrictions/?bp-attachment=Justifying-Blanket-Restrictions-May-2020-GH.pdf

Holmes, D., Kennedy, S. L., & Perron, A. (2004). The mentally ill and social exclusion: A critical examination of the use of seclusion from the patient's perspective. *Issues in Mental Health Nursing, 25*(6), 559–578. https://doi.org/10.1080/01612840490472101

Huber, C. G., Schneeberger, A. R., Kowalinski, E., Fröhlich, D., von Felten, S., Walter, M., et al. (2016). Suicide risk and absconding in psychiatric hospitals with and without open door policies: A 15 year, observational study. *The Lancet Psychiatry, 3*(9), 842–849. https://doi.org/10.1016/S2215-0366(16)30168-7

Insel, P. M., & Moos, R. H. (1974). Psychological environments: Expanding the scope of human ecology. *American Psychologist, 29*(3), 179.

Jansen, G. (1994). *Safety culture: A study of permanent way staff at British Rail.* Vrije Universiteit.

Jansson, J.-Å., & Eklund, M. (2002). Stability of perceived ward atmosphere over time, diagnosis and gender for patients with psychosis. *Nordic Journal of Psychiatry, 56*(6), 407–412.

Johnson, M. E., & Delaney, K. R. (2006). Keeping the unit safe: A grounded theory study. *Journal of the American Psychiatric Nurses Association, 12*(1), 13–21. https://doi.org/10.1177/1078390306286440

Jones, C. B., Sousane, Z., & Mossburg, S. E. (2023). *Addressing workplace violence and creating a safer workplace.* Patient Safety Network. https://psnet.ahrq.gov/perspective/addressing-workplace-violence-and-creating-safer-workplace

Joyce, A., Moussa, B., Elmes, A., Campbell, P., Suchowerska, R., Buick, F., et al. (2022). Organisational structures and processes for health and well-being: Insights from work integration social enterprise. *BMC Public Health, 22*(1), 1624. https://doi.org/10.1186/s12889-022-13920-4

Kagawa-Singer, M., & Chung, R. C.-Y. (1994). A paradigm for culturally based care in ethnic minority populations. *Journal of Community Psychology, 22*(2), 192–208. https://doi.org/10.1002/1520-6629(199404)22:2<192::AID-JCOP2290220213>3.0.CO;2-H

Kaur, M., De Boer, R. J., Oates, A., Rafferty, J., & Dekker, S. (2019). Restorative just culture: A study of the practical and economic effects of implementing restorative justice in an NHS trust. *MATEC Web of Conferences, 273*, 01007. https://doi.org/10.1051/matecconf/201927301007

Laker, C., Cella, M., Callard, F., & Wykes, T. (2020). The impact of ward climate on staff perceptions of barriers to research-driven service changes on mental health wards: A cross-sectional study. *Journal of Psychiatric and Mental Health Nursing, 27*(3), 281–295. https://doi.org/10.1111/jpm.12577

Lang, U. E., Hartmann, S., Schulz-Hartmann, S., Gudlowski, Y., Ricken, R., Munk, I., et al. (2010). Do locked doors in psychiatric hospitals prevent patients from absconding? *The European Journal of Psychiatry, 24*, 199–204.

Lendemeijer, B., & Shortridge-Baggett, L. (1997). The use of seclusion in psychiatry: A literature review. *Scholarly Inquiry for Nursing Practice, 11*(4), 299–306, 308–315.

Lepping, P., Masood, B., Flammer, E., & Noorthoorn, E. O. (2016). Comparison of restraint data from four countries. *Social Psychiatry and Psychiatric Epidemiology, 51*(9), 1301–1309. https://doi.org/10.1007/s00127-016-1203-x

Lo, S. B., Gaupp, R., Huber, C., Schneeberger, A., Garic, G., Voulgaris, A., et al. (2018). Influence of an "open door policy" on ward climate: Impact on treatment quality. *Psychiatrische Praxis, 45*(03), 133–139. https://doi.org/10.1055/s-0042-121784

Martin, J. (1992). *Cultures in organizations: Three perspectives.* Oxford University Press.

Martin, J., Sitkin, S., & Boehm, M. (1985). Founders and the elusiveness of a cultural legacy. In J. Martin (Ed.), *Organizational culture* (pp. 99–124). Sage.

Mearns, K., Flin, R., Gordon, R., & Fleming, M. (1998). Measuring safety climate on offshore installations. *Work & Stress, 12*(3), 238–254. https://doi.org/10.1080/02678379808256864

Moos, R. (1973). Conceptualizations of human environments. *American Psychologist, 28*(8), 652–665.

Moos, R. (1974). *Evaluating treatment environments: A social ecological approach.* Wiley.

National Institute for Health and Care Excellence. (2015). *Violence and aggression: Short-term management in mental health, health and community settings (NICE Guideline NG10).* https://www.nice.org.uk/guidance/ng10/evidence/full-guideline-pdf-70830253

Nesset, M. B., Rossberg, J. I., Almvik, R., & Friis, S. (2009). Can a focused staff training programme improve the ward atmosphere and patient satisfaction in a forensic psychiatric hospital? A pilot study. *Scandinavian Journal of Caring Sciences, 23*(1), 117–124. https://doi.org/10.1111/j.1471-6712.2008.00597.x

NHS England. (2017). *The fifteen steps challenge.* https://www.england.nhs.uk/wp-content/uploads/2017/11/15-steps-inpatient.pdf

NHS Resolution. (2023). *Being fair 2.* https://resolution.nhs.uk/wp-content/uploads/2023/03/Being-fair-2-final-1.pdf

Nicholls, D., Kidd, K., Threader, J., & Hungerford, C. (2015). The value of purpose built mental health facilities: Use of the Ward Atmosphere Scale to gauge the link between milieu and physical environment. *International Journal of Mental Health Nursing, 24*(4), 286–294.

Norton, K. (2004). Re-thinking acute psychiatric inpatient care. *International Journal of Social Psychiatry, 50*(3), 274–284.

Ouchi, W. G., & Wilkins, A. L. (1985). Organizational culture. *Annual Review of Sociology, 11*(1), 457–483. https://doi.org/10.1146/annurev.so.11.080185.002325

Paradiso, L., & Sweeney, N. (2019). Just culture: It's more than policy. *Nursing Management, 50*(6), 38–45.

Parish, C. (2013). Change ward culture to cut violence and aggression. *Mental Health Practice, 16*(10), 6–7.

Patterson, B., Leadbetter, D., & Miller, G. (2005). Beyond Zero Tolerance: A varied approach to workplace violence. *British Journal of Nursing, 14*(15), 810–815. https://doi.org/10.12968/bjon.2005.14.15.18598

Pelto-Piri, V., Wallsten, T., Hylén, U., Nikban, I., & Kjellin, L. (2019). Feeling safe or unsafe in psychiatric inpatient care, a hospital-based qualitative interview study with inpatients in Sweden. *International Journal of Mental Health Systems, 13*(1), 23. https://doi.org/10.1186/s13033-019-0282-y

Peters, T. J., & Waterman, R. H. J. (1982). *In search of excellence. Lessons from America's best-run companies.* Harper Row.

Philo, C. (1997). Across the water: Reviewing geographical studies of asylums and other mental health facilities. *Health & Place, 3*(2), 73–89. https://doi.org/10.1016/S1353-8292(97)00002-6

Price, O., Baker, J., Bee, P., Grundy, A., Scott, A., Butler, D., et al. (2018). Patient perspectives on barriers and enablers to the use and effectiveness of de-escalation techniques for the management of violence and aggression in mental health settings. *Journal of Advanced Nursing, 74*(3), 614–625. https://doi.org/10.1111/jan.13488

Rabab, S., Tomlin, J., Huband, N., & Völlm, B. (2020). Care Quality Commission inspections of high-security hospitals. *The Journal of Forensic Practice, 22*(2), 83–96. https://doi.org/10.1108/JFP-09-2019-0044

Reader, T. W., & O'Connor, P. (2014). The Deepwater Horizon explosion: Non-technical skills, safety culture, and system complexity. *Journal of Risk Research, 17*(3), 405–424. https://doi.org/10.1080/13669877.2013.815652

Rousseau, D. (1988). The construction of climate in organizational research. In I. Robertson (Ed.), *International review of industrial and organizational research.* Wiley.

Safewards. (2024). *Clear mutual expectations.* https://safewards.net/interventions/clear-mutual-expectations

Schalast, N., & Redies, M. (2005). *Development of an assessment questionnaire (handout).* Paper presented at the The Sixth Nordic Symposium on Forensic Psychiatry, Vaasa, Finland.

Schalast, N., Redies, M., Collins, M., Stacey, J., & Howells, K. (2008). EssenCES, a short questionnaire for assessing the social climate of forensic psychiatric wards. *Criminal Behaviour and Mental Health, 18*(1), 49–58.

Schein, E. H. (2004). *Organizational culture and leadership.* Jossey-Bass.

Schneeberger, A. R., Kowalinski, E., Fröhlich, D., Schröder, K., von Felten, S., Zinkler, M., et al. (2017). Aggression and violence in psychiatric hospitals with and without open door policies: A 15-year naturalistic observational study. *Journal of Psychiatric Research, 95*, 189–195. https://doi.org/10.1016/j.jpsychires.2017.08.017

Schreiber, L. K., Metzger, F. G., Flammer, E., Rinke, H., Fallgatter, A. J., & Steinert, T. (2022). Open doors by fair means: A quasi-experimental controlled study on the effects of an open-door policy on acute psychiatric wards. *BMC Health Services Research, 22*(1), 941. https://doi.org/10.1186/s12913-022-08322-6

Scott, T., Mannion, R., Marshall, M., & Davies, H. (2003). Does organisational culture influence health care performance? A review of the evidence. *Journal of Health Services Research & Policy, 8*(2), 105–117. https://doi.org/10.1258/135581903321466085

Secker, J., Benson, A., Balfe, E., Lipsedge, M., Robinson, S., & Walker, J. (2004). Understanding the social context of violent and aggressive incidents on an inpatient unit. *Journal of Psychiatric and Mental Health Nursing, 11*(2), 172–178. https://doi.org/10.1111/j.1365-2850.2003.00703.x

Sequeira, H., & Halstead, S. (2002). Control and restraint in the UK: Service user perspectives. *The British Journal of Forensic Practice, 4*(1), 9–18. https://doi.org/10.1108/14636646200200003

Smircich, L. (1983). Concepts of culture and organizational analysis. *Administrative Science Quarterly, 28*(3), 339–358. https://doi.org/10.2307/2392246

Smith, S. B. (1995). Restraints: Retraumatization for rape victims? *Journal of Psychosocial Nursing and Mental Health Services, 33*(7), 23–28. https://doi.org/10.3928/0279-3695-19950701-06

Swuste, P., van Gulijk, C., Groeneweg, J., Zwaard, W., Lemkowitz, S., & Guldenmund, F. (2020). From Clapham Junction to Macondo, Deepwater Horizon: Risk and safety management in high-tech-high-hazard sectors: A review of English and Dutch literature: 1988–2010. *Safety Science, 121*, 249–282. https://doi.org/10.1016/j.ssci.2019.08.031

Tan, K. H., Pang, N. L., Siau, C., Foo, Z., & Fong, K. Y. (2019). Building an organizational culture of patient safety. *Journal of Patient Safety and Risk Management, 24*(6), 253–261. https://doi.org/10.1177/2516043519878979

Tomlin, J., Bartlett, P., & Völlm, B. (2018). Experiences of restrictiveness in forensic psychiatric care: Systematic review and concept analysis. *International Journal of Law and Psychiatry, 57*, 31–41. https://doi.org/10.1016/j.ijlp.2017.12.006

Tonkin, M. (2015). A review of questionnaire measures for assessing the social climate in prisons and forensic psychiatric hospitals. *International Journal of Offender Therapy and Comparative Criminology, 60*(12), 1376–1405. https://doi.org/10.1177/0306624X15578834

Tuvesson, H., & Eklund, M. (2017). Nursing staff stress and individual characteristics in relation to the ward atmosphere in psychiatric in-patient wards. *Issues in Mental Health Nursing, 38*(9), 726–732. https://doi.org/10.1080/01612840.2017.1324929

van Baarle, E., Hartman, L., Rooijakkers, S., Wallenburg, I., Weenink, J.-W., Bal, R., et al. (2022). Fostering a just culture in healthcare organizations: Experiences in practice. *BMC Health Services Research, 22*(1), 1035. https://doi.org/10.1186/s12913-022-08418-z

van der Merwe, M., Bowers, L., Jones, J., Simpson, A., & Haglund, K. (2009). Locked doors in acute inpatient psychiatry: A literature review. *Journal of Psychiatric and Mental Health Nursing, 16*(3), 293–299. https://doi.org/10.1111/j.1365-2850.2008.01378.x

van der Schaaf, P. S., Dusseldorp, E., Janssen, W. A., Keuning, F. M., & Noorthoorn, E. O. (2013). Impact of the physical environment of psychiatric wards on the use of seclusion. *British Journal of Psychiatry, 202*(2), 142–149. https://doi.org/10.1192/bjp.bp.112.118422

Weltens, I., Bak, M., Verhagen, S., Vandenberk, E., Domen, P., van Amelsvoort, T., et al. (2021). Aggression on the psychiatric ward: Prevalence and risk factors. A systematic review of the literature. *PLoS One, 16*(10), e0258346. https://doi.org/10.1371/journal.pone.0258346

Wilkins, A. L. (1983). The culture audit: A tool for understanding organizations. *Organizational Dynamics, 12*(2), 24–38. https://doi.org/10.1016/0090-2616(83)90031-1

World Health Organization. (1953). *The community mental hospital: Third report of the expert committee on mental health*. World Health Organization.

World Health Organization. (2019). *Strategies to end seclusion and restraint: WHO quality rights specialized training*. World Health Organization.

World Health Organization. (2021). *Global patient safety action plan 2021–2030: Towards eliminating unavoidable harm in health care*. World Health Organization.

Wynn, R. (2004). Psychiatric inpatients' experiences with restraint. *Journal of Forensic Psychiatry & Psychology, 15*(1), 124–144. https://doi.org/10.1080/14789940410001655187

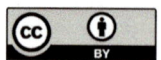

# Trauma-Informed Care

Alina Haines-Delmont, Joy A. Duxbury, Veenu Gupta,
and Tella Lantta

## 1 Introduction: A Paradigm Shift Towards Trauma-Informed Thinking

Trauma was declared a global public health concern when the World Health Organisation (Kessler et al., 2017)[1] found that 70% of the world's population have experienced at least one lifetime traumatic event ranging from threatened death, serious injury or sexual violence to the unexpected death of a loved one. Of these, approximately 13% of the population report experiencing four or more traumatic events in their life. Factors at individual, relationship, community and societal levels

---

[1] Based on an analysis of data captured in the WHO World Mental Health (WMH) surveys. The WMH Surveys are a series of community epidemiological surveys that used this weighting scheme to generate a representative sample of trauma occurrences in the general population of participating countries.

---

A. Haines-Delmont (✉)
School of Nursing and Public Health, Manchester Metropolitan University, Manchester, UK
e-mail: a.haines@mmu.ac.uk

J. A. Duxbury
Institute of Health, University of Cumbria, Lancaster, UK
e-mail: Joy.duxbury@cumbria.ac.uk

V. Gupta
Department of Psychology, Institute for Medical Humanities, University of Durham, Durham, UK
e-mail: veenu.gupta@durham.ac.uk

T. Lantta
Department of Nursing Science, University of Turku, Turku, Finland

Centre for Forensic Behavioural Science, Swinburne University of Technology, Melbourne, VIC, Australia
e-mail: tella.lantta@utu.fi

© The Author(s) 2024
N. Hallett et al. (eds.), *Coercion and Violence in Mental Health Settings*,
https://doi.org/10.1007/978-3-031-61224-4_13

have been identified as explanatory factors in both the occurrence of trauma and its sequelae. The trauma experienced in childhood (i.e. adverse childhood experiences—ACEs) has been identified as a key risk factor for poor mental and physical health in adulthood (Alvarez et al., 2011; Anderson et al., 2016; Kessler et al., 2010).

In this chapter, we refer to trauma as 'an event, series of events, or set of circumstances that is experienced by an individual as physically or emotionally harmful or life-threatening and that has lasting adverse effects on the individual's functioning and mental, physical, social, emotional, or spiritual well-being' (Substance Abuse and Mental Health Services Administration [SAMHSA], 2012, p. 2). The experience of a mental health crisis in itself can have a long-term traumatic effect, with the potential for retraumatisation through the use of coercive practices (Nizum et al., 2020).

A large proportion of people with mental health problems who access services present with high rates of trauma (Anderson et al., 2016), especially complex trauma (i.e. multiple or prolonged traumatic events) (Beckett et al., 2017). Women report higher odds of lifetime trauma/post-traumatic stress disorder (PTSD) than men (Valentine et al., 2019). Black people are more likely to experience PTSD than other ethnic groups (Roberts et al., 2011). Black men in particular are more likely to be subject to detention under mental health legislation (NHS Digital, 2019), thus more likely to be involuntarily hospitalised in mental health settings (Barnett et al., 2019) and potentially retraumatised (Mohan et al., 2006; Morgan et al., 2004). Racial and socio-economic inequalities are of key concern when it comes to trauma. One would think, therefore that services are designed in a way to acknowledge these inequalities with the view to aid recovery. However, as argued in this chapter, while there are key developments in this area, mental health services have been slow in embracing and implementing approaches to care dealing directly with trauma, by recognising this important link or responding appropriately, especially with regard to socio-demographic and key cultural differences.

The trauma-informed paradigm/philosophy—also referred to as trauma-informed care (TIC), trauma-informed approach (TIA) or trauma-informed care and practice (TICP) (Muskett, 2014)—is a system development model grounded in a holistic understanding of how trauma exposure affects one's neurological, biological, psychological and social development (Paterson, 2014), using an adapted definition of TIC, from SAMHSA (2014). This means that all people at all levels within an organisation have a basic understanding that trauma affects people's experiences and behaviour in the context of coping strategies in response to childhood or past adversity and circumstances as well as current events. It represents a paradigm shift within inpatient mental health services, challenging the early twentieth century institutional practices—blaming the individual, explaining behaviour as a consequence of a mental illness rather than a response/coping mechanism to trauma—which unfortunately are still common in some services. At a fundamental level, it is a shift from a service that asks 'What is wrong with you?' to considering 'What happened to you?'; a process of organisational change supporting environments and relationships that promote recovery and reduce or prevent retraumatisation (Sweeney et al., 2018). Trauma-informed approaches encourage services to reframe behaviour seen as challenging as a functional, innately developed survival technique for trauma developed under acute distress. It contextualises trauma based on each individual's social and political background to understand how these impact past and current presentations (Sweeney et al., 2018). Trauma-informed key principles include safety, collaboration, empowerment, trustworthiness and choice (Isobel & Edwards, 2017).

Its principles are therefore particularly pertinent to inpatient mental health services—where the biomedical model of psychiatry is still predominant. People are admitted at times of crisis, sometimes without pre-existing trauma histories but experiencing high distress, loss of autonomy, social belonging and dislocation from normal support and family/friends (Muskett, 2014), sometimes with significant trauma histories, and often subject to involuntary treatment, psychotropic medication and the use of coercive practices. If trauma goes unrecognised, there is the risk that they can be retraumatised by ward practices (Walsh & Benjamin, 2020). Thus, approaches with a trauma-informed philosophy at their core include the recognition of the high rates of trauma amongst people with mental health problems (well documented in the literature (e.g. Anderson et al., 2016)) and the need to both understand the impact of trauma and respond appropriately.

However, while there is momentum in the uptake of trauma-informed approaches, there are still many barriers to their implementation. Trauma-informed care is a widely accepted philosophical model/framework within mental health settings but it is not always clear on how to operationalise it. As highlighted further in this chapter, more needs to happen to reach a consensus and allow the articulation of this guiding philosophy/framework to inform clinical practice.

## 2    The Impact of Coercive Practices on Trauma and the Concept of Retraumatisation

Mental health services run the risk of retraumatising trauma survivors. The use of coercive practices within mental health settings can trigger the same physiological responses associated with the original trauma and subsequently retraumatise the individual. Retraumatisation within services affects both staff and patients. The act of regularly practising restraint can have a physical and emotional toll such as injury, chronic stress and burnout.

Since their inception, the use of coercive interventions such as seclusion and restraint and more recently broader restrictive practices have received increasing criticism. Concerns over their negative impact have continued to grow. This is especially true when one looks at the experiences of service users and how they perceive these practices and their damaging effects. Since the 1980s, the number of high-profile cases resulting in physical and psychological trauma has risen significantly and been reported widely and globally. The negative impact on those who are cared for in services is palpable. This has not only been reported upon in the media but also in day-to-day practice and the increasing research conducted in this area.

Historically, however, there is a dearth of literature on the trauma associated with coercion and issues which do tend to be reported upon largely revolve around the use of seclusion and restraint; the 'harder end' of the spectrum of restrictions. Furthermore, there is a scarcity of literature dedicated specifically to the perspective of the patient.

Persons with mental health problems are undoubtedly vulnerable to additional traumatic or iatrogenic experiences that occur within mental health settings. It is reported that many of those diagnosed with mental disorders have been exposed to some sort of trauma historically (Mueser et al., 2004). The long-term effects of trauma can then in turn result in vulnerable hospitalised patients exhibiting distress and negative approaches to coping, often inappropriately referred to as 'challenging'.

## 2.1    Cycle of Trauma

It has been argued by some that a cycle of trauma for hospitalised patients can be inadvertently perpetuated by mental health professionals who respond to escalating and threatening behaviour by using coercive practices that subsequently retraumatise individuals (Huckshorn, 2006; National Association of State Mental Health Program Directors [NASMHPD], 2005). Admission to mental health services can then be traumatic for patients without pre-existing trauma histories as a result of loss of autonomy and dislocation from normal supports and family (Muskett, 2014). Using coercive methods exacerbates the impact of these experiences (Borckardt et al., 2007). This can result in fear, mistrust, depression and negative coping behaviours, such as self-harm, dissociative behaviour and aggression (Saakvitne et al., 2000).

Trauma symptoms and the absence of perceived safe and supportive inpatient environments create obstacles to effective treatment and care for those in mental health services (Muskett, 2014). Providers may have no definitive way of knowing who has a history of trauma; Elliott et al. (2005) suggest accordingly that 'universal trauma precautions' should be applied to all; that is, nurses routinely using practices that are growth-promoting and recovery-focused and less likely to retraumatise those already exposed to significant interpersonal trauma.

## 2.2    Spectrum of Coercion

The iatrogenic harm caused by coercive practices is still poorly recognised yet the spectrum of coercion and its impact can be wide-reaching. O'Brien and Golding (2003) argue that we should understand coercion as 'any use of authority to override the choice of another' (p. 168). Szmukler and Appelbaum (2008) later conceptualised coercion as ranging from harder types, such as legal measures, seclusion, restraint and enforced medication, to softer types. Soft coercion is defined as a perceived threat of punishment or force (Gilburt et al., 2010; Lloyd-Evans et al., 2010).

The term 'softer' coercion is often used to capture the meaning of both soft and subtle coercion (Anderson et al., 2020).

When exposed to the formal harder type of coercive care, patients might be subject to forced medication, seclusion or physical restraint. During such circumstances, coercion is explicit, more likely to be documented in patients' records and is largely regulated within legal frameworks. In contrast, soft coercion could be perceived to be less obvious (O'Brien & Golding, 2003). This can include actions where health professionals use their power to put pressure on patients to behave in a certain way and comply with treatment plans. This kind of softer coercion is more implicit, is less subject to formal decisions and documentation and can also be described by some as informal coercion or more recently blanket restrictions (Anderson et al., 2020). Many examples of informal coercion exist and mental health professionals tend to underestimate the impact of their use.

Despite patients reporting harrowing experiences related to hard coercion (Hughes et al., 2009; Paksarian et al., 2014), less attention is given in the literature to softer coercion and 'the "heterogeneity of coercion" remains poorly understood' (Molodynski et al., 2016, p. 1). Szmukler (2015) calls for a more precise understanding to advance thinking and research into the broader spectrum of coercive practice (Allison & Flemming, 2019). The differences between and impact of hard and soft coercion are outlined more fully below.

### 2.2.1 Hard Coercion and Trauma

A plethora of studies in mental health settings over the years has cast light on the negative and complex aspects regarding, in particular, the use of seclusion with or without restraint and many patients are left with negative views of the events (Larue et al., 2013; Wilson et al., 2017). Whilst there are recommendations reporting the safe use of these practices (NICE, 2015), they remain contentious areas of mental health care. Existing literature suggests that there are serious physical and psychological implications surrounding approaches associated with 'hard coercion' for both mental health patients and nurses alike. There is growing evidence that such approaches are not compatible with the values of recovery in mental health care (Douglas et al., 2022).

Concerns associated with the use of restraint and seclusion specifically include reports of psychological trauma, physical injuries and even death (Douglas et al., 2022; Knowles et al., 2015; Wilson et al., 2017). According to the literature, the experience of restraint can have a profound physical and psychological impact on individuals, and few are likely to remain neutral about it (Bigwood & Crowe, 2008; Frueh et al., 2005). With regard to the physical impact, there is a clear evidence base that highlights issues pertaining to injuries and in some cases death (Duxbury et al., 2011; Kersting et al., 2019; Lazarus, 2001).

The psychological effects can be wide-ranging and include trauma, fear, dissatisfaction, stigma and perceptions of punishment. Some studies suggest that participants report feelings of anger (Donat, 2002; Frueh et al., 2005; Kontio et al., 2012), recall traumatic memories or experiences of trauma (Haw et al., 2011) and express feelings of abandonment and isolation (Bonner et al., 2002; Holmes et al., 2004;

Larue et al., 2013; Mayers et al., 2010). Furthermore, restraint creates the potential for corrupted cultures of care, diminishes the care experience and tends to undermine the development of a trusting relationship between staff and patients (Douglas et al., 2022).

In a concerning number of studies, patients have reported that they felt restraint had been employed abusively and that staff had applied undue force. In a study by Haw et al. (2011), for example, 84% of forensic inpatients experienced the use of seclusion and restraint negatively, saying it reminded them of a 'prison cell', and believed it was a consequence of disobedience to staff. Keski-Valkama et al. (2010) found that 66.3% of patients perceived seclusion as a punitive measure; this proportion was significantly higher in the forensic group (73.1%) than in the general psychiatric group (54.1%). Patients also reported that the imposition of seclusion and/or restraint was the consequence of 'bad behaviour'.

In contrast, research on practitioners' views tends to focus on the management of safety and less so on the impact on the patient. For example, various studies focus on an increase in violent acts and risk of injury for both patients and staff during SR episodes (Paterson & Duxbury, 2007). Furthermore, whilst there are some reports of restraint being experienced in a positive light providing patients with a sense of security when they have lost control of their actions (Iversen et al., 2011; Wynn, 2004), evidence suggests that the practice is largely experienced by those receiving it as negative.

### 2.2.2  Soft Coercion and Trauma

There is increasing evidence today of the negative impact of practices referred to as soft, subtle or informal coercion, blanket restrictions and/or broader restrictive practices as described above. Allison and Flemming (2019) conducted a qualitative evidence synthesis to obtain an overview regarding experiences related to softer coercion. They concluded that it is important for practitioners to have a greater understanding of how the clinical environment has an impact on their role and the power of coercion within 'caring relationships'.

The impact of the environment and ward culture has been reported upon for some time (Duxbury, 2002). Studies, for example, have provided important insights into patients' perceptions of a range of contributory factors including the physical and atmospheric milieu of an environment, the culture of wards and levels of aggression and acuity in psychiatric settings. Yet their impact with regard to trauma is often overlooked. Many practices and procedures, such as ward rounds, ward rules, search procedures, locked doors and mixed-sex patient populations are retraumatising, as they are experienced by patients as emotionally unsafe and disempowering practices (Borge & Fagermoen, 2008; Clark et al., 2008; Cleary, 2003).

The potential negative impact of restrictions such as unit rules is also evident. The Mental Health Act Code of Practice (Code) defines blanket restrictions as rules or policies that restrict a patient's liberty and other rights, which are routinely applied to all patients, or classes of patients, or within a service, without individual risk assessments to justify their application. Studies suggest that the overarching experience of psychiatric hospitalisation may be distressing, harmful, or traumatic to many patients, and patients report that coercion is incompatible with expectations of care and that it is 'anti-recovery' (Frueh et al., 2005). Consequently, patients may express feelings of animosity towards staff due to the diminishment of trust.

The impact of soft coercion in the form of blanket restrictions is gaining growing attention and their role in exacerbating trauma outcomes cannot be underestimated. Deveau and McDonnell (2009) argued some time back that the practice of blanket restrictions has the potential to cause immediate and lasting harm whilst breaching people's human rights. They further suggested that the misapplication of BR can disrupt the delivery of care that is respectful and responsive to people's preferences, needs and values, and therefore needs to be addressed.

## 3    Trauma-Informed Care Approaches and Interventions

Trauma-informed care (TIC) approaches and care systems are seen as an essential component in reducing the use of seclusion and restraint, and other types of coercive measures in mental health settings (Huckshorn, 2004). This approach assists professionals in gaining insight into the causes of violence and aggression and understanding factors that may trigger violent episodes. On an organisational level, this approach requires being conscious that their services can retraumatise admitted patients by the use of coercive measures (Aremu et al., 2018). In this section, we provide an overview of existing TIC-based approaches and interventions to reduce coercive measures and their impact on health outcomes and practice.

Trauma-informed interventions have been explored in different mental health settings, including acute inpatient units for adults (Aremu et al., 2018; Blair et al., 2017; Blair & Moulton-Adelman, 2015; Duxbury et al., 2019), forensic inpatient mental health care for adults (Maguire et al., 2012; Putkonen et al., 2013 [men only]), children and adolescent units (Azeem et al., 2011), substance abuse units (Borckardt et al., 2011), geriatric units (Borckardt et al., 2011) and community-based services (Craig & Sanders, 2018). To establish the impact or effectiveness of using trauma-informed approaches, various study designs have been adopted including quality improvement (e.g. Aremu et al., 2018; Blair et al., 2017; Blair & Moulton-Adelman, 2015), quasi-experimental (e.g. Azeem et al., 2011; Borckardt et al., 2011; Duxbury et al., 2019), experimental (Putkonen et al., 2013) and retrospective evaluation (Guzman-Parra et al., 2016).

TIC approaches related to the aim of decreasing the use of coercive measures in inpatient settings have been most widely studied about the Six Core Strategies, originating from TIC (e.g. Azeem et al., 2011; Craig & Sanders, 2018; Guzman-Parra et al., 2016). These six strategies include the use of restraint and seclusion reduction tools, consumer roles in inpatient settings, debriefing techniques, leadership towards organisational change, use of data to inform practice and workforce development. The strategy related to the leadership is seen as a mandatory core intervention, including defining and articulating a vision, values and philosophy that expects the reduction of coercive measures, creating an action plan to implement that vision and holding staff accountable to that plan. TIC is an essential part of the strategies, such as workforce development on service and staff education levels. The use of tools includes measurement of trauma, and debriefing techniques take into account the potentially traumatising effects of coercive measures (Huckshorn, 2008).

In the UK, an adapted version of the Six Core Strategies, 'REsTRAIN YOURSELF', was developed and implemented (Duxbury et al., 2019). This version also includes six main strategies: Setting team goals for the reduction of restraint, reflecting upon the use of restraint and personal communication styles, using approaches to help patients and staff ascertain needs and challenges with regard to aggression on the ward, employing partnership working strategies to reduce restraint such as 'advance directives' (my safety plan), and positive communication, exploring environmental challenges to make appropriate changes, and debriefing following incidents or near misses of restraint. These six are further divided into smaller interventions (Table 1). It is mentioned that 'REsTRAIN YOURSELF' notices the impact of trauma for both staff and service users, and by clinical supervision seeks solutions to reduce it (Duxbury et al., 2019).

Another multicomponent model based on TIC is the engagement model (Blair & Moulton-Adelman, 2015; Borckardt et al., 2011; Hardesty et al., 2007), with its origins in the Sanctuary approach (Bloom, 1997; Sanctuary Institute, 2022). The model aims to provide a safe and healing environment founded on trauma-informed care. It has two main components, key clinical interventions and leadership approach, which are divided into smaller interventions (Table 1). In the engagement model, trauma history is screened during admission, to better understand individual

**Table 1** Components of different TIC-based interventions

| Six Core Strategies[a] | REsTRAIN YOURSELF[a] | Engagement model |
|---|---|---|
| Use of restraint and seclusion reduction tools | My safety plan sensory/comfort/low-stimulus rooms | *Key clinical interventions* admission process Minimising the power differential: a culture shift physical environment |
|  | Visible nurse |  |
| Consumer roles in inpatient settings | Community meetings advocacy and peer support |  |
| Debriefing techniques | Debriefing tool | *Leadership approaches* |
| Leadership towards organisational change | Identified and agreed on targets and philosophy | Shared decision-making: Empowering staff to own their practice staff education and quality review rewards and recognition |
|  | Use of ward champions |  |
|  | Executive walk rounds |  |
| Use of data to inform practice | Visual display data including safety crosses and mood boards |  |
| Workforce development | Trauma- and prevention-orientated training |  |

[a]*REsTRAIN Yourself* has its origins in Six Core Strategies and their similar components are in the same row

triggers and to provide helpful strategies to cope. A trauma-informed approach is present also, for example, in staff education (Blair & Moulton-Adelman, 2015).

The components of these TIC-based interventions are described in Table 1. While these interventions share similar components, albeit with various names, they are also unique in what they comprise. For example, the Six Core Strategies include a component called 'Use of Restraint and Seclusion Reduction Tools'. In 'REsTRAIN Yourself', this component has been divided into three smaller interventions: My Safety Plan, Sensory/Comfort/low stimulus rooms and Visible Nurse (Duxbury et al., 2019). They all include clinical interventions to reduce the use of coercive measures, leadership activities and organisational-level changes.

The TIC approach has also been used together with other interventions to reduce coercive measures. These interventions have included brief solution-focused therapy (Aremu et al., 2018) and different intervention packages. For example, Blair et al. (2017) combined TIC-based training for staff with the use of the Brøset Violence Checklist (BVC), crisis intervention course, changes in hospital policy and procedures, and environmental enhancements. Aremu et al. (2018) focused on increasing staff's engagement with service users, and Blair et al. (2017) on staff behaviour (Risking Connections® training).

## 3.1 Outcomes of Trauma-Informed Care (TIC) Approaches and Interventions Related to Coercive Measures

Multiple intervention studies have been conducted worldwide on TIC approaches and the reduction of coercive measures. TIC interventions have had a positive impact on the reduction of coercion.

The use of the TIC approach to reduce the use of coercive measures has been studied in the USA (e.g. Aremu et al., 2018; Blair & Moulton-Adelman, 2015; Borckardt et al., 2011), Australia (Maguire et al., 2012) and Europe (Finland, Putkonen et al., 2013; Spain, Guzman-Parra et al., 2016; UK, Duxbury et al., 2019). The Six Core Strategies, a trauma-informed intervention, have spread in clinical practice in many countries, including Canada, Australia, New Zealand, Germany, Turkey, Sweden, Finland, the United Kingdom and the Czech Republic (LeBel et al., 2014).

Studies evaluating the impact of TIC approaches have reported results related to the use of physical restraint (Duxbury et al., 2019), mechanical restraint (Guzman-Parra et al., 2016; Guzmán-Parra et al., 2022; Putkonen et al., 2013), seclusion rooms (Putkonen et al., 2013), involuntary medication (Aremu et al., 2018) and observation (Putkonen et al., 2013). Other outcomes measured have included physical violence towards others or self (Putkonen et al., 2013), injuries of staff and patients (Putkonen et al., 2013), attitudes towards patient aggression and engagement with patients (Aremu et al., 2018).

Results related to the reduction of mechanical restraint events by implementing TIC have been mixed. In the USA, when using Six Core Strategies, the length, events and percentage of patients experiencing mechanical restraint declined

(Conley, 2004). In Spain, in a small-scale study conducted in one unit using four of the Six Core Strategies, a significant reduction was seen in mechanical restraint events (Guzman-Parra et al., 2016), while on a larger scale, with 20 units, implementation did not have an impact; however, the length of the events decreased (Guzmán-Parra et al., 2022). In Finland, the length of mechanical restraint events decreased significantly after implementing the Six Core Strategies (Putkonen et al., 2013).

For seclusion and observation events, the effect of Six Core Strategies in Finland in units with men with schizophrenia was a significant decrease in the length of mechanical restraint (Putkonen et al., 2013). In Australia, a project following Six Core Strategies resulted in a significant decrease in seclusion events and hours (Maguire et al., 2012). A quality improvement project conducted in the USA found a decrease in the use of involuntary medication after implementing the TIC approach together with brief solution-focused therapy (Aremu et al., 2018).

A declining trend in the use of seclusion and restraint after the introduction of TIC approaches has been established in both adult (Borckardt et al., 2011) and children and adolescent psychiatric care settings (Azeem et al., 2011). Beyond the impact on the level of coercive measures, evidence suggests that implementing TIC approaches, for example, the Six Core Strategies did not affect physical violence (Putkonen et al., 2013), nor attitudes towards patient aggression or engagement with patients from the staff perspectives (Aremu et al., 2018).

Existing evidence about impact points to the fact that, as with other types of complex interventions aiming to reduce the use of coercive measures, implementation and achieving sustainability can be an issue (Wieman et al., 2014). Currently, there is a lack of studies showing the long-term impact or effectiveness of TIC-based interventions. However, there are some results showing reduction of the use of coercive measures could be sustained over time, possibly benefiting from the use of a structured implementation model, such as the Iowa Model for Evidence-Based Practice–Revised (Hale & Wendler, 2023). Such a model could give a structure for translating research evidence to clinical practice in a way that an intervention would be permanently integrated into care. In addition, current research on the TIC approach in reducing the use of coercive measures does not give clear answers on whether this approach works for all genders equally or for people with different ethnic backgrounds. One of the few randomised-controlled trials in this area, for example, conducted within forensic mental health wards for men, indicated an over-representation of white Finnish Caucasians (Putkonen et al., 2013), limiting the generalisability with regard to other genders, nations and ethnicities. As the TIC approach has been, in general, tested in organisational and ward contexts without individual randomisation (e.g. Duxbury et al., 2019; Maguire et al., 2012), there is a lack of information about whom this intervention might work best.

In studies aiming to reduce the use of coercive measures, the main outcomes have self-evidently focused on seclusion, restraint and involuntary medication. So far, there is a lack of knowledge about patient experience, namely if the intervention has an impact at an individual level on post-traumatic symptoms, retraumatisation or psychological symptoms. We propose that future research should focus on the perspective of people with lived experiences, patients and family members. To help us contextualise and better understand trauma histories/journeys, the next section incorporates the accounts, views and reflections of one of the authors with lived experience of psychosis.

## 4    Emerging from the Depths of Trauma: A Lived Experience Account

### 4.1    The Circle of Trauma: Between a Rock and a Hard Place

I was travelling in Thailand on my own and feeling free with independence. I'd stopped taking my psychiatric medication as no one was monitoring me on it anymore. I had trouble sleeping, I wasn't eating or drinking properly and I began to feel unsafe travelling on my own. This was the perfect storm that meant I became consumed by my psychosis. I was uncovering the mysteries of the universe laying in a hammock on the beach, realising the moon in the night sky was responsible for the formation of waves I saw lapping the sea. Everything was mesmerising until my thoughts became terrifying and instead of seeing a beautiful reality, my world was consumed by terror and delusion. Slowly over time, I thought people were trying to poison me, there were conspiracies going on through the news I saw on TV, and I thought I was the only one who knew the truth.

I was swimming and the sea was so grand and overwhelming. I was hurt and felt stuck between the crashing waves pushing me against the rocks. My experiences of delusion led me to feel unsafe, feel out of control and think that bad things were happening to me. These were manifestations of a previous trauma I suffered in my childhood where I experienced bullying. This circle of trauma was repeating itself and what I was experiencing in Thailand was me reliving that trauma in a different way. Maybe it was bubbling to the surface as I had not dealt with my childhood trauma. I couldn't recognise that these experiences were replications of my past and so I became consumed by my psychosis.

I had overstayed my visa and needed to return home to the UK, but I had to navigate Thai Airways. I thought the people in the airport were sending dangerous people to different countries via their different airlines. It was my duty to alert people of this risk to the world. I found it difficult to get home, I was taken off an aeroplane as I was considered a risk and driven in the back of a car outside the airport with a bag over my head. On reflection, I don't understand the need for this; the only sense I can make now is they did this to calm me down. I needed a medical check that was communicated to me by the British Embassy. Eventually, I returned home after a long flight during which I remained hypervigilant and terrified throughout the whole journey. I thought that as soon as we landed, I would be killed. As the plane landed, nothing happened, and I didn't need to stay longer on the plane or be handcuffed by anyone. At the airport gate, I fell into my mother's arms and cried and cried.

We eventually reached home, but my psychosis followed me. Over the next few days, I thought my mother and family were imposters taken over by Thai people who were out to get me and poison me. I couldn't eat or drink anything or leave home as I thought everyone wanted to harm me. My family realised I was unwell and called the GP. Two GPs came and went, and then some others arrived to assess me, but I didn't trust them. They said they were social workers that were there to help. But were they going to harm me? Why was my mum listening to everything they said? Did she not believe me that they were sent here by someone to kill me? Or were they the ones that were going to help me alert the world to danger? They told my mum to pack a bag for me. My mum told me to go with them. I did what my mum said, even though I believed they were going to kill me, but I walked to my death.

I got to the hospital and was there for 4 weeks. I was detained under the Mental Health Act[2] against my will. The Mental Health Act (1983) in the UK is where a patient is identified as suffering from a mental health disorder and can be detained against their will by mental health professionals if the patient is considered to be a risk to themselves and/or others. This detention is for the purpose of assessment and/or treatment. Multiple independent mental health professionals must be in agreement about the decision to detain. This meant I had to be there, I didn't have a choice, and again I felt as though I was not in control or safe. The first week I refused all treatment as I didn't trust their intentions, and I became angry as I felt unsafe and didn't know why I was there; they were delaying my mission. I became angry and the rapid response team started running towards me, there were a dozen or so of them, against only me. I was forcibly restrained and injected with an intra-muscular injection. I went into a deep sleep. Over the next few days, I slowly returned to reality, and I didn't feel as scared, and the delusions were slowly dissi-pating. Despite the benefits of this forced treatment, at the time I still experienced terror, violence and coercion.

My family were also traumatised by my experiences. They didn't know what was happening in Thailand, just through snapshots of phone calls with them at different times and stages in my trauma. They had no control over my situation while I was abroad. Then my mum was having to navigate visiting me in hospital whilst looking after my younger sister and my dad who was ill with cancer at the time. My family and I went through a shared trauma, but I was the only one who got help with this at the time. It felt like everything around me was consumed in trauma, I was between a rock and a hard place. I needed support and cushioning from the constant blows happening both in reality and what I thought was reality.

## 4.2    Recycling Trauma

There is much talk on trauma-informed care, but how can forcible treatment ever be considered trauma-informed? For it to be trauma-informed, it requires learning from accounts and experiences of trauma that may run the risk of retraumatising

---

[2] Add brief info about the MHA for non-UK readers.

individuals through reliving that experience and asking them to reflect on it. There are ways to make the process much less harmful, through drawing on effective communication strategies, understanding the history and triggers of the patient, ensuring they have as much choice and control over the situation, and kind and compassionate care. This all seems incompatible with forced treatment and detention under the Mental Health Act. Although, in order to prevent those who have experienced trauma from additionally experiencing iatrogenic harm at the hands of service providers, listening and learning from patient experience are essential. Although reflections of those with lived experiences of trauma are beneficial and can better inform clinical practice. It may however run the risk of retraumatising patients. Therefore, there is an opportunity to inform clinical practice by those who work as experts by experience, who are more likely to be in recovery and be more distanced from their traumatic experiences. Often contexts in which the medical model is re-enacted can be triggering for those who have experienced coercion or trauma. This might also occur for those who work in expert-by-experience roles. For example, displays of power imbalances, and lack of choice and control in everyday life, may be especially triggering for those who have experienced trauma. It is essential to find ways to process trauma and make sense of our experiences, but it is not to justify or make sense of why others were violent towards us as we may never understand this and it feels wrong to justify or humanise any kind of violence.

## 4.3    Trauma-Informed Care: The Calm After the Storm and the Warmth of the Sun

Following my 4 weeks under detention of the Mental Health Act, I was discharged to the early intervention in psychosis team (EIP). This team lay in contrast to the risk and medically informed approach of inpatient treatment. The EIP team felt like it was enveloping me in safety and support across all areas of my life. I was emotionally validated, and I had continuous consistent compassionate support for 3 years. My needs were met across those years in a number of areas such as psychological, psychiatric, social, employment, family and physical health support. I was able to understand my experiences, the trauma I went through and how to manage my health needs going forward. The support was also extended to my family, so they could understand my experiences. The treatment felt like the calm after the storm, I was at peace, and I could feel the warmth of the sun, trust my experiences and understand my reality as it was. I was able to understand my experiences through the narrative I constructed. I started writing a blog called 'The Teal Tiger' (Gupta, 2022), which embodied my experiences of psychosis, in which I share my experiences, with creative license, which gives me control over the meanings I want those experiences to have. The trauma remains in that body of work, and so I can leave it there, and be free of it in my own world.

## 4.4 Post-Traumatic Growth and Emerging Identity: Weathering the Storm

To help me understand my own experiences and learn ways to move forward, I completed a BSc in Psychology, a PGDip in Mental Health Nursing and an MSc in Psychological Research Methods. I have now currently completed my PhD in psychology and am working as a Research Associate on the EXTEND EIP study to understand how to personalise the duration of EIP care for people with psychosis. It feels as though I have moved forward from my own lived experiences to conduct research that can support others with similar experiences. I have been able to make sense of my experiences through psychological and conceptual models of mental health and disability that I identify with and I have created my own ways to understand my experiences.

Having worked as an expert by experience, where I use my experiences to help inform the training of clinical psychologists, I became interested in understanding how my identity was affected by my experiences of working in roles that related to my lived experiences. I developed the EMERGES framework (Gupta et al., 2023) through a systematic narrative review. The framework has helped me understand the trajectory of my own experiences and it is a framework that embodies my lived experience. It explains the identity of lived experience researchers and providers, which identifies influencing factors through the acronym of EMERGES: of Empowerment, Motivation to integrate our lived experiences, Empathy of the self and others that occurs through sharing and constructing narratives that we understand our own experiences through learning through the experiences of others, Recovery model and medical model, Growth and Transformation, discussing experiences of Exclusion and our historical experiences of Survivor roots. This conceptual model helps me understand my experiences of trauma and who I am now, having moved through the stages of the framework.

For example, having been a survivor, this is the root of all my experiences and the foundation on which my interests and professional experience are based. Through exclusion from social networks and society due to the stigma of my diagnosis, I have been supported to get through these experiences with support from Early Intervention in Psychosis care. Through engaging in expert-by-experience work, I have been able to grow and transform into someone who is much more than someone who has been a service user, and I have much more to offer, and my experiences can be learned from, supporting service providers and services to also grow. The different models in psychology such as the recovery model, medical model and the EMERGES framework help me to understand my own experiences and the power imbalances in my trauma, and experiences of healthcare. It also makes me realise the complexity of recovery, which does not just limit someone to being symptom-free but being able to live alongside difficulties and traumatic experiences, that are so prominent. It seems unfair and invalidates the severity of the trauma experienced if we are expected to overcome these experiences completely. I have gained empathy and a shared understanding of others with similar experiences. This extends to survivors of different types of traumas, but the violence and boundaries crossed in personal relationships and experiences with the mental health system are something each of us can understand, relate to and which connect us as survivors. These experiences motivate me to want to integrate my own lived experiences into the work I do and ensure that the training of healthcare professionals is informed by lived experience and trauma-informed approaches. These experiences of survivorship inform the perspectives I bring to my expert-by-experience role and the things I advocate for to make services safer spaces for people with mental health experiences. Although, those in expert-by-experience roles also require support due to their increased risk of being triggered when drawing on and reliving their lived experiences.

My professional experiences in mental health have been empowering, and I feel I have come a long way from what I consider my survivor roots and the raw and emotional experiences I have gone through. I have weathered the storm and emerged whole. I previously lost myself in my psychosis and experiences of trauma, but through trauma-informed care, and seeking to understand my experiences through more compassionate psychological models and trauma-informed models, I have built myself up through a better understanding of my own experiences, building resilience and fostering aspects of myself such as my professional skills that move me further away from my survivor roots.

It is difficult to not be self-defined by trauma, but it is empowering knowing I have emerged on the other side and can help inform trauma-informed services from a more distanced position as a professional with expertise in the area. This perspective from which I approach trauma-informed work helps me maintain a distance from the raw and emotional burden of these experiences that I might experience writing this from a survivor's point of view. Instead, the expert-by-experience role helps me articulate these experiences from a distance and in ways that can be tolerated by myself and others. I encourage other survivors to understand their own traumas in ways they find helpful to process what has happened to them.

That trauma I experienced is submerged, and whilst there may be triggers that raise it to the surface, I know I can remain afloat. I have emerged from the depths of trauma despite aspects of myself that have eroded away but with the remnants of the strongest, and most resilient aspects of myself that have weathered the storms, as my basic needs of warmth and compassionate care have been met.

## 5    What Next?

This chapter has brought together evidence, reflection and lived experience to raise awareness about the importance and impact of trauma and retraumatisation for people accessing mental health services internationally, the range and effectiveness of trauma-informed interventions used to reduce coercive measures, and key shortfalls within both research and practice in this area.

The evidence suggests that traumatic and harmful experiences within mental health settings are wide-ranging and warrant greater attention. Whether coercion is deemed to be hard or soft, formal or informal, it is a complex phenomenon with harmful repercussions and outcomes. It has been described as a necessary evil by some (Wilson et al., 2017) and without doubt remains challenging for nurses who struggle between a wish to do good and a desire to stay within the norms of existing nontherapeutic cultures of 'care'. According to Iversen et al. (2011), maintaining the therapeutic alliance and being mindful of the objectives of person-centredness, safety and comfort during, prior to and following incidents including the use of restrictive practices can positively influence perceptions of the experience of coercion (Larue et al., 2013). Nonetheless, Hodas (2006) states that trauma-informed organisations, programmes and services are those that are cognisant that their services can retraumatise those with significant trauma histories through the indiscriminate application of any coercive practice. A trauma-informed approach to inpatient care provides an alternate lens by understanding the negative effects of trauma history on patients so that staff can develop a milieu that anticipates and responds to those who feel distressed and out of control. To develop a culture of safety, staff perceptions, approaches and policies need to change in a myriad of ways.

Firstly, the importance of collaboration between staff and patients needs to be recognised and the issue of trauma placed at centre stage and at the heart of all aspects of policy, procedures and workforce development (Douglas et al., 2022). To influence the clinical practice that governs the use of coercion and to address resulting trauma, it is essential to explore and listen to patients' experiences, and concerns of, and about the use of coercive practices. The call for meaningful involvement of people with lived experience, patients and family members/carers resonates in all sections of this chapter. Veenu's story takes us to experiences of a multiplicity of traumas and retraumatisation but highlights that, when services are trauma-informed, compassionate and person-centred, they can aid recovery. It also alludes to the idea that survivors need to understand their traumas in their own ways, in contrast to forced formulations from service providers, to enable them to make sense of their own experiences of trauma and survivorship in ways they personally identify with, consequently giving them more control over their experiences. Much anecdotal evidence on service user involvement identifies that experts-by-experience have emphasised the importance of introducing trauma-informed models of care in service provision, but that service providers are slow to implement changes in service provision. Veenu's account identifies how learning from lived experiences can help inform trauma-informed services and justifies and provides a rationale to introduce trauma-informed services as a matter of urgency. It also identifies that learning from lived experience may be a process that is retraumatising, and so the emphasis is placed on learning from service users who work in expert-by-experience roles, where they may be more distanced from their survivorship. This can support services to become trauma-informed, without inflicting more harm on survivors to re-live their experiences. Although, increasing support for those in these roles is important through, for example, supervision, reflective or trauma-informed practices that may be important for them in their roles.

Secondly, there is a need to foster and implement data-informed practice, exploring the extent and nature of disproportionality with regard to trauma to better understand the intersectionality between socio-cultural historically embedded traumas such as racism, poverty, colonialism, disability, sexism and gender-based abuse (Sweeney et al., 2018). We stress the importance of hearing from minorities who are trauma survivors yet who are under-represented in coercive practice-related data. While future research should aim to un-silence these communities to address significant gaps, using innovative inclusive methodologies and approaches, services should strive to address disproportionality through a wide range of strategies beyond data-informed practice, including the involvement of people with lived experience in staff training.

Evidence presented in this chapter suggests that, while a number of trauma-informed interventions have been found to be effective in different mental health settings, leading to substantial reductions in the use of coercive measures, more research is still warranted to understand if these interventions work in different populations (taking into account gender, ethnicity, sexuality, religion, etc.,) and whether they create positive and sustainable change, beyond the reduction of coercion, to individual outcomes, such as post-traumatic symptoms. In some studies, there has not been any significant effect on the use of coercion by TIC-based interventions. These contradictory findings suggest that there is room to explore for whom and in which circumstances these interventions actually work.

The literature exploring trauma in relation to coercion is not comprehensive and to a certain extent dated. More importantly, it lacks diversity, especially with regard to ethnicity and other key protected characteristics. This is probably due to the legacy of longstanding 'whiteness' in academia (and implicitly the people who undertake the research in this field) and in psychiatry in general. These implicit biases and gaps in evidence need to be addressed to adequately explore the relationship between trauma and coercion in mental health settings and the response to this, especially given the drive to use evidence-based practice.

Thirdly, we argue that there are limitations and gaps in knowledge regarding the implementation of trauma-informed interventions in mental health settings and the sustainability of their impact in the long term. When aiming to transform research findings into practice, a more detailed description of intervention fidelity, feasibility, sustainability and the implementation process is warranted. As previous research has been conducted in high-income countries, it would be invaluable to also understand the costs of implementation. Low- and middle-income countries may not have, for example, the same resources as high-income countries in their mental facilities to support clinical leadership to implement and sustain complex TIC-based interventions. Knowing the costs of implementation could help these countries to plan if the implementation is feasible or not.

The final argument, however, reiterates the principle of 'universal precautions,' whereby all inpatients are treated as if they have been traumatised (Walsh & Benjamin, 2020). This would mean that trauma does not necessarily need to be diagnosed, as the principles of collaboration, engagement, compassion, etc., are implemented for all individuals, given the distress during the admission process, in addition to their own suffering from mental health problems (Sweeney et al., 2018). While trauma-informed care is highly pertinent to mental health inpatient settings where there are high levels of trauma amongst patients, its principles are relevant to all inpatients, regardless of their experience of trauma, providing a theoretical framework for understanding and implementing many approaches to care. For mental health nurses, for example, it is not necessarily about identifying or treating complex trauma, but acknowledging and being mindful of its presence, neurobiological and psychological effects on people, and the relevance of past trauma on current presentation and interactions, including the potential for retraumatisation (Isobel & Edwards, 2017). While it might not be possible to eradicate all coercive practices (and implicit traumatisation), given the paradox of custodial care, there is a need for all services to use a model of care that is transparent and that places the patient at the centre of care, enabling individual care plans, choice and flexibility (Muskett, 2014). This might be a useful approach going forward, where all people accessing inpatient mental health services are treated as if they have already been traumatised (Walsh & Benjamin, 2020), thus diminishing the importance of diagnosing trauma in the first place.

These arguments are closely linked to those for and against using solely the DSM-5 or ICD-11 frameworks to define and recognise or diagnose trauma (Sweeney et al., 2018); especially the arguments against the over-medicalisation of human experience (Frances, 2013) and the conceptualisation of responses to trauma as symptoms specific disorders rather than natural human reactions to extreme adversity (McHugh & Treisman, 2007). Alternative conceptualisations of trauma acknowledging the role of social traumas overlooked by DSM-5 or ICD-11 might be better placed, given that a higher likelihood of trauma experience is linked to social inequalities such as poverty and racial discrimination—especially for Black people. These include the psycho-social narrative-based 'Power Threat Meaning Framework' alternative to the psychiatric diagnostic approach (Johnstone et al., 2018) and SAMHSA's (2014) conceptualisation of trauma response, acknowledging the life-threatening trauma event, as well as the way one experiences that event (i.e. intra- and interpersonal context) and its effects (SAMHSA, 2014).

Research exploring in-depth trauma survivors' cases and experiences advocates for these alternative approaches (Sweeney et al., 2018). They argue that trauma-informed care should not need validation or diagnosis, but the principle of same engagement for all at its core; a process of organisational change that creates recovery and compassionate-based environments for all, acknowledging that experiences of trauma go beyond the patient, and are common to staff, family members, friends and others (Sweeney et al., 2018, p. 321). Trauma-informed care should not be an afterthought, an add-on to existing mental health services, services should be developed following a trauma-informed approach from the start.

## References

Allison, R., & Flemming, K. (2019). Mental health patients' experiences of softer coercion and its effects on their interactions with practitioners: A qualitative evidence synthesis. *Journal of Advanced Nursing, 75*(11), 2274–2284.

Alvarez, M. J., Roura, P., Osés, A., Foguet, Q., Solà, J., & Arrufat, F. X. (2011). Prevalence and clinical impact of childhood trauma in patients with severe mental disorders. *The Journal of Nervous and Mental Disease, 199*(3), 156–161. https://doi.org/10.1097/NMD.0b013e31820c751c

Anderson, F., Howard, L., Dean, K., Moran, P., & Khalifeh, H. (2016). Childhood maltreatment and adulthood domestic and sexual violence victimisation among people with severe mental illness. *Social Psychiatry and Psychiatric Epidemiology, 51*(7), 961–970. https://doi.org/10.1007/s00127-016-1244-1

Anderson, U., Fathollahi, J., & Gustin, L. W. (2020). Nurses' experiences of informal coercion on adult psychiatric wards. *Nursing Ethics, 27*(3), 741–753.

Aremu, B., Hill, P. D., McNeal, J. M., Petersen, M. A., Swanberg, D., & Delaney, K. R. (2018). Implementation of trauma-informed care and brief solution-focused therapy: A quality improvement project aimed at increasing engagement on an inpatient psychiatric unit. *Journal of Psychosocial Nursing and Mental Health Services, 56*(8), 16–22. https://doi.org/10.3928/02793695-20180305-02

Azeem, M. W., Aujla, A., Rammerth, M., Binsfeld, G., & Jones, R. B. (2011). Effectiveness of Six Core Strategies based on trauma informed care in reducing seclusions and restraints at a child and adolescent psychiatric hospital. *Journal of Child and Adolescent Psychiatric Nursing, 24*(1), 11–15. https://doi.org/10.1111/j.1744-6171.2010.00262.x

Barnett, P., Mackay, E., Matthews, H., Gate, R., Greenwood, H., Ariyo, K., et al. (2019). Ethnic variations in compulsory detention under the Mental Health Act: A systematic review and meta-analysis of international data. *The Lancet Psychiatry, 6*(4), 305–317. https://doi.org/10.1016/S2215-0366(19)30027-6

Beckett, P., Holmes, D., Phipps, M., Patton, D., & Molloy, L. (2017). Trauma-informed care and practice: Practice improvement strategies in an inpatient mental health ward. *Journal of Psychosocial Nursing and Mental Health Services, 55*(10), 34–38. https://doi.org/10.3928/02793695-20170818-03

Bigwood, S., & Crowe, M. (2008). 'It's part of the job, but it spoils the job': a phenomenological study of physical restraint. *International Journal of Mental Health Nursing, 17*(3), 215–222.

Blair, M., & Moulton-Adelman, F. (2015). The Engagement Model for reducing seclusion and restraint: 13 years later. *Journal of Psychosocial Nursing and Mental Health Services, 53*(3), 39–45. https://doi.org/10.3928/02793695-20150211-01

Blair, E. W., Woolley, S., Szarek, B. L., Mucha, T. F., Dutka, O., Schwartz, H. I., Wisniowski, J., & Goethe, J. W. (2017). Reduction of seclusion and restraint in an inpatient psychiatric setting: A pilot study. *The Psychiatric Quarterly, 88*(1), 1–7. https://doi.org/10.1007/s11126-016-9428-0

Bloom, S. L. (1997). *Creating sanctuary: Toward the evolution of sane societies.* Routledge.

Bonner, G., Lowe, T., Rawcliffe, D., & Wellman, N. (2002). Trauma for all: A pilot study of the subjective experience of physical restraint for mental health inpatients and staff in the UK. *Journal of Psychiatric and Mental Health Nursing, 9*(4), 465–473. https://doi.org/10.1046/j.1365-2850.2002.00504.x

Borckardt, J. J., Grubaugh, A. L., Pelic, C. G., et al. (2007). Enhancing patient safety in psychiatric settings. *Journal of Psychiatric Practice, 13*, 355–361.

Borckardt, J. J., Madan, A., Grubaugh, A. L., Danielson, C. K., Pelic, C. G., Hardesty, S. J., Hanson, R., Herbert, J., Cooney, H., Benson, A., & Frueh, B. C. (2011). Systematic investigation of initiatives to reduce seclusion and restraint in a state psychiatric hospital. *Psychiatric Services (Washington, D.C.), 62*(5), 477–483. https://doi.org/10.1176/ps.62.5.pss6205_0477

Borge, L., & Fagermoen, M. S. (2008). Patients' core experiences of hospital treatment: Wholeness and self-worth in time and space. *Journal of Mental Health, 17*(2), 193–205. https://doi.org/10.1080/09638230701505996

Clark, C., Young, M., Jackson, E., et al. (2008). Consumer perceptions of integrated trauma-informed services among women with co-occurring disorders. *Journal of Behavioral Health Services & Research, 35*(1), 71–90.

Cleary, M. (2003). The challenges of mental health care reform for contemporary mental health nursing practice: Relationships, power and control. *International Journal of Mental Health Nursing, 12*(2), 139–147.

Conley, J. (2004). The NTAC training curriculum for the reduction of seclusion and restraint. *Evaluation Fast Facts from the Evaluation Center at HSRI, 3*(1), 1–4.

Craig, J. H., & Sanders, K. L. (2018). Evaluation of a program model for minimizing restraint and seclusion. *Advances in Neurodevelopmental Disorders, 2*, 344–352. https://doi.org/10.1007/s41252-018-0076-2

Deveau, R., & McDonnell, A. (2009). As the last resort: Reducing the use of restrictive physical interventions using organisational approaches. *British Journal of Learning Disabilities, 37*(3), 172–177.

Donat, D. C. (2002). Impact of improved staffing on seclusion/restraint reliance in a public psychiatric hospital. *Psychiatric Rehabilitation Journal, 25*, 413–416.

Douglas, L., Donohue, G., & Morrissey. (2022). Patient experience of physical restraint in the acute setting: A systematic review of the qualitative research evidence. *Issues in Mental Health Nursing, 43*(5), 473–481. https://doi.org/10.1080/01612840.2021.1978597

Duxbury, J. (2002). An evaluation of staff and patient views of and strategies employed to manage inpatient aggression and violence on one mental health unit: A pluralistic design. *Journal of Psychiatric and Mental Health Nursing, 9*(3), 325–337. https://doi.org/10.1046/j.1365-2850.2002.00497.x

Duxbury, J., Aiken, F., & Dale, C. (2011). Deaths in custody: The role of restraint. *Journal of Learning Disabilities and Offending Behaviour, 2*(4), 178–190.

Duxbury, J., Baker, J., Downe, S., Jones, F., Greenwood, P., Thygesen, H., McKeown, M., Price, O., Scholes, A., Thomson, G., & Whittington, R. (2019). Minimising the use of physical restraint in acute mental health services: The outcome of a restraint reduction programme ('REsTRAIN YOURSELF'). *International Journal of Nursing Studies, 95*, 40–48. https://doi.org/10.1016/j.ijnurstu.2019.03.016

Elliott, D. E., Bjelajac, P., Fallot, R. D., Markoff, L. S., & Reed, B. (2005). Trauma-informed or trauma denied: Principles and implementation of trauma-informed services for women. *Journal of Community Psychology, 33*(4), 461–477. https://doi.org/10.1002/jcop.20063

Frances, A. (2013). Saving normal: An insider's revolt against out-of-control psychiatric diagnosis, DSM-5, big pharma and the medicalization of ordinary life. *Psychotherapy in Australia, 19*(3), 14–18.

Frueh, B. C., Knapp, R. G., Cusack, K. J., Grubaugh, A. L., Sauvageot, J. A., Cousins, V. C., & Hiers, T. G. (2005). Patients' reports of traumatic or harmful experiences within the psychiatric setting. *Psychiatric Services, 56*(9), 1123–1133. https://doi.org/10.1176/appi.ps.56.9.1123

Gilburt, H., Slade, M., Rose, D., Lloyd-Evans, B., Johnson, S., & Osborn, D. (2010). Service users' experiences of residential alternatives to standard acute wards: Qualitative study of similarities and differences. *The British Journal of Psychiatry, 197*(Suppl. 53), s26–s31.

Gupta, V. (2022). *The Teal Tiger*. WordPress blog. https://tealtigerblog.wordpress.com

Gupta, V., Eames, C., Golding, L., et al. (2023). Understanding the identity of lived experience researchers and providers: A conceptual framework and systematic narrative review. *Research Involvement and Engagement, 9*, 26. https://doi.org/10.1186/s40900-023-00439-0

Guzman-Parra, J., Aguilera Serrano, C., García-Sánchez, J. A., Pino-Benítez, I., Alba-Vallejo, M., Moreno-Küstner, B., & Mayoral-Cleries, F. (2016). Effectiveness of a multimodal intervention program for restraint prevention in an acute Spanish Psychiatric ward. *Journal of the American Psychiatric Nurses Association, 22*(3), 233–241. https://doi.org/10.1177/1078390316644767

Guzmán-Parra, J., Aguilera-Serrano, C., Huizing, E., Bono Del Trigo, A., Villagrán, J. M., Hurtado Melero, V., García-Sanchez, J. A., & Mayoral-Cleries, F. (2022). Factors associated with prolonged episodes of mechanical restraint in mental health hospitalization units in Andalusia. *Journal of Psychiatric and Mental Health Nursing, 29*(6), 873–882. https://doi.org/10.1111/jpm.12824

Hale, R., & Wendler, M. C. (2023). Evidence-based practice: Implementing trauma-informed care of children and adolescents in the inpatient psychiatric setting. *Journal of the American Psychiatric Nurses Association, 29*(2), 161–170. https://doi.org/10.1177/1078390320980045

Hardesty, S., Borckardt, J. J., Hanson, R., Grubaugh, A. L., Danielson, C. K., Madan, A., Weinstein, B. L., Hogarth, C. R., Pelic, C., Hazy, J., & Shoemaker, M. L. (2007). Evaluating initiatives to reduce seclusion and restraint. *Journal for Healthcare Quality, 29*(4), 46–55. https://doi.org/10.1111/j.1945-1474.2007.tb00205.x

Haw, C., Stubbs, J., Bickle, A., & Stewart, I. (2011). Coercive treatments in forensic psychiatry: A study of patients' experiences and preferences. *Journal of Forensic Psychiatry & Psychology, 22*(4), 564–585.

Hodas, G. (2006). *Responding to childhood trauma: The promise and practice of trauma informed care*. http://www.dpw.state.pa.us/ucmprd/groups/public/documents/manual/s_001585.pdf

Holmes, D., Kennedy, S. L., & Perron, A. (2004). The mentally ill and social exclusion: A critical examination of the use of seclusion from the patient' perspective. *Issues in Mental Health Nursing, 25*, 559–578.

Huckshorn, K. A. (2004). Reducing seclusion restraint in mental health use settings: Core strategies for prevention. *Journal of Psychosocial Nursing and Mental Health Services, 42*(9), 22–33. https://doi.org/10.3928/02793695-20040901-05

Huckshorn, K. A. (2006). Redesigning state mental health policy to prevent the use of seclusion and restraint. *Administration and Policy in Mental Health, 3*, 482–491.

Huckshorn, K. A. (2008). *Six Core Strategies for reducing seclusion and restraint use*. https://www.nasmhpd.org/sites/default/files/2022-08/Consolidated%2520Six%2520Core%2520Strategies%2520Document.pdf

Hughes, R., Hayward, M., & Finlay, W. M. L. (2009). Patients' perceptions of the impact of involuntary inpatient care on self, relationships and recovery. *Journal of Mental Health, 18*(2), 152–160. https://doi.org/10.1080/09638230802053326

Isobel, S., & Edwards, C. (2017). Using trauma informed care as a nursing model of care in an acute inpatient mental health unit: A practice development process. *International Journal of Mental Health Nursing, 26*(1), 88–94. https://doi.org/10.1111/inm.12236

Iversen, V. C., Sallaup, T., Vaaler, A. E., Helvik, A. S., Morken, G., & Linaker, O. (2011). Patients' perceptions of their stay in a psychiatric seclusion area. *Journal of Psychiatric Intensive Care, 7*(1), 1–10.

Johnstone, L., Boyle, M., Cromby, J., et al. (2018). *The power threat meaning framework: Towards the identification of patterns in emotional distress, unusual experiences and troubled or troubling behaviour, as an alternative to functional psychiatric diagnosis*. British Psychological Society.

Kersting, X. A. K., Hirsch, S., & Steinert, T. (2019). Physical harm and death in the context of coercive measures in psychiatric patients: A systematic review. *Frontiers in Psychiatry, 10*, 400. https://doi.org/10.3389/fpsyt.2019.00400

Keski-Valkama, A., Koivisto, A. M., Eronen, M., & Kaltiala-Heino, R. (2010). Forensic and general psychiatric patients' view of seclusion: A comparison study. *The Journal of Forensic Psychiatry and Psychology, 21*(3), 446–461.

Kessler, R. C., McLaughlin, K. A., Green, J. G., Gruber, M. J., Sampson, N. A., Zaslavsky, A. M., et al. (2010). Childhood adversities and adult psychopathology in the WHO World Mental Health Surveys. *The British Journal of Psychiatry, 197*(5), 378–385. https://doi.org/10.1192/bjp.bp.110.080499

Kessler, R. C., Aguilar-Gaxiola, S., Alonso, J., Benjet, C., Bromet, E. J., Cardoso, G., et al. (2017). Trauma and PTSD in the WHO world mental health surveys. *European Journal of Psychotraumatology, 8*(Suppl. 5), 1353383. https://doi.org/10.1080/20008198.2017.1353383

Knowles, S. F., Hearne, J., & Smith, I. (2015). Physical restraint and the therapeutic relationship. *The Journal of Forensic Psychiatry & Psychology, 26*(4), 461–475. https://doi.org/10.1080/14789949.2015.1034752

Kontio, R., Joffe, G., Putkonen, H., Kuosmanen, L., Hane, K., Holi, M., & Välimäki, M. (2012). Seclusion and restraint in psychiatry: Patients' experiences and practical suggestions on how to improve practices and use alternatives. *Perspectives in Psychiatric Care, 48*(1), 16–24.

Larue, C., Dumais, A., Boyer, R., Goulet, M. H., Bonin, J. P., & Baba, N. (2013). The experience of seclusion and restraint in psychiatric settings: Perspectives of patients. *Issues in Mental Health Nursing, 34*(5), 317–324. https://doi.org/10.3109/01612840.2012.753558

Lazarus, A. (2001). Physical restraint, thromboembolism, and death in 2 patients. *Journal of Clinical Psychiatry, 62*, 207–208.

LeBel, J. L., Duxbury, J. A., Putkonen, A., Sprague, T., Rae, C., & Sharpe, J. (2014). Multinational experiences in reducing and preventing the use of restraint and seclusion. *Journal of Psychosocial Nursing and Mental Health Services, 52*(11), 22–29. https://doi. org/10.3928/02793695-20140915-01

Lloyd-Evans, B., Johnson, S., Slade, M., Barrett, B., Byford, S., Gilburt, H., & Skinner, R. (2010). *In-patient alternatives to traditional mental health acute in-patient care.* Queen's Printer and Controller of HMSO.

Maguire, T., Young, R., & Martin, T. (2012). Seclusion reduction in a forensic mental health setting. *Journal of Psychiatric and Mental Health Nursing, 19*(2), 97–106. https://doi. org/10.1111/j.1365-2850.2011.01753.x

Mayers, P., Keet, N., Winkler, G., & Flisher, A. J. (2010). Mental health service users' perceptions and experiences of sedation, seclusion and restraint. *The International Journal of Social Psychiatry, 56*(1), 60–73. https://doi.org/10.1177/0020764008098293

McHugh, P., & Treisman, G. (2007). PTSD: A problem diagnostic category. *Journal of Anxiety Disorders, 21*, 211–222.

Mohan, R., McCrone, P., Szmukler, G., Micali, N., Afuwape, S., & Thornicroft, G. (2006). Ethnic differences in mental health service use among patients with psychotic disorders. *Social Psychiatry and Psychiatric Epidemiology, 41*(10), 771–776. https://doi.org/10.1007/ s00127-006-0094-7

Molodynski, A., Khazaal, Y., & Callard, F. (2016). Coercion in mental healthcare: Time for a change in direction. *BJPsych International, 13*(1), 1–3.

Morgan, C., Mallett, R., Hutchinson, G., & Leff, J. (2004). Negative pathways to psychiatric care and ethnicity: The bridge between social science and psychiatry. *Social Science & Medicine, 58*(4), 739–752. https://doi.org/10.1016/s0277-9536(03)00233-8

Mueser, K. T., Salyers, M. P., Rosenberg, S. D., et al. (2004). Interpersonal trauma and posttraumatic stress disorder in patients with severe mental illness: Demographic, clinical, and health correlates. *Schizophrenia Bulletin, 30*, 45–57.

Muskett, C. (2014). Trauma-informed care in inpatient mental health settings: A review of the literature. *International Journal of Mental Health Nursing, 23*(1), 51–59. https://doi.org/10.1111/ inm.12012

National Association of State Mental Health Program Directors. (2005). *Position statement on services and supports to trauma survivors.* Alexandria.

National Institute for Health and Care Excellence. (2015). *Violence and aggression: Short-term management in mental health, health and community settings.* NICE guideline [NG10]. https:// www.nice.org.uk/guidance/ng10/chapter/1-recommendations

NHS Digital. (2019). *Detentions Under the Mental Health Act. Ethnicity Facts and Figures.* https://www.ethnicity-facts-figures.service.gov.uk/health/mental-health/ detentions-under-the-mental-health-act/latest

Nizum, N., Yoon, R., Ferreira-Legere, L., Poole, N., & Lulat, Z. (2020). Nursing interventions for adults following a mental health crisis: A systematic review guided by trauma-informed principles. *International Journal of Mental Health Nursing, 29*(3), 348–363. https://doi.org/10.1111/ inm.12691. PMID: 31904178.

O'Brien, A. J., & Golding, C. G. (2003). Coercion in mental healthcare: The principle of least coercive care. *Journal of Psychiatric and Mental Health Nursing, 10*(2), 167–173.

Paksarian, D., Mojtabai, R., Kotov, R., Cullen, B., Nugent, K. L., & Bromet, E. J. (2014). Perceived trauma during hospitalization and treatment participation among individuals with psychotic disorders. *Psychiatric Services (Washington, D.C.), 65*(2), 266–269. https://doi.org/10.1176/ appi.ps.201200556

Paterson, B. (2014). *Mainstreaming trauma.* In Conference paper, Psychological Trauma Informed Care, Stirling.

Paterson, B., & Duxbury, J. (2007). Restraint and the question of validity. [Point de vue ethique face a la contention]. *Nursing Ethics, 14*(4), 535–545.

Putkonen, A., Kuivalainen, S., Louheranta, O., Repo-Tiihonen, E., Ryynänen, O. P., Kautiainen, H., & Tiihonen, J. (2013). Cluster-randomized controlled trial of reducing seclusion and restraint in secured care of men with schizophrenia. *Psychiatric Services (Washington, D.C.)*, *64*(9), 850–855. https://doi.org/10.1176/appi.ps.201200393

Roberts, A., Gilman, S., Breslau, J., Breslau, N., & Koenen, K. (2011). Race/ethnic differences in exposure to traumatic events, development of post-traumatic stress disorder, and treatment-seeking for post-traumatic stress disorder in the United States. *Psychological Medicine, 41*(1), 71–83. https://doi.org/10.1017/S0033291710000401

Saakvitne, K., Gamble, S., Pearlman, L. A., & Lev, B. T. (2000). *Risking connection: A training curriculum for working with survivors of childhood abuse*. Sidran.

Sanctuary Institution. (2022). *Sanctuary model*. https://www.thesanctuaryinstitute.org/about-us/the-sanctuary-model/

Substance Abuse and Mental Health Services Administration. (2014). *SAMHSA's concept of trauma and guidance for a trauma-informed approach. SAMHSA's trauma and justice strategic initiative*. U.S. Department of Health and Human Services Substance Abuse and Mental Health Services Administration, Office of Policy Planning and Innovation. https://www.nasmhpd.org/sites/default/files/SAMHSA_Concept_of_Trauma_and_Guidance.pdf

Substance Abuse and Mental Health Services Administration [SAMHSA], Trauma and Justice Strategic Initiative. (2012). *SAMHSA's working definition of trauma and guidance for trauma-informed approach*. Substance Abuse and Mental Health Services Administration.

Sweeney, A., Filson, B., Kennedy, A., Collinson, L., & Gillard, S. (2018). A paradigm shift: Relationships in trauma-informed mental health services. *BJPsych Advances, 24*(5), 319–333. https://doi.org/10.1192/bja.2018.29

Szmukler, G. (2015). Compulsion and "coercion" in mental health care. *World Psychiatry, 14*(3), 259–261.

Szmukler, G., & Appelbaum, P. S. (2008). Treatment pressures, leverage, coercion, and compulsion in mental health care. *Journal of Mental Health, 17*, 233–244.

Valentine, S. E., Marques, L., Wang, Y., Ahles, E. M., Dixon De Silva, L., & Alegría, M. (2019). Gender differences in exposure to potentially traumatic events and diagnosis of posttraumatic stress disorder (PTSD) by racial and ethnic group. *General Hospital Psychiatry, 61*, 60–68. https://doi.org/10.1016/j.genhosppsych.2019.10.008

Walsh, K., & Benjamin, R. (2020). Using participatory methods to engage multidisciplinary clinical staff in the embedding of trauma-informed care and practice principles in a sub-acute mental health inpatient unit. *Journal of Multidisciplinary Healthcare, 13*, 485–494. https://doi.org/10.2147/jmdh.S240240

Wieman, D. A., Camacho-Gonsalves, T., Huckshorn, K. A., & Leff, S. (2014). Multisite study of an evidence-based practice to reduce seclusion and restraint in psychiatric inpatient facilities. *Psychiatric Services (Washington, D.C.), 65*(3), 345–351. https://doi.org/10.1176/appi.ps.201300210

Wilson, C., Rouse, L., Rae, S., & Kar Ray, M. (2017). Is restraint a 'necessary evil' in mental health care? Mental health inpatients' and staff members' experience of physical restraint. *International Journal of Mental Health Nursing, 26*(5), 500–512. https://doi.org/10.1111/inm.12382

Wynn, R. (2004). Psychiatric inpatients' experiences with restraint. *Journal of Forensic Psychiatry & Psychology, 15*(1), 124–144. https://doi.org/10.1080/14789940410001655187

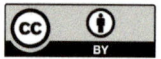

# Part IV

# Interventions

# Preventing and Managing Challenging Behaviour: Staff Training

Jakub Lickiewicz, Nutmeg Hallett, Jaroslav Pekara, and Nico Oud

## 1    Introduction

Workplace violence, which encompasses violence, aggression and sexual harassment, has been shown to negatively affect the organisation (e.g. staff turnover, higher absenteeism, reduced job commitment and job dissatisfaction), the mental and physical health of healthcare providers, and the quality of healthcare delivery (Liu et al., 2019). Similarly, the restrictive interventions that are used to manage workplace violence and behaviours that are challenging to manage can have a negative impact on the staff who utilise them and the patients who experience and witness them. Patient and staff safety is paramount and a priority to organisations (Hassiotis et al., 2022); reducing workplace violence and restrictive practices are key to achieve a safe environment. Negative factors such as lack of information, insufficient personnel and equipment, and communication breakdowns can increase the risk of violent behaviour and restrictive interventions in healthcare services (Mento et al., 2020). Therefore, the problem of workplace violence and restrictive interventions in the healthcare system must be addressed at all organisational levels and should lead to a consistent and coordinated organisational response.

J. Lickiewicz (✉)
Faculty of Health Sciences, Jagiellonian University Medical College, Krakow, Poland
e-mail: Jakub.lickiewicz@uj.edu.pl

N. Hallett
School of Nursing and Midwifery, University of Birmingham, Birmingham, UK
e-mail: n.n.hallett@bham.ac.uk

J. Pekara
Paramedic Department, Medical College, Prague, Czech Republic
e-mail: pekara@vszdrav.cz

N. Oud
Oud Consultancy, Amsterdam, The Netherlands
e-mail: nico.oud@freeler.nl

Violence prevention comprises three tiers, according to the public health model (Paterson et al., 2004). Primary prevention of violence is those actions which are taken to stop violence in advance of its occurrence. Secondary violence prevention is the actions that are taken to halt imminent violence. In tertiary violence prevention, interventions occur during and after an episode of violence to reduce its impact and minimise the harm to the individuals involved (Hallett et al., 2014).

Some actions can be taken to counteract the negative impact of workplace violence. One preventive method is to educate healthcare staff, training them specifically to deal with behaviours that can be challenging to manage (Morphet et al., 2018). While there is no universal methodology for such training, the focus has shifted from physical defence to preventive techniques over time. The ultimate goal is not to deliver skills to deal with challenging behaviour but rather to develop knowledge and skills to prevent such behaviour from occurring in the first place. The main focus is to teach proactive behaviour.

Patient violence and restrictive practices are intrinsically linked; studies will often use one as the proxy for the other. This is reflected in the Restraint Reduction Network Training Standards (Ridley & Leitch, 2021), which provide 'ethical training standards to protect human rights and minimise restrictive practices'. In England, it is a statutory requirement that the standards must be met by all organisations delivering training on restrictive practices. This demonstrates the shift in focus away from managing patient violence and towards reducing practices. Goulet et al. (2017) reviewed seclusion and restraint reduction programmes. They found they had six key components: (1) leadership, (2) training, (3) post-seclusion and restraint review, (4) patient participation, (5) prevention tools and (6) the therapeutic environment. The first should be a core element of seclusion and restraint reduction programmes.

Reducing restrictive practices needs a comprehensive and integrated approach directed at all factors and stakeholders. A measure that has been shown to decrease risks to staff is the provision of training in the prevention, recognition and management of work-related aggression and violence (Geoffrion et al., 2020).

Staff must have the appropriate skills to prevent aggressive and violent behaviour and to reduce the conditions that lead to it in mental health settings. However, service users should play an essential role in the prevention process, including being involved in developing and delivering training (Ridley & Leitch, 2021). Aggression management training programmes should be recovery-focused, trauma-informed and person-centred care. This approach should provide the basis for a reduction in restrictive practices in mental health settings (Muir-Cochrane, 2022; Cross et al., 2022).

This chapter reviews the current knowledge on staff training on aggression and violence prevention in clinical mental health care. The scope of this chapter is to focus on the general rules based on creating and providing this type of training. Besides a literature review, we share our thoughts on the goal of the training and factors that might influence its effectiveness. Furthermore, based on the literature review, we suggest the content of the training. We end this chapter with our thoughts on evaluating the training using different types of tools and questionnaires.

## 2   Aims of Training

Training must be provided with explicit reference to supporting an overall human rights-based approach, focusing on minimising the use of restrictive interventions and ensuring any use of restrictive interventions and other restrictive practices is rights-respecting (Ridley & Leitch, 2021). Training aims might differ depending on the individual and organisational perspective. The goal might be related to learning new knowledge (cognitive goal) and skills or changing attitudes and self-efficacy (psychological/affective goal).

Staff training should be comprehensive. The 'Colton, 2004 Checklist for Assessing Your Organization's Readiness for Reducing Seclusion and Restraint' is a comprehensive tool developed from a literature review and is based on nine recurring themes, one of which is orientation and training. The checklist states that the most effective training programmes tend to cover a wide range of topics rather than focusing primarily on behavioural interventions. However, some attempts were to teach a training module to provide a credible tertiary strategy based on 'spontaneous reaction' (Mott et al., 2012). Comprehensive (interdisciplinary) educational training for all staff members should guide them toward the goal, structure and content of a complete safety and health programme to recognise, prevent and manage workplace violence to be effective. It should provide staff with the knowledge, skills and competencies to implement such programmes consistently across their work shifts (Bowers et al., 2009; Colton, 2004).

According to the RRN standards (Ridley & Leitch, 2021), strategies need to be explicit about the learning outcomes in relation to the three following factors: the experience of people who use services, trauma-informed care and core skills in building therapeutic relationships, and the principles of positive behaviour support (or equivalent interventions aimed at understanding, safety and therapeutically supporting behaviour). There are also crucial legal and ethical issues (including duties of services under the Human Rights Act), risks associated with restrictive interventions, safety planning tools and advanced decisions. Among other related factors are the thoughts and feelings of the staff about being exposed to disturbing behaviour. Alternatives to restrictive interventions, effective de-escalation techniques or conflict resolution styles should be included.

## 3   Recommended Content for Training

### 3.1   General Guidelines Regarding Training

According to Maguire et al. (2022), optimal training should be place-based, responsive to local needs, and include relevant clinical, cultural, consumer/caregiver and contextual factors. Training may benefit from a focus on applying the learned knowledge, skills and attitudes, and there is a need for ongoing training reinforcement in the clinical setting beyond the initial introduction and provision of information and orientation to relevant skills (Maguire et al., 2022).

Interventions within training should be aimed at primary, secondary and tertiary levels of prevention. Primary interventions should aim to improve quality of life and reduce the likelihood of behaviours of concern (Ridley & Leitch, 2021). They should be used as part of everyday working practice and based on good quality person-centred support to meet the needs before problems arise. Secondary interventions, such as person-centred de-escalation strategies, should be used when early warning signs of behaviours of concern appear. Tertiary interventions should be applied to bring resolution and to re-establish/restore safety for everyone. They are used when an actual behaviour of concern occurs and in the aftermath and may include physical, chemical or mechanical restraints, seclusion, or enhanced observation (Ridley & Leitch, 2021). Personnel should be trained at all these levels of interventions. Focusing on the three levels of prevention within a theoretical nursing framework may promote a positive violence prevention and management climate (Björkdahl et al., 2013; Efkemann et al., 2019).

Ethical issues must be included in the creation of the training curriculum. Four principles must be covered in such training: respect for autonomy or free choice, care and support of people in a social environment, prohibiting pain or suffering and ethical distribution (Kramer & Walter, 2019). Integrating ethical principles into training supports high-quality and respectful patient care. Moreover, training should cover staff duties under human rights law and relevant legislation and how these legal standards underpin other laws and policies pertinent to restrictive interventions (Cross et al., 2022).

Different aspects should be stressed when working with adults with psychiatric problems, children or people with dementia. Therefore, different services will have different training needs (NICE, 2015; Ridley & Leitch, 2021). For this reason, a training needs analysis (TNA) should be completed before training (Cross et al., 2022). It should include the topics in which staff must be trained, their content, level, frequency, duration and results. Preparing a TNA allows a training programme to be tailored to the personnel's needs. Training should be contextualised to the environment and the type of patient/client (Baig et al., 2018). Non-physical intervention training in the positive and proactive prevention and therapeutic management of aggression and violence is informed by a risk assessment and needs-based approach to ensure that the training is 'fit for purpose' (Cross et al., 2022). The training content for restrictive interventions should also refer to any elevated risks identified in the TNA (Ridley & Leitch, 2021).

Multidisciplinary team members must attend relevant training programmes and refresher training, as informed by the standards of their continuous professional development (Cross et al., 2022). All new staff should receive initial training in reducing restrictive interventions and managing patient violence. Refresher training, which is usually shorter than initial training, is designed to equip an organisation's existing employees with the most up-to-date skills, methods and processes required to enhance their performance in dealing with behaviours that can be challenging to manage. It assumes that the skills of the existing employees might be outdated because of the advancement in knowledge and the human tendency to forget things. Thus, refresher training is conducted to keep employees updated with the latest skills and knowledge. This training type should occur approximately every 6 months (Baig et al., 2018). Training providers must develop refresher training curricula that consider the current needs of the organisation, service or individuals, using information from the TNA (Ridley & Leitch, 2021). Training updates could include changes to legislation, national guidance, supporting organisational policy and procedure; lessons learned and reinforcing non-physical intervention elements (Cross et al., 2022).

The training organisation must maintain the training records for each delivered programme (Ridley & Leitch, 2021). Training providers must have a policy for dealing with concerns that arise during training. Training providers must have internal quality assurance systems and be able to provide evidence that they effectively monitor the quality and consistency of their training services.

Another critical issue is the duration of the training. Geoffrion et al. (2020) found that training had different duration times, from a couple of hours to a few weeks. The RRN training standards do not stipulate the total time required for training but do include guidelines for some elements; primary strategies and preventative approaches should be given 'proportional time' (no less than 1 day or 6 h) (Ridley & Leitch, 2021). Similarly, secondary strategies should typically be given at least 3 h.

## 3.2    Content of the Training Programme

In a culture that seeks to minimise the risk of workplace violence through effective organisational, environmental and clinical risk assessment, the primary focus should be on recognition, prevention and de-escalation (Cross et al., 2022). This approach should promote therapeutic engagement, collaboration with service users (patients/clients) and advanced directives. All stakeholders have the right to work or to be treated in the safest and least restrictive healthcare setting. Solutions to the issue of aggression, violence and sexual harassment cannot be found without taking the service user seriously and having them actively involved. The problem of aggression and violence needs to be managed with a multifaceted approach. This section describes the key topics that should be included in the training curriculum.

### 3.2.1    Causes and Vulnerabilities Associated with the Risk of Developing Distressed Behaviour

To prevent distressed behaviour, violence and the associated restrictive interventions, it is necessary to understand the context in which such behaviours can occur. Training should provide reference to evidence-based frameworks for understanding the root causes of distress (Ridley & Leitch, 2021). Hastings et al. (2013) created a framework, updated by Bowring et al. (2019), to understand why challenging behaviours occur, see Fig. 1. While the framework was developed for people with intellectual disabilities, it holds true for people with mental illness as well (Ridley & Leitch, 2021) and can be used in training to support participants' understanding.

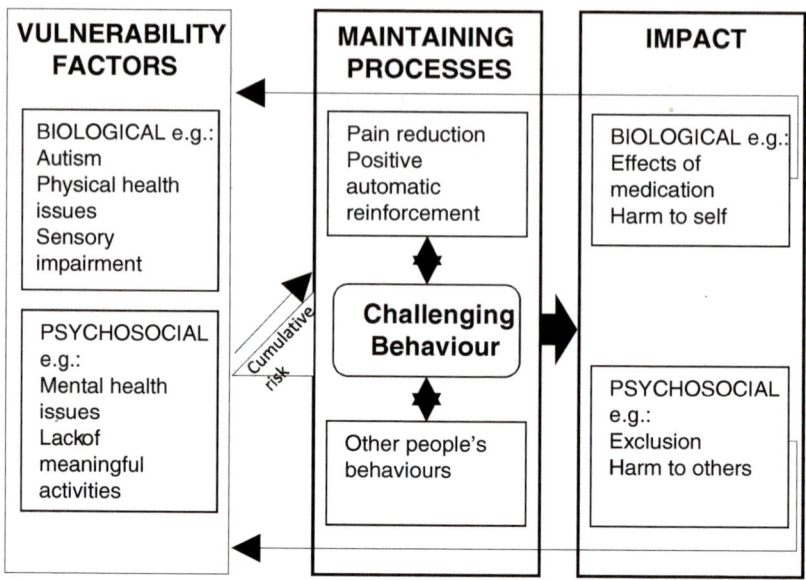

**Fig. 1** Framework for understanding challenging behaviour. Adapted from Bowring et al. (2019)

When managing individual risk factors, staff need to be made aware of early recognition of escalating behaviour, or recognition of warning signs or situations that may lead to distress or violence. This should include recognising, preventing and diffusing volatile situations or aggressive behaviour. Responses should include appropriate use of medication, proper use of safe rooms and knowledge of the standard response action plan for potentially violent situations (including the availability of assistance, response to alarm systems and communication procedures) (Ridley & Leitch, 2021).

Training should empower staff to develop a person-centred, values-based approach to care, in which personal relationships, continuity of care and a positive approach to promote health underpin the therapeutic relationship. Training must contain an understanding of the relationship between mental health problems and distress among patients. Risk assessment tools, such as the Brøset Violence Checklist (BVC) or Dynamic Appraisal of Situational Aggression (DASA) can be helpful.

### 3.2.2   Primary Strategies and Preventative Approaches

To aid in the understanding of the root causes of distress, training should include evidence-based frameworks such as Positive Behaviour Support or Safewards (Ridley & Leitch, 2021). Participants must learn to recognise potential triggers and vulnerabilities contributing to distressed behaviours, such as communication issues, sensory differences, mental and physical health concerns, social isolation and past trauma (Hastings et al., 2013). The training should promote a culture of support and implement primary strategies that proactively address individual needs, reducing the likelihood of harmful behavioural issues. Additionally, it is crucial to explore how the environment affects both those the people receiving support and the staff within that environment, emphasising the link between improving quality of life and reducing restrictive practices (Ridley & Leitch, 2021). The training should also cover the significance of building healthy therapeutic relationships in meeting individual needs. Lastly, participants should be encouraged to identify specific triggers and events leading to distress in those they support. Personalised approaches to recognise and manage these triggers should be a focus, along with self-reflection on staff members' own triggers and responses.

### 3.2.3   Communication Skills and De-Escalation

According to the National Institute for Health and Care Excellence (NICE, 2015), health and social care organisations should train staff in de-escalation. Furthermore, the RRN training standards require that a proportional time (at least 3 h) is given to the use of secondary strategies (Ridley & Leitch, 2021), which mostly comprise person-centred de-escalation strategies.

Key components of de-escalation training should provide a blend of staff skills and intervention processes (Brenig et al., 2023). Staff skills include verbal skills (negotiating, tactful language, calm tone of voice, sensitive use of humour), non-verbal skills (attentive posture and body language, active listening, appropriate eye contact), the ability to maintain personal control in the face of aggression, and the capacity to express a positive, empathetic, supportive and non-authoritarian therapeutic attitude.

Process-related skills include engaging with the patient, making reasonable assessments (e.g. necessity and timing of intervention, level of staff support needed, the safety of the area) and implementing de-escalation strategies (shared problem-solving, facilitating expression, offering alternatives to aggression, limit-setting).

### 3.2.4   Restrictive Interventions

Training on restrictive interventions should align with a commitment to reduce their overall use and focus on person-centred support (Ridley & Leitch, 2021). Training should include teaching the use of restrictive interventions, which may include physical restraint, clinical holding (a secure comfort position that helps the patient feel safe and secure during medical procedures) or mechanical restraint. Specific restrictive interventions taught must be suitable for the population being served, and training should incorporate additional safeguards if the TNA identifies increased risks. The RRN standards stipulate the following (Ridley & Leitch, 2021):

- Blanket training of restrictive techniques is discouraged, especially for emergency admission services.
- Training should clearly define the restrictive intervention's purpose and context.
- Trainers must be competent and formally assessed to deliver specific interventions, with clinical experience being beneficial.
- Training should cover the lawful circumstances for using the intervention, including an overarching definition of restraint.

- It should also address legislation, guidance, local policies and the importance of consent or consultation when using the intervention.
- Training must emphasise the least restrictive approach, avoiding threats or punishment.
- Risks associated with the intervention, warning signs of distress and actions to take should be covered in training.
- Safety concerns during training and potential risks within the training environment should be addressed.
- Training sessions should allow sufficient time for practice and competence assessments.
- The use of the specific restrictive intervention should occur within a therapeutic or supportive relationship.
- The training content should highlight the importance of complying with reporting requirements and participating in review processes to reduce the need for future restrictive interventions.

Medication to control behaviour (chemical restraint) and isolation must be discussed as essential knowledge for any employee. Chemical restrictions and isolation increase vulnerability to violence (Ridley & Leitch, 2021).

Physical techniques can be understood as hands-on methods that can be used to neutralise, de-escalate, escape from and survive actual violence. They include self-defence and patient restraint methods, as well as assault response and avoidance techniques, breakaway techniques and personal safety training (Miller, 2010).

Professional codes of practice clearly define that the deliberate application of pain is unacceptable and should not be taught. Training providers must not include teaching any restrictive intervention that uses pain to force an individual to comply (Ridley & Leitch, 2021). Individual practitioners are professionally and personally accountable for applying restrictive interventions. They must report any actions that cause concern, such as using physical techniques in life-threatening situations, for example, in case of preventing a suicidal attempt (Cross et al., 2022).

Attitudes are crucial in decision-making (Doedens et al., 2020; Laukkanen et al., 2019). There is a risk that personnel might perceive coercive measures as the best solution for challenging behaviours, without understanding their negative consequences. Understanding proper attitudes should be implemented before teaching physical techniques. The personnel must understand what motivates patients and develop their empathy before physical techniques will be provided. Methods should be based on adequately understanding the patient's challenging behaviours and should be an element of the process, with the right approach and relationship. The physical skills included in training must be selected carefully to assure the safety of all parties involved (Bleetman & Lifshitz, 2022).

According to the RRN standards, when teaching and assessing competence in practical (e.g. physical) skills with a restrictive component, the ratio of trainers to participants must not be more than 1:12; a minimum of two trainers is required if the cohort size is greater than 12 (Ridley & Leitch, 2021). The trainer-to-participant ratio must be risk assessed according to the activity that occurs and the rationale for the agreed ratio outlined in the course risk assessment and TNA (Cross et al., 2022; RNAO, 2019). Furthermore, the training environment should be risk assessed and fit for purpose, any emerging environmental risks should be clearly described to the participants, and the safety protocols should be described.

Training reinforces that physical interventions should be used if failure to intervene will result in harm that is judged likely more significant than that caused by using the intervention. The risks associated with using physical intervention are clearly articulated in the training manual; this must include both physical and psychological risks.

The use of simulated resistance during training can pose significant risks. Only trainers must role-play resistance in such simulations (Cross et al., 2022). Role plays must be directly managed by a separate trainer who should immediately stop the scenario if there is evidence of risk. Trainers ensure that any injuries, incidents, and near-misses during education and training programmes are accurately recorded and reported through established reporting systems.

When restrictive procedures are used, staff must be fully aware of the rights and risks involved. These must be addressed in training syllabuses that place them within the relevant legal, ethical and professional context. Training standards to reduce restraint must be seen in learning about human rights and duty of care (Cross et al., 2022).

### 3.2.5 Post-Incident Procedures and Patient/Personnel Well-being

Training must reference the importance of required procedures related to post-incident review and have content that allows participants to understand the meaning of 'trauma' and how it can impact people's experience of restrictive interventions (RNAO, 2019). Post-incident procedures have two parts (Ridley & Leitch, 2021):

1. Post-incident support.
2. Post-incident reflection and learning.

The former should pay attention to the well-being of all involved, including witnesses; the latter provides a space for learning and reduces the risk of subsequent incidents. Training should stress the importance of both elements.

It is common for employees to show distress after the application of restrictive interventions and the events that led to their use; they may need counselling and employee assistance programmes (EAP) to recover from the experience. In recognition of the circular nature of prevention, with post-incident review feeding into primary prevention strategies, training for staff in approaches such as mindfulness or other means of regulating their well-being and mental state can help them maintain reflective practice under stress (Cross et al., 2022). Adding this topic to the programme could reduce the risk of burnout, which may affect the staff's relationship with a patient.

### 3.2.6   Leadership and Teamwork

Leadership training should be provided to supervisors. This includes training in recognising conflicts and conflict resolution skills, the importance of early intervention, and supervisory/coaching skills (Wang et al., 2008). According to Fricke et al. (2023), strong leadership that cultivates a culture of support and respect is a prerequisite for a successful workplace violence prevention programme. Training that encourages the team to train together promotes the culture of safety and can teach managers about follow-up, communication and preventive actions.

## 4     Assessment of Training

Training programmes should include a system of competency assessment for participants and a reporting structure that informs line managers of individual training results. Evaluation procedures establish the efficacy of training (Cross et al., 2022). According to the RRN standards, training must include a competency-based assessment within each programme, with participants assessed for knowledge and skills (Ridley & Leitch, 2021). Participants should be able to clearly articulate the rationale for using restrictive interventions and the knowledge that must be acquired related to the legal and ethical implications of using restrictive interventions.

Various measures of training effectiveness have been developed. Participants' ability to de-escalate can be assessed at an individual level. The De-escalating Aggressive Behaviour Scale (DABS) can measure participants' performance in managing aggressive behaviour (Nau et al., 2009). Initially designed for nursing students, this scale contains seven items based primarily on communication, negotiation and collaboration. Developed in German originally, the DABS has been translated into English (Mavandadi et al., 2016).

Training effectiveness can also be assessed by virtual scenarios in which participants must deal with a potentially violent situation according to the training curriculum (Stephen et al., 2022). Other methods of measuring effectiveness might include:

- Comparing the number of episodes of aggression based on assault logs, reports of incidents or percentage of participants who have been a victim of aggression. A workplace violence questionnaire might also be used (Geoffrion et al., 2020).
- Assessing knowledge about aggression, using knowledge tests or self-perceived improvements in knowledge, such as the confidence in Coping With Patient Aggression Instrument (de la Fuente et al., 2019; Thackrey, 1987).
- Participant's attitudes and perceptions, using standardised scales such as the Perception of Aggression Scale (POAS) (Palmstierna & Barredal, 2006), Impact of Aggression Scale (IMPACS) (Needham et al., 2005), Attitudes Towards Aggression Scale (ATAS) (Jansen et al., 2005) or Staff Attitudes to Coercion Scale (SACS) (Husum et al., 2008).

Measurement of the environment for preventing and managing violence in the wards could also be helpful. Significantly, the patient may also be involved in this process, giving valuable feedback on training effectiveness from the service user perspective (Björkdahl et al., 2013).

More generally, rates of incidents or restrictive interventions, injuries or lost workdays could be recorded before and after the training. Other, more subjective methods might be personnel satisfaction with the training course or its relevance for the work on the ward (Richter et al., 2006).

In the evaluation process, cultural differences could be included. Teaching personnel in different economic and historical settings could have different attitudes toward aggression. Culture affects different perceptions and approaches to patients, treatment and workplace violence concerning personnel attitudes, terminology and forms of workplace violence. Those factors are crucial in the case of multicultural countries, where patients and personnel members rise in, e.g. different ethnical groups or have other experiences from their country of origin (Kumari et al., 2020; Lickiewicz et al., 2019).

Changes in approach and attitudes towards aggression might be the consequence of the thinking process and might result in a more positive direction in the personnel relationship.

## 5    Training Effectiveness

The effectiveness of education programmes in preventing and managing workplace violence (WPV) has been demonstrated through various studies, as Morphet et al. (2018) identified in their scoping review of workplace violence prevention in healthcare. The studies they identified primarily focus on two approaches: recognising at-risk behaviours and triggers, and communication and de-escalation. Several studies reported decreased violence following staff education in identifying at-risk behaviours and implementing communication and de-escalation strategies (Ching et al., 2010; Deans, 2004; Fernandes et al., 2002; Gillam, 2014; Magnavita, 2011). This suggests that education can play a significant role in reducing actual occurrences of WPV. Education in recognising at-risk behaviours and communication and de-escalation significantly enhanced the ability of student nurses to identify risk factors for violence (Beech & Leather, 2003). This improved recognition is a critical step in preventing violent situations from escalating. In simulated environments, nurses demonstrated an increased ability to de-escalate potentially violent situations (Deans, 2004; Nau et al., 2010). This indicates that the skills acquired through education are transferable to real-world scenarios, albeit in controlled settings.

In contrast, the efficacy of evasive self-defence or break-away training was less clear. Studies found that participants often could not apply the self-defence techniques they learned during training when tested in simulated settings (Dickens et al., 2009; Rogers et al., 2006). Additionally, there was no evidence to suggest that self-defence training effectively reduced the incidence of WPV in healthcare settings. Overall, the evidence supports the use of educational programmes focusing on recognising at-risk behaviours and communication and de-escalation as effective methods for managing and preventing WPV, particularly in healthcare environments.

A Cochrane review of training for preventing and minimising workplace aggression towards healthcare workers found that the effect of training on the reduction of aggressive episodes might be low in the long term (Geoffrion et al., 2020). However, the authors suggest that training could lead to more frequent reporting of aggressive incidents by staff, which might otherwise be underreported. There is a concern that increased self-confidence from training may lead staff to become more involved in confrontational situations than before. The study also notes a possible short-term increase in knowledge without sustained long-term effects. Geoffrion et al. (2020) conclude that these findings are affected by the low quality of the included studies.

The evidence is similarly weak when examining de-escalation training. A multidisciplinary review of de-escalation training of 64 studies, including 55 studies from nursing or psychiatry, noted varied outcomes (Engel et al., 2020). Survey-based outcomes suggest slight to moderate improvements in attitudes and behaviours post-training, emphasising the potential for individual and organisational benefits. Behavioural outcomes, however, present a less clear impact on reducing aggressive episodes long-term. The mixed results highlight the complexity of measuring the effectiveness of de-escalation training and call for higher-quality research to conclusively determine its impact on reducing aggression and enhancing safety in interactions.

A further notable limitation of the literature on the effectiveness of education programmes in preventing and managing WPV is the age of the evidence. Many of the key studies, such as those by Dickens et al. (2009), Rogers et al. (2006), Beech and Leather (2003) and others, were conducted more than a decade ago. This temporal gap raises concerns about their findings' current relevance and applicability to today's workplace environments, which may have evolved significantly due to changes in healthcare practices, technological advancements and shifts in workplace dynamics and culture. Given the rapid evolution of workplace settings and the emergence of new challenges and risks, it is possible that the strategies, techniques and outcomes identified in these older studies may not fully align with the present-day context of WPV.

One factor that needs further exploration is the gender of the participants. Before aggression training, Lickiewicz et al. (2020) observed differences in perceptions of aggression between males and women. Before the training, both groups negatively perceived aggressive behaviour. After the training, women saw aggressive behaviour as a defence of territory and behaviour that served a particular purpose, which hadn't been noted before. The changing perception may have resulted from a better understanding of the motivation and causes of aggression. No such effect was observed in the male group (Lickiewicz et al., 2020).

# 6    Conclusion

This chapter has comprehensively examined the role of staff education in reducing distressed behaviours and mitigating WPV. It has delineated the three-pronged approach to education: recognising at-risk behaviours, honing communication and de-escalation skills, and training in physical techniques. The efficacy of these methods in reducing the occurrence of WPV incidents has been substantiated, albeit with varying degrees of success. The education programmes, combining recognition of potential risks and effective communication strategies, have shown significant promise in curtailing violent episodes.

However, the applicability and success of evasive self-defence or break-away training remain ambiguous. While theoretically beneficial, these techniques often fall short in practical application, as evidenced in simulated scenarios. This inconsistency highlights a gap between training and real-world exigencies. Furthermore, this chapter highlights a notable limitation of the extant literature, much of which is over a decade old. Given the dynamic and evolving nature of healthcare environments, contemporary research is urgently needed. Such research should reassess the existing training modules and explore innovative strategies. The research on training effectiveness needs stronger methodological approaches as previous studies might be affected by risk of bias.

The advent of artificial intelligence (AI) and its recent exponential growth will open new avenues in training. It is important to note that the integration of artificial intelligence in the context of this chapter has not been addressed. This omission may quickly date the content presented, as the field is rapidly evolving with technological advancements. AI will likely be able to facilitate personalised learning, catering to individual styles and knowledge levels. Through simulations and virtual reality, it will offer safe, realistic training scenarios for de-escalation and self-defence. AI may provide continuous learning opportunities and immediate feedback, enhancing skill development. Its predictive analysis capabilities may help anticipate potential incidents, allowing for proactive training. Moreover, AI's scalability will ensure wide-reaching, accessible and consistent training across diverse locations.

While staff education programmes have shown effectiveness in managing WPV, there is an undeniable need for ongoing refinement and evolution of these programmes. Continuous evaluation, updated training content and the incorporation of new learning methodologies are imperative to maintain their relevance and effectiveness. The chapter calls for a sustained commitment to research and development in this field, ensuring that the strategies employed are grounded in current evidence and adaptable to workplace environments' changing landscapes. This approach is crucial for safeguarding the well-being of staff and maintaining a safe and productive workplace.

# References

Baig, L., Tanzil, S., Shaikh, S., Hashmi, I., Khan, M. A., & Polkowski, M. (2018). Effectiveness of training on de-escalation of violence and management of aggressive behavior faced by health care providers in a public sector hospital of Karachi. *Pakistan Journal of Medical Sciences, 34*(2), 294.

Beech, B., & Leather, P. (2003). Evaluating a management of aggression unit for student nurses. *Journal of Advanced Nursing, 44*(6), 603–612.

Björkdahl, A., Hansebo, G., & Palmstierna, T. (2013). The influence of staff training on the violence prevention and management climate in psychiatric inpatient units. *Journal of Psychiatric and Mental Health Nursing, 20*(5), 396–404.

Bleetman, A., & Lifshitz, S. (2022). Physical interventions and restraint. In J. Gall & J. Payne-James (Eds.), *Current practice in forensic medicine*. John Wiley & Sons.

Bowers, L., Allan, T., Simpson, A., Jones, J., Van Der Merwe, M., & Jeffery, D. (2009). Identifying key factors associated with aggression on acute inpatient psychiatric wards. *Issues in Mental Health Nursing, 30*(4), 260–271. https://doi.org/10.1080/01612840802710829

Bowring, D. L., Painter, J., & Hastings, R. P. (2019). Prevalence of challenging behaviour in adults with intellectual disabilities, correlates, and association with mental health. *Current Developmental Disorders Reports, 6*(4), 173–181. https://doi.org/10.1007/s40474-019-00175-9

Brenig, D., Gade, P., & Voellm, B. (2023). Is mental health staff training in de-escalation techniques effective in reducing violent incidents in forensic psychiatric settings? A systematic review of the literature. *BMC Psychiatry, 23*, 246. https://doi.org/10.1186/s12888-023-04714-y

Ching, H., Daffern, M., Martina, T., & Thomasa, S. (2010). Reducing the use of seclusion in a forensic psychiatric hospital: Assessing the impact on aggression, therapeutic climate and staff confidence. *Journal of Forensic Psychiatry and Psychology, 21*(5), 737–760. https://doi.org/10.1080/14789941003681361

Colton, D. (2004). *Checklist for assessing your organisation's readiness for reducing seclusion and restraint*. Commonwealth Center for Children and Adolescence.

Cross, G., Kay, G., Johnston, A., Paterson, B., Reid, K., & Thomas, B. (2022). *Towards safer services. Minimum standards for organisational restraint reduction plans*. Restraint Reduction Network.

de la Fuente, M., Schoenfisch, A., Wadsworth, B., & Foresman-Capuzzi, J. (2019). Impact of behavior management training on nurses' confidence in managing patient aggression. *The Journal of Nursing Administration, 49*(2), 73–78. https://doi.org/10.1097/NNA.0000000000000713

Deans, C. (2004). The effectiveness of a training program for emergency department nurses in managing violent situations. *Australian Journal of Advanced Nursing, 21*(4), 17–22.

Dickens, G., Rogers, G., Rooney, C., Mc Guinness, A., & Doyle, D. (2009). An audit of the use of breakaway techniques in a large psychiatric hospital: A replication study. *Journal of Psychiatric and Mental Health Nursing, 16*(9), 777–783.

Doedens, P., Vermeulen, J., Boyette, L. L., Latour, C., & de Haan, L. (2020). Influence of nursing staff attitudes and characteristics on the use of coercive measures in acute mental health services—A systematic review. *Journal of Psychiatric and Mental Health Nursing, 27*(4), 446–459.

Efkemann, S. A., Bernard, J., Kalagi, J., Otte, I., Ueberberg, B., Assion, H. J., Zeiß, S., Nyhuis, P. W., Vollmann, J., Juckel, G., & Gather, J. (2019). Ward atmosphere and patient satisfaction in psychiatric hospitals with different ward settings and door policies. Results from a mixed methods study. *Frontiers in Psychiatry, 10*, 576. https://doi.org/10.3389/fpsyt.2019.00576

Engel, R. S., McManus, H. D., & Herold, T. D. (2020). Does de-escalation training work? A systematic review and call for evidence in police use-of-force reform. *Criminology and Public Policy, 19*(3), 721–759. https://doi.org/10.1111/1745-9133.12467

Fernandes, C. M. B., Raboud, J. M., Christenson, J. M., Bouthillette, F., Bullock, L., Ouellet, L., & Moore, C. F. (2002). The effect of an education program on violence in the emergency department. *Annals of Emergency Medicine, 39*(1), 47–55. https://doi.org/10.1067/mem.2002.121202

Fricke, J., Siddique, S. M., Douma, C., Ladak, A., Burchill, C. N., Greysen, R., & Mull, N. K. (2023). Workplace violence in healthcare settings: a scoping review of guidelines and systematic reviews. *Trauma, Violence, & Abuse, 24*(5), 3363–3383.

Geoffrion, S., Hills, D. J., Ross, H. M., Pich, J., Hill, A. T., Dalsbø, T. K., et al. (2020). Education and training for preventing and minimizing workplace aggression directed toward healthcare workers. *The Cochrane Database of Systematic Reviews, 9*(9), CD011860. https://doi.org/10.1002/14651858.CD011860.pub2

Gillam, S. W. (2014). Nonviolent crisis intervention training and the incidence of violent events in a large hospital emergency department: An observational quality improvement study. *Advanced Emergency Nursing Journal, 36*(2), 177–188. https://doi.org/10.1097/TME.0000000000000019

Goulet, M. H., Larue, C., & Dumais, A. (2017). Evaluation of seclusion and restraint reduction programmes in mental health: A systematic review. *Aggression and Violent Behavior, 34*, 139–146.

Hallett, N., Huber, J. W., & Dickens, G. L. (2014). Violence prevention in inpatient psychiatric settings: Systematic review of studies about the perceptions of care staff and patients. *Aggression and Violent Behavior, 19*(5), 502–514. https://doi.org/10.1016/j.avb.2014.07.009

Hassiotis, A., Almvik, R., & Fluttert, F. (2022). Coercion as a response to violence in mental health-care settings. *Lancet Psychiatry, 9*(1), 6–8.

Hastings, R. P., Allen, D., Baker, P., Gore, H. J., Hughes, J. C., McGill, P., Noone, S. J., & Toogood, S. (2013). A conceptual framework for understanding why challenging behaviours occur in people with developmental disabilities. *International Journal of Positive Behavioural Support, 3*(2), 5–13.

Husum, T. L., Finset, A., & Ruud, T. (2008). The staff attitude to coercion scale (SACS): Reliability, validity and feasibility. *International Journal of Law and Psychiatry, 31*(5), 417–422.

Jansen, G. J., Middel, B., & Dassen, T. W. (2005). An international comparative study on the reliability and validity of the attitudes towards aggression scale. *International Journal of Nursing Studies, 42*(4), 467–477.

Kramer, G., & Walter, G. (2019). Arbeitsschutz, Recht, Ethik. In J. Nau, G. Walter, & N. Oud (Eds.), *Aggression, Gewalt und Aggressionsmanagement: Lehr- und Praxishandbuch zur Gewaltprävention für Pflege-, Gesundheits- und Sozialberufe* (pp. 417–447). Hogrefe.

Kumari, A., Kaur, T., Ranjan, P., Chopra, S., Sarkar, S., & Baitha, U. (2020). Workplace violence against doctors: Characteristics, risk factors, and mitigation strategies. *Journal of Postgraduate Medicine, 66*(3), 149.

Laukkanen, E., Vehviläinen-Julkunen, K., Louheranta, O., & Kuosmanen, L. (2019). Psychiatric nursing staffs' attitudes towards the use of containment methods in psychiatric inpatient care: An integrative review. *International Journal of Mental Health Nursing, 28*(2), 390–406.

Lickiewicz, J., Jagielski, P., Hughes, P. P., & Makara-Studzińska, M. (2020). The gender-related impact of a violence management training programme on medical school students—Preliminary results. *International Journal of Environmental Research and Public Health, 17*(19), 7130.

Lickiewicz, J., Nag, T., Ravnanger, C., Jagielski, P., & Makara-Studzińska, M. (2019). The Perception of aggression towards the medical personnel of psychiatric wards in Poland and in Norway—A comparative analysis. *Archives of Psychiatry and Psychotherapy, 3*, 61–70. https://doi.org/10.12740/APP/110698

Liu, J., Gan, Y., Jiang, H., Li, L., Dwyer, R., Lu, K., Yan, S., Sampson, O., Xu, H., Wang, C., Zhu, Y., Chang, Y., Yang, Y., Yang, T., Chen, Y., Song, F., & Lu, Z. (2019). Prevalence of workplace violence against healthcare workers: A systematic review and meta-analysis. *Occupational and Environmental Medicine, 76*(12), 927–937.

Magnavita, N. (2011). Violence prevention in a small-scale psychiatric unit: Program planning and evaluation. *International Journal of Occupational and Environmental Health, 17*(4), 336–344. https://doi.org/10.1179/oeh.2011.17.4.336

Maguire, T., McKenna, B., & Daffern, M. (2022). Establishing best practice in violence risk assessment and violence prevention education for nurses working in mental health units. *Nurse Education in Practice, 61*, 103335. https://doi.org/10.1016/j.nepr.2022.103335

Mavandadi, V., Bieling, P. J., & Madsen, V. (2016). Effective ingredients of verbal de-escalation: validating an English modified version of the 'De-Escalating Aggressive Behaviour Scale'. *Journal of Psychiatric and Mental Health Nursing, 23*(6-7), 357–368.

Mento, C., Silvestri, M. C., Bruno, A., Muscatello, M. R. A., Cedro, C., Pandolfo, G., et al. (2020). Workplace violence against healthcare professionals: A systematic review. *Aggression and Violent Behavior, 51*, 101381. https://doi.org/10.1016/j.avb.2020.101381

Miller, J. M. (2010). Incident control, attack avoidance, escape and physical self-protection trainings in healthcare settings. In M. R. Privitera (Ed.), *Workplace violence in mental and general healthcare settings*. Bartlett.

Morphet, J., Griffiths, D., Beattie, J., Velasquez Reyes, D., & Innes, K. (2018). Prevention and Management of Occupational Violence and Aggression in Healthcare: A scoping review. *Collegian, 25*, 621–632.

Mott, A., Walton, J., Harries, L., Highfield, P., Bleetman, A., & Dobson, P. (2012). Personal defence training in a medium secure unit—A pilot study. *The Journal of Mental Health Training, Education, and Practice, 7*(4), 200–213. https://doi.org/10.1108/17556221211287217

Muir-Cochrane E.C. (2022). *Restrictive mental health practices in the management of acutely unwell patients* [PhD thesis, College of Medicine and Public Health, Flinders University, Adelaide, South Australia].

National Institute of Health and Social Care Excellence. (2015). *Violence and aggression: short-term management in mental health, health and community settings*. NICE guideline (NG10). https://www.nice.org.uk/guidance/ng10/chapter/1-Recommendations

Nau, J., Halfens, R., Needham, I., & Dassen, T. (2009). The de-escalating aggressive behaviour scale: Development and psychometric testing. *Journal of Advanced Nursing, 65*(9), 1956–1964.

Nau, J., Halfens, R., Needham, I., & Dassen, T. (2010). Student nurses' de-escalation of patient aggression: A pretest–posttest intervention study. *International Journal of Nursing Studies, 47*(6), 699–708. https://doi.org/10.1016/j.ijnurstu.2009.11.011

Needham, I., Abderhalden, C., Halfens, R. J., Dassen, T., Haug, H. J., & Fischer, J. E. (2005). The impact of patient aggression on Carers scale: Instrument derivation and psychometric testing. *Scandinavian Journal of Caring Sciences, 19*(3), 296–300.

Palmstierna, T., & Barredal, E. (2006). Evaluation of the perception of aggression scale (POAS) in Swedish nurses. *Nordic Journal of Psychiatry, 60*(6), 447–451.

Paterson, B., Leadbetter, D., & Miller, G. (2004). *Workplace violence in health and social care as an international problem: A public health perspective on the 'Total Organisational Response'*. http://www.nm.stir.ac.UK/documents/ld-integrated-response.pdf

Registered Nurses' Association of Ontario. (2019). *Preventing violence, harassment and bullying against health workers* (2nd ed.). RNAO.

Richter, D., Needham, I., & Kunz, S. (2006). The effects of aggression management training for mental health care and disability care staff: A systematic review. In *Violence in mental health settings* (pp. 211–227). Centre for Reviews and Dissemination.

Ridley, J., & Leitch, S. (2021). *Restraint reduction network: Training standards* (1st ed.). BILD Publications.

Rogers, P., Ghroum, P., Benson, R., Forward, L., & Gournay, K. (2006). Is breakaway training effective? An audit of one medium secure unit. *The Journal of Forensic Psychiatry & Psychology, 17*(4), 593–602. https://doi.org/10.1080/14789940600893056

RRN relates to Cross, G., Kay, G., Johnston, A., Paterson, B., Reid, Thomas, B. (2022) Towards safer services. Minimum standards for organisational restraint reduction plans.

Stephen, T., King, K., Taylor, M., Jackson, M., & Hilario, C. A. (2022). Virtual, simulated code white for undergraduate nursing students. *Canadian Journal of Nursing Research, 54*(3), 320–330. https://doi.org/10.1177/08445621221101290

Thackrey, M. (1987). Clinician confidence in coping with patient aggression: Assessment and enhancement. *Professional Psychology: Research and Practice, 18*(1), 57–60. https://doi.org/10.1037/0735-7028.18.1.57

Wang, S., Hayes, L., & O'Brien-Pallas, L. L. (2008). *A review and evaluation of workplace violence prevention programmes in the health sector.* Nursing Health Services Research Unit.

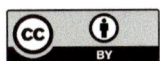

# De-Escalation in Mental Health Care Settings

Mary Lavelle, António Luís Ferreira, Søren Dixen, and Lene Lauge Berring

## 1    Introduction

De-escalation is defined as

> A collective term for a range of interwoven staff-delivered components comprising communication, self-regulation, assessment, actions, and safety maintenance, which aims to extinguish or reduce patient aggression/agitation irrespective of its cause, and improve staff-patient relationships while eliminating or minimizing coercion or restriction. (Hallett & Dickens, 2017)

For many decades, mental health staff used mainly physical techniques to manage aggressive and violent situations. Mechanical or physical restraint and/or seclusion were the interventions that staff were trained in. De-escalation emerged more implicitly through the intuition of selected nurses and doctors. The physical

Søren Dixen: Lived experience author.

M. Lavelle (✉)
School of Psychology, Queen's University Belfast, Belfast, UK
e-mail: mary.lavelle@qub.ac.uk

A. L. Ferreira
Unidade Local de Saúde São José, Clínica 1, Lisbon, Portugal
e-mail: antonio.ferreira@ulssjose.min-saude.pt

S. Dixen
Maskine Maskine Amager, Copenhagen, Denmark
e-mail: dixen@mmamager.dk

L. L. Berring
Department of Regional Health Research, University of Southern Denmark, Odense, Denmark
e-mail: lberring@health.sdu.dk

© The Author(s) 2024
N. Hallett et al. (eds.), *Coercion and Violence in Mental Health Settings*,
https://doi.org/10.1007/978-3-031-61224-4_15

component of aggression management was reinforced by distinctive training programs for (more or less violent) self-defence (Gertz, 1980).

In recent years, we have seen a move towards the introduction of de-escalation techniques in aggression management training. De-escalation relies on mental health staff skilfully employing verbal and nonverbal communication to redirect the client towards a calmer personal space (Berring et al., 2016a, b). Internationally, de-escalation has been identified as the first-line intervention in the management of aggression in mental health settings by the World Health Organization (2017).

Despite its prominence in policy and practice, empirical evidence to support de-escalation as a technique is currently lacking. De-escalation training has evolved from staff anecdotal reports of what works, rather than empirical evidence (Gaynes et al., 2017). There is limited evidence that current training in de-escalation techniques is effective in improving staff's ability to de-escalate violent and aggressive behaviour (Johnston et al., 2022; Price et al., 2015) and practice varies significantly by ward even when patient populations remain similar (Renwick et al., 2016). When used, de-escalation is estimated to be effective in halting the escalation sequence in approximately two-thirds of cases, with early intervention associated with better outcomes (Lavelle et al., 2016).

Nurses, doctors and other mental health workers need adequate options for every stage of the escalation curve. In recent years, de-escalation practice has received increasing attention from a qualitative research perspective. These studies employ in-depth observations of practice alongside analysis of staff and client perspectives of aggression management intending to develop an empirical understanding of de-escalation. This research has advanced our understanding of these complex social interactions, highlighting a number of factors that support, or conversely hinder, effective de-escalation. For example, stressful working environments and/or the impact of client trauma (Beattie et al., 2018). The qualitative findings alongside the direct experience of staff have led to the emergence of de-escalation principles, approaches and interventions. Furthermore, de-escalation has been integrated into complex models of care including Safewards (Bowers, 2014; Bowers et al., 2015) trauma-informed care (Huang et al., 2014; Muskett, 2014) and recovery (Slade et al., 2014).

This chapter provides the reader with state-of-the-art information on conflict management and interpersonal de-escalation in mental health settings and an overview of the practical approaches to implementing it in practice.

## 2    Situational Dynamics and Conflict Escalation

Many aggression management approaches refer to an escalation curve that illustrates the increasing emotional arousal in the conflict situation. Although the notion of a curve simplifies the complexity of aggressive situations, the curve highlights the empirically well-known fact that most violent situations, inside and outside of psychiatry, grow out of a situational escalation. The empirically based Safewards model (Bowers et al., 2014; Bowers et al., 2015) describes domains that influence the frequency of conflict on mental health wards including, but not limited to, patient characteristics, the staff team and the physical environment. The model illustrates how these domains naturally give rise to '*flashpoints*', which can trigger conflict and/or containment events and how patient and staff factors can influence and modify this link.

## 2.1    Patient Factors

The majority of research to date has focused on patient characteristics and behaviours; schizophrenia, young age, alcohol use, drug misuse, a history of violence and hostile-dominant interpersonal styles were found to be the predictors of patient violence (d'Ettorre & Pellicani, 2017). Although it is important to identify risk factors associated with patient behaviour, this is only one aspect. Recently, there has been an increased focus on how post-traumatic experiences can trigger a violent response (Beattie et al., 2018).

## 2.2    Ward Environment

Ward environment and design have been found to play a role in aggression and it can be perceived as a threat to physical and psychological safety for staff and patients (Beattie et al., 2018).

The customs and practices of staff on a ward including the clarity of, and adherence to, patient rules, the cleanliness and tidiness of the ward and the ward ideology have also been shown to influence rates of conflict on wards (Bowers et al., 2014; Bowers, 2009). Wards designed specifically to reduce environmental stress by reducing ward social density, reducing noise, improving access to nature and designing spaces to conduct unobtrusive observations have been beneficial in reducing the use of restrictive practice (Ulrich et al., 2018).

## 2.3    Staff–Patient Interactions

In mental health care, several studies have shown that violence is often preceded by staff–patient interactions and patient behavioural cues (Papadopoulos et al., 2012a, b). A meta-analysis revealed that patient–staff interactions accounted for 39% of the variance in patient violence (Bowers et al., 2011). Specifically three circumstances are frequently identified in literature as antecedents to escalation: staff denial of a patient request, staff suggesting that a patient act in a particular way and staff requesting that the patient desist from some action (limit setting) (Bowers et al., 2011). This can be experienced as psychological pressure (Potthoff et al., 2022), even though psychological pressure aims to improve treatment adherence it can be seen as informal coercion, this can escalate a situation as the patient's legal rights are violated.

Innovate research studies mapping incidents on wards reveal that most incidents occur in places where interactions between staff, patients and visitors take place (i.e. staff office, ward entrance and the day rooms), people get close to each other and conflicts arise out of 'normal' encounters (e.g. asking for medication) (Nijman et al., 1997; Papadopoulos et al., 2012a, b).

Another well-established fact is that the events and situations that lead to violence in psychiatric institutions are viewed quite differently by staff and patients (Duxbury & Whittington, 2005; Fletcher et al., 2021). Whereas staff attribute aggressive behaviour mainly to the mental illness itself, patients are more likely to see situational aspects and staff behaviour as precursors (Fletcher et al., 2021; Price et al., 2018). Taken together, this research suggests that staff behaviour may be as important as a precursor to violent incidents as patient behaviour.

Negative emotional reactions of staff towards patients may be another factor in triggering angry, hostile and potentially violent reactions (Haugvaldstad & Husum, 2016). Staff displaying a dominant style (i.e. dominance orientation) can become dangerous for two reasons. First, it may shape the ward milieu so that aggression and counter-aggression set the tone of the ward (Haugvaldstad & Husum, 2016; Nijman et al., 1999). Second, staff who are prone to dominance orientation are likely to react more aggressively and violently toward even minor hostile behaviour (Omer, 2021). This is in no way meant to blame staff for aggression and violence with which they are confronted, it just means that staff should be aware of their own reactions and behaviour.

As mental health workers who are trained in psychology and psychiatry, they can be biased toward an individualistic perspective that looks only to cognitions and emotions. However, communication interactionists who have specialised in the field of conflict management try to see the 'relational logic' (Donohue, 2003) that emerges from the interaction of the parties involved. Escalation, in this sense, means that hostile and aggressive behaviour tends to be mutually reinforcing so that each party's reactions lead to greater harm with each new round of actions. The escalation from interaction to violence might take several hours, but it also might only take seconds. This is the reason why an escalation curve is misleading when you try to apply it to real situations. The escalation curve suggests an ideal type of interaction with a steady increase of tension, which usually is not the case.

Escalating behaviours can be triggered by diverging goals and intentions of the interacting parties. Whereas staff try to fulfil their therapeutic and safety roles, patients often have short-term goals that support their subjective quality of life and, most importantly, their subjective needs and identity. Some authors argue that striving for needs and identity are the main causes that trigger violence, regardless of the social context and institution. John Burton, a leading violence theorist stated, after reviewing the general literature on violence causation:

*'The conclusion to which we are coming is that seemingly different and separate social problems, from street violence to industrial frictions, to ethnic and international conflicts, are symptoms of the same cause: institutional denial of needs of recognition and identity and the sense of security when they are satisfied, despite losses through violent conflict'.* (Burton, 1997, p. 38)

This is also true for interpersonal conflicts in mental health care. When the incompatibility of staff and patient intentions becomes clearer to both sides, the escalation is fuelled by emotions (e.g. anger) and cognitions (e.g. prior experiences). In general, expectations shape our behaviour as well as the observation of the other party involved (Haugvaldstad & Husum, 2016). Therefore, the incompatibility of the two parties' expectations can be regarded as the key factor for conflict escalation. Mental Health workers can expect a patient to comply with orders, and a patient will expect a nurse to show caring (and not security) behaviour (Engström et al., 2020; Fletcher et al., 2021). When these or other expectations are violated, distrust can occur. Distrust is a key cognition that can lead to increased aggression. Both sides, staff and patient, experience being aversively stimulated by the other's behaviour (Haugvaldstad & Husum, 2016; Whittington & Richter, 2005; Whittington & Wykes, 1996).

The feeling of being provoked by the other party will, in many cases, lead to aggressive reactions which will stimulate the opponent in return (Haugvaldstad & Husum, 2016). Distrust and aversive stimulation can lead both parties into the above-mentioned relational logic of escalation, where inflammatory language is only the overt signal of underlying cognitions and emotions. Being trapped in this logic of escalation will, then, lead to more or less fixed expectations about the other party's behaviour: *This nurse wants to harm me and I have to defend myself.* Cognitive processes turn to narrowness and rigidity the more the interaction escalates (Omer, 2021).

Questioning participating staff and patients after a violent incident, Benson et al. (2003) found discourses of blame on both sides. In conflict theory, this expectation and its connected rigidity are regarded to be some of the most powerful cognitive frames that make resolving conflict so difficult. Breaking this logic and its expectation frame is, therefore, a key task for nonviolent conflict resolution.

At this point, it is important to stress the role of the patient's psychopathology. The symptoms of the actual mental disorder surely shape the patient's observational and appraisal abilities. Further, the control of impulsivity and conflict-solving skills are impaired by the disorder. Experimental psychological research has shown that subjects who score highly on trait hostility (persistent over time) will also express higher levels of state hostility (temporary condition, present for short periods of time) (Lindsay & Anderson, 2000). However, the basic conflict situation is still based on an interaction. Without a triggering event from the social environment of the patient, which has been regarded as an aversive stimulus, the escalation would not have begun. Thus so far, violence by psychiatric patients is not materially different from violence committed by healthy subjects. For a common-sense approach to research on interpersonal violence in general, risk factors can be divided into the following categories: predisposing factors and processes, situational elements and triggering events (Reiss & Roth, 1993). To prevent a violent escalation, staff have only minimal chances to affect the predisposing psychopathology in the short term. Even the situation of the often involuntary admission cannot be changed easily. What staff can do is to learn from previous situations, such as within a trauma-informed perspective, where the focus is on learning from the service providers. For

example, programmes exist where service providers educate healthcare professionals in how to create safety by reducing seclusion and restraints (US Department of
Health and Human Services 2014).

## 3    Staff Stress and Emotion Regulation

Staff behaviour is one of the crucial points where the prevention of violence is initiated. If patients feel aversively stimulated by staff, this usually does not happen by
the staff's intention, rather it will happen unintentionally.

Many mental health workers who work in psychiatric institutions have to face
traumatic events, such as violence and the use of coercive measures, an overwhelming work-load and organisational pressure and, thus, feel highly distressed (Beattie
et al., 2018; Johnson et al., 2017; Siegrist et al., 2003). Working conditions affect the
encounters between staff and patients. Staff may not be able to react as calmly and
therapeutically as they intend to. Current working conditions in mental health care,
and the stressful situations associated with aggression itself, mean staff must be able
to manage their own distress in order to behave in a way that reduces the risk of
aggression and violence (Haugvaldstad & Husum, 2016). Therefore, stress management and emotion regulation are the basis for applying de-escalation skills effectively.

There is some indirect positive effect from dedicated training programs in relation to staff stress and emotional regulation especially when the training targets the
whole organisation such as Trauma-Informed Care (TIC (see Chap. Trauma
Informed Care)). TIC aims to promote a safe environment for everybody and
thereby minimise conflict by changing organisational cultures to respond appropriately to the effects of trauma at all levels (Fernández et al., 2023; Keesler, 2020).

Staff can, for example, be trained in mindfulness as this has the potential to
reduce symptoms of burn-out and thereby increase safety as this may raise nurses'
self-awareness (Wampole & Bressi, 2019). The key to managing emotions is self-
awareness, being able to share stressful emotions with colleagues (Nay, 2004) and
engaging in reflective practice or debriefing following stressful events (Asikainen
et al., 2023; Scott et al., 2022). As mental health workers, we have to know the personal signs that indicate stress and arousal. These indicators might be physical (e.g.
sweating, elevated heart frequency) or psychological (e.g. polarised thinking, labelling). Because such indicators are highly individualistic, anger therapists recommend setting up a personal anger scale that includes the whole range of reactions in
connection with experienced anger (see Nay, 2004). However, we also need to know
how to prevent violence.

## 4    Basic Rules of Conflict Management

De-escalation alone is not an option for all aggressive and potentially violent incidents. In some situations, physical techniques against aggressive patients are
unavoidable. However, even in such circumstances, supportive and reassuring

communication is still required. Which option to choose depends on several contextual factors: the current situation on the ward, the patient's psychiatric symptoms, the patient's conflict-solving skills and impulsivity control, staff experience of conflict management, and, of course, the intensity of the conflict. The type of aggression or violence is also highly relevant. Instrumental violence (acts that are related to specific goals) has to be handled differently than emotional violence (behaviour that emerges from interpersonal tension) (Dutschmann, 2000, 2003). For instrumental violence, general cognitive behavioural interventions are more appropriate than specific body language or rhetoric skills, which are better applied to situations with high arousal.

Generally, verbal interventions are possible for patients who are not highly delusional or disorganised (e.g. patients with dementia) (Alpert & Spillmann, 1997). Quite common, but difficult to master, are triggered displaced aggressions. Patients sometimes feel more provoked by fellow patients, relatives or other mental health workers than the one who becomes the target of the aggression. Triggered displaced aggressions are a combination of two aversive stimulations by different people where a minor stimulus can lead to an excessive violent outburst (Miller et al., 2003).

The types of conflict and the contexts within which they happen are so diverse and specific, that it is generally recommended to first consider and learn several basic rules rather than to stick to highly ambitious skills or techniques which may only be appropriate in special situations. That is not to say that mastery of such skills may not be advantageous, and we provide details of specific skills below.

The following recommendations are mainly about general attitudes toward conflict, staff involvement in such conflicts, and the adequate timing of interventions. These recommendations are informed by the findings of a substantial thematic synthesis of key components of de-escalation techniques conducted by Price and Baker (2012) and previously published similar recommendations including Safewards (Paterson & Leadbetter, 1999; Stevenson, 1991).

Before going into details of conflict management and de-escalation, two important warnings must be given. First, the reader has to be aware that the following recommendations must not be used in a cookbook manner. It is possible that the same intervention applied to the same patient works successfully in one situation but not in another. Don't stick to the rules too tightly. A well-known example from experience for many psychiatric nurses is that the appearance of an authoritarian doctor can, in some situations, change an aggressive patient into a calm and compliant one. Sometimes it is possible to enforce a conflict resolution, namely when the force is associated with capability, legitimacy and credibility (Schellenberg, 1996).

Second, the reader should be aware that they are not able to apply effective de-escalation techniques from reading this or other printed matter on the topic. De-escalation requires in-depth training. Experience from several training programs has further shown that it is beneficial to train personnel from one ward together so that every staff member receives the same knowledge and each one can rely on their colleagues. However, a very important way of learning is to receive feedback from the service users (Slade et al., 2019), this will give mental health care workers a concrete experience of what to do better the next time.

## 4.1     Respect, Empathy and Concern for Patients

The first basic rule stresses the general attitude towards the patient and his or her aggression. Effective de-escalators are open and sincere, and display empathy, concern, respect and fairness (Engström et al., 2020; Price & Baker, 2012). Staff have to be aware that, apart from patients with specific personality disorders, human beings and, therefore, patients, are usually not voluntarily aggressive or violent. In general, aggression and violence are triggered by the subjective notion that one has to defend oneself against another's intimidations, provocations or unjust behaviour (Anderson & Bushman, 2002; Haugvaldstad & Husum, 2016); however, justified these accusations might be from a different perspective.

Patients who violently try to abscond from the ward, understandably, see their quality of life severely reduced by the closed door. Thus, aggressive and potentially violent patients subjectively face a serious problem that they cannot cope with in any other way. The attitude of empathy and respect may in many cases help to find out which problem it is that triggers the patient's aggression and, at the same time, is the basis for interpersonal conflict resolution in so far as the patient can feel more accepted and understood by staff (Price & Baker, 2012).

## 4.2     Assess the Risks

The second rule of conflict management is to assess the risks, this may be achieved using tools such as theBrøset Violence Checklist (Woods & Almvik, 2002). This will enable staff members to be prepared and better able to initiate a de-escalation intervention (Hvidhjelm et al., 2023). It is important that expectations are realistic. Staff must ask themselves *'Can this situation be managed without physical intervention?'* Because of the situation's acuity and variability this question, in many cases, must be answered by intuition. If staff don't feel safe enough to manage this situation using nonphysical options alone, they should switch over to plan B, i.e. the preparation of physical interventions.

## 4.3     Control the Situation, Not the Patient

Third, the next basic rule is not to control the patient but to control the situation. Conflict management within an interaction has the goal of getting the best out of the situation for both parties, a win-win situation as it is commonly termed in game theory (Davidson & Wood, 2004). The goal of avoiding violence depends on both parties' reactions. However, it is impossible to predict the outcome of an interaction in advance. If the patient has the impression that staff are trying to control or even coerce him or her into specific behaviour, hostile reactions are very likely to emerge. The use of power usually contradicts a therapeutic relationship (Engström et al., 2020; Fletcher et al., 2021).

Staff appearing calm and in control of the situation are thought to facilitate patients' ability to manage their own feelings and emotions alongside showing a degree of trust in the patient (Duperouzel, 2008; Price & Baker, 2012). Techniques staff use to remain calm include focusing on the assessment of patients or acknowledging feelings of anxiety when they arise rather than denying them (Price & Baker, 2012).

## 4.4    Teamwork—Share Thinking, Decisions and Responsibilities with Colleagues

In cases where this is possible, risk assessment, decision-making, responsibilities and actions should be shared with colleagues and if possible, the patient. Several reasons make this rule obligatory. Conflict situations are associated with high emotional tension, and staff decisions might be biased by their own emotional involvement.

Although de-escalation works better within a one-to-one interaction, fellow staff can create safety for the person who is responsible for the one-to-one interaction, by scaffolding their interaction; ensuring other patients nearby are calm and that the environment is optimised. Furthermore, colleagues will be attuned to pivotal moments in the de-escalation interaction, where the patient begins to calm down or when crisis interventions need to be used (e.g. physical interventions) helping to save patients and staff from injuries.

## 4.5    Early Intervention

De-escalation works more successfully when it is done as an early intervention (Lavelle et al., 2016; Price & Baker, 2012). This is illustrated by the escalation curve. The more both parties' behaviour and tensions are similar to 'normal' dimensions, the better they are able to plan and respond to a nonviolent intervention. In other words, de-escalation may be less appropriate in situations that are accompanied by high risks and tensions.

## 4.6    Slow Things Down

One of the main subgoals in de-escalation is to gain time. Very often, aggressive interpersonal communication, e.g. accusations and shouting, proceeds quickly. Emotional arousal makes quick responses highly likely, and participants feel subjectively under pressure to respond so that the opponent will not get the impression that one has given in. Experimental psychological research has, however, shown that time pressure leads to less thorough information processing and, consequently, to inadequate decisions (De Dreu, 2003; Van Kleef et al., 2004). A gain in time may not only lead to better decisions, but it may reduce interpersonal tension.

## 4.7    Spatial Awareness

Spatial considerations are equally important. A balance must be struck between being close enough to the patient to develop rapport but not invading their personal space (Price & Baker, 2012). Although some patients may have a preference for touch and find it calming, it may lead to further escalation in others. As with most aspects of de-escalation, an understanding of the specific preferences and needs of the individual will inform the approach. However, keeping a distance between staff and patients will safeguard against immediate hits or blows.

## 4.8    Confidence and Certainty without Provocation

De-escalation interventions have to be applied with apparent self-confidence and certainty, without being provocative. Like several other principles and techniques in this regard, this rule asks for a balanced procedure. If staff show too much complacency, it may be regarded as arrogant and provocative. No, or too little, self-confidence may give the impression that staff are not able to codetermine the outcome of difficult situations. This problem is known from research on aggressive children, where parents who permanently give in are known to increase the demands and aggressive actions of their children. Omer (2001, 2021) uses the term 'complementary escalation' for this kind of escalation which stands in contrast to the well-known type of reciprocal escalation.

## 4.9    Avoid Power Plays

Power plays between staff and patients have to be avoided. Quite often, major conflicts grow out of minor disputes or misunderstandings. The question of whose perspective is right or wrong can lead to an argument. Conflicts are fuelled by each party's notion that one cannot give in because this might show weakness. Apparently unimportant differences become issues of personal identity and honour.

For experienced and self-confident staff, this kind of conflict should not be necessary in many cases. Effective de-escalation should facilitate autonomy and empower the patient to feel they are choosing to de-escalate (Duperouzel, 2008; Price & Baker, 2012). Face-saving alternatives can be offered to patients to achieve this. Of course, staff cannot make promises or concessions that will lead to conflict in later situations.

## 4.10    Safety Awareness

Staff should be aware of general safety issues. Aggressive situations often occur in ward environments where there are several other people. The safety of fellow patients or inexperienced staff should always be kept in mind. As one does not know the outcome of a de-escalation attempt from the start, the place of such an intervention should be carefully considered. Where possible, an open way to flee should be within reach and potentially dangerous objects should be removed.

## 5  De-Escalation Practical Principles and Interventions

Duperouzel (2008) described how good de-escalators explained their strategies and illustrated how they initially tried to discover the reasons for the patient's behaviour in order to help them solve their problems. Furthermore, good de-escalators invest a lot of time in developing relationships with patients. Studies employing grounded theory approaches (Delaney & Johnson, 2006; Johnson & Delaney, 2007) investigated different dimensions of de-escalation in two psychiatric units and described escalation and de-escalation as unpredictable as non-linear processes. The authors emphasised the dilemmas staff faced when deciding how and when to intervene: too early and too dramatic intervention might be perceived by patients as over-controlling, and too late intervention might endanger the safety of staff and patients (Johnson & Delaney, 2007, p. 50). Hallett and Dickens' (2015) survey showed a consensus on the nature of de-escalation among clinical staff in a low- and medium-security mental health setting, including expressing empathy, care, humour and calmness.

In a thematic synthesis, based on 11 papers, Price and Baker (2012) extracted key characteristics of effective de-escalators and key components of de-escalation techniques. Some of these characteristics are presented in other sections of this chapter where relevant (see Sects. 4 and 6) but the overall findings are summarised here. Characteristics of effective de-escalators include an ability to empathise with the patient, communicate in an open, honest, supportive, coherent, non-judgemental, confident and genuine manner; effective de-escalators maintain control, appearing calm when met with aggression; effective de-escalators present with a calm, gentle and soft voice, use tactful language, sensitive use of humour and an awareness of their body language as a way of expressing concern and empathy for the patient and developing rapport. Early intervention was recommended, although acknowledged that this depends on the specific circumstances; a de-escalation strategy requires flexibility and creativity to try to understand the reasons for the patient's behaviour and intervene in a way that meets the specific needs of the patient while balancing safety with patient autonomy (Price & Baker, 2012).

### 5.1  De-Escalation Interventions

De-escalation is difficult to describe, anyhow, it has become an important part of complex violence and restraint reduction models such as Safewards (Bowers et al., 2014; Bowers et al., 2015), six core strategies (Huckshorn et al., 2006) and recovery (Slade et al., 2014). A literature search using de-escalation, violence and psychiatry as search terms, identified several references describing de-escalation practices based on literature reviews, expert accounts and consensus statements (DelBel, 2003; Fauteux, 2010; Richmond et al., 2012). Definitions of de-escalation are most often based on theoretical descriptions; for example, Stevenson (1991, p. 6) defined de-escalation as *'a complex interactive process in which the patient is directed toward a calmer personal space'*. Stevenson's account identifies four important aspects of de-escalation:

1. Knowing yourself.
2. Knowing the patient.
3. Knowing the situation.
4. Knowing how to communicate.

These four themes are generally recognised by other authors as being central to de-escalation (DelBel, 2003; Paterson & Leadbetter, 1999; Stubbs & Dickens, 2008).

The de-escalation component of the Safewards intervention is called 'Talk Down' (Bowers, 2014; Bowers et al., 2015). This is a three-step process, which draws on a range of previously developed techniques and details the three steps staff should take when interacting with a patient who is agitated, angry or upset. The steps are summarised in a poster:

1. Delimiting—establishing safety and getting started.
2. Clarifying—eliciting and hearing the patient, establishing the nature of the problem.
3. Resolving—addressing the issue via appeal negotiation, comprise or providing choices.

Staff qualities required for this process are also displayed including self-control, respect and empathy. Wards using the talk-down component of Safewards are required to display the talk-down poster in a prominent position on the ward and nominate a 'talk-down champion' who is a ward staff member already identified as someone who is skilled at de-escalation. As champions, they will explain the techniques to their fellow team members and facilitate the implementation of this method in practice (Bowers, 2014; Bowers et al., 2015).

The de-escalation component of the six core strategies includes a trauma-informed care (Huang et al., 2014; Muskett, 2014) approach and is related to the use of language, e.g. learning how to ask and debriefing (Riahi et al., 2016). Within this approach, violence and restraint are viewed as critical incidents that must be avoided in the future, using debriefing techniques such as formal post-incident review to support this goal.

An example of a de-escalation approach, which was underpinned by these principles and co-created with experts by experience, can be seen in Table 1 (Berring et al., 2016a). The de-escalation components were co-created based on real-life situations in acute mental health care settings. This de-escalation approach includes two phases: (i) an acute phase and (ii) a relationships phase. In the *acute phase*, a feeling of safety must be established; this is achieved when personal space is respected and only *one* staff member is engaging and communicating with the patient, while other

**Table 1** De-escalation divided into seven components

| Acute phase | |
| --- | --- |
| Respect personal space | To make a dialogue possible, it is important not to violate the patient's personal space. The space within which the patient feels safe, and to which she/he can withdraw to regain self-control. Personal space is established by the staff keeping their distance and signal plenty of time. This also demonstrates that the staff are willing to spend the time needed to help the patient. |
| Create focus | The patient must feel that there is one person present who wants to help him/her. This is achieved through focused attention from the caregiver, which means that the caregiver interacts with nobody but the patient. With the caregiver focusing only on helping the patient, it becomes possible to engage the patient in a dialogue. |
| Change context | Changing context means creating a new situation. This can be done by creating a diversion, but also by giving a new meaning to the situation. A change of context can take a patient by surprise and lead to a turning point. |
| *Relationship phase* | |
| Show empathy | Empathy is a pre-condition for a successful de-escalation. You show empathy by putting yourself in the patient's shoes. Empathy can take a variety of forms, but supporting autonomy must be included. |
| Understand the patient | Once the patient is in a state that allows dialogue, you must make a determined effort to understand the patient's perspective. In this interpretative process, the most important thing is to keep on listening to the patient's experience. In this process, you must be open and curious. |
| Align expectations | The goal of de-escalation is to support a common solution to the problem. Before the process is finalised, it is important to align expectations. The basis for an alignment of mutual expectations lies in involving the patient in shared decision-making. |
| Evaluate the process | Evaluation is the last and most important part of the de-escalation process. It is important to create an atmosphere in which staff and patients can reflect on what happened, thus turning it into a learning situation. Do not interpret the behaviour of others. Stay focused on your own actions while the patient is processing the experience. |

staff members stand by in order to have an overview of the situation, thereby protecting both patients and staff, against physical and psychological injuries. Before the *relationship phase* can start, staff members must establish a trusting relationship in order to continue the de-escalation process. In the *relationship phase,* staff start to know the patient, listen to the patient's point of view, and understand the situation from the patient's perspective. This de-escalation approach requires teamwork to meet the patient's needs. This collaborative approach focuses attention on skills related to the whole community rather than individual mental health workers only. In both phases, staff must be aware of their own reactions and feelings. This collaborative de-escalation approach offers a potential turning point in violence management because the problem will be solved together with the patient (i.e. in aligning expectations). Immediate validation of the encounter is provided in the final step of the process where all parties give feedback in the final debriefing/evaluation step. This is where staff and patients process their experience and achieve learning (Berring et al., 2016b).

## 5.2    De-Escalation Training

Health and social care provider organisations should train staff who work in services, where restrictive interventions may be used, in psychosocial methods to avoid or minimise restrictive interventions. Many countries have guidelines to achieve this and have adopted the BILD/Restraint Reduction Network Training Standards recommendations (citation needed):

- De-escalation training should aim to facilitate culture change and improve the quality of life of those being restrained and those supporting them.
- Reduce reliance on restrictive practices by promoting a positive culture and practice that focuses on prevention, de-escalation and reflective practice.
- Increase understanding of the root causes of behaviour and recognition that many behaviours are the result of distress due to unmet needs.
- Where required, the de-escalation training should focus on the safest and most dignified use of restrictive interventions, including physical restraint.

  A training curriculum could include:

- A person-centred, values-based approach to care, in which personal relationships, continuity of care and a positive approach to promote health underpin the therapeutic relationship.
- An understanding of the relationship between mental health problems, early childhood traumatic experiences and the risk of violence and aggression.
- Skills to assess why a behaviour is likely to become violent or aggressive, including personal, constitutional, mental, physical, environmental, social, communicational, functional and behavioural factors.
- Skills, methods and techniques to reduce or avert imminent violence and defuse aggression when it arises (for example, verbal de-escalation).
- Skills, methods and techniques to undertake restrictive interventions safely when these are required.
- Skills to undertake an immediate post-incident debrief.
- Skills to undertake a formal external post-incident review in collaboration with experienced service users who are not currently using the service.

## 6    Communication Skills

The de-escalation interventions described in the previous section state the importance of verbal communication during de-escalation in understanding and clarifying the concern from the patients' perspective and negotiating a solution. However, verbal de-escalation techniques do not occur in isolation but are intrinsically linked with the gestural and physical (nonverbal) communication of the de-escalator.

The mastering of body language and related physical features is one of the most important and at the same time one of the most difficult tasks when learning conflict management. Verbal communication is usually overemphasised in de-escalation training. This emphasis on verbal communication is in stark contrast to research findings which stem from the 1960s, but still hold true today, where nonverbal communication was found to be more important for sending social cues and emotional signals (De Gelder, 2009; Hall et al., 2019; Mehrabian & Ferris, 1967; Mehrabian & Wiener, 1967; Roter et al., 2006). Related to the overemphasis of words in interactions is the common notion that humans are rational beings who calculate their decisions and actions thoroughly in order to make the best out of each situation. During periods of high arousal, e.g. during an escalation phase, our attentional scope is narrowed (Gable et al., 2015). With diminished cognitive resources, greater reliance is placed on interpretation and communication via the nonverbal channel. The spoken word alone does not fully capture the complexity of the interaction (Turner, 2002).

Considering the importance of the interaction, it cannot be overstated that the outcome of the situation does not depend solely on patient behaviour. As discussed previously, staff are very likely to attribute aggression and violence to the mental disorder and to underestimate contextual and personal factors that may contribute to the outcome (Fletcher et al., 2021). Related to this problem are two further common misunderstandings. Many interpersonal conflicts are based on different notions about what has been said or done. Current sociological and communication research stresses the point that communication is not just a message from A to B. Communicative messages are co-constructed by both sender and receiver (Clark & Brennan, 1991; Hall et al., 2019; Kessler, 2013). This means that a communicative *'message'* is encoded by A and has to be decoded by B. This includes verbal speech alongside nonverbal cues such as body language, facial expression, gestures, vocal pitch, and tone. Equal to, or even more important than the sender's intentions, is the receiver's perception and interpretation of the sender and their message. Therefore, the verbal and nonverbal presentation of staff to the patient is highly important.

It must be cautioned at this stage that both staff and patients may fall into the trap of self-fulfilling prophecies. When I, as a mental health worker, have had experience with specific patients who are not able to comply with nonviolent interventions, I might be reluctant to apply them next time. The opposite is also true: when I, as a patient, have had only bad or even victimising experiences during my previous admissions, I will expect that the next nurse I encounter will also behave like that, regardless of how they actually behave. Friendly or therapeutically positive signals viewed through this lens may be interpreted by the patient as a *'trick'*.

As mental health workers who try to de-escalate interpersonal tensions, we have, therefore, to be aware that our bodies are communicating our emotions and feelings, regardless of what we are trying to express verbally. Facial expressions, gestures and other aspects of body language that can be observed by others make it impossible not to communicate (Watzlawick et al., 2017). Therefore, the most important task in this regard is to know what we look like when we are heightened emotionally due to interpersonal conflict. As we normally do not walk in front of a mirror during a dispute with our partner, most of us do not know what kind of body language we present to others.

Role plays recorded on video may give the first impression of what our body reveals to others. Some mental health hospitals are now using body-worn cameras to record de-escalation to support staff reflection and learning (Wilson et al., 2022). While trying to master our body language, the next task is to avoid incongruent impressions towards the other party in the conflict (Stevenson, 1991). Our body language should give the same message as our verbal communication. If verbal and nonverbal channels contradict, an observer will most likely regard the nonverbal expression as 'true' and the verbal signals as faked. Furthermore, incongruent messaging has been shown to increase distress in other healthcare contexts (Gorawara-Bhat et al., 2017). Nevertheless, although nonverbal cues arise naturally and automatically, it is possible to suppress or alter their expression (Ekman, 1997).

The goal of nonverbal communication displayed during de-escalation is to give the distressed interacting partner a feeling of comfort and safety. Details of nonverbal communication depend on the (multi-)cultural settings and the ethnic origins of all the people involved. Staff have to be aware that some aspects of nonverbal communication are culture-bound. Nonverbal behaviour is likely to lead to misunderstandings on both sides. Thus, the following recommendations, which are thought to be effective on the European continent in general, have to be considered carefully when translated into local mental health settings. These recommendations are largely based on research exploring patient and staff perceptions of what communication is effective rather than analysis of what works in practice.

In line with our verbal communication, body language should minimise threats and give a clear signal of openness about the patient's concerns. The calm, gentle and soft tone of voice alongside tactful and sensitive language should be used (Price & Baker, 2012). Hand and arm gestures are a powerful vehicle to provide signals of threat. Lowered, uncrossed arms with open hands show that we are not aggressive (Troisi, 1999). A relaxed appearance is also presented through body posture, of the head and the gaze of the eyes (Bannerman et al., 2009; Troisi, 1999). An upright position of the head, combined with subtle tilts to the left and right may induce the observation that one is interested in the other person and actively listening (Price & Baker, 2012). Active or empathic listening is further supported by head nodding and maintaining eye contact without staring. All gestures should be slow and gentle. Sudden movements toward another person may be regarded as an attack (Troisi, 1999) and should be avoided. Sufficient spatial distance should also be provided (see Sect. 4).

Although nonverbal communication plays an important role in the management of interpersonal conflict in mental health care, mastering these features is not trivial. Having an awareness of your communicative signals and an understanding of how they might be perceived by others is a great first step but may not necessarily lead to an adequate use of techniques in practice. Artificial manipulations of nonverbal signals (e.g. facial expressions) may end up sending mixed messages because basic emotions and associated expressions are difficult to mask. Professional stage actors can surely talk about this problem. However, studies beyond mental health settings have shown body language may be one factor in preventing assaults, as it affects perceptions of vulnerability and submissiveness (Blaskovits & Bennell, 2019). More successful than just manipulating one's expression is changing the thinking about conflicts and their solutions. Thus, technique alone doesn't make for successful conflict management; stress management and basic conflict management rules (see Sect. 4) are equally important.

## 7    Situation-Intervention-Rationale: A Clinical Example of De-Escalation Practice

The purpose of this final section is to assimilate the key themes presented in this chapter and apply them to a clinical example. Here a description of each stage in the de-escalation process is provided detailing three important aspects of information at each stage:

- **The situation**: the scenario context and the behaviour of the patient and staff.
- **The intervention:** the actions employed by the staff to actively de-escalate the patient.
- **The rationale**: the beliefs and assumptions that underpin the actions taken by staff.

The clinical example used here is adapted from Berring et al. (2016b, p. 501). To summarise the scenario, the patient felt cheated because staff members forgot to take him to the fitness room. The patient responded by entering the dining room, pulling down his trousers and 'mooning' at the other patients. He expected to be subjected to physical interventions and was surprised when a staff member instead helped him gain control by stating that she understood his frustration and worked with him to achieve his goal through a compromised approach.

### 7.1    Situation Part 1

Tristan was irritable and upset because staff members forgot to take him to the fitness room, as they usually would. It was a busy shift and the staff simply forgot. When staff saw Tristan at lunchtime, he appeared tense and irritable.

Staff called Tristan and the other patients to dinner. When they were entering the dining area, Tristan entered and responded by pulling down his trousers and 'mooning' at the other patients. Some of the patients told Tristan to stop, asking the staff to intervene. Tristan stated, 'If my will doesn't count for anything I don't care, even if they put me in mechanical restraints…'.

**Principles of Intervention**

Respect personal space and pay attention to the patient's needs. Observation and early intervention.

Attention to angry and aggressive behaviour manifested by the patient.

Focus on preventive measures instead of behaviour management measures intervening as early as possible, (prevention in early stages, always).

**Rationale**

Minimisation of angry behaviours and ineffective limit setting are the most frequent factors contributing to the escalation of behaviour and violence.

Respecting personal space is key to assessing and implementing de-escalation measures.

## 7.2    Situation Part 2

The nurse who was in the dining area, approached Tristan and asked him, 'Could I invite you to come with me to somewhere more private so we can have a chat and try to understand why you are upset?'

Tristan hesitated for a moment but then followed the nurse to a space known as a 'comfort room'.

**Principles of Intervention**

Assess the therapeutic milieu.

Ensure safe conditions for de-escalation.

Suggest the patient accompanies a professional to a space that guarantees privacy.

**Rationale**

Pay attention to the therapeutic milieu or service environment:

- Choose a quiet place or a comfort room, but one that is visible to staff. When going to this space, always let others know that you are there with the patient, leaving the door open.
- Have other staff members nearby.
- Ensure you, and the patient, can exit quickly if necessary.
- The angrier the patient, the more space needed to feel comfortable (pay attention to the communication being displayed and the physical distance between you and the patient).
- Ask how you can help the patient.
- Never turn your back on an angry patient.
- Leave immediately if there are signs that behaviour is escalating beyond what is manageable

## 7.3 Situation Part 3

The nurse, adopted a comforting and quiet posture and, engaging with Tristan, asked him, *'Do you want to sit down and speak about what has happened?'*

Tristan hesitated for a moment and said, 'I think that I prefer to stay on my feet'.

Nurse: 'Okay Tristan, but I'm going to sit down. It is more comfortable if you sit…'.

Tristan agreed and sat down.

Nurse: 'I felt that you were tense and irritable… Is something bothering or concerning you at the moment?'

### Principles of Intervention

Focus on your own emotions (self-awareness): Appear calm and in control.

Position in the room: If the patient agrees, both nurse and patient should sit at a 45-degree angle.

Attention to non-verbal communication: Do not tower over or stare at the patient.

Use clarification with the patient: When he begins to talk, listen actively.

Manage silences in the interaction and let the patient talk without interrupting.

### Rationale

The perception that someone is in control of the situation can be comforting and calming to an individual who is beginning to lose control of managing their emotions/behaviours.

Sitting at a 45-degree angle puts you both on the same level but allows for frequent breaks in eye contact. Towering over or staring can be interpreted as threatening or controlling by paranoid individuals.

Clarification and active listening allow patients to feel heard and understood. It helps build rapport, and energy can be channelled productively.

## 7.4 Situation Part 4

Tristan said, 'The only thing that I ask every day is to go to the fitness room for a bit and today no one remembers it.'

The nurse calmly said, 'You are right, I am sorry we didn't tell you about this earlier, but today we were very busy. I know this is not a reason. Can I help you see how we can get you to the fitness room some other way'.

**Principles of Intervention**
Understand the patient's perspective and respect the interaction: Listen to the patient even if they are yelling.
Use a non-provocative and non-judgmental approach with the patient.

**Rationale**

Behaviour generates behaviour:

- Loudly arguing with the patient will only escalate anger and violence.
- When the tone of voice is low and calm and the words are spoken slowly, anxiety levels in others may decrease.

## 7.5    Situation Part 5

Nurse: 'What do you think would help now since it was not possible to take you to go to the fitness room?'

**Principles of Intervention**
Displaying empathy and genuineness is a way of being present and engaged in the intervention (e.g. 'I'm here for you'):
Do not treat the individual in a humiliating manner.
Give back control (e.g. 'what will help now?')

**Rationale**

Even patients with more severe psychopathology may respond to non-provocative interpersonal contact and genuine expressions of concern and caring.

## 7.6    Situation Part 6

Tristan said, 'I don't know because the only thing that I wanted to do was go to the fitness room…'.
Nurse: 'I understand your frustration, your anger, but it's not ok to moon the other patients, do you agree… If you need help controlling those feelings we could help at any time'.

### Principles of Intervention

Align expectations: clear, consistent, and enforceable expectations about behaviour (e.g. empathise with feelings and emotions and not with behaviours: 'It's okay to be angry, but it is not okay to threaten him'.)

Offer help and availability to the patient: 'if you are having trouble controlling your anger we will help you'.

### Rationale

Gives the patient a better understanding of the expectations and consequences of not adhering to those limits on behaviour (i.e. empathise with emotions and not behaviours).

## 7.7    Situation Part 6

Nurse: 'Next time, do you think that it would be possible for you to approach us and ask us to remember that you want to go to the fitness room? If it's not possible could we negotiate another time of the day to go to the fitness room? For instance, how do you feel about going to the fitness room in the evening? Another important aspect is to do that without 'mooning' other patients... Do you think that is also possible? If not, try to imagine yourself in the other patients' place, and imagine yourself being mooned when they don't have something that they want...'.

Tristan thinks about the nurse's suggestions and agrees.

Tristan: 'Okay, since the staff cannot go with me to the fitness room now, the evening seems fine'.

Both parties apologise for what has happened and Tristan returns to dinner.

### Principles of Intervention

Acknowledge the patient's needs

Listen to a patient's expressed needs, regardless of whether they are rational or irrational.

Give choices: Suggest other options and work with the patient to identify one that suits both.

### Rationale

This contributes to the individual's perception that the nurse is trying to understand, and tries to understand the reason at the core of their behaviour. Determine how some of the patient's needs can be met productively.

Evaluating the incidents helps staff and patients to learn what caused the situation and learn how to prevent this in the future.

# 8    Conclusions

De-escalation is often an individual technique, scaffolded by team efforts aiming to meet patients' needs while protecting both patients and staff against physical and psychological injuries. Although de-escalation remains an under-researched area, there have been positive steps forward and de-escalation is now a central feature of many current complex models of care (e.g. Safewards). De-escalation is an important tool for mental health workers who stand between two dangers: using too much force or doing nothing when faced with violent behaviour. Good de-escalation skills help staff to cope actively with difficult situations without using physical force.

## References

Alpert, J. E., & Spillmann, M. K. (1997). Psychotherapeutic approaches to aggressive and violent patients. *Psychiatric Clinics of North America, 20*(2), 453–472.

Anderson, C. A., & Bushman, B. J. (2002). Human aggression. *Annual Review of Psychology, 53*(1), 27–51.

Asikainen, J., Vehviläinen-Julkunen, K., Repo-Tiihonen, E., & Louheranta, O. (2023). Use of debriefing following restrictive practices in forensic psychiatric care. *The Journal of Forensic Practice, 25*(1), 46–56.

Bannerman, R. L., Milders, M., De Gelder, B., & Sahraie, A. (2009). Orienting to threat: Faster localization of fearful facial expressions and body postures revealed by saccadic eye movements. *Proceedings of the Royal Society B: Biological Sciences, 276*(1662), 1635–1641.

Beattie, J., Innes, K., Griffiths, D., & Morphet, J. (2018). Healthcare providers' neurobiological response to workplace violence perpetrated by consumers: Informing directions for staff Well-being. *Applied Nursing Research, 43*, 42–48.

Benson, A., Secker, J., Balfe, E., Lipsedge, M., Robinson, S., & Walker, J. (2003). Discourses of blame: Accounting for aggression and violence on an acute mental health inpatient unit. *Social Science & Medicine, 57*(5), 917–926.

Berring, L. L., Hummelvoll, J. K., Pedersen, L., & Buus, N. (2016a). A co-operative inquiry into generating, describing, and transforming knowledge about de-escalation practices in mental health settings. *Issues in Mental Health Nursing, 37*(7), 451–463.

Berring, L. L., Pedersen, L., & Buus, N. (2016b). Coping with violence in mental health care settings: Patient and staff member perspectives on de-escalation practices. *Archives of Psychiatric Nursing, 30*(5), 499–507.

Blaskovits, B., & Bennell, C. (2019). Are we revealing hidden aspects of our personality when we walk? *Journal of Nonverbal Behavior, 43*, 329–356.

Bowers L. (2009). Association between staff factors and levels of conflict and containment on acute psychiatric wards in England. *Psychiatric services. 60*(2), 231–239.

Bowers, L. (2014). A model of de-escalation. *Mental Health Practice, 17*(9), 36–37.

Bowers, L., Alexander, J., Bilgin, H., Botha, M., Dack, C., James, K., et al. (2014). Safewards: The empirical basis of the model and a critical appraisal. *Journal of Psychiatric and Mental Health Nursing, 21*(4), 354–364.

Bowers, L., James, K., Quirk, A., Simpson, A., Stewart, D., & Hodsoll, J. (2015). Reducing conflict and containment rates on acute psychiatric wards: The Safewards cluster randomised controlled trial. *International Journal of Nursing Studies, 52*(9), 1412–1422. https://doi.org/10.1016/j.ijnurstu.2015.05.001

Bowers, L., Stewart, D., Papadopoulos, C., Dack, C., Ross, J., Khanom, H., et al. (2011). *Inpatient violence and aggression: A literature* (Report from the Conflict and Containment Reduction Research Programme, Kings College, London).

Burton, J. W. (1997). Violence explained: The sources of conflict, violence and crime and their prevention. Manchester University Press.

Clark, H. H., & Brennan, S. E. (1991). Grounding in communication. In *Perspectives on socially shared cognition* (pp. 127–149). American Psychological Association.

d'Ettorre, G., & Pellicani, V. (2017). Workplace violence toward mental healthcare workers employed in psychiatric wards. *Safety and Health at Work, 8*(4), 337–342.

Davidson, J., & Wood, C. (2004). A conflict resolution model. *Theory Into Practice, 43*(1), 6–13.

De Dreu, C. K. (2003). Time pressure and closing of the mind in negotiation. *Organizational Behavior and Human Decision Processes, 91*(2), 280–295.

De Gelder, B. (2009). Why bodies? Twelve reasons for including bodily expressions in affective neuroscience. *Philosophical Transactions of the Royal Society B: Biological Sciences, 364*(1535), 3475–3484.

Delaney, K. R., & Johnson, M. E. (2006). Keeping the unit safe: Mapping psychiatric nursing skills. *Journal of the American Psychiatric Nurses Association, 12*(4), 198–207.

DelBel, J. C. (2003). De-escalating workplace aggression. *Nursing Management, 34*(9), 30–34.

Donohue, W. A. (2003). The promise of an interaction-based approach to negotiation. *International Journal of Conflict Management, 14*(3/4), 167–176.

Duperouzel, H. (2008). It's OK for people to feel angry' the exemplary management of imminent aggression. *Journal of Intellectual Disabilities, 12*(4), 295–307.

Dutschmann, A. (2000). *Verhaltenssteuerung bei aggressiven Kindern und Jugendlichen* (Manual zum Typ A des ABPro'). DGVT.

Dutschmann, A. (2003). *Aggressionen und Konflikte unter emotionaler Erregung: Deeskalation und Problemlösung (Das Aggressions-Bewältigungs-Programm ABPro)*. DGVT-Verlag.

Duxbury, J., & Whittington, R. (2005). Causes and management of patient aggression and violence: Staff and patient perspectives. *Journal of Advanced Nursing, 50*(5), 469–478.

Ekman, P. (1997). Expression or communication about emotion. In *Uniting psychology and biology: Integrative perspectives on human development* (pp. 315–338). American Psychological Association.

Engström, I., Engström, K., & Sellin, T. (2020). Adolescents' experiences of the Staff's different interaction styles in coercive youth Care in Sweden: A qualitative study. *Issues in Mental Health Nursing, 41*(11), 1027–1037. https://doi.org/10.1080/01612840.2020.1757794

Fauteux, K. (2010). De-escalating angry and violent clients. *American Journal of Psychotherapy, 64*(2), 195–213.

Fernández, V., Gausereide-Corral, M., Valiente, C., & Sánchez-Iglesias, I. (2023). Effectiveness of trauma-informed care interventions at the organizational level: A systematic review. *Psychological Services, 20*(4), 849–862.

Fletcher, A., Crowe, M., Manuel, J., & Foulds, J. (2021). Comparison of patients' and staff's perspectives on the causes of violence and aggression in psychiatric inpatient settings: An integrative review. *Journal of Psychiatric and Mental Health Nursing, 28*(5), 924–939.

Gable, P. A., Poole, B. D., & Harmon-Jones, E. (2015). Anger perceptually and conceptually narrows cognitive scope. *Journal of Personality and Social Psychology, 109*(1), 163.

Gaynes, B. N., Brown, C. L., Lux, L. J., Brownley, K. A., Van Dorn, R. A., Edlund, M. J., et al. (2017). Preventing and de-escalating aggressive behavior among adult psychiatric patients: A systematic review of the evidence. *Psychiatric Services, 68*(8), 819–831.

Gertz, B. (1980). Training for prevention of assaultive behavior in a psychiatric setting. *Psychiatric Services, 31*(9), 628–630.

Gorawara-Bhat, R., Hafskjold, L., Gulbrandsen, P., & Eide, H. (2017). Exploring physicians' verbal and nonverbal responses to cues/concerns: Learning from incongruent communication. *Patient Education and Counseling, 100*(11), 1979–1989.

Hall, J. A., Horgan, T. G., & Murphy, N. A. (2019). Nonverbal communication. *Annual Review of Psychology, 70*, 271–294.

Hallett, N., & Dickens, G. L. (2015). De-escalation: A survey of clinical staff in a secure mental health inpatient service. *International Journal of Mental Health Nursing, 24*(4), 324–333.

Hallett, N., & Dickens, G. L. (2017). De-escalation of aggressive behaviour in healthcare settings: Concept analysis. *International Journal of Nursing Studies, 75*, 10–20.

Haugvaldstad, M. J., & Husum, T. L. (2016). Influence of staff's emotional reactions on the escalation of patient aggression in mental health care. *International Journal of Law and Psychiatry, 49*, 130–137.

Huang, L. N., Flatow, R., Biggs, T., Afayee, S., Smith, K., Clark, T., et al. (2014). *SAMHSA's concept of truama and guidance for a trauma-informed approach*. https://ncsacw.acf.hhs.gov/userfiles/files/SAMHSA_Trauma.pdf

Huckshorn, K. A., CAP, I., & Director, N. (2006). *Six core strategies for reducing seclusion and restraint use*. https://www.nasmhpd.org/sites/default/files/Consolidated%20Six%20Core%20Strategies%20Document.pdf

Hvidhjelm, J., Berring, L. L., Whittington, R., Woods, P., Bak, J., & Almvik, R. (2023). Short-term risk assessment in the long term: A scoping review and meta-analysis of the Brøset Violence Checklist (BVC). *Journal of Psychiatric and Mental Health Nursing, 30*(4), 637–648.

Johnson, J., Panagioti, M., Bass, J., Ramsey, L., & Harrison, R. (2017). Resilience to emotional distress in response to failure, error or mistakes: A systematic review. *Clinical Psychology Review, 52*, 19–42.

Johnson, M. E., & Delaney, K. R. (2007). Keeping the unit safe: The anatomy of escalation. *Journal of the American Psychiatric Nurses Association, 13*(1), 42–52.

Johnston, I., Price, O., McPherson, P., Armitage, C. J., Brooks, H., Bee, P., et al. (2022). De-escalation of conflict in forensic mental health inpatient settings: A Theoretical Domains Framework-informed qualitative investigation of staff and patient perspectives. *BMC Psychology, 10*(1), 1–17.

Keesler, J. M. (2020). Promoting satisfaction and reducing fatigue: Understanding the impact of trauma-informed organizational culture on psychological wellness among Direct Service Providers. *Journal of Applied Research in Intellectual Disabilities, 33*(5), 939–949.

Kessler, G. (2013). Collaborative language learning in co-constructed participatory culture. *CALICO Journal, 30*(3), 307–322.

Lavelle, M., Stewart, D., James, K., Richardson, M., Renwick, L., Brennan, G., et al. (2016). Predictors of effective de-escalation in acute inpatient psychiatric settings. *Journal of Clinical Nursing, 25*(15–16), 2180–2188.

Lindsay, J. J., & Anderson, C. A. (2000). From antecedent conditions to violent actions: A general affective aggression model. *Personality and Social Psychology Bulletin, 26*(5), 533–547.

Mehrabian, A., & Ferris, S. R. (1967). Inference of attitudes from nonverbal communication in two channels. *Journal of Consulting Psychology, 31*(3), 248.

Mehrabian, A., & Wiener, M. (1967). Decoding of inconsistent communications. *Journal of Personality and Social Psychology, 6*(1), 109.

Miller, N., Pedersen, W. C., Earleywine, M., & Pollock, V. E. (2003). A theoretical model of triggered displaced aggression. *Personality and Social Psychology Review, 7*(1), 75–97.

Muskett, C. (2014). Trauma-informed care in inpatient mental health settings: A review of the literature. *International Journal of Mental Health Nursing, 23*(1), 51–59.

Nay, W. R. (2004). *Taking charge of anger: How to resolve conflict, sustain relationships, and express yourself without losing control*. Guilford Press.

Nijman, H. L., Allertz, W. F., Merckelbach, H. L., & Ravelli, D. P. (1997). Aggressive behaviour on an acute psychiatric admissions ward. *The European Journal of Psychiatry, 11*(2), 106–114.

Nijman, H. L., Muris, P., Merckelbach, H. L., Palmstierna, T., Wistedt, B., Vos, A., et al. (1999). The staff observation aggression scale–revised (SOAS-R). *Aggressive Behavior, 25*(3), 197–209.

Omer, H. (2001). Helping parents deal with children's acute disciplinary problems without escalation: The principle of nonviolent resistance. *Family Process, 40*(1), 53–66.

Omer, H. (2021). *Non-violent resistance: A new approach to violent and self-destructive children*. Cambridge University Press.

Papadopoulos, C., Bowers, L., Quirk, A., & Khanom, H. (2012a). Events preceding changes in conflict and containment rates on acute psychiatric wards. *Psychiatric Services, 63*(1), 40–47.

Papadopoulos, C., Ross, J., Stewart, D., Dack, C., James, K., & Bowers, L. (2012b). The antecedents of violence and aggression within psychiatric in-patient settings. *Acta Psychiatrica Scandinavica, 125*(6), 425–439.

Paterson, B., & Leadbetter, D. (1999). De-escalation in the management of aggression and violence: Towards evidence-based practice. In *Aggression and violence: Approaches to effective management* (pp. 95–123). Springer.

Potthoff, S., Gather, J., Hempeler, C., Gieselmann, A., & Scholten, M. (2022). "Voluntary in quotation marks": a conceptual model of psychological pressure in mental healthcare based on a grounded theory analysis of interviews with service users. *BMC psychiatry, 22*(1), 186.

Price, O., & Baker, J. (2012). Key components of de-escalation techniques: A thematic synthesis. *International Journal of Mental Health Nursing, 21*(4), 310–319.

Price, O., Baker, J., Bee, P., Grundy, A., Scott, A., Butler, D., et al. (2018). Patient perspectives on barriers and enablers to the use and effectiveness of de-escalation techniques for the management of violence and aggression in mental health settings. *Journal of Advanced Nursing, 74*(3), 614–625.

Price, O., Baker, J., Bee, P., & Lovell, K. (2015). Learning and performance outcomes of mental health staff training in de-escalation techniques for the management of violence and aggression. *The British Journal of Psychiatry, 206*(6), 447–455.

Reiss, A., & Roth, J. (1993). *Understanding and preventing violence: Panel on the understanding and control of violent behavior.* National Academy Press.

Renwick, L., Lavelle, M., Brennan, G., Stewart, D., James, K., Richardson, M., et al. (2016). Physical injury and workplace assault in UK mental health trusts: An analysis of formal reports. *International Journal of Mental Health Nursing, 25*(4), 355–366. https://doi.org/10.1111/inm.12201

Riahi, S., Dawe, I. C., Stuckey, M. I., & Klassen, P. E. (2016). Implementation of the six core strategies for restraint minimization in a specialized mental health organization. *Journal of psychosocial nursing and mental health services, 54*(10), 32–39.

Richmond, J. S., Berlin, J. S., Fishkind, A. B., Holloman, G. H., Jr., Zeller, S. L., Wilson, M. P., et al. (2012). Verbal de-escalation of the agitated patient: Consensus statement of the American Association for Emergency Psychiatry Project BETA De-escalation Workgroup. *Western Journal of Emergency Medicine, 13*(1), 17.

Roter, D. L., Frankel, R. M., Hall, J. A., & Sluyter, D. (2006). The expression of emotion through nonverbal behavior in medical visits: Mechanisms and outcomes. *Journal of General Internal Medicine, 21*, 28–34.

Schellenberg, J. A. (1996). *Conflict resolution: Theory, research, and practice.* Suny Press.

Scott, Z., O'Curry, S., & Mastroyannopoulou, K. (2022). The impact and experience of debriefing for clinical staff following traumatic events in clinical settings: A systematic review. *Journal of Traumatic Stress, 35*(1), 278–287.

Siegrist, K., Rödel, A., & Siegrist, J. (2003). A theory-based study on psychosocial workload as an instrument of health promotion in a hospital. *Gesundheitswesen (Bundesverband der Arzte des Offentlichen Gesundheitsdienstes (Germany)), 65*(11), 612–619.

Slade, M., Amering, M., Farkas, M., Hamilton, B., O'Hagan, M., Panther, G., et al. (2014). Uses and abuses of recovery: Implementing recovery-oriented practices in mental health systems. *World Psychiatry, 13*(1), 12–20.

Slade, M., Rennick-Egglestone, S., Blackie, L., Llewellyn-Beardsley, J., Franklin, D., Hui, A., et al. (2019). Post-traumatic growth in mental health recovery: qualitative study of narratives. *BMJ open, 9*(6), e029342.

Stevenson, S. (1991). *Heading off violence with verbal de-escalation.* SLACK Incorporated.

Stubbs, B., & Dickens, G. (2008). Prevention and management of aggression in mental health: An interdisciplinary discussion. *International Journal of Therapy and Rehabilitation, 15*(8), 351–357.

Troisi, A. (1999). Ethological research in clinical psychiatry: The study of nonverbal behavior during interviews. *Neuroscience & Biobehavioral Reviews, 23*(7), 905–913.

Turner, J. H. (2002). *Face to face: Toward a sociological theory of interpersonal behavior.* Stanford University Press.

Ulrich, R. S., Bogren, L., Gardiner, S. K., & Lundin, S. (2018). Psychiatric ward design can reduce aggressive behavior. *Journal of Environmental Psychology, 57*, 53–66.

US Department of Health and Human Services. (2014). SAMHSA's concept of trauma and guidance for a traumainformed approach.

Van Kleef, G. A., De Dreu, C. K., & Manstead, A. S. (2004). The interpersonal effects of emotions in negotiations: A motivated information processing approach. *Journal of Personality and Social Psychology, 87*(4), 510.

Wampole, D. M., & Bressi, S. K. (2019). Exploring strategies for promoting trauma-informed care and reducing burnout in acute care psychiatric nursing. *Journal of Nursing Education and Practice, 9*(5), 110.

Watzlawick, P., Beavin, J., & Jackson, D. (2017). Some tentative axioms of communication. In *Communication theory* (pp. 74–80). Routledge.

Whittington, R., & Richter, D. (2005). Interactional aspects of violent behaviour on acute psychiatric wards. *Psychology, Crime & Law, 11*(4), 377–388.

Whittington, R., & Wykes, T. (1996). Aversive stimulation by staff and violence by psychiatric patients. *British Journal of Clinical Psychology, 35*(1), 11–20.

Wilson, K., Eaton, J., Foye, U., Ellis, M., Thomas, E., & Simpson, A. (2022). What evidence supports the use of body worn cameras in mental health inpatient wards? A systematic review and narrative synthesis of the effects of body worn cameras in public sector services. *International Journal of Mental Health Nursing, 31*(2), 260–277.

Woods, P., & Almvik, R. (2002). The Brøset violence checklist (BVC). *Acta Psychiatrica Scandinavica, 106*, 103–105.

World Health Organization. (2017). *Strategies to end seclusion and restraint: WHO QualityRights specialized training.* https://iris.who.int/bitstream/handle/10665/329605/9789241516754-eng.pdf?sequence=1

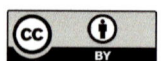

# Pharmacological Approaches for Managing Inpatient Aggression

Lisa A. Mistler, John A. Baker, and Adriana Mihai

## 1   Introduction

Agitation and aggression in psychiatry have a multitude of potential causes. Some underlying causes may be internal to the patient, such as having a comorbid medical illness or substance use, and some causes may be external, such as being in a noisy, crowded or confusing environment or having a difficult interpersonal interaction with others. Prevention of aggression is paramount and cannot be overemphasised. However, when prevention fails, ideal treatment should involve and include patients as partners as early in the process as possible, for ethical reasons as outlined in other chapters, as well as to minimise the risk of harm to patients and others.

Dr. Mistler is supported by the Health Resources and Services Administration (HRSA) of the US Department of Health and Human Services (HHS) as part of an award T32HP32520 totalling $2,496,422 (2021–2026) with 0% financed with non-governmental sources. The contents are those of the author(s) and do not necessarily represent the official views of, nor an endorsement by, HRSA, HHS or the US Government.

L. A. Mistler (✉)
Geisel School of Medicine, Hanover, NH, USA

Dartmouth-Hitchcock Medical Center, Lebanon, NH, USA
e-mail: lisa.a.mistler@hitchcock.org

J. A. Baker
Leeds and York Partnership NHS Foundation Trust, Leeds, UK

School of Healthcare, University of Leeds, Leeds, UK
e-mail: j.baker@leeds.ac.uk

A. Mihai
Psychiatric Department, University of Medicine, Pharmacy, Science and Technology George Emil Palade, Targu Mures, Romania

Institute of Psychotherapy and Personal Development (IPPD), Tirgu Mures, Romania
e-mail: adriana.mihai@umfst.ro

© The Author(s) 2024
N. Hallett et al. (eds.), *Coercion and Violence in Mental Health Settings*,
https://doi.org/10.1007/978-3-031-61224-4_16

Several treatment approaches regarding inpatient aggressive behaviour exist, including psychopharmacological and behavioural methods (Bak et al., 2019). Specific brain circuits have been proposed to underlie aggressive behaviour, particularly the amygdala, limbic prefrontal regions and the connection between the two (Aleyasin et al., 2018). Additionally, multiple neurotransmitters, including serotonin and dopamine, have been hypothesised to be involved, based on animal and human models of aggression (Yanowitch & Coccaro, 2011). Given the magnitude of the problem and the limitations of our knowledge, a broad range of medications has been investigated for anti-aggressive properties (Bak et al., 2019). However, despite the high prevalence of the use of medications to address psychiatric inpatient aggression, evidence for the efficacy of the pharmacological management of aggressive behaviour is currently lacking (Gaynes et al., 2017).

In this chapter, we begin with a brief overview of medication use in psychiatric emergencies. We then concisely describe the neurobiology, neurophysiology and anatomy of aggression. Subsequently, we summarise recent systematic reviews, meta-analyses and national guidelines addressing the pharmacotherapy of aggression in general adult psychiatry. We conclude the chapter with a description of the experience of rapid tranquillisation written by a person with lived experience and make recommendations for the conduct of future research.

In this chapter, the person with lived experience was not involved in the writing of the rest of the chapter. However, their balanced description of their experiences, at the end of the chapter, reflects many of the key points raised. They state that it is not unreasonable to become agitated when one has lost some rights and freedoms, and that with a well-trained and led staff, giving the person space can result in them calming themselves without need for medication. Further they state that prn meds and rapid tranquillisation should be used only in the most extreme situations, once all other options have been tried, and that the use of such methods should be well-thought-out and reasoned. We are grateful for their contribution.

## 2  Overview of Medication Use in Psychiatric Emergencies

Using pharmacologic agents to reduce acute agitation in patients living with psychiatric illnesses remains controversial because they are often given without a patient's consent. When parenteral, rather than oral, medication is used (Hirsch & Steinert, 2019; Kim et al., 2021), this practice is sometimes called 'rapid tranquillisation' (RT) (Zareifopoulos & Panayiotakopoulos, 2019). RT should be reserved only for patients in acute distress who are agitated, combative or otherwise at risk for violent behaviour *and* unable to engage in or benefit from de-escalation attempts. The indication for immediate intervention such as RT is that there is a high potential risk to the patient and others around them. Clinicians should maintain awareness that RT may be harmful as it could lead to undesirable medical or psychological side effects and legal conflicts and could undermine the clinician–patient relationship. Deciding whether or not to use RT must also take into account the patient's underlying psychiatric illness(es) and physical health status, as well as the need for timely resolution of the situation, due to the emergent risk of harm to the patient or others. As such, all clinicians should be familiar with available RT options, the side effects associated with each, the duration of action, routes of administration and the empirical evidence regarding their use in such a setting (Zareifopoulos & Panayiotakopoulos, 2019). Furthermore, the legal and ethical conditions under which RT may be implemented differ from country to country, and because there is limited evidence regarding the efficacy of specific agents, is largely dependent on clinical judgement and what medications are available (Hirsch & Steinert, 2019).

## 3     Neurobiology of Aggression

The literature proposes that violence is a heterogeneous behavioural response to the interpretation of environmental stimuli and threats, a response that is also influenced by the social, neurobiological and environmental context of the individual (Manchia et al., 2020). Current knowledge suggests that reactive and proactive violence depends on the activation of different brain circuits and neurotransmitter systems (Romero-Martínez et al., 2022). Among them, the more solid evidence points towards the serotonin (5-HT) system in terms of changes in 5-HT levels and 5-HT receptor function, but also genetic and epigenetic modifications at the level of the enzymes involved in the synthesis, degradation and/or reuptake of 5-HT (Pavlov et al., 2012; Romero-Martínez et al., 2022). However, no definitive predictive biomarkers of violent behaviour have yet been identified (Manchia et al., 2020; Pinna & Manchia, 2017). For this reason, future studies in large and controlled clinical and community populations examining genetic and epigenetic markers as well as behavioural-cognitive, brain imaging and metabolomics signatures of violence are needed (Caruso et al., 2021).

### 3.1     Neuroanatomy

Studies on the neuroanatomical substrates of aggression have proposed possible alterations in brain areas also involved with the formation of psychotic symptoms and affective regulation, including frontotemporal circuitry, the amygdala-orbitofrontal system, prefrontal cortex and hippocampus (Fjellvang et al., 2018; Manchia et al., 2017; Pompili et al., 2017; Widmayer et al., 2018, 2019). The corticolimbic network has been suggested to play an important role in aggression and violence, as the amygdala plays a key role in perceiving and interpreting threat stimuli in the surrounding environment (Manchia et al., 2020). This network represents the connection between brain areas in the cortical region, such as the anterior cingulate cortex (ACC), the prefrontal cortex (PFC) and the insula and amygdala.

### 3.2     Neurotransmitters

Several decades of preclinical and clinical research have demonstrated a central role for different neurotransmitters and neuromodulators in the neurobiology of violence. Biogenic amines including serotonin (5-HT), norepinephrine (NE), dopamine (DA), glutamate and GABA, as well as neuropeptides such as substance P, vasopressin and oxytocin, all appear to play a key modulating function in violent behaviour (Manchia et al., 2020). Multiple lines of evidence have shown dysfunction in the serotonin (5-HT) system in aggressive and in mentally ill subjects, with reduced 5-HT activity associated with depression as well as with impulsive aggression (Comai et al., 2016; Gowin et al., 2013). Central nervous 5-HT has been studied using challenge techniques; such techniques have been demonstrated to alter amygdala activity in response to threatening stimuli, or stimuli that may elicit violence. Responses from the amygdala then activate or dampen activity in the surrounding cortices; however, such responses differ, depending on the type of violence being exhibited (Manchia et al., 2020).

The contributing role of steroid hormones is another focus of recent research. In a multiple regression model including abuse/neglect history, psychopathy and impulsivity, baseline cortisol explained 58% of the variance in trait aggression (a chronic, long-standing personality characteristic) and 26% of the variance in state aggression (temporary, short-lasting outbursts of anger) (Gowin et al., 2013). These findings support the hypothesis that adverse childhood experiences may predict a reduced hypothalamus-pituitary-adrenal (HPA)-axis reactivity, leading to the possibility that a history of child maltreatment, psychopathy and an impaired HPA-axis reactivity might act synergistically in the production of aggressive behaviour (Haller et al., 2014; Toth et al., 2011). Recently, pathological appetitive aggression, in which positive feelings are associated with perpetrating violent behaviour, has been hypothesised to result from excessive activation of evolutionarily conserved reward circuits, also mediating the rewarding effects of addictive drugs (Golden & Shaham, 2018). The authors suggest that inappropriate appetitive aggression shares core features with addiction: aggression is often sought despite adverse consequences, and relapse rates among aggressive offenders are as high as relapse rates in drug addiction (Golden & Shaham, 2018). Pathological appetitive aggression is distinguished from defensive aggression, which is a fear response to a perceived threatening situation, and there are no positive feelings associated with the aggressive act.

## 3.3    Genetics

Several genes have been investigated to explore a possible correlation with aggressive behaviour. The most intensively studied is the catechol-O-methyltransferase (COMT) gene on chromosome 22. COMT is involved in the metabolism of dopamine, one of the neurotransmitters hypothesised to be involved in the production of the symptoms of schizophrenia. A meta-analysis involving 2370 individuals showed that male patients with schizophrenia who carried the low-activity methionine allele in the COMT gene had an increase in aggression risk of approximately 50% compared with homozygous valine patients (Singh et al., 2012). A more recent Swedish cohort study was concordant with the hypothesis that COMT genotypes modify the sensitivity to the environment that confers either risk (methionine allele) or protection (valine allele) for aggressive behaviour (Tuvblad et al., 2016).

## 4      Brief Review of Most Common Medications Used

There are various reasons why the evidence base for the most effective pharmacologic management of acute aggression is sparse. First, because of the potential dangers associated with violence, gold-standard randomised-controlled trials (RCTs), especially RCTs with large numbers of participants, evaluating new treatments, are few. Second, there is no consensus regarding outcome measures when treating violence, leading to considerable heterogeneity in existing studies. Thus, while neurotransmitters are the putative targets of pharmacologic treatment of aggression, current practice is still somewhat a matter of trial and error, with broad guidelines for classes of medications to use. In this section, we summarise the most commonly used types of medications, the ways that they are used, and describe systematic reviews and published guidelines for their use. Finally, based on these reviews and guidelines, we offer general recommendations for the use of psychopharmacologic agents in addressing acute aggression.

### 4.1      Benzodiazepines

Benzodiazepines are a class of medications used primarily as anxiolytics and soporifics; they are also used acutely to treat seizures. They facilitate the binding of GABA, an inhibitory neurotransmitter, throughout the central nervous system, essentially 'slowing down' activity in the brain. At lower doses, most benzodiazepines will cause some sedation, and at higher doses, can induce sleep. The differences between the various benzodiazepines are primarily in metabolism; longer-acting medications such as diazepam have half-lives between 40 and 250 h, intermediate-acting medications such as lorazepam have half-lives between 12 and 40 h, and shorter-acting medications such as midazolam have half-lives between 1 and 12 h (Griffin et al., 2013). Lorazepam is often used for rapid tranquillisation in part because of its safety profile; while several other benzodiazepines continue to have an effect in the body for up to days after administration, lorazepam has a relatively shorter time of effect, in particular with those who have liver disease. Lorazepam is available in injectable form (intravenous, or IV, and intramuscular, or IM), sublingual and in liquid or pill form.

### 4.2      Antipsychotic Medications

First- and second-generation neuroleptic medications, also called antipsychotic medications, belong to classes of medications that block dopamine receptors in the brain (first-generation) or combinations of dopamine and serotonin (second-generation). They are used to treat symptoms of psychosis, often in the context of schizophrenia, bipolar disorder and depression. They can be used acutely to treat mania and adjunctively in the treatment of bipolar disorder and major depression. The major difference between first- and second-generation antipsychotic medications is in their likelihood of causing certain side effects. First-generation medications are more likely to lead to movement disorders such as tardive dyskinesia and extrapyramidal symptoms. Second-generation medications, with a couple of exceptions, are more likely to lead to metabolic dysfunction—hyperlipidemia, weight gain and type II diabetes mellitus. In addition to pill and liquid forms, many antipsychotic medications are available for acute and long-acting intramuscular (IM) administration. While antipsychotic medications such as haloperidol are commonly used to manage acute agitation and aggression in psychiatric settings, the mechanism of action is unknown. Hypothetical mechanisms include sedation leading to the reduction of agitation, dopamine blockade leading to the reduction of underlying psychosis, and at higher doses, first-generation antipsychotic medications are similar in structure to GABA, thereby slowing brain activity (Wilson et al., 2012).

## 4.3    Anticholinergic and Antihistaminergic Medications

Anticholinergic and antihistaminergic medications such as benztropine and diphenhydramine are frequently used in the context of the management of aggression as adjunctive medication to antipsychotic medications in order to prevent or manage extrapyramidal symptoms, such as dystonia, akathisia and parkinsonism. They are sometimes used on their own to manage aggression, although the mechanism of action is primarily through sedation and reduction of involuntary muscle movement due to acetylcholine blockade. These medications can have side effects of sedation, dry mouth and blurred vision, among others. Many anticholinergic and antihistaminic medications are available in pill, liquid and IM form.

## 4.4    Additional Medications

Droperidol is a dopamine antagonist related to haloperidol that is used to prevent and treat postoperative nausea and vomiting. It has been used primarily in the ED as a sedative or tranquilliser via the IM or IV route in patients with acute agitation, as it has a more rapid onset and shorter duration of action than haloperidol. In 2001, the FDA issued a black box warning about the risk of QT prolongation, and the drug fell out of common use. However, two large retrospective studies showed no increase in mortality or morbidity for droperidol when used at doses of 5–10 mg (Perkins et al., 2015).

## 4.5    Summary of Systematic Reviews

In order to update their 2015 guidelines for the treatment of acute agitation, the National Institute of Health and Care Excellence (NICE) identified nine systematic reviews of medication comparisons (NICE, 2019). Of these, six were Cochrane Reviews, all of which included people with agitation in the context of psychosis. The only study citing high-quality evidence was by Khokhar and Rathbone (2016), in which they concluded that IM droperidol was more effective than placebo in achieving tranquillisation after 30 min, with comparable side effects to placebo. The remaining studies reported mostly low and low to medium quality evidence, largely due to problems with bias. The remaining studies are summarised in the following paragraph.

Haloperidol plus promethazine was reported as more effective at causing sedation at 30 min as compared to lorazepam or haloperidol alone, with no significant difference between the effects of haloperidol plus promethazine, ziprasidone or olanzapine (Huf et al., 2016). No difference was found regarding efficacy or adverse effects of IM risperidone versus IM haloperidol and IM olanzapine after 24 h; there was no difference between aripiprazole and haloperidol but aripiprazole required more injections to achieve sedation; and aripiprazole was more effective than placebo and less effective than olanzapine at 2 h post-IM (Ostinelli et al. 2017, 2018b, b). Another review concluded there was no significant difference between benzodiazepine, placebo or haloperidol IM in the short term, and in the medium term, benzodiazepine IM was more effective than placebo. Also, while there was no significant difference in the effectiveness of a benzodiazepine plus haloperidol versus either benzodiazepine or haloperidol alone in the short term, sedation was more likely in the group that received benzodiazepine plus haloperidol versus haloperidol alone (Zaman et al., 2017). One review found a difference between treatments: haloperidol plus promethazine, olanzapine and droperidol were the safest and most effective at reducing agitation within 2 h, although there were more adverse effects with haloperidol and haloperidol plus lorazepam (Bak et al., 2019). Neither of the two remaining papers showed any difference in efficacy or adverse effects of haloperidol, olanzapine, aripiprazole, loxapine and lorazepam IM (Dundar et al., 2016; Kousgaard et al., 2017).

## 4.6    Guidelines for the Pharmacotherapy of Aggression

In our efforts to compile the most up-to-date guidelines for the pharmacotherapy of aggression, we searched recent systematic reviews and meta-analyses, and hand-searched references from each to find listed guidelines (Bak et al., 2019; Cowman et al., 2017; Muir-Cochrane et al. 2020a, b; NICE, 2015, 2019; Roppolo et al., 2020). We selected guidelines for the pharmacologic management of aggression based on available research evidence when possible, and on consensus when research was limited. These guidelines were authored by experts from various regions, including North America, Europe, the UK and Latin America.

The 2005 *Expert Consensus Guidelines: Treatment of Behavioral Emergencies,* aimed at clinicians who work with clients who become aggressive or agitated, were derived from survey responses from 48 leading American experts on psychiatric emergency medicine (Allen et al., 2005). According to the guidelines, an ideal medication to treat agitation would be 'non-invasive and easy to administer, have a rapid onset, calm without sedating, address underlying symptoms and have a favourable tolerability and safety profile' (Allen et al., 2005; Martínez-Raga et al., 2018). In general, guidelines recommend initially assessing for any underlying medical cause of agitation and aggression and treating if possible (Garriga et al., 2016; Roppolo et al., 2020). Benzodiazepines are recommended for patients with undifferentiated agitation and aggression due to alcohol withdrawal, while antipsychotic medication is recommended for clients exhibiting psychotic symptoms and low-dose antipsychotics for delirious agitated patients (Roppolo et al., 2020).

The first International Experts' Meeting on Agitation in October 2016 in Madrid was attended by 20 experts from Europe and Latin America who had clinical experience managing acute agitation (Martínez-Raga et al., 2018). This group identified the lack of universal protocols or guidelines, lack of education and training of providers and limited available clinical data as considerable barriers to treating agitation properly. A poll of attendees found that antipsychotic medications were used more than 50% of the time, with benzodiazepines second most common. An increasing trend in the use of inhaled antipsychotic medications was noted, although their use was not yet widespread (Martínez-Raga et al., 2018). Most importantly, this group emphasised focusing on client-centred care and the service user experience, indicating that medication should be non-traumatic/non-coercive and that whenever possible, client preference should guide choice (Martínez-Raga et al., 2018). This group of international experts agreed that the ideal time to intervene with medications would be as early as possible in the cycle of increasing agitation, between the low-moderate to mid-moderate level of severity; however, they noted that client and caregiver preference was for pharmacologic intervention during mild agitation (Martínez-Raga et al., 2018). They concluded that the benefits of early intervention outweigh the risks, and strongly recommended this as a course of action (Martínez-Raga et al., 2018).

The National Institute for Health and Care Excellence (NICE) in the UK has written guidelines for short-term management of acute agitation in psychiatric settings that were developed by a multidisciplinary team of healthcare professionals, clients with a personal experience of aggressive behaviour, their caregivers and guideline methodologists (NICE, 2015). NICE performed a systematic review of rapid tranquillisation based on data from a series of Cochrane reviews (NICE, 2015) with permission from the publisher, and with assistance from the Cochrane Schizophrenia Group, into one review which was analysed according to the strategy in the review protocol. Their recommendations are to use lorazepam IM alone or with IM haloperidol plus IM promethazine for RT in adults (NICE, 2015). They state that the choice of medication should be driven by the service user's preferences, comorbid physical health issues, possible intoxication, previous response to medications, the potential for interactions with other medications and the total daily dose of medications that the person has taken (NICE, 2015).

## 5    Recommended Pharmacologic Strategies to Address Acute Aggression

### 5.1    Pro Re Nata (PRN) Medication

Oral and parenteral medications can be used as preventatives as well as for acute treatment of agitation and aggression. Often referred to as PRN (for the Latin term pro re nata, meaning 'as the circumstance arises'), such medications and their route of administration should be agreed upon in advance in collaboration with the patient

(McDougall et al., 2022). However, in practice, such medications are often prescribed routinely without consulting patients, as prophylaxis to prevent aggressive and violent incidents in hospitals (Mardani et al., 2022). Unfortunately, these can be used in a coercive manner—e.g. 'either you take this med or go into seclusion'—or to 'medicate' understandable behaviours that could be addressed through other means (McDougall et al., 2022). While the use of PRN medication is widespread in psychiatry, there is little evidence in the literature regarding its effectiveness (McDougall et al., 2022; Patel et al., 2019); this may be because performing randomised-controlled trials with this population for acute aggression is difficult.

Given the prevalence of PRN use, we present a summary of the NICE guidelines that have been written regarding prescribing PRN medication as part of a strategy to de-escalate or prevent situations that may lead to violence and aggression. NICE recommends that PRN medication should not be prescribed routinely or automatically on admission and should be individualised to the specific needs of the client after discussion with the client if possible. When PRN medication is prescribed, it should be clearly written in the care plan and the prescription itself under what circumstances it is to be offered, with specific intervals between doses, identifying the maximum daily dose. The NICE guidelines state that the maximum daily dose should not exceed that specified by the British National Formulary when combined with the person's standard dose or their dose for rapid tranquillisation and should be exceeded only if this is planned to achieve an agreed therapeutic goal, documented and carried out under the direction of a senior prescribing individual. Further, NICE recommends that the clinical team should review PRN medication at least once a week including a written rationale for continuation. If PRN medication has not been used since the last review, NICE recommends consideration of stopping (NICE, 2015).

## 5.2 Recommended Strategies for Pharmacotherapy in Acute Agitation

Rapid tranquillisation (RT) is defined as the administration of sedative medication by injection (Hirsch & Steinert, 2019; Zareifopoulos & Panayiotakopoulos, 2019). Most reviews describe a lack of sufficient evidence to support any particular approaches to treat aggression via medications, explaining that most studies remain descriptive or compare a small number of agents (de Almeida et al., 2017; de Souza et al., 2022; Hirsch et al., 2021). They also noted that reported outcomes were not consistent across studies, using a variety of measures and criteria. While there were differences in specific algorithms and recommendations between guidelines, there were some common principles. These included paying attention to the service user experience and working in partnership with service users and their carers, adopting approaches to care that respect service users' independence, choice and human rights, and increasing social inclusion by decreasing exclusionary practices, such as the use of seclusion. In the best of situations, a service user would be able to create an individualised pharmacological strategy to reduce the risk of, or address directly, violence and aggression. This would be in collaboration with a multidisciplinary team that develops the specific plan, with doses, timing, target symptoms and regular reviews of the plan, taking into account the service user's preferences and values (NICE, 2015). As there is no evidence showing clear superiority for any specific medication or combination, individualised treatment needs to be emphasised, taking into account the service user's view, pre-existing physical health problems, previous response to medications including adverse effects, the potential for interactions with other medications and the total daily dose of medications prescribed and administered (NICE, 2015). Per NICE guidelines, IM lorazepam is recommended for service users who have not taken antipsychotic medication before because it is an effective intervention that is likely to be acceptable to most people. Prescribing an initial, single dose ensures that any subsequent treatment options can be individualised, taking account of both response and any emergent adverse effects of the initial treatment choice (NICE, 2015).

The NICE (2015) algorithm recommends first taking into account the client's preference for medication and route of administration in the context of RT. If the client has no experience with antipsychotic medication, NICE recommends the use of lorazepam. If there is a partial response to lorazepam, consider another dose; if there is no response, consider IM haloperidol plus IM promethazine. If the client has a partial response to haloperidol plus promethazine, consider another dose if needed. If there is no response to IM haloperidol plus promethazine, consider IM lorazepam if that has not already been used. If IM lorazepam has already been used, then further review with the team and expert opinion should be sought. In the case of prolonged QT interval, or no electrocardiogram results, avoid IM haloperidol plus promethazine and use IM lorazepam. NICE further recommends that after RT, side effects, vital signs and levels of hydration and consciousness should be monitored at least hourly until there are no further physical health concerns (NICE, 2015). They also recommend increasing monitoring to every 15 min if the maximum dose has been exceeded, the service user is sedated, is suspected of having taken illicit substances or alcohol, has a pre-existing health condition or has previously experienced harm resulting from any restrictive intervention.

# 6    Special Populations and Situations

## 6.1    Older Adults

The European Academy of Neurology recommends that when agitation and aggression exist when someone has a form of dementia, this should only be treated with atypical antipsychotic medications after non-pharmacologic methods have been exhausted or there is an imminent risk of severe self-harm/harm to others (Frederiksen et al., 2020). They also make a 'weak recommendation' to stop antipsychotic medications as soon as possible, citing this as good practice.

## 6.2    Violence in the Emergency Department

The very small number of research studies involving the management of aggression in emergency department settings has been summarised as not adequate to provide a framework for evidence-based practice in these settings (Fricke et al., 2022; Taylor & Rew, 2011). However, we found an additional review and network meta-analysis studying the most optimal medication treatment of acute agitation in the emergency department. Their concerns were safety and time to tranquillisation, and they concluded that while ketamine and droperidol have intermediate effectiveness, high-quality evidence is lacking to support either one as safer or more effective (de Souza et al., 2022).

# 7 Personal Experience with Medication, Chris Munt

Many patients who are admitted to mental health units have personal experience or knowledge as to the use of PRN and rapid tranquillisation medications. The management of such interventions appears to many who have been detained or admitted on a voluntary basis to be unclear, inconsistent and used primarily to make patients docile and compliant. There is a consensus that such arrangements at best are an example of care through control; at worst it's exploiting those who lack the resources to challenge such decisions. Taking into account the natural emotions associated with being removed from society, your liberty suspended, rights curtailed, and placed into an environment that appears somewhat clinical, with non-negotiable routines and procedures, is it no wonder that sometimes these individuals will express their shock, frustration, confusion in a loud, animated and disturbing manner? It is entirely possible that with the right environment, with a skilled, experienced and well-led workforce, these natural responses might be viewed as natural given the context, and even part of a healing process, rather than internalising those feelings and emotions. I have experienced different teams on the same ward having vastly different tolerances to such behaviours, and from my observations, the teams that will not defer to PRN as the first or second response will have a similar outcome for the patient, which is a gradual reduction of behaviours of concern whether PRN is dispensed or not.

Over two decades, I experienced multiple admissions to such institutions. I experienced countless incidents of being given PRN medication. Most of the time I complied, but whenever I refused, it was made clear that to do so would result in my detention, even though I was always admitted as a voluntary patient and had the right to choose whether or not to take medication. On too many occasions, I observed this abuse of power taking place with other patients, through explicit or implicit threats. Though thankfully not routine, I was witness to incidents of physical restraint on patients followed by rapid tranquillisation. Such events are not easily erased from my memory, and the trauma experienced by the victim is an anathema in the context of therapeutic and humane treatments.

Many patients in my experience maintain that some staff take an enthusiastic part in such restrictive interventions, while some will conduct themselves professionally, with the patient front and centre of their concerns. I have observed patients taking 24 h to recover from tranquillisation with no clear memory of what happened and what led to the incident. Therefore, there is no learning for that individual other than a legacy of fear and suspicion.

I'm not anti-medication and recognise that it has its place in what should be a suite of options for both the patient and the professional. But they should be tailored to the individual and closely scrutinised and managed. We should have more concordance in prescribing medications, as a key flaw in the arguments for compliance is that under such regimes, patients tend to stop taking their meds when unsupervised. If we engage patients in the prescribing progress and understand their fears or resistance, we might find that patients will take their medications in both supervised and non-supervised conditions.

In summary, we should better demonstrate the use of PRN and rapid tranquillisation only when other approaches have been considered and deployed. In addition, those dispensing these medications must articulate a rationale for doing so and such incidences should be properly scrutinised to establish trends and patterns associated with different staff and different teams.

## 8    Recommendations for Future Research

This chapter shows that the body of evidence accumulated from RCTs is lacking. Statistical power is low in many studies due to the small number of participants and the generalisability of results to daily clinical practice can be difficult, due to the limited inclusion criteria for studies. We recommend that future large-scale pragmatic trials will be conducted which include people with lived experience as research partners in the endeavour. Further, we suggest the following as particular topics to be explored:

1. Is the use of medication more effective than other methods in promoting de-escalation in people who are identified as likely to demonstrate significant violence?
2. What forms of management of violence and aggression do service users prefer and what roles do advance statements and decisions have in management and prevention?
3. What guideline and algorithm adaptations are needed in the management of aggression and violence in the context of substance use and withdrawal?
4. What guideline and algorithm adaptations are needed for specific health settings, such as in the emergency department, on a general hospital ward or in a secure psychiatric facility?
5. What are novel methods for the delivery of medications in acute agitation (for example, intranasal or epidermal administration)?
6. What are the long-term effects and side effects of RT?
7. How useful is PRN medication in preventing violence or in aiding the ability of the service user to engage in de-escalation more readily?

## References

Aleyasin, H., Flanigan, M., & Russo, S. (2018). Neurocircuitry of aggression and aggression seeking behavior: Nose poking into brain circuitry controlling aggression. *Current Opinion in Neurobiology, 49*, 184–191. https://doi.org/10.1016/J.CONB.2018.02.013

Allen, M. H., Currier, G. W., Carpenter, D., Ross, R. W., & Docherty, J. P. (2005). The expert consensus guideline series. Treatment of behavioral emergencies. *Journal of Psychiatric Practice, 11*(Suppl 1), 5–25. https://doi.org/10.1097/00131746-200511001-00002

Bak, M., Weltens, I., Bervoets, C., De Fruyt, J., Samochowiec, J., Fiorillo, A., Sampogna, G., Bienkowski, P., Preuss, W. U., Misiak, B., Frydecka, D., Samochowiec, A., Bak, E., Drukker, M., & Dom, G. (2019). The pharmacological management of agitated and aggressive behaviour: A systematic review and meta-analysis. *European Psychiatry, 57*, 78–100. https://doi.org/10.1016/j.eurpsy.2019.01.014

Caruso, R., Antenora, F., Riba, M., Belvederi Murri, M., Biancosino, B., Zerbinati, L., & Grassi, L. (2021). Aggressive behavior and psychiatric inpatients: A narrative review of the literature with a focus on the European experience. *Current Psychiatry Reports, 23*, 1–12. https://doi.org/10.1007/S11920-021-01233-Z/TABLES/1

Comai, S., Bertazzo, A., Vachon, J., Daigle, M., Toupin, J., Côté, G., Turecki, G., & Gobbi, G. (2016). Tryptophan via serotonin/kynurenine pathways abnormalities in a large cohort of aggressive inmates: Markers for aggression. *Progress in Neuropsychopharmacology & Biological Psychiatry, 70*, 8–16. https://doi.org/10.1016/J.PNPBP.2016.04.012

Cowman, S., Björkdahl, A., Clarke, E., Gethin, G., & Maguire, J. (2017). A descriptive survey study of violence management and priorities among psychiatric staff in mental health services, across seventeen European countries. *BMC Health Services Research, 17*, 1–10. https://doi.org/10.1186/S12913-017-1988-7/TABLES/9

de Almeida, C. G., Del Grossi Moura, M., Barberato-Filho, S., de Sá Del Fiol, F., Motta, R. H. L., & de Cássia Bergamaschi, C. (2017). Rapid tranquilization for psychiatric patients with psychomotor agitation: What is known about it? *Psychiatric Quarterly, 88*, 885–895. https://doi.org/10.1007/s11126-017-9504-0

de Souza, I. S., Thode, H. C., Shrestha, P., Allen, R., Koos, J., & Singer, A. J. (2022). Rapid tranquilization of the agitated patient in the emergency department: A systematic review and network meta-analysis. *The American Journal of Emergency Medicine, 51*, 363–373. https://doi.org/10.1016/J.AJEM.2021.11.011

Dundar, Y., Greenhalgh, J., Richardson, M., & Dwan, K. (2016). Pharmacological treatment of acute agitation associated with psychotic and bipolar disorder: A systematic review and meta-analysis. *Human Psychopharmacology, 31*, 268–285. https://doi.org/10.1002/HUP.2535

Fjellvang, M., Grøning, L., & Haukvik, U. K. (2018). Imaging violence in schizophrenia: A systematic review and critical discussion of the MRI literature. *Frontiers in Psychiatry, 9*, 333. https://doi.org/10.3389/fpsyt.2018.00333

Frederiksen, K. S., Cooper, C., Frisoni, G. B., Olich, D. L., Georges, J., Kramberger, M. G., Nilsson, C., Passmore, P., Mantoan Ritter, L., Religa, D., Schmidt, R., Stefanova, E., Verdelho, A., Vandenbulcke, M., Winblad, B., & Waldemar, G. (2020). A European academy of neurology guideline on medical management issues in dementia. *European Journal of Neurology, 2020*, 1805–1820. https://doi.org/10.1111/ene.14412

Fricke, J., Siddique, S. M., Douma, C., Ladak, A., Burchill, C. N., Greysen, R., & Mull, N. K. (2022). Workplace violence in healthcare settings: A scoping review of guidelines and systematic reviews. *Trauma, Violence and Abuse, 24*(5), 3363–3383. https://doi.org/10.1177/15248380221126476

Garriga, M., Pacchiarotti, I., Kasper, S., Zeller, S. L., Allen, M. H., Vázquez, G., Baldaçara, L., San, L., McAllister-Williams, R. H., Fountoulakis, K. N., Courtet, P., Naber, D., Chan, E. W., Fagiolini, A., Möller, H. J., Grunze, H., Llorca, P. M., Jaffe, R. L., Yatham, L. N., Hidalgo-Mazzei, D., Passamar, M., Messer, T., Bernardo, M., & Vieta, E. (2016). Assessment and management of agitation in psychiatry: Expert consensus. *World Journal of Biological Psychiatry, 17*, 86–128. https://doi.org/10.3109/15622975.2015.1132007

Gaynes, B. N., Brown, C. L., Lux, L. J., Brownley, K. A., van Dorn, R. A., Edlund, M. J., Coker-Schwimmer, E., Palmieri Weber, R., Sheitman, B., Zarzar, T., Viswanathan, M., & Lohr, K. N. (2017). Preventing and de-escalating aggressive behavior among adult psychiatric patients: A systematic review of the evidence. *Psychiatric Services, 68*, 819–831. https://doi.org/10.1176/APPI.PS.201600314

Golden, S. A., & Shaham, Y. (2018). Aggression addiction and relapse: A new frontier in psychiatry. *Neuropsychopharmacology, 43*, 224–225. https://doi.org/10.1038/NPP.2017.173

Gowin, J. L., Green, C. E., Alcorn, J. L., Swann, A. C., Moeller, F. G., & Lane, S. D. (2013). The role of cortisol and psychopathy in the cycle of violence. *Psychopharmacology, 227*, 661–672. https://doi.org/10.1007/S00213-013-2992-1

Griffin, C. E., Kaye, A. M., Rivera Bueno, F., & Kaye, A. D. (2013). Benzodiazepine pharmacology and central nervous system–mediated effects. *The Ochsner Journal, 13*, 214.

Haller, J., Harold, G., Sandi, C., & Neumann, I. D. (2014). Effects of adverse early-life events on aggression and anti-social behaviours in animals and humans. *Journal of Neuroendocrinology, 26*, 724–738. https://doi.org/10.1111/JNE.12182

Hirsch, S., & Steinert, T. (2019). The use of rapid tranquilization in aggressive behavior. *Deutsches Ärzteblatt International, 116*, 445. https://doi.org/10.3238/ARZTEBL.2019.0445

Hirsch, S., Thilo, N., Steinert, T., & Flammer, E. (2021). Patients' perception of coercion with respect to antipsychotic treatment of psychotic disorders and its predictors. *Social Psychiatry and Psychiatric Epidemiology, 56*, 1381–1388. https://doi.org/10.1007/s00127-021-02083-z

Huf, G., Alexander, J., Gandhi, P., & Allen, M. H. (2016). Haloperidol plus promethazine for psychosis-induced aggression. *Cochrane Database of Systematic Reviews, 11*(11), CD005146. https://doi.org/10.1002/14651858.CD005146.pub3

Khokhar, M. A., & Rathbone, J. (2016). Droperidol for psychosis-induced aggression or agitation. *Cochrane Database of Systematic Reviews, 12*(12), CD002830. https://doi.org/10.1002/14651858.CD002830.PUB3/REFERENCES

Kim, H. K., Leonard, J., Corwell, B., Connors, N. J., Leonard, J. B., & Corwell, B. N. (2021). Safety and efficacy of pharmacologic agents used for rapid tranquilization of emergency department patients with acute agitation or excited delirium. *Expert Opinion on Drug Safety, 20*(2), 123–138. https://doi.org/10.1080/14740338.2021.1865911

Kousgaard, S. J., Licht, R. W., & Nielsen, R. E. (2017). Effects of intramuscular midazolam and Lorazepam on acute agitation in non-elderly subjects—A systematic review. *Pharmacopsychiatry, 50*, 129–135. https://doi.org/10.1055/s-0043-100766

Manchia, M., Booij, L., Pinna, F., Wong, J., Zepf, F., & Comai, S. (2020). Neurobiology of violence. In B. Carpiniello, A. Vita, & C. Mencacci (Eds.), *Violence and mental disorders* (Comprehensive approach to psychiatry) (Vol. 1, pp. 25–47). Springer. https://doi.org/10.1007/978-3-030-33188-7_2

Manchia, M., Carpiniello, B., Valtorta, F., & Comai, S. (2017). Serotonin dysfunction, aggressive behavior, and mental illness: Exploring the link using a dimensional approach. *ACS Chemical Neuroscience, 8*, 961–972. https://doi.org/10.1021/ACSCHEMNEURO.6B00427

Mardani, A., Paal, P., Weck, C., Jamshed, S., & Vaismoradi, M. (2022). Practical considerations of PRN medicines management: An integrative systematic review. *Frontiers in Pharmacology, 13*, 759998. https://doi.org/10.3389/fphar.2022.759998

Martínez-Raga, J., Amore, M., Di Sciascio, G., Florea, R. I., Garriga, M., Gonzalez, G., Kahl, K. G., Karlsson, P. A., Kuhn, J., Margariti, M., Pacciardi, B., Papageorgiou, K., Pompili, M., Rivollier, F., Royuela, Á., Safont, G., Scharfetter, J., Skagen, B., Tajima-Pozo, K., & Vidailhet, P. (2018). 1st international experts' meeting on agitation: Conclusions regarding the current and ideal management paradigm of agitation. *Frontiers in Psychiatry, 9*, 54. https://doi.org/10.3389/FPSYT.2018.00054/BIBTEX

McDougall, T., Pickup, J., Clarke, S., Baker, J., & Alderson, S. (2022). Promoting alternatives to PRN medicines in secure inpatient mental health services. *Mental Health Practice, 25*(2), 13–19. https://doi.org/10.7748/mhp.2021.e1589

Muir-Cochrane, E., Oster, C., Gerace, A., Dawson, S., Damarell, R., & Grimmer, K. (2020b). The effectiveness of chemical restraint in managing acute agitation and aggression: A systematic review of randomized controlled trials. *International Journal of Mental Health Nursing, 29*, 110–126. https://doi.org/10.1111/INM.12654

Muir-Cochrane, E., Oster, C., & Grimmer, K. (2020a). International research into 22 years of use of chemical restraint: An evidence overview. *Journal of Evaluation in Clinical Practice, 26*, 927–956. https://doi.org/10.1111/JEP.13232

National Institute of Health and Care Excellence. (2015). *Violence and aggression: Short-term management in mental health, health and community settings NICE guideline.* https://www.nice.org.uk/guidance/ng10

National Institute of Health and Care Excellence. (2019). *2019 surveillance of Violence and aggression: Short-term management in mental health, health and community settings NICE guideline NG10—summary of evidence.* https://www.nice.org.uk/guidance/ng10/resources/2019-surveillance-of-violence-and-aggression-shortterm-management-in-mental-health-health-and-community-settings-nice-guideline-ng10-pdf-9097015205365

Ostinelli, E. G., Brooke-Powney, M. J., Li, X., & Adams, C. E. (2017). Haloperidol for psychosis-induced aggression or agitation (rapid tranquillisation). *Cochrane Database of Systematic Reviews, 7*, CD009377. https://doi.org/10.1002/14651858.CD009377.pub3

Ostinelli, E. G., Hussein, M., Ahmed, U., Rehman, F., Miramontes, K., & Adams, C. E. (2018b). Risperidone for psychosis-induced aggression or agitation (rapid tranquillisation). *Cochrane Database of Systematic Reviews, 4*, CD009412. https://doi.org/10.1002/14651858.CD009412.PUB2

Ostinelli, E. G., Jajawi, S., Spyridi, S., Sayal, K., & Jayaram, M. B. (2018a). Aripiprazole (intramuscular) for psychosis-induced aggression or agitation (rapid tranquillisation). *Cochrane Database of Systematic Reviews, 1*(1), CD008074. https://doi.org/10.1002/14651858.CD008074.PUB2

Patel, J., Frankel, S., & Tampi, R. R. (2019). Evidence for using PRN pharmacotherapy to treat undifferentiated acute agitation or aggression. *Annals of Clinical Psychiatry, 31*, 54–69.

Pavlov, K. A., Chistiakov, D. A., & Chekhonin, V. P. (2012). Genetic determinants of aggression and impulsivity in humans. *Journal of Applied Genetics, 53*, 61–82. https://doi.org/10.1007/s13353-011-0069-6

Perkins, J., Ho, J. D., Vilke, G. M., & Demers, G. (2015). American Academy of Emergency Medicine position statement: Safety of droperidol use in the emergency department. *The Journal of Emergency Medicine, 49*, 91–97. https://doi.org/10.1016/J.JEMERMED.2014.12.024

Pinna, M., & Manchia, M. (2017). Preventing aggressive/violent behavior: A role for biomarkers? *Biomarkers in Medicine, 11*(9), 701–704. https://doi.org/10.2217/bmm-2017-0135

Pompili, E., Carlone, C., Silvestrini, C., & NicolÒ, G. (2017). Focus on aggressive behaviour in mental illness. *Rivista di Psichiatria, 52*, 175–179. https://doi.org/10.1708/2801.28344

Romero-Martínez, Á., Sarrate-Costa, C., & Moya-Albiol, L. (2022). Reactive vs proactive aggression: A differential psychobiological profile? Conclusions derived from a systematic review. *Neuroscience and Biobehavioral Reviews, 136*, 104626. https://doi.org/10.1016/J.NEUBIOREV.2022.104626

Roppolo, L. P., Morris, D. W., Khan, F., Downs Pharmd, R., Metzger, J., Carder, T., Wong, A. H., & Wilson, M. P. (2020). Improving the management of acutely agitated patients in the emergency department through implementation of project BETA (best practices in the evaluation and treatment of agitation). *J Am Coll Emerg Physicians Open, 1*, 898–907. https://doi.org/10.1002/emp2.12138

Singh, J. P., Volavka, J., Czobor, P., & van Dorn, R. A. (2012). A meta-analysis of the Val158Met COMT polymorphism and violent behavior in schizophrenia. *PLoS One, 7*, e43423. https://doi.org/10.1371/JOURNAL.PONE.0043423

Taylor, J. L., & Rew, L. (2011). A systematic review of the literature: Workplace violence in the emergency department. *Journal of Clinical Nursing, 20*, 1072–1085. https://doi.org/10.1111/J.1365-2702.2010.03342.X

Toth, M., Mikics, E., Tulogdi, A., Aliczki, M., & Haller, J. (2011). Post-weaning social isolation induces abnormal forms of aggression in conjunction with increased glucocorticoid and autonomic stress responses. *Hormones and Behavior, 60*(1), 28–36. https://doi.org/10.1016/j.yhbeh.2011.02.003

Tuvblad, C., Narusyte, J., Comasco, E., Andershed, H., Andershed, A. K., Colins, O. F., Fanti, K. A., & Nilsson, K. W. (2016). Physical and verbal aggressive behavior and COMT genotype: Sensitivity to the environment. *American Journal of Medical Genetics Part B: Neuropsychiatric Genetics, 171*, 708–718. https://doi.org/10.1002/AJMG.B.32430

Widmayer, S., Borgwardt, S., Lang, U. E., Stieglitz, R. D., & Huber, C. G. (2019). Functional neuroimaging correlates of aggression in psychosis: A systematic review with recommendations for future research. *Frontiers in Psychiatry, 10*, 777. https://doi.org/10.3389/FPSYT.2018.00777/FULL

Widmayer, S., Sowislo, J. F., Jungfer, H. A., Borgwardt, S., Lang, U. E., Stieglitz, R. D., & Huber, C. G. (2018). Structural magnetic resonance imaging correlates of aggression in psychosis: A systematic review and effect size analysis. *Frontiers in Psychiatry, 9*, 217. https://doi.org/10.3389/FPSYT.2018.00217/FULL

Wilson, M. P., Pepper, D., Currier, G. W., Holloman, G. H., & Feifel, D. (2012). The psychopharmacology of agitation: Consensus statement of the American association for emergency psychiatry project BETA psychopharmacology workgroup. *Western Journal of Emergency Medicine, 13*, 26–34. https://doi.org/10.5811/WESTJEM.2011.9.6866

Yanowitch, R., & Coccaro, E. F. (2011). The neurochemistry of human aggression. *Advances in Genetics, 75*, 151–169. https://doi.org/10.1016/B978-0-12-380858-5.00005-8

Zaman, H., Sampson, S. J., Beck, A. L. S., Sharma, T., Clay, F. J., Spyridi, S., Zhao, S., & Gillies, D. (2017). Benzodiazepines for psychosis-induced aggression or agitation. *Cochrane Database of Systematic Reviews, 12*(12), CD003079. https://doi.org/10.1002/14651858.CD003079.pub4

Zareifopoulos, N., & Panayiotakopoulos, G. (2019). Treatment options for acute agitation in psychiatric patients: Theoretical and empirical evidence. *Cureus, 11*, e6152. https://doi.org/10.7759/cureus.6152

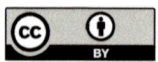

# Alternatives to Coercion

Enric Garcia Torrents and Anna Björkdahl

## 1   Introduction

Coercion in mental healthcare has been a longstanding issue, with roots tracing back to the early days of institutionalised care. Historically, mental health treatment was often characterised by a paternalistic approach, where healthcare professionals made decisions on behalf of patients, sometimes resorting to forceful and invasive interventions. This approach was largely driven by a perceived need to protect both the individual and society, with the autonomy and dignity of the individual often being overlooked.

Coercion in mental healthcare can take various forms, including involuntary hospitalisation, forced medication and the use of physical restraints or seclusion. These practices have been shown to have profound implications for the autonomy, dignity and well-being of individuals receiving care. The use of coercive practices often results in a significant loss of autonomy for these individuals, which can be detrimental to their recovery process.

Moreover, coercion and violence are intrinsically linked. The imposition of coercive measures often requires some form of violence or force, and the experience of being coerced can lead to violent reactions. This cycle of violence and coercion can exacerbate mental health symptoms and hinder the recovery process. Over the years, there has been a growing recognition of the need for alternatives to coercion in mental healthcare. This shift in perspective has been driven by a number of factors, including advances in our understanding of mental health and recovery,

E. G. Torrents (✉)
Medical Anthropology Research Centre, Universitat Rovira I Virgili, Tarragona, Spain
e-mail: enric.garcia@urv.cat

A. Björkdahl
Centre for Psychiatric Research, Karolinska Institutet, Solna, Sweden
e-mail: anna.bjorkdahl@ki.se

© The Author(s) 2024
N. Hallett et al. (eds.), *Coercion and Violence in Mental Health Settings*,
https://doi.org/10.1007/978-3-031-61224-4_17

increased awareness of human rights, and the lived experiences of individuals who have been subjected to coercive practices.

In the rest of the chapter, we explore inpatient, community-based and treatment-wide alternatives, aiming to help transform traditional practices. In the inpatient context, alternative methods create therapeutic environments that respect patients' autonomy and comfort. These solutions strive to replace coercive measures with patient-controlled interventions, such as sensory rooms and open door policies, fostering an atmosphere of trust and safety. Community-based alternatives focus on social support and inclusive care. By providing resources like recovery colleges and peer support services, individuals are empowered to actively engage in their journey to mental well-being. Treatment-wide alternatives promote patient agency and active participation in decision-making processes. These approaches foster collaborative communication between patients and healthcare providers, ensuring that treatment plans align with individual preferences and needs.

To end with, we provide real-world examples to underscore the effectiveness of these alternatives, while emphasising the importance of cultural and socioeconomic factors in shaping mental healthcare practices. By showcasing how alternatives can be put into practice, this chapter aims to inspire transformative changes, promoting compassionate and patient-centred mental healthcare worldwide.

## 2    Need for Alternatives

Coercion in mental healthcare is a complex and multifaceted issue with profound implications for the autonomy, dignity, and well-being of individuals receiving care (Golay et al., 2019). The use of coercive practices often results in a significant loss of autonomy for these individuals, which, according to numerous studies, can be detrimental to their recovery process (Chieze et al., 2019). Autonomy, the capacity to make informed, uncoerced decisions about one's own life and well-being, is a fundamental human right. It is particularly crucial in healthcare settings, where individuals should have the right to make informed decisions about their treatment and care (Puras & Gooding, 2019).

However, in many mental healthcare settings, the choices and decisions of individuals are often overridden by healthcare professionals (Chapman et al., 2020). Research has shown that this can lead to a sense of disempowerment and helplessness, which can exacerbate mental health symptoms and hinder the recovery process (Cusack et al., 2018; Herrman et al., 2022). The individual's sense of self-efficacy and control over their own life can be undermined, potentially leading to feelings of hopelessness and despair. This is particularly concerning given that a sense of self-efficacy and control is often a key factor in recovery from mental health conditions (Sashidharan et al., 2019). Moreover, the use of coercion in mental healthcare can lead to stigmatisation and labelling, further compounding the challenges faced by individuals with mental health conditions (Steiger et al., 2023). Societal stigma and discrimination are significant barriers to recovery and social inclusion for these individuals (Tyerman et al., 2021). When individuals are subjected to coercion, they can be labelled and stereotyped, further marginalising them within society.

This can lead to social isolation, reduced opportunities and poorer mental health outcomes (Puras, 2022). The individual's identity can become defined by their mental health condition and their experiences of coercion, rather than their strengths, abilities and potential (Mckeown et al., 2019).

Coercive practices can also cause significant psychological distress. Being subjected to such practices can lead to increased anxiety and depression, and a heightened sense of helplessness and fear (Verbeke et al., 2019). This can be particularly harmful for individuals with a history of trauma (Torrents, 2022). Coercive practices can potentially re-traumatise these individuals, triggering past traumas and exacerbating their mental health symptoms (Hennessy et al., 2023). This highlights the importance of trauma-informed care, which recognises and responds to the effects of trauma, in mental healthcare settings (Hennessy et al., 2023). Trauma-informed care emphasises physical, psychological and emotional safety for both consumers and providers, and helps survivors rebuild a sense of control and empowerment (Sweeney et al., 2018).

Trust is a cornerstone of any therapeutic relationship, and yet, coercive practices can severely damage the trust between mental health professionals and individuals receiving care. When individuals are subjected to coercion, they may feel betrayed and violated (Bolsinger et al., 2020). This can make it difficult to establish a therapeutic alliance, a collaborative partnership that is often a key factor in successful mental health treatment. The individual may become wary of mental health professionals and services, potentially leading to disengagement from care and poorer mental health outcomes (Hachtel et al., 2019).

Therefore, it is essential to find alternatives to coercion that respect individuals' autonomy, dignity and rights, and promote their recovery and social inclusion (Moro et al., 2022). This includes promoting shared decision-making, where individuals and healthcare professionals collaborate to make decisions about care. Shared decision-making respects the individual's autonomy and expertise in their own life and experiences, and can help to build trust and a therapeutic alliance (Zinkler & von Peter, 2019). It also includes implementing trauma-informed care, which can help prevent re-traumatisation and promote safety and empowerment (Mihelicova et al., 2018). Finally, it includes challenging stigma and discrimination, both within mental healthcare settings and in society more broadly, to promote social inclusion and opportunities for individuals with mental health conditions (Perers et al., 2022).

## 3    Inpatient Alternative Approaches

Inpatient settings, such as hospitals or clinics, often present unique challenges in the field of mental health care. Individuals admitted to these settings are frequently in the midst of a severe crisis, experiencing high levels of distress and potentially exhibiting violent behaviour. These circumstances can lead to an increased reliance on coercive measures, such as physical restraints or forced medication, in an attempt to manage the situation. However, such practices can exacerbate feelings of distress and powerlessness, potentially hindering the recovery process.

Recognising these challenges, this section explores innovative inpatient alternatives that aim to transform the traditional approach to mental health care within these settings. These alternatives, which include sensory rooms, open doors policy, AD and patient-controlled admissions, are designed to reduce coercion, promote autonomy and dignity and facilitate recovery even in the midst of a crisis. Each of these alternatives offers unique strategies to navigate the complexities of inpatient care, providing more humane, compassionate and effective treatment options. In the following subsections, we will delve into each of these inpatient alternatives in detail, discussing their principles, methods and the evidence supporting their effectiveness.

Moreover, we will examine the challenges and opportunities associated with implementing these alternatives, providing a comprehensive overview of the current landscape of inpatient mental health care. By exploring these inpatient alternatives, we aim to shed light on the potential of these approaches to transform the inpatient experience, reduce coercion and promote the well-being of individuals with mental health issues, even in the most challenging circumstances.

## 3.1    Sensory Rooms

Sensory rooms (SRs), also known as multisensory environments, are therapeutic spaces designed to stimulate or soothe the senses. They provide a calming and safe environment for individuals experiencing mental health crises. These rooms are an innovative approach to mental health care, offering a non-pharmacological method for managing distress and promoting relaxation.

The concept of sensory rooms originated in the Netherlands in the 1970s, initially designed for individuals with intellectual disabilities. Recognising the broader therapeutic potential of sensory rooms, they have since been adapted for use in various mental health settings, including hospitals, clinics and community centres across the globe (Brown et al., 2019).

SRs are equipped with a variety of sensory tools, such as soft lighting, calming music, comfortable furniture and tactile objects. The goal is to create an environment that can be tailored to the unique sensory needs of each individual, whether that involves stimulating the senses, soothing the senses or a combination of both. Individuals are encouraged to explore the room and use the sensory tools in ways that are comforting and calming to them. This could involve listening to calming music, watching a lava lamp, feeling the texture of a weighted blanket or smelling a favourite scent. The focus is on promoting a sense of safety, comfort and control, reducing distress and promoting relaxation (Alvarsson et al., 2010). SRs can significantly reduce coercion in mental health care. By providing a calming and soothing environment, SRs can help individuals manage distress and prevent crises, reducing the need for coercive interventions such as seclusion and restraint (Hirsch & Steinert, 2019). This can have a profound impact on the individual's well-being, promoting a sense of calm, comfort and recovery (Hedlund Lindberg et al., 2019).

Research has shown that SRs can reduce distress, aggression and self-harm, and increase feelings of calm and relaxation (Björkdahl et al., 2016). Individuals report feeling more in control of their emotions and more able to cope with stress and distress (Grinde & Grindal Patil, 2009). Staff members report a decrease in the use of coercive interventions and an improvement in the therapeutic environment (Haig & Hallett, 2023). Despite these promising results, further research is needed to fully understand the effectiveness of SRs across different settings and populations, and to establish best practices for their implementation.

## 3.2   Open Doors Policy

The open doors policy signifies a paradigm shift in mental health care, underpinned by the principles of transparency, openness and a deep respect for patient autonomy. This policy advocates for the doors of mental health facilities to remain unlocked as much as possible, marking a substantial deviation from traditional practices that often involve containment and control (Hochstrasser et al., 2018a). The inception of the open doors policy was a response to the mounting concerns about the prevalent use of coercion in mental health care, especially the practices of seclusion and restraint. These methods, which typically involve confining individuals in locked rooms or physically restraining them, have been widely criticised for violating individuals' rights and dignity (Kowalinski et al., 2019). The open doors policy introduces an alternative approach that upholds individuals' autonomy and freedom of movement (Steinert et al., 2019).

Implementing an open doors policy necessitates a cultural and procedural transformation within mental health facilities. Rather than relying on locked doors and physical barriers to manage behaviour and avert crises, facilities that adopt this policy concentrate on fostering positive relationships, enhancing communication and cultivating a therapeutic environment (Compton et al., 2023). Staff members receive training in de-escalation techniques and conflict resolution, equipping them to handle crises without resorting to coercion (Gather et al., 2019).

Transparency is a cornerstone of the open doors policy. Individuals are kept informed about the policy and its implications for their care. They are encouraged to move freely within the facility and participate actively in decision-making processes related to their care. This level of openness and transparency can engender trust and foster collaboration between individuals and staff members, thereby promoting a therapeutic environment that is less coercive (Hochstrasser et al., 2018b).

By championing freedom of movement and respect for patient autonomy, this policy can diminish the use of seclusion, restraint and other coercive interventions. This can profoundly impact individuals' well-being, fostering a sense of autonomy, dignity and recovery (Kowalinski et al., 2019). Facilities that have adopted this policy have reported a decrease in the use of seclusion and restraint, a reduction in violent incidents and an enhancement in the therapeutic environment. Individuals have reported feeling more respected and empowered, while staff members have noted a more positive and collaborative working environment (Steinert et al., 2019), pointing to the fact that the open doors policy can significantly curtail the use of coercion in mental health care.

## 3.3    Advance Directives and Informed Consent

Advance Directives (ADs) are legal instruments that allow individuals to express their preferences for future mental health treatment in the event they become unable to make decisions for themselves. This innovative approach to mental health care is rooted in the principles of autonomy, self-determination and respect for individual rights (Tinland et al., 2022).

The implementation of ADs involves a formal process in which individuals express their treatment preferences in a written document (Campbell & Kisely, 2009). This document may include preferences regarding medication, hospitalisation, use of seclusion or restraint and other aspects of care. The document also typically designates a trusted person to make decisions on the individual's behalf if they become unable to do so. The AD is then shared with the individual's mental health care provider and becomes part of their medical record. Informed consent is a critical component of ADs. It ensures that individuals are fully aware of the potential risks and benefits of their chosen treatment options and that they have the opportunity to ask questions and receive satisfactory answers before making a decision.

This process respects the individual's autonomy and right to make informed decisions about their care (Murray & Wortzel, 2019). ADs and informed consent reduce coercion in mental health care by giving individuals control over their future treatment. Studies have shown that these practices can reduce the use of coercive measures, improve patient satisfaction and enhance the therapeutic alliance between patients and mental health professionals (Barbui et al., 2021). Patients often report feeling more respected, and mental health professionals report a more collaborative and trusting therapeutic relationship (Braun et al., 2023), thus proving to be an essential intervention in the reduction of coercive measures.

## 3.4    Patient-Controlled Admissions

Patient-controlled admissions (PCAs) are a progressive approach in mental health care that empowers patients by placing the decision-making authority regarding hospital admission directly in their hands. This approach is firmly rooted in the principle of patient autonomy, recognising that individuals with mental health issues are often the best judges of their own mental health needs (Lindkvist et al., 2019). PCAs represent a significant shift in power dynamics, giving patients the authority to decide when hospitalisation is necessary. This approach necessitates a high level of trust and collaboration between patients and mental health professionals, fostering a more equitable and respectful therapeutic relationship (Olsø et al., 2016).

The implementation of a PCA involves a formal agreement between the patient and the mental health care provider. Under this agreement, the patient has the right to admit themselves to the hospital or clinic when they feel it's necessary, without the need for a professional's approval. The duration of the stay is also typically decided by the patient, within certain agreed-upon limits. This approach respects the patient's autonomy and self-knowledge, while also ensuring that the hospital resources are used responsibly (Ellegaard et al., 2017). By giving patients control over their admissions, this approach can prevent crises and reduce the need for involuntary hospitalisation (Strand & von Hausswolff-Juhlin, 2015). This can have a profound impact on the patient's well-being, promoting a sense of autonomy, control and recovery (Smitmanis-Lyle et al., 2022).

Studies have shown that PCAs have the potential to reduce the number of involuntary admissions, improve patient satisfaction and enhance the therapeutic alliance between patients and mental health professionals (Thomsen et al., 2018). Patients report feeling more respected and empowered, and mental health professionals report a more collaborative and trusting therapeutic relationship (Skott et al., 2021), showcasing the potential impact of PCA on reducing coercion in mental health care.

## 3.5 Comparative Overview of Inpatient Alternatives

The above-described alternatives to coercion in mental health inpatient settings represent promising interventions to reduce the use of coercive practices. A common factor is the promotion of different aspects of patient autonomy and person-centred care. At the same time, they may not be suitable for all patients and could present challenges to clinical implementation. It is also important to realise that the interventions are supported by different levels of evidence. An overview of the advantages, disadvantages and evidence in support of the interventions is shown in Table 1.

## 4 Community Alternatives

This section delves into the realm of community alternatives, which are innovative approaches to mental health care that are implemented outside of traditional inpatient settings. These alternatives are rooted in the belief that mental health care should be integrated into the community, promoting social inclusion, autonomy and recovery.

Community alternatives encompass a wide range of interventions, from Recovery Colleges and Peer Support Services to Crisis Intervention Teams and Soteria and respite houses. Each of these alternatives offers unique strategies to reduce coercion in mental health care, providing more humane, compassionate and effective treatment options.

**Table 1** Comparative overview of inpatient alternatives

| Intervention | Advantages | Disadvantages | Support by evidence |
|---|---|---|---|
| Sensory rooms | Provides a calming environment | Requires resources to set up and maintain | Emerging: Early studies show promise, the body of research is still growing |
| | Non-pharmacological method for managing distress | May not be suitable for all patients | |
| Open doors policy | Promotes freedom and autonomy | Requires staff training to manage potential risks | Mixed: Some studies show reduced use of seclusion and restraint, yet results vary across different settings |
| | Can reduce feelings of confinement and distress | May not be suitable for all settings or patients | |
| Advance directives | Respects patient's preferences and autonomy | Requires patient to anticipate future needs and preferences | Established: Numerous studies support the use of AD, although implementation can be challenging |
| | Can guide care during crises when the patient may be unable to communicate preferences | May be difficult to implement if patient's condition changes rapidly | |
| Patient-controlled admissions | Gives patients' control over the admission process | Requires resources and flexible bed management | Preliminary: Initial studies show reduced hospital stays and improved patient satisfaction, further research is needed to confirm findings |
| | Can prevent crises and reduce involuntary admissions | May not be suitable for all patients or situations | |

In the following subsections, we will explore each of these community alternatives in detail, discussing their principles, methods and the evidence supporting their effectiveness. We will also examine the challenges and opportunities associated with implementing these alternatives, providing a comprehensive overview of the current landscape of community-based mental health care.

By exploring these community alternatives, we aim to shed light on the potential of community-based approaches to transform mental health care, reduce coercion and promote the well-being of individuals with mental health issues.

## 4.1    Recovery Colleges

Recovery colleges represent an innovative approach to mental health care, grounded in the principles of education, co-production and empowerment. These institutions provide a range of courses about mental health and recovery, designed and delivered collaboratively by individuals with lived experience of mental health issues and mental health professionals (Repper et al., 2022).

The concept of recovery colleges originated in the United Kingdom in the early twenty-first century, as part of the broader recovery movement in mental health care. This movement recognised the value of education as a powerful tool for recovery, and the unique insights and knowledge that individuals with lived experience can bring to the educational process (Thériault et al., 2020).

Recovery colleges operate on several key principles. Firstly, they embrace the concept of co-production, with courses being jointly designed and delivered by individuals with lived experience and mental health professionals. This collaborative approach fosters a sense of equality and mutual respect, and ensures that the courses are relevant, practical and grounded in real-life experiences (Bourne et al., 2018). Secondly, recovery colleges offer a diverse range of courses, covering topics such as understanding mental health issues, coping strategies and principles of recovery. This diversity ensures that individuals can find courses that are relevant to their needs and interests, and that they can continue to learn and grow throughout their recovery journey. Thirdly, recovery colleges are open to anyone interested in learning about mental health and recovery. This includes individuals with mental health issues, their families and friends, and mental health professionals. This inclusivity fosters a sense of community and mutual understanding, and helps to break down barriers and stigma associated with mental health (Crowther et al., 2019).

The implementation of recovery colleges can significantly reduce coercion in mental health care. By promoting education and empowerment, these institutions enable individuals to take control of their mental health and recovery, reducing the need for coercive interventions. This can have a profound impact on individuals' well-being, fostering a sense of empowerment, hope and recovery (Thériault et al., 2020).

As of the current date, there are over 100 recovery colleges worldwide, with the majority located in the United Kingdom, Australia and Canada. These institutions vary in size and scope, but all share a commitment to the principles of co-production, education and empowerment. The operation of these colleges typically involves a team of staff members, including coordinators, educators and peer support workers, who work together to develop and deliver the courses. Funding for these colleges often comes from a combination of government funding, grants and course fees (Repper et al., 2022).

Research has shown that recovery colleges can have a positive impact on individuals' mental health and well-being. Participants report increased knowledge and understanding of mental health, improved self-confidence and self-efficacy, and enhanced hope and optimism about the future. However, further research is needed to fully understand the impact of these colleges on individuals' mental health outcomes and experiences, and to identify best practices for their implementation (Hayes et al., 2023). By fostering a sense of empowerment, hope and recovery, these institutions can play a crucial role in transforming mental health care and reducing coercion.

## 4.2    Peer Support Services

Peer support services represent a transformative approach in mental health care, predicated on the mutual exchange of experiences and knowledge between individuals who have encountered similar mental health challenges. This paradigm shift towards peer-led support has been instrumental in fostering a sense of community, empowerment and recovery among individuals navigating their mental health journeys (Shalaby & Agyapong, 2020).

The genesis of peer support lies in the consumer/survivor/ex-patient (C/S/X) movement that emerged in the 1970s and 1980s. This movement was a response to the often dehumanising and coercive practices of traditional mental health care. Advocates of the movement sought to challenge these practices and promote alternatives that respect individuals' autonomy, dignity and lived experiences (Ibrahim et al., 2020). Peer support services are grounded in the principles of empathy, mutual aid and experiential knowledge. Peer supporters are individuals who have lived experience of mental health conditions and recovery, and who have received training to support others on their recovery journey. They offer a unique perspective, understanding and empathy that can be profoundly validating and empowering for those they support (Kinane et al., 2022).

The role of peer supporters is multifaceted. They provide emotional support, share coping strategies, offer practical advice and advocate for individuals within the mental health system. They also serve as role models, demonstrating that recovery is possible and inspiring hope. Importantly, peer support is based on mutual respect and equality, with the peer supporter and the individual they support learning and growing together (Easter et al., 2021). Peer support services can be provided in various settings, including mental health services, community organisations and online platforms. They can take various forms, including one-on-one support, group support, peer-run services and peer-led education and advocacy initiatives. The flexibility and diversity of peer support services make them accessible and relevant to a wide range of individuals (Kent, 2019). Implementing peer support services requires a shift in the traditional power dynamics of mental health care. It involves recognising and valuing the expertise of lived experience and creating spaces where this expertise can be shared and honoured. It also requires resources and training to ensure that peer supporters are supported in their role and that the services are safe and effective (Sanchez-Moscona & Eiroa-Orosa, 2021).

Despite these challenges, the benefits of peer support services are significant. Research has shown that they can reduce the use of coercive measures, enhance patient satisfaction and improve mental health outcomes. They can also promote a sense of empowerment and self-efficacy, which are key factors in recovery from mental health conditions (Johnson & Rogers, 2020), offering a supportive and empowering approach that respects the individual's autonomy and lived experiences.

## 4.3      Crisis Intervention Teams

Crisis Intervention Teams (CITs) represent a community-based approach to mental health crises, offering an alternative to traditional law enforcement responses. These teams consist of specially trained police officers who collaborate with mental health professionals and community agencies to provide a compassionate, effective response to individuals experiencing mental health crises (Marcus & Stergiopoulos, 2022). The CIT model was first developed in Memphis, Tennessee, in the 1980s, in response to a tragic incident where a man experiencing a mental health crisis was fatally shot by police. The model has since been adopted by many law enforcement agencies across the United States and internationally, reflecting a growing recognition of the need for a more humane and effective response to mental health crises (Rogers et al., 2019).

The primary goal of CITs is to ensure the safety and well-being of all involved parties during a mental health crisis. CIT officers receive specialised training in recognising and understanding mental health conditions, de-escalation techniques and crisis intervention strategies. They work closely with mental health professionals and community agencies to connect individuals with appropriate services and support, aiming to divert them from the criminal justice system whenever possible (Kane et al., 2018).

CITs also play a crucial role in reducing stigma and improving community relations. By promoting understanding and compassion towards individuals with mental health conditions, CITs can help to challenge negative stereotypes and foster a more inclusive and supportive community environment (Hogan & Goldman, 2021). However, the implementation of CITs is not without its challenges. It requires a significant investment in training and resources, as well as a strong commitment from law enforcement agencies, mental health services and the community. It also requires a shift in attitudes and practices, moving away from a punitive approach towards a more compassionate and supportive response to mental health crises (Haigh et al., 2020).

Despite these challenges, the benefits of CITs are significant. Research has shown that CITs can reduce the use of force, improve officer safety and increase access to mental health services. They can also reduce the criminalisation of individuals with mental health conditions, promoting a more just and humane approach to mental health crises (Marcus & Stergiopoulos, 2022). By promoting safety, compassion and access to services, CITs can transform the way our communities respond to mental health crises.

## 4.4      Soteria and Respite Houses

Soteria and respite houses represent a community-based alternative to traditional mental healthcare, providing a supportive and non-coercive environment for individuals experiencing mental health crises. These facilities are grounded in the principles of respect, empowerment and recovery, offering a transformative approach to mental health care (Friedlander et al., 2022).

The Soteria model was first developed in the 1970s by psychiatrist Loren Mosher as a response to the often coercive and institutional nature of mental healthcare. Soteria houses provide a residential setting where individuals experiencing acute mental health crises, particularly those with psychosis, can live and receive support from a team of non-professional staff. The focus is on creating a therapeutic environment that respects the individual's experience and autonomy, rather than relying on medication and coercion (Croft et al., 2021). Respite houses, on the other hand, offer a temporary place of refuge for individuals experiencing mental health crises. They provide a calm and supportive environment where individuals can take a break from their usual surroundings, receive peer support and develop coping strategies. Respite houses aim to prevent the escalation of crises and reduce the need for hospitalisation, promoting recovery and autonomy (Cooper et al., 2021).

Both Soteria and respite houses emphasise the importance of a supportive and understanding community in facilitating recovery. They provide a space where individuals can explore their experiences, develop self-understanding and build resilience. The focus is on the individual's strengths and potential, rather than their symptoms or diagnosis (Calton et al., 2008). However, implementing the Soteria and respite house models is not without its challenges. It requires a shift in the traditional power dynamics of mental healthcare, with non-professional staff and peers taking on significant roles. It also requires resources and training to ensure that staff can provide appropriate support and manage potential risks. Furthermore, these models may not be suitable for all individuals or situations, and further research is needed to understand how they can be most effectively implemented (Nischk & Rusch, 2019).

Despite these challenges, the benefits of Soteria and respite houses are significant. Research has shown that they can reduce the use of coercive measures, enhance patient satisfaction and improve mental health outcomes. They can also promote a sense of empowerment and self-efficacy, which are key factors in recovery from mental health conditions (Stupak & Dobroczyński, 2019), representing a promising alternative to traditional mental healthcare, offering a supportive and non-coercive approach that respects the individual's autonomy and promotes their recovery.

## 4.5    Comparative Overview of Community Alternatives

The described alternatives are implemented outside of inpatient settings and promote mental health care integration into the community, social inclusion, autonomy and recovery. Similarly to inpatient alternatives to coercive practices, these interventions may not be suitable for all persons and some require substantial resources from the community. Table 2 shows an overview of the advantages, disadvantages and evidence in support of the community alternatives.

**Table 2** Comparative overview of community alternatives

| Intervention | Advantages | Disadvantages | Support by evidence |
|---|---|---|---|
| Recovery colleges | Provides education and skills training | Requires resources and staffing | Established: Numerous studies show improved self-management skills and recovery outcomes |
| | Promotes self-management and recovery | Effectiveness may depend on curriculum and teaching quality | |
| Peer support services | Provides support from someone with lived experience | Requires careful recruitment and training | High: A substantial body of research supports the effectiveness of peer support services |
| | Can reduce feelings of isolation | Role and responsibilities need to be clearly defined | |
| Crisis intervention teams | Provides immediate, intensive support | Requires significant resources and staffing | Mixed: While some studies show reduced hospital admissions and improved patient satisfaction, results vary across different settings and populations |
| | Can prevent hospitalisation | May not be available in all areas | |
| | Promotes dialogue | | |
| Soteria and respite houses | Provides a non-medical, home-like environment | Requires resources to maintain | Emerging: Early studies show promise, particularly in reducing hospitalisation rates and improving quality of life, but more research is needed |
| | Can provide respite for individuals and families | May not be suitable for individuals with severe symptoms | |

## 5 Treatment-Wide Alternatives

This section explores treatment-wide alternatives, which are innovative approaches to mental health care that can be applied across various settings, from inpatient to community-based environments:

### 5.1 Shared and Supported Decision-Making

Shared decision-making has its roots in the patient-centred care movement, which emerged in the 1950s, advocating for the active involvement of patients in their healthcare. Historically, mental healthcare was characterised by a paternalistic approach, where healthcare professionals made decisions on behalf of patients, sometimes resorting to forceful and invasive interventions. This approach was largely driven by a perceived need to protect both the individual and society, often overlooking the autonomy and dignity of the individual (Duffy et al., 2023).

However, over the years, there has been a paradigm shift towards shared and supported decision-making, a cornerstone of patient-centred care. This approach fosters a collaborative relationship between patients and healthcare providers, respecting the autonomy of the patient, acknowledging their unique insights into their own experiences and needs, and actively involving them in the decision-making process. This is particularly crucial in mental healthcare, where decisions can have profound implications for the patient's autonomy, dignity and well-being (Drake et al., 2022).

Shared decision-making can empower patients, enhancing their sense of control over their own lives and their healthcare journey. This can contribute to a sense of self-efficacy, which is often a key factor in recovery from mental health conditions (Hughes et al., 2018). By fostering a sense of partnership and trust, shared decision-making can also enhance the therapeutic alliance, a collaborative partnership that is often a key factor in successful mental health treatment (del Barrio et al., 2013).

Supported decision-making goes a step further, providing additional support to individuals who may have difficulty making decisions due to their mental health condition. This can involve a trusted person who helps the individual understand their options and make decisions, or structured decision-making tools that guide the individual through the decision-making process (Burns & Rose, 2013). However, shared and supported decision-making is not without its challenges. It requires a shift in power dynamics, with healthcare professionals needing to relinquish some of their traditional authority and control. It also requires resources and training to implement effectively, and may not be suitable for all patients or situations (Knight et al., 2018).

Despite these challenges, the benefits of shared and supported decision-making are significant. Research has shown that it can enhance patient satisfaction, improve treatment adherence and lead to better health outcomes (Penzenstadler et al., 2020). It can also reduce the use of coercion in mental healthcare, promoting a more respectful and dignified approach to care (Stone et al., 2020). Further research is needed to understand how to implement this approach effectively in different contexts and to evaluate its impact on patient outcomes and experiences (Sugiura et al., 2020).

## 5.2    Open Dialogue Teams

Open Dialogue (OD) is a transformative approach to mental health care that originated in Western Lapland, Finland, in the 1980s. OD teams represent a transformative approach to mental health care, focusing on fostering open, respectful and inclusive communication between individuals with mental health issues, their families and mental health professionals. OD has garnered significant attention for its emphasis on dialogical communication and its potential to reduce coercion in mental health treatment. The approach emerged as a response to the limitations of traditional mental health care, which often relied on individualised treatment plans and medical authority (Alakare & Seikkula, 2021). OD seeks to create a more inclusive and dialogical approach to mental health treatment, emphasising the importance of involving patients and their support networks in the decision-making process ((Olson et al., 2014). The key principles of OD include:

- Immediate response: The team responds to a mental health crisis as soon as possible, often within 24 h. This immediate response is crucial in building a therapeutic alliance and preventing unnecessary hospitalisation.
- Social network perspective: OD involves a network of professionals, including mental health nurses, psychiatrists, psychologists and social workers, working together with the patient and their social network. This approach acknowledges that mental health issues are embedded in social contexts and require a holistic response.
- Flexibility and mobility: The OD team is flexible and mobile, meeting in places where the patient feels most comfortable. This could be at home, in a community centre or a hospital.
- Continuity: The same team is responsible for the entire treatment process, from the initial crisis to outpatient care. This continuity of care is essential in building trust and understanding.

The implementation of OD involves several core principles and practices:

- First contact: When a person experiences a mental health crisis, a team, including mental health nurses, immediately responds and initiates contact. This rapid response is crucial for building a therapeutic alliance and preventing unnecessary hospitalisation.
- Multifamily meetings: Multifamily meetings form the core of OD. These meetings involve the patient, their family, friends and other relevant individuals, coming together with the treatment team to discuss the crisis and potential solutions.
- Open communication: Participants are encouraged to express their perspectives openly and respectfully. Mental health nurses facilitate the dialogue, ensuring that everyone's voice is heard and valued.
- Network approach: OD involves a network of professionals, including mental health nurses, psychiatrists, psychologists, and social workers, working together with the patient and their social network. This approach acknowledges that mental health issues are embedded in social contexts and require a holistic response.
- Flexibility in treatment planning: Treatment plans are not predetermined; instead, they emerge from the ongoing dialogue during the multifamily meetings. The focus is on finding a solution that aligns with the patient's preferences and social context.

Implementing OD requires a shift in the traditional hierarchical relationship between patients and healthcare providers. Mental health professionals must be trained in the principles of OD and must be willing to work collaboratively with patients and their social networks. One of the main challenges in implementing OD is the need for a significant shift in mindset and practice for mental health professionals. This includes moving away from a medical model of care, where the professional is the expert, to a dialogical model, where the patient's voice is central (von Peter et al., 2019). OD teams are characterised by their emphasis on immediate help, a social network perspective and flexibility and mobility. The approach encourages immediate meetings with individuals and their social networks at the onset of a crisis, often within 24 h. These meetings, which are typically held in the individual's home or another familiar environment, involve a team of mental health professionals who are trained in the principles of OD.

The OD teams approach is rooted in the belief that mental health issues are not isolated phenomena, but rather are deeply intertwined with an individual's social context. Therefore, the approach emphasises the importance of including the individual's social network, such as family members and friends, in the treatment process. This can help to foster a sense of understanding, support and shared responsibility, which can be crucial for recovery (Freeman et al., 2019).

The OD teams approach is also characterised by its flexibility and mobility. The treatment process is not rigidly structured but rather is adapted to meet the unique needs and preferences of the individual and their social network. The team is also mobile, able to meet with individuals and their social networks in a variety of settings (Galbusera & Kyselo, 2018). This method has been shown to reduce the use of coercive measures in mental health care. By fostering open, respectful and inclusive communication, the approach can help to de-escalate crises, prevent the need for involuntary hospitalisation and promote recovery. This can have a profound impact on the individual's well-being, promoting a sense of autonomy, dignity and recovery (Bergström et al., 2018).

Studies have shown that the approach can reduce the use of coercive measures, improve patient satisfaction and enhance the therapeutic alliance between patients and mental health professionals. Patients report feeling more respected and empowered, and mental health professionals report a more collaborative and trusting therapeutic relationship (Sunthararajah et al., 2022). The impact of the OD teams approach on mental health care, in the light of current evidence, appears to be profound and several international research projects are currently underway to test the approach (HopenDialogue, 2023).

## 5.3    Trauma-Informed Care

Trauma-informed care (TIC) is a transformative approach to mental health care that acknowledges the pervasive impact of trauma and strives to prevent re-traumatisation within healthcare settings. This approach is grounded in an understanding of the widespread impact of trauma and promotes environments of healing and recovery rather than practices that may inadvertently re-traumatise individuals (Sweeney et al., 2018).

TIC is not a specific therapeutic technique but rather an organisational structure and treatment framework that involves understanding, recognising and responding to the effects of all types of trauma. It emphasises physical, psychological and emotional safety for both consumers and providers and helps survivors rebuild a sense of control and empowerment. The principles of TIC include safety, trustworthiness and transparency, peer support, collaboration and mutuality, empowerment, voice and choice, and sensitivity to cultural, historical and gender issues. These principles guide the behaviour of staff and the organisation as a whole, shaping the approach to providing care and managing services.

Implementing TIC requires a shift in organisational culture towards recognising the prevalence and impact of trauma and incorporating this understanding into all aspects of service delivery (Sweeney & Taggart, 2018). This involves training staff to recognise signs of trauma, integrating trauma-informed practices into policies and procedures, and creating safe and supportive environments that prevent re-traumatisation. TIC has the potential to reduce the use of coercive measures in mental health care (Molloy et al., 2020). By fostering an environment of understanding and support, TIC can help to de-escalate situations that might otherwise lead to the use of coercion. Furthermore, by helping individuals understand and manage their trauma-related symptoms, TIC can empower individuals to take control of their recovery, reducing the need for coercive interventions (Aremu et al., 2018).

The effectiveness of TIC in reducing coercion and promoting recovery is supported by a growing body of evidence. Several studies have found that trauma-informed approaches can lead to reductions in the use of seclusion and restraint, improvements in patient satisfaction and engagement, and better mental health outcomes (Norman, 2022). However, implementing TIC can be challenging, requiring a commitment to organisational change and ongoing staff training (Mihelicova et al., 2018). Despite these challenges, the potential benefits of TIC for reducing coercion and promoting recovery make it a promising alternative to traditional approaches in mental health care.

## 5.4    Registry of Coercive Measures

The establishment of a Registry of Coercive Measures (RCM) represents a crucial step towards transparency and accountability in mental health care. This registry serves as a comprehensive database, documenting instances of coercive practices within mental health facilities. By systematically recording these incidents, the registry provides valuable insights into the prevalence and nature of coercion, thereby informing efforts to reduce its use.

The RCM is not merely a tool for data collection, but a catalyst for change. It encourages mental health facilities to critically examine their practices and identify areas for improvement. By making coercion visible, the registry fosters a culture of accountability and continuous improvement, driving efforts to minimise the use of coercive practices (Flammer et al., 2020). The data collected in the registry can be used to monitor trends, identify patterns and evaluate the effectiveness of interventions aimed at reducing coercion. This evidence-based approach is crucial for informing policy and practice, ensuring that efforts to reduce coercion are grounded in a solid understanding of the current landscape. Moreover, the registry can serve as a tool for advocacy and awareness-raising. By shedding light on the extent and nature of coercive practices, the registry can help to raise awareness about the issue and advocate for change. This can contribute to a broader societal dialogue about coercion in mental health care, fostering a culture of respect for human rights and dignity. The implementation of an RCM requires a commitment to transparency, accountability and continuous improvement. It involves the systematic collection and analysis of data, as well as the use of this data to inform policy and practice. While this can be a complex and challenging process, the potential benefits in terms of reducing coercion and promoting human rights make it a worthwhile endeavour (Välimäki et al., 2019).

The effectiveness of the RCM in reducing coercion is yet to be fully established (Steinert & Flammer, 2019). However, preliminary evidence suggests that it can contribute to a reduction in the use of coercive practices by promoting transparency, accountability and evidence-based decision-making (Välimäki et al., 2019). Further research is needed to fully understand the impact of the registry and to identify best practices for its implementation.

## 5.5 Comparative Overview of Treatment-Wide Alternatives

Treatment-wide alternatives have the advantage that they can be applied in both inpatient and community-based environments. The alternatives described in this section promote patient inclusion and autonomy, empowerment and systematic and informed practices. Challenges to implementation could be related to available resources and required shifts in care culture. An overview of the advantages, disadvantages and evidence support is shown in Table 3.

## 6 Real-World Examples

The following section provides an in-depth exploration of real-world examples where alternatives to coercion in mental health care have been successfully implemented. These examples span a range of countries and contexts, demonstrating the diversity and adaptability of these approaches. Each subsection focuses on a specific case, detailing the unique challenges, strategies and outcomes associated with implementing these alternatives.

From the OD approach in Lapland, Finland, to the Inclúyete programme in Almería, Spain, these examples provide valuable insights into the practical application of the alternatives discussed in previous sections. They demonstrate the potential of these approaches to reduce coercion, promote autonomy and improve patient outcomes in mental health care. In each case, the text will explore the specifics of the approach, its implementation, the challenges faced and the outcomes achieved. This will provide a comprehensive understanding of how these alternatives work in practice and the potential they hold for transforming mental health care.

It is important to note, however, that each of these examples is unique, shaped by its specific cultural, social and institutional context. Therefore, while they provide valuable lessons, these examples should not be seen as one-size-fits-all solutions,

**Table 3** Comparative overview of treatment-wide alternatives

| Intervention | Advantages | Disadvantages | Support by evidence |
|---|---|---|---|
| Shared and supported decision-making | Promotes patient autonomy and engagement | Requires time and effort from both patients and providers may be challenging if the patient has severe cognitive impairment | High: Numerous studies support the effectiveness of shared decision-making in improving patient satisfaction and treatment outcomes |
| | Can improve treatment outcomes | | |
| Open dialogue (both in- and outpatient) | Inclusive and dialogical approach | Requires a shift in traditional power dynamics | Mixed: Some studies show positive outcomes, yet results vary across different settings and populations |
| | Involves patient's social network | Requires extensive training for staff | |
| Trauma-informed care | Prevents re-traumatisation promotes safety and empowerment | Requires extensive training for staff | Promising: Early studies show promise in reducing the use of seclusion and restraint, more research is needed |
| | | May require changes to the physical environment | |
| Registry of coercive measures | Provides a systematic way to track and reduce coercive measures | Requires resources to set up and maintain | Preliminary: Initial studies suggest that registries help reduce the use of coercive measures |
| | Can inform policy and practice | Effectiveness depends on accurate reporting | |

but rather as sources of inspiration and learning for the development of context-specific strategies to reduce coercion in mental health care.

## 6.1    Open Dialogue in Lapland, Finland

In Western Lapland, the OD approach was developed in response to the limitations of traditional mental health care, which often relied heavily on medical authority and individualised treatment plans. The Finnish team, led by psychotherapist and researcher Jaakko Seikkula, sought to create a more inclusive and dialogical approach to mental health treatment, emphasising the importance of involving patients and their support networks in the decision-making process (Alakare & Seikkula, 2021).

The implementation of OD in Lapland has been characterised by several key principles and practices. The approach is characterised by an immediate response to mental health crises, often within 24 h. This rapid response is crucial for building a therapeutic alliance and preventing unnecessary hospitalisation. The Lapland OD team is also flexible and mobile, meeting patients where they are most comfortable, whether at home, in a community centre or hospital. Continuity of care is also a critical aspect of the approach, with the same team responsible for the entire treatment process, from the initial crisis to outpatient care. It has been shown that the implementation of OD requires a significant change in the mindset and practice of mental health professionals (Putman & Martindale, 2021). Moving from a medical model of care, where the professional is the expert, to a dialogical model, where the patient's voice is central, has been challenging. However, the Finnish team has shown that this shift is not only possible but also beneficial for patient outcomes (Martindale, 2021).

Despite the challenges, the OD approach in Lapland has led to improved outcomes for people with mental health problems. Studies have shown reduced medication use, lower hospitalisation rates and improved social functioning among patients treated with this approach in Lapland (Woods & Haynes, 2022). However, it is important to note that more research is needed to fully understand the effectiveness of OD and to identify the best ways to implement it in different contexts. The OD approach in Lapland has also shown remarkable results in reducing coercion and promoting well-being. By actively involving patients in their care, the approach promotes a deep sense of empowerment and autonomy. This patient-centred approach enables individuals to play an active role in shaping their treatment plans, leading to a greater sense of agency and reduced feelings of powerlessness, ultimately contributing to an improvement in the patient's overall well-being and drastically reducing any chance of a coercive approach being asked for (Schubert et al., 2021).

The OD approach in Lapland places a strong emphasis on crisis prevention. By intervening promptly in distressing situations, this approach effectively prevents crises from escalating to the point where coercive measures may become necessary. Timely and comprehensive intervention at the onset of crises minimises the need for coercive treatment, promotes a more compassionate and humane approach to mental health care (von Peter et al., 2019) and serves as a model for other regions and countries seeking to implement similar approaches in their mental health care systems. However, it is important to remember that the successful implementation of OD requires a significant change in the mindset and practice of mental health professionals, as well as the necessary resources and support, and further research to establish the approach as best practice is essential (Ebbert, 2019).

## 6.2 Inclúyete Program in Almería, Spain

The Inclúyete programme, a pioneering initiative based in Almería, Spain, is a testament to the power of voluntary participation in reducing the use of coercion in the treatment of severe mental disorders. Launched half a decade ago, the programme is the result of a collaboration between the University of Almería, the Public Foundation for the Social Integration of People with Mental Disorders (FAISEM), the Clinical Management Unit for Mental Health at the University Hospital of Torrecardenas and the Mental Health Advocacy Board of Almería (Cangas et al., 2023).

The main objective of the Inclúyete programme is to promote social inclusion and reduce the social stigma associated with mental disorders. In doing so, the programme aims to minimise the need for coercive measures in mental health treatment. This is achieved through a series of workshops open to anyone interested in the subject. These workshops, held in public spaces throughout the city, offer practical activities that encourage social interaction and personal development. The voluntary nature of participation in these workshops demonstrates the programme's commitment to reducing coercion (Gil García, 2019).

The programme's focus on social inclusion, active participation and recovery is in direct contrast to traditional, often coercive, methods of mental health treatment. By encouraging active participation in a wide range of activities, the programme offers individuals the opportunity to explore their interests, develop new skills and engage with the wider community. This approach not only reduces the need for coercion but also helps to challenge and change societal attitudes towards mental health (Vielma-Aguilera et al., 2021). In its 5 years of existence, the Inclúyete programme has organised around 20 activities, including nautical sports, animal-assisted exercise, radio and podcasts, physical training (athletics), literary expression, art and emotion, and pickleball. These activities are carefully designed to engage participants, promote social interaction and reduce the isolation often experienced by people with mental health disorders (Cerezuela et al., 2023).

The programme's impact on reducing coercion in mental health treatment is evident in the high attendance rates and significant improvements in participants' symptoms. All participants with mental health disorders maintain high attendance rates, over 80% at 1 year. There were also statistically significant improvements in negative symptomology, changes in positive symptomology and improvements in functional autonomy (Casado et al., 2020). These results suggest that the programme's non-coercive, inclusive approach is effective in engaging people with mental health problems and promoting their recovery (Díaz-Garrido et al., 2023).

## 6.3   Hugarafl Centre in Reykjavík, Iceland

The Hugarafl Centre in Reykjavík, Iceland, is a testament to the potential of community-based alternatives in mental health care. The centre takes a comprehensive approach to mental health care, integrating different therapeutic modalities to meet the diverse needs of its service users. Hugarafl, which means 'mind power' in Icelandic, encapsulates the centre's philosophy of empowering individuals to take charge of their mental health. The centre's services are designed to foster self-efficacy and resilience in its service users, promoting a sense of agency and control over their mental health journey (Council of Europe, 2021).

The centre offers a range of services including individual and group therapy, vocational training and social activities. These services are tailored to the needs and preferences of the individual, ensuring a person-centred approach to care. The centre's therapeutic modalities include cognitive behavioural therapy, mindfulness-based interventions and art therapy. These therapies aim to equip individuals with the skills and strategies to manage their mental health symptoms and improve their overall well-being. Vocational training at Hugarafl aims to improve the employability of its service users. By providing opportunities for skills development and work experience, the centre supports individuals in their transition to employment, promoting social inclusion and economic independence (Council of Europe, 2021). Social activities at the centre, such as group outings and shared meals, promote a sense of community among service users. These activities provide opportunities for social interaction and mutual support, helping to combat the social isolation often associated with mental illness.

The Hugarafl centre's comprehensive approach to mental health care has shown promising results. Service users have reported improvements in their mental health symptoms, increased self-efficacy and improved social functioning. In addition, the centre's emphasis on empowerment and self-determination is in line with the principles of recovery-oriented care, reducing the need for coercive interventions (Hugarafl, 2023). However, it is important to note that the centre's approach requires significant resources, including a multidisciplinary team of mental health professionals and a well-equipped facility. In addition, the success of the centre depends on the active involvement of service users and their commitment to their mental health journey. Therefore, while the Hugarafl centre serves as an inspiring example of a community-based alternative to coercion, its approach may not be feasible or appropriate for all contexts.

By integrating different therapeutic modalities and promoting empowerment and self-determination, the centre effectively reduces the need for coercive interventions. However, more research is needed to evaluate the effectiveness of this approach in different contexts and populations.

## 6.4    Soteria House in Jerusalem, Israel

Soteria House in Jerusalem, Israel, is a unique community-based alternative to traditional psychiatric hospitalisation. It was founded in the 1970s, inspired by the original Soteria House in California, USA. The Soteria model is based on the belief that people experiencing acute psychosis can recover in a supportive, non-restrictive environment without the extensive use of antipsychotic medication (Friedlander et al., 2022).

The Soteria House in Jerusalem provides a home-like environment for its residents, offering a safe and supportive space for people experiencing acute psychosis. The house is staffed by a multidisciplinary team, including mental health professionals and people with lived experience of mental health problems. The team provides 24-h support to help residents manage their symptoms and cope with their daily lives. One of the key principles of the Soteria model is the minimisation of antipsychotic medication. Instead of relying on medication as the primary form of treatment, Soteria House emphasises the importance of interpersonal relationships, community integration and self-determination. Residents are encouraged to participate in daily activities, such as cooking, cleaning and socialising, which can help foster a sense of normalcy and autonomy (Soteria Israel, 2023).

The Soteria House in Jerusalem has been the subject of several studies which have shown promising results. Research has shown that residents of Soteria House have lower rates of hospitalisation and use less antipsychotic medication compared to individuals in traditional psychiatric care (Calton et al., 2008). In addition, residents have reported high levels of satisfaction with the care they receive at Soteria House, particularly appreciating the supportive and non-restrictive environment (Jacobs, 2019). However, it is important to note that the Soteria model may not be suitable for everyone. Some people may require more intensive medical intervention, particularly in the case of severe or treatment-resistant psychosis (Cooper et al., 2021). In addition, the implementation of the Soteria model requires significant resources, including well-trained and dedicated staff and a suitable living environment. Despite these challenges, the Soteria House in Jerusalem serves as a valuable example of a community-based alternative to traditional psychiatric care, demonstrating the potential benefits of a supportive, non-coercive approach to the treatment of acute psychosis.

## 6.5    MindFreedom Ghana and International

MindFreedom International is a non-profit organisation that advocates for human rights in the area of mental health. It operates worldwide, with a significant presence in Ghana, where it is known as MindFreedom Ghana. This section provides a detailed examination of the organisation's work, focusing on its efforts to reduce coercion in mental health care and promote alternatives. MindFreedom International's mission is to protect the right to self-determination in mental health care. The organisation advocates for a mental health system that is recovery-based, person-centred and respects the autonomy and dignity of the individual. MindFreedom International promotes alternatives to coercive practices such as involuntary hospitalisation and forced medication that is often used in traditional mental health care. The organisation believes that these practices can be harmful and counterproductive, leading to a loss of autonomy and dignity and hindering the recovery process.

In Ghana, MindFreedom operates under the name MindFreedom Ghana. The organisation works closely with local communities, mental health professionals and people with lived experience of mental health problems (MindFreedom, 2023). MindFreedom Ghana's activities include advocacy, education and support for individuals and families affected by mental health issues. The organisation also works with local and national government bodies to influence mental health policy and practice (Stastny & Lehmann, 2007). One of MindFreedom Ghana's key strategies is the promotion of community-based mental health care. The organisation believes that mental health care should be provided in the community, where individuals can receive support in a familiar and supportive environment. Community-based care can help reduce the use of coercive practices, such as involuntary hospitalisation, that are often associated with institutional care (Ward, 2022).

MindFreedom Ghana also advocates the use of SSDM in mental health care. Shared decision-making is a collaborative process in which individuals and healthcare professionals work together to make informed decisions about care. This approach respects individual autonomy and promotes patient-centred care, making it a valuable alternative to coercive practices (Stastny & Lehmann, 2007).

Despite the significant contributions of MindFreedom International and MindFreedom Ghana, there are challenges facing the organisation. These include limited resources, social stigma associated with mental health issues and resistance from traditional mental health systems. To overcome these challenges, the organisation relies on the support of its members, donors and partners, and continues to advocate for systemic change in mental health care. Through its advocacy, education and support activities, it contributes to the transformation of mental health systems towards more respectful, person-centred and recovery-oriented models of care. However, more research is needed to evaluate the impact of their work and to identify strategies to address the challenges they face.

## 7    Concluding Remarks

In conclusion, the issue of coercion in mental health care is complex and multifaceted, with profound implications for the autonomy, dignity and well-being of people receiving care. The use of coercive practices often results in a significant loss of autonomy for these individuals, which can be detrimental to their recovery process. However, there is growing recognition of the need for alternatives to restraint in mental health care. These alternatives, which include SSDM, trauma-informed care, OD teams and sensory rooms, can help to promote patients' autonomy, dignity and well-being while reducing the use of coercive practices.

The implementation of alternative approaches to mental health care requires a collaborative effort involving various stakeholders, such as nurses, psychiatrists, social workers, family members, support and user groups, and people with lived experience. To successfully integrate these alternatives, education and training programmes for mental health professionals are essential to familiarise them with the principles and evidence supporting these interventions. Policy reform within mental health systems can be advocated by stakeholders to prioritise the integration of alternative interventions, requiring collaboration with mental health organisations, policymakers and government agencies. Investment in research to provide evidence of the effectiveness of alternative approaches is essential to gain wider acceptance and support.

User groups and family members should be involved in decision-making processes to ensure that patients' perspectives and preferences are taken into account. Peer support specialists can provide valuable insights into the design and delivery of alternative interventions through their lived experience. Starting with pilot programmes or small-scale initiatives can effectively introduce alternatives into mental health practice and pave the way for wider implementation.

Nurses, psychiatrists and social workers can advocate for the inclusion of CAM in individualised treatment plans, complementing traditional approaches for a more holistic and person-centred approach to care. Collaborative development of guidelines and best practices ensures consistency and quality of care. Creating a culture of collaboration and dialogue among stakeholders fosters a supportive and non-hierarchical environment that promotes continuous improvement and innovation in mental health care. By applying these strategies, alternative approaches can be effectively integrated into mental health practice, contributing to patient autonomy, reduced coercion and a recovery-oriented model of care.

**Acknowledgements** We would like to express our sincere gratitude to our colleagues, the HOPEnDialogue network of open dialogue research, the experts by experience from the Soteria network and the Mad In America international network, the International Institute Psychiatric Withdrawal, the EU COST FOSTREN Fostering and Strengthening Approaches to Reducing Coercion in European Mental Health Services, the International Society for Psychological and Social Approaches to Psychosis (ISPS), the users and practitioners of Trieste's mental health services and the Inclúyete programme in Almería for the invaluable insights and information they provided. Their contributions, along with those of many others who also provided feedback despite not being mentioned in this brief note, have helped to shape the depth and quality of our research, and their commitment to advancing mental health practice is truly commendable.

# References

Alakare, B., & Seikkula, J. (2021). The historical development of Open Dialogue in Western Lapland. In *Open dialogue for psychosis: Organising mental health services to prioritise dialogue, relationship and meaning*. Routledge.

Alvarsson, J., Wiens, S., & Nilsson, M. (2010). Stress recovery during exposure to nature sound and environmental noise. *International Journal of Environmental Research and Public Health, 7*, 1036–1046.

Aremu, B., Hill, P. D., McNeal, J. M., Petersen, M. A., Swanberg, D., & Delaney, K. R. (2018). Implementation of trauma-informed care and brief solution-focused therapy: A quality improvement project aimed at increasing engagement on an inpatient psychiatric unit. *Journal of Psychosocial Nursing and Mental Health Services, 56*(8), 16–22.

Barbui, C., Purgato, M., Abdulmalik, J., Caldas-de-Almeida, J. M., Eaton, J., Gureje, O., et al. (2021). Efficacy of interventions to reduce coercive treatment in mental health services: Umbrella review of randomised evidence. *The British Journal of Psychiatry, 218*(4), 185–195.

Bergström, T., Seikkula, J., Alakare, B., Mäki, P., Köngäs-Saviaro, P., Taskila, J. J., Tolvanen, A., & Aaltonen, J. (2018). The family-oriented open dialogue approach in the treatment of first-episode psychosis: Nineteen–year outcomes. *Psychiatry Research, 270*, 168–175.

Björkdahl, A., Perseius, K. I., Samuelsson, M., & Lindberg, M. H. (2016). Sensory rooms in psychiatric inpatient care: Staff experiences. *International Journal of Mental Health Nursing, 25*(5), 472–479.

Bolsinger, J., Jaeger, M., Hoff, P., & Theodoridou, A. (2020). Challenges and opportunities in building and maintaining a good therapeutic relationship in acute psychiatric settings: A narrative review. *Frontiers in Psychiatry, 10*, 965.

Bourne, P., Meddings, S., & Whittington, A. (2018). An evaluation of service use outcomes in a recovery college. *Journal of Mental Health, 27*(4), 359–366.

Braun, E., Gaillard, A. S., Vollmann, J., Gather, J., & Scholten, M. (2023). Mental health service users' perspectives on psychiatric advance directives: A systematic review. *Psychiatric Services, 74*(4), 381–392.

Brown, A., Tse, T., & Fortune, T. (2019). Defining sensory modulation: A review of the concept and a contemporary definition for application by occupational therapists. *Scandinavian Journal of Occupational Therapy, 26*(7), 515–523.

Burns, T., & Rose, D. (2013). How can the service user voice be best heard at psychiatric meetings? *The British Journal of Psychiatry, 203*(2), 88–89.

Calton, T., Ferriter, M., Huband, N., & Spandler, H. (2008). A systematic review of the Soteria paradigm for the treatment of people diagnosed with schizophrenia. *Schizophrenia Bulletin, 34*(1), 181–192.

Campbell, L. A., & Kisely, S. R. (2009). Advance treatment directives for people with severe mental illness. *Cochrane Database of Systematic Reviews, 2009*(1), CD005963. https://doi.org/10.1002/14651858.CD005963.pub2

Cangas, A. J., Sánchez, E., de Lemus, M. L., & López-Pardo, A. (2023). The "Incluyete"(get involved) program: A socio-educational experience for social inclusion in mental health. In *Psychological interventions for psychosis: Towards a paradigm shift* (pp. 453–464). Springer International Publishing.

Casado, D. G., Ruano, Á. M., Cangas, A. J., & López-Pardo, A. (2020). Comparativa entre dos programas de actividad física con personas con Trastorno Mental Grave: El espacio como herramienta terapéutica. *Revista de Estilos de Aprendizaje, 13*(25), 55–69.

Cerezuela, J. L., Lirola, M. J., & Cangas, A. J. (2023). Pickleball and mental health in adults: A systematic review. *Frontiers in Psychology, 14*, 1137047.

Chapman, A., Williams, C., Hannah, J., & Pūras, D. (2020). Reimagining the mental health paradigm for our collective well-being. *Health and Human Rights, 22*(1), 1.

Chieze, M., Hurst, S., Kaiser, S., & Sentissi, O. (2019). Effects of seclusion and restraint in adult psychiatry: A systematic review. *Frontiers in Psychiatry, 10*, 491.

Compton, M. T., Kelley, M. E., Anderson, S., Graves, J., Broussard, B., Pauselli, L., Zern, A., Pope, L. G., Johnson, M., & Haynes, N. L. (2023). Opening doors to recovery: A randomized controlled trial of a recovery-oriented community navigation service for individuals with serious mental illnesses and repeated hospitalizations. *The Journal of Clinical Psychiatry, 84*(2), 45068.

Cooper, R. E., Mason, J. P., Calton, T., Richardson, J., & Moncrieff, J. (2021). Opinion piece: The case for establishing a minimal medication alternative for psychosis and schizophrenia. *Psychosis, 13*(3), 276–285.

Council of Europe. (2021). *Compendium report: good practices in the Council of Europe to Promote Voluntary Measures in Mental Health*. Council of Europe.

Croft, B., Weaver, A., & Ostrow, L. (2021). Self-reliance and belonging: Guest experiences of a peer respite. *Psychiatric Rehabilitation Journal, 44*(2), 124.

Crowther, A., Taylor, A., Toney, R., Meddings, S., Whale, T., Jennings, H., Pollock, K., Bates, P., Henderson, C., Waring, J., & Slade, M. (2019). The impact of Recovery Colleges on mental health staff, services and society. *Epidemiology and Psychiatric Sciences, 28*(5), 481–488.

Cusack, P., Cusack, F. P., McAndrew, S., McKeown, M., & Duxbury, J. (2018). An integrative review exploring the physical and psychological harm inherent in using restraint in mental health inpatient settings. *International Journal of Mental Health Nursing, 27*(3), 1162–1176.

del Barrio, L. R., Cyr, C., Benisty, L., & Richard, P. (2013). Gaining Autonomy & Medication Management (GAM): New perspectives on well-being, quality of life and psychiatric medication. *Ciência & Saúde Coletiva, 18*, 2879–2887.

Díaz-Garrido, J. A., Zúñiga, R., Laffite, H., & Morris, E. (Eds.). (2023). *Psychological interventions for psychosis: Towards a paradigm shift*. Springer.

Drake, R. E., Cimpean, D., & Torrey, W. C. (2022). Shared decision making in mental health: Prospects for personalized medicine. *Dialogues in Clinical Neuroscience, 11*(4), 455–463.

Duffy, R. M., Sidhu, D. S., & Kelly, B. D. (2023). Optimising patient care in psychiatry with autonomy and choice. In *Handbook on optimizing patient care in psychiatry* (pp. 110–123). Routledge.

Easter, M. M., Swanson, J. W., Robertson, A. G., Moser, L. L., & Swartz, M. S. (2021). Impact of psychiatric advance directive facilitation on mental health consumers: Empowerment, treatment attitudes and the role of peer support specialists. *Journal of Mental Health, 30*(5), 585–593.

Ebbert, N. E. (2019). Open dialogue: The evidence and further research. *Psychiatric Services, 70*(6), 530–531.

Ellegaard, T., Mehlsen, M., Lomborg, K., & Bliksted, V. (2017). Use of patient-controlled psychiatric hospital admissions: Mental health professionals' perspective. *Nordic Journal of Psychiatry, 71*(5), 362–369.

Flammer, E., Frank, U., & Steinert, T. (2020). Freedom restrictive coercive measures in forensic psychiatry. *Frontiers in Psychiatry, 11*, 146.

Freeman, A. M., Tribe, R. H., Stott, J. C., & Pilling, S. (2019). Open dialogue: A review of the evidence. *Psychiatric Services, 70*(1), 46–59.

Friedlander, A., Tzur Bitan, D., & Lichtenberg, P. (2022). The Soteria model: Implementing an alternative to acute psychiatric hospitalization in Israel. *Psychosis, 14*(2), 99–108.

Galbusera, L., & Kyselo, M. (2018). The difference that makes the difference: A conceptual analysis of the open dialogue approach. *Psychosis, 10*(1), 47–54.

Gather, J., Scholten, M., Henking, T., Vollmann, J., & Juckel, G. (2019). What replaces the locked door? Conceptual and ethical considerations regarding open door policies, formal coercion and treatment pressures. *Der Nervenarzt, 90*, 690–694.

Gil García, S. (2019). *Programa Inclúyete: La Inclusión Social Frente al Estigma en Salud Mental a Través del Deporte.* Universidad de Almería.

Golay, P., Morandi, S., Silva, B., Devas, C., & Bonsack, C. (2019). Feeling coerced during psychiatric hospitalization: Impact of perceived status of admission and perceived usefulness of hospitalization. *International Journal of Law and Psychiatry, 67*, 101512.

Grinde, B., & Grindal Patil, G. (2009). Biophilia: Does visual contact with nature impact on health and well-being? *International Journal of Environmental Research and Public Health, 6*, 2332–2343.

Hachtel, H., Vogel, T., & Huber, C. G. (2019). Mandated treatment and its impact on therapeutic process and outcome factors. *Frontiers in Psychiatry, 10*, 219.

Haig, S., & Hallett, N. (2023). Use of sensory rooms in adult psychiatric inpatient settings: A systematic review and narrative synthesis. *International Journal of Mental Health Nursing, 32*(1), 54–75.

Haigh, C. B., Kringen, A. L., & Kringen, J. A. (2020). Mental illness stigma: Limitations of crisis intervention team training. *Criminal Justice Policy Review, 31*(1), 42–57.

Hayes, D., Camacho, E. M., Ronaldson, A., Stepanian, K., McPhilbin, M., Elliott, R. A., Repper, J., Bishop, S., Stergiopoulos, V., Brophy, L., & Giles, K. (2023). Evidence-based Recovery Colleges: Developing a typology based on organisational characteristics, fidelity and funding. *Social Psychiatry and Psychiatric Epidemiology, 59*(5), 759–768.

Hedlund Lindberg, M., Samuelsson, M., Perseius, K. I., & Björkdahl, A. (2019). The experiences of patients in using sensory rooms in psychiatric inpatient care. *International Journal of Mental Health Nursing, 28*(4), 930–939.

Hennessy, B., Hunter, A., & Grealish, A. (2023). A qualitative synthesis of patients' experiences of re-traumatization in acute mental health inpatient settings. *Journal of Psychiatric and Mental Health Nursing, 30*(3), 398–434.

Herrman, H., Allan, J., Galderisi, S., Javed, A., Rodrigues, M., & WPA Task Force on Implementing Alternatives to Coercion in Mental Health Care. (2022). Alternatives to coercion in mental health care: WPA position statement and call to action. *World Psychiatry, 21*(1), 159–160.

Hirsch, S., & Steinert, T. (2019). Measures to avoid coercion in psychiatry and their efficacy. *Deutsches Ärzteblatt International, 116*(19), 336.

Hochstrasser, L., Fröhlich, D., Schneeberger, A. R., Borgwardt, S., Lang, U. E., Stieglitz, R. D., & Huber, C. G. (2018a). Long-term reduction of seclusion and forced medication on a hospital-wide level: Implementation of an open-door policy over 6 years. *European Psychiatry, 48*(1), 51–57.

Hochstrasser, L., Voulgaris, A., Möller, J., Zimmermann, T., Steinauer, R., Borgwardt, S., Lang, U. E., & Huber, C. G. (2018b). Reduced frequency of cases with seclusion is associated with "opening the doors" of a psychiatric intensive care unit. *Frontiers in Psychiatry, 9*, 57.

Hogan, M. F., & Goldman, M. L. (2021). New opportunities to improve mental health crisis systems. *Psychiatric Services, 72*(2), 169–173.

HopenDialogue. (2023). *The project.* https://www.hopendialogue.net/the-project/

Hugarafl. (2023). *About Hugarafl.* https://hugarafl.is/about-hugarafl/

Hughes, T. M., Merath, K., Chen, Q., Sun, S., Palmer, E., Idrees, J. J., Okunrintemi, V., Squires, M., Beal, E. W., & Pawlik, T. M. (2018). Association of shared decision-making on patient-reported health outcomes and healthcare utilization. *The American Journal of Surgery, 216*(1), 7–12.

Ibrahim, N., Thompson, D., Nixdorf, R., Kalha, J., Mpango, R., Moran, G., Mueller-Stierlin, A., Ryan, G., Mahlke, C., Shamba, D., & Puschner, B. (2020). A systematic review of influences on implementation of peer support work for adults with mental health problems. *Social Psychiatry and Psychiatric Epidemiology, 55*, 285–293.

Jacobs, Y. (2019). Soteria: Reflections on "Being With" finding ones way through psychosis. *Journal of Humanistic Psychology, 59*(5), 681–685.

Johnson, A. H., & Rogers, B. A. (2020). "We're the normal ones here": Community involvement, peer support, and transgender mental health. *Sociological Inquiry, 90*(2), 271–292.

Kane, E., Evans, E., & Shokraneh, F. (2018). Effectiveness of current policing-related mental health interventions: A systematic review. *Criminal Behaviour and Mental Health, 28*(2), 108–119.

Kent, M. (2019). Developing a strategy to embed peer support into mental health systems. *Administration and Policy in Mental Health and Mental Health Services Research, 46*(3), 271–276.

Kinane, C., Osborne, J., Ishaq, Y., Colman, M., & MacInnes, D. (2022). Peer supported Open Dialogue in the National Health Service: Implementing and evaluating a new approach to mental health care. *BMC Psychiatry, 22*(1), 138.

Knight, F., Kokanović, R., Ridge, D., Brophy, L., Hill, N., Johnston-Ataata, K., & Herrman, H. (2018). Supported decision-making: The expectations held by people with experience of mental illness. *Qualitative Health Research, 28*(6), 1002–1015.

Kowalinski, E., Hochstrasser, L., Schneeberger, A. R., Borgwardt, S., Lang, U. E., & Huber, C. G. (2019). Six years of open-door policy at the University Psychiatric Hospital Basel. *Der Nervenarzt, 90*, 705–708.

Lindkvist, R. M., Landgren, K., Liljedahl, S. I., Daukantaitė, D., Helleman, M., & Westling, S. (2019). Predictable, collaborative and safe: Healthcare provider experiences of introducing brief admissions by self-referral for self-harming and suicidal persons with a history of extensive psychiatric inpatient care. *Issues in Mental Health Nursing, 40*(7), 548–556.

Marcus, N., & Stergiopoulos, V. (2022). Re-examining mental health crisis intervention: A rapid review comparing outcomes across police, co-responder and non-police models. *Health & Social Care in the Community, 30*(5), 1665–1679.

Martindale, B. (2021). Research from Western Lapland of Open Dialogue for psychosis. In *Open dialogue for psychosis: Organising mental health services to prioritise dialogue, relationship and meaning.* Routledge.

Mckeown, M., Scholes, A., Jones, F., & Aindow, W. (2019). Coercive practices in mental health services: Stories of recalcitrance, resistance and legitimation. In *Madness, violence, and power: A critical collection* (pp. 263–285). University of Toronto Press.

Mihelicova, M., Brown, M., & Shuman, V. (2018). Trauma-informed care for individuals with serious mental illness: An avenue for community psychology's involvement in community mental health. *American Journal of Community Psychology, 61*(1–2), 141–152.

MindFreedom International. (2023). *About MFI.* https://mindfreedom.org/about-mfi/

Molloy, L., Fields, L., Trostian, B., & Kinghorn, G. (2020). Trauma-informed care for people presenting to the emergency department with mental health issues. *Emergency Nurse, 28*(2), 30–35.

Moro, M. F., Pathare, S., Zinkler, M., Osei, A., Puras, D., Paccial, R. C., & Carta, M. G. (2022). The WHO QualityRights initiative: Building partnerships among psychiatrists, people with lived experience and other key stakeholders to improve the quality of mental healthcare. *The British Journal of Psychiatry, 220*(2), 49–51.

Murray, H., & Wortzel, H. S. (2019). Psychiatric advance directives: Origins, benefits, challenges, and future directions. *Journal of Psychiatric Practice, 25*(4), 303–307.

Nischk, D., & Rusch, J. (2019). What makes Soteria work? On the effect of a therapeutic milieu on self-disturbances in the schizophrenia syndrome. *Psychopathology, 52*(4), 213–220.

Norman, S. (2022). Trauma-informed guilt reduction therapy: Overview of the treatment and research. *Current Treatment Options in Psychiatry, 9*(3), 115–125.

Olsø, T. M., Gudde, C. B., Moljord, I. E. O., Evensen, G. H., Antonsen, D. Ø., & Eriksen, L. (2016). More than just a bed: Mental health service users' experiences of self-referral admission. *International Journal of Mental Health Systems, 10*, 1–7.

Olson, M., Seikkula, J., & Ziedonis, D. (2014). *The key elements of dialogic practice in open dialogue: Fidelity criteria*. University of Massachusetts Medical School.

Penzenstadler, L., Molodynski, A., & Khazaal, Y. (2020). Supported decision making for people with mental health disorders in clinical practice: A systematic review. *International Journal of Psychiatry in Clinical Practice, 24*(1), 3–9.

Perers, C., Bäckström, B., Johansson, B. A., & Rask, O. (2022). Methods and strategies for reducing seclusion and restraint in child and adolescent psychiatric inpatient care. *Psychiatric Quarterly, 93*(1), 107–136.

Puras, D. (2022). Report of the special rapporteur on the right of everyone to the enjoyment of the highest attainable standard of physical and mental health. *Philippine Law Journal, 95*, 274.

Puras, D., & Gooding, P. (2019). Mental health and human rights in the 21st century. *World Psychiatry, 18*(1), 42.

Putman, N., & Martindale, B. (Eds.). (2021). *Open dialogue for psychosis: Organising mental health services to prioritise dialogue, relationship and meaning*. Routledge.

Repper, J., Brewin, J., Meddings, S., McPhilbin, M., Yeo, C., & Slade, M. (2022). Recovery Colleges Characterisation and Testing in England (RECOLLECT): Rationale and protocol. *BMC Psychiatry, 22*, 627.

Rogers, M. S., McNiel, D. E., & Binder, R. L. (2019). Effectiveness of police crisis intervention training programs. *The Journal of the American Academy of Psychiatry and the Law, 47*(4), 414–421.

Sanchez-Moscona, C., & Eiroa-Orosa, F. J. (2021). Training mental health peer support training facilitators: A qualitative, participatory evaluation. *International Journal of Mental Health Nursing, 30*(1), 261–273.

Sashidharan, S. P., Mezzina, R., & Puras, D. (2019). Reducing coercion in mental healthcare. *Epidemiology and Psychiatric Sciences, 28*(6), 605–612.

Schubert, S., Rhodes, P., & Buus, N. (2021). Transformation of professional identity: An exploration of psychologists and psychiatrists implementing Open Dialogue. *Journal of Family Therapy, 43*(1), 143–164.

Shalaby, R. A. H., & Agyapong, V. I. (2020). Peer support in mental health: Literature review. *JMIR Mental Health, 7*(6), e15572.

Skott, M., Durbeej, N., Smitmanis-Lyle, M., et al. (2021). Patient-controlled admissions to inpatient care: A twelve-month naturalistic study of patients with schizophrenia spectrum diagnoses and the effects on admissions to and days in inpatient care. *BMC Health Services Research, 21*, 598. https://doi.org/10.1186/S12913-021-06617-8

Smitmanis-Lyle, M., Allenius, E., Salomonsson, S., et al. (2022). What are the effects of implementing patient-controlled admissions in inpatient care? A study protocol of a large-scale implementation and naturalistic evaluation for adult and adolescent patients with severe psychiatric conditions throughout Region Stockholm. *BMJ Open, 12*, e065770. https://doi.org/10.1136/bmjopen-2022-065770

Soteria Israel. (2023). *About Soteria Israel*. https://www.soteria.org.il/english

Stastny, P., & Lehmann, P. (Eds.). (2007). *Alternatives beyond psychiatry*. Peter Lehmann Publishing.

Steiger, S., Moeller, J., Sowislo, J. F., Lieb, R., Lang, U. E., & Huber, C. G. (2023). General and case-specific approval of coercion in psychiatry in the public opinion. *International Journal of Environmental Research and Public Health, 20*(3), 2081.

Steinert, T., & Flammer, E. (2019). Frequency of coercive measures as a quality indicator for psychiatric hospitals? *Der Nervenarzt, 90*, 35–39.

Steinert, T., Schreiber, L., Metzger, F. G., & Hirsch, S. (2019). Open doors in psychiatric hospitals: An overview of empirical findings. *Der Nervenarzt, 90*, 680–689.

Stone, M., Kokanovic, R., Callard, F., & Broom, A. F. (2020). Estranged relations: Coercion and care in narratives of supported decision-making in mental healthcare. *Medical Humanities, 46*(1), 62–72.

Strand, M., & von Hausswolff-Juhlin, Y. (2015). Patient-controlled hospital admission in psychiatry: A systematic review. *Nordic Journal of Psychiatry, 69*(8), 574–586.

Stupak, R., & Dobroczyński, B. (2019). The Soteria project: A forerunner of "a third way" in psychiatry. *Psychiatria Polska, 53*(6), 1351–1364.

Sugiura, K., Mahomed, F., Saxena, S., & Patel, V. (2020). An end to coercion: Rights and decision-making in mental health care. *Bulletin of the World Health Organization, 98*(1), 52.

Sunthararajah, S., Clarke, K., Razzaque, R., Chmielowska, M., Brandrett, B., & Pilling, S. (2022). Exploring patients' experience of peer-supported open dialogue and standard care following a mental health crisis: Qualitative 3-month follow-up study. *BJPsych Open, 8*(4), e139.

Sweeney, A., & Taggart, D. (2018). (Mis) understanding trauma-informed approaches in mental health. *Journal of Mental Health, 27*(5), 383–387.

Sweeney, A., Filson, B., Kennedy, A., Collinson, L., & Gillard, S. (2018). A paradigm shift: Relationships in trauma-informed mental health services. *BJPsych Advances, 24*(5), 319–333.

Thériault, J., Lord, M. M., Briand, C., Piat, M., & Meddings, S. (2020). Recovery colleges after a decade of research: A literature review. *Psychiatric Services, 71*(9), 928–940.

Thomsen, C. T., Benros, M. E., Maltesen, T., Hastrup, L. H., Andersen, P. K., Giacco, D., & Nordentoft, M. (2018). Patient-controlled hospital admission for patients with severe mental disorders: A nationwide prospective multicentre study. *Acta Psychiatrica Scandinavica, 137*(4), 355–363.

Tinland, A., Loubière, S., Mougeot, F., Jouet, E., Pontier, M., Baumstarck, K., et al. (2022). Effect of psychiatric advance directives facilitated by peer workers on compulsory admission among people with mental illness: A randomized clinical trial. *JAMA Psychiatry, 79*(8), 752–759.

Torrents, E. G. (2022). Pathogenic societies and collective madness: A critical look at normalcy. *African Journal of Humanities and Social Sciences, 2*(1), 1–6.

Tyerman, J., Patovirta, A. L., & Celestini, A. (2021). How stigma and discrimination influences nursing care of persons diagnosed with mental illness: A systematic review. *Issues in Mental Health Nursing, 42*(2), 153–163.

Välimäki, M., Yang, M., Vahlberg, T., Lantta, T., Pekurinen, V., Anttila, M., & Normand, S. L. (2019). Trends in the use of coercive measures in Finnish psychiatric hospitals: A register analysis of the past two decades. *BMC Psychiatry, 19*, 1–15.

Verbeke, E., Vanheule, S., Cauwe, J., Truijens, F., & Froyen, B. (2019). Coercion and power in psychiatry: A qualitative study with ex-patients. *Social Science & Medicine, 223*, 89–96.

Vielma-Aguilera, A., Castro-Alzate, E., Saldivia Bórquez, S., & Grandón-Fernández, P. (2021). Interventions to reduce stigma toward people with severe mental disorders in Ibero-America: A systematic review. *Revista Ciencias de la Salud, 19*(1), 5–31.

von Peter, S., Aderhold, V., Cubellis, L., Bergström, T., Stastny, P., Seikkula, J., & Puras, D. (2019). Open dialogue as a human rights-aligned approach. *Frontiers in Psychiatry, 10*, 387.

Ward, N.E. (2022). *An inquiry into the role of social movements and patient activism in shaping the field of mental health.* Doctoral dissertation, Adelphi University.

Woods, D., & Haynes, J. (2022). The eradication of schizophrenia in Western Lapland and Open Dialogue in the work of Ridiculusmus. In *The big anxiety: Taking care of mental health in times of crisis.* Bloomsbury Publishing (p. 69). https://www.torrossa.com/gs/resourceProxy?an=5213273&publisher=FZ0661#page=88

Zinkler, M., & von Peter, S. (2019). End coercion in mental health services—Toward a system based on support only. *Laws, 8*(3), 19.

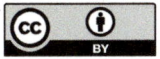

# Post-occurrence Review

Kevin McKenna, Brodie Paterson, Nutmeg Hallett, and Lene Lauge Berring

## 1    Introduction

Fearful or threatening experiences can have long-term psychological and emotional consequences. Being subjected to coercive measures, such as seclusion and restraint, is an intrusive experience which and can lead to negative psychological consequences such as distress and fear for all involved. Following the application of coercive measures, patients have reported feelings of dehumanisation and being 'retraumatised' by the evoking memories of previous traumatic events (Cusack et al., 2018; Nyttingnes et al., 2016). Nurses report role conflicts and decreased job satisfaction (Jansen et al., 2020; Krieger et al., 2021). Intervening after coercive interventions, or indeed any occurrence that has the potential to result in harm, is essential for reducing the impact of such experiences. This is true for patients who experience or witness them and for the staff who apply them. Being given space to revisit the event creates an opportunity to make sense of what happened and why, and to discuss how to avoid similar situations in the future. For decades, post-occurrence procedures have been recommended to reduce the harms caused by coercive measures (Nolan, 2000).

K. McKenna (✉)
Dundalk Institute of Technology, Dundalk, County Louth, Ireland
e-mail: kevin.mckenna@dkit.ie

B. Paterson
Queen Mary University of London, London, UK

N. Hallett
School of Nursing and Midwifery, University of Birmingham, Birmingham, UK
e-mail: n.n.hallett@bham.ac.uk

L. L. Berring
Psychiatric Research Unit, Region Zealand, Slagelse, Denmark
e-mail: lelb@regionsjaelland.dk

Professional and regulatory reports consistently identify violence towards personnel as a complex occupational hazard within mental healthcare (Iozzino et al., 2015; US Bureau of Labor Statistics, 2022). Exposure to such violence involves risks of potentially serious physical injury and a broad range of emotional, cognitive, behavioural, social and vocational impacts (Gillespie et al., 2013; National Institute of Health and Care Excellence [NICE], 2015; Needham et al., 2005).

Attention to managing the aftermath of negative experiences has traditionally been framed dichotomously within approaches that seek either to prevent aggression and violence or to eliminate or minimise the use of restrictive interventions. This dichotomy is at odds with the reality in inpatient mental settings in which aggression, violence and restrictive coercive practices involves a series of complex bidirectional relationships (Baker et al., 2021).

Johnson (2010) proposed that these traditionally distinct bodies of knowledge be integrated so that the findings of one could inform the other. Bowers (2014) proposed such an integrated approach based upon the proposition of unit-specific associations between rates of 'conflict' behaviours, including all manifestations of aggression and 'containment' interventions, including all restrictive practices. Bowers (2014) suggested that, because of the dynamic reciprocal relationship between containment and conflict, addressing common contributory factors could effectively reduce both.

This chapter explores the psychological and emotional effects that coercive measures, such as seclusion and restraint, have on patients and healthcare staff within mental health settings. Furthermore, it explores how other occurrences, including but not limited to patient violence, can be harmful. It argues that a feasible means of addressing these impacts is by employing post-occurrence reviews as an approach which reconceptualises occurrences as opportunities to foster understanding, learning and prevention, rather than as occasions to apportion blame. In doing so, the chapter considers the nomenclature, regulatory context and historical lineage of debriefing, and the evidence base pertaining to its effectiveness in order to provide a balanced analysis of the place of post-occurrence reviews in mental healthcare settings. The chapter advocates for a reflective and proactive approach in the aftermath of coercive occurrences that can serve both to improve patient care and to secure the well-being of the staff charged with its provision.

## 2    The Significance of Terminology

There has recently been a growing recognition that the actions taken in the aftermath of coercive interventions (e.g. seclusion, restraint, forced medication) or occurrences of patients' challenging behaviour may play an important role in prevention. Throughout this chapter, we refer to these actions collectively as 'post-occurrence reviews', with this terminology having been chosen deliberately. The term occurrence is used in preference to 'incident' which can carry the connotation of negativity or blame, suggesting that something went wrong or was mishandled, and we propose 'occurrence', as a more neutral term, with the focus shifted towards understanding and learning from the event rather than attributing fault. The term review is purposefully employed to convey a proactive formal assessment of something incorporating comprehensive critical appraisal and exploration with the 'intention of instituting change if necessary' with emphasis on 'the whole' rather than component activities (Oxford English Dictionary, 2024). Review is preferred to 'debrief' due to the definitional uncertainty and emotively laden perceptions of 'debrief' as 'formal, militaristic and impersonal' (Restraint Reduction Network [RRN], 2019, p. 4) and preferred to 'support', based on the understanding of support needs as being a singular component of a more comprehensive review.

## 3    Regulatory Frameworks and Current Best Practices

'Debriefing' or 'post-incident review' which are widely mandated across professional and regulatory guidelines, seek to alleviate immediate distress and to prevent future incidents, as evidenced by directives from the US Occupational Safety and Health Administration (OSHA, 2016), the Joint Commission (2022) and the National Institute of Mental Health England (NIMHE, 2004). These measures, necessitate trauma-informed medical and psychological supports, for individuals who have either experienced or witnessed violent episodes, a structured assessment of each incident to pinpoint contributory factors, with necessary preventive measures implemented within a 'culture of learning' (NIMHE, 2004).

The UK offers an illustrative example of regulations regarding post-occurrence reviews. According to the Department of Health (DOH, 2014) 'Positive and Proactive Care' guidance, post-incident reviews after restrictive practices are mandatory, to evaluate and address both physical and emotional impacts, encourage reflection and devise preventative strategies. Guiding principles include voluntary service user involvement post-recovery, engagement of an external reviewer and distinct reviews for staff and service users, emphasising the revision of care plans following the review. This guidance mentions a 'more in-depth review process' (DOH, 2014), typically happening the day after, triggered by the severity of an incident or at an individual's request, with a flexible structure that might include a facilitated reflective session akin to the post-incident review.

The UK's NICE (2015) violence guidelines distinguish between immediate 'post-incident debrief' and 'formal review' following seclusion and/or restraint episodes. A debrief, in the presence of a 'nurse and doctor' enables the service user involved to discuss the incident, offers other witnesses the opportunity to express their experiences and allows all staff to share their insights. The subsequent external post-incident review, conducted ideally within 72 hours led by an external service user and staff trained for such reviews, aims to assess the physical and emotional impact on all participants, including witnesses. The process supports the identification of contributory/causative factors, the evaluation of the effectiveness of any interventions utilised and the development of future prevention or response strategies. It also identifies any service barriers and corrective actions, culminating in a report for the involved unit.

These guidelines are supported by regulatory enforcement. The Care Quality Commission (CQC, 2015) requires that inspection teams review evidence of engagement with service users post-restraint, in addition to appraising the debriefing conducted with staff and reflective reviews of the occurrence by a multidisciplinary team. Evidence is required to demonstrate how the debriefing process has informed preventive measures, with actions clearly documented in care plans and are subject to regular monitoring and review.

Professional and regulatory guidelines collectively acknowledge the responsibility of organisations to address the needs of all affected individuals post-occurrence, including mitigating distress, facilitating reflective processing and learning, and revising preventative measures continually. However, there is a need for clarity on the implementation of these mandates. While there is consensus on the 'if and when', the 'how' and 'why' aspects are less explored, potentially complicating the practical application of these obligations within health and safety legislation, aggression and violence prevention policies, and organisational strategies aimed at reducing or eliminating coercive practices.

Despite the many regulatory and professional mandates that require post-occurrence reviews to be undertaken, there is a pressing need for greater clarity on their specific role, purpose and function. This clarity is particularly crucial because of suggestions, albeit contested, that some post-occurrence interventions have been associated with harm to participants (Kagee, 2002).

## 4    A Brief History of 'Debriefing'

'Debriefing' has its roots in the United States (US) military; 'after combat interviews' were used in World War 2 to accurately capture the events of a battle soon after it had ended (Samter et al., 1993). Military debriefing was later expanded to provide an opportunity for soldiers injured in combat to talk about their experiences. For soldiers, the process of factually retelling the traumatic incident was viewed as a way of preventing the long-term consequences of suppressing the incident. In the 1960s and adjacent to military developments, crisis-intervention models were being developed for use with otherwise healthy individuals experiencing psychological crises, i.e. life events that could cause significant stress such as bereavement or major illness (Murphy et al., 2015). Crisis-intervention models were adapted for people experiencing psychiatric crises, and for people involved in civilian disasters.

'Critical incident stress debriefing', the first psychological debriefing intervention, described by Mitchell in 1983, was originally developed as a group intervention for workers in high-risk occupations such as the police and fire services, to manage stress (Mitchell et al., 2003). Taking ideas from military debriefing, crisis-intervention models and psychoeducational theory, the aim of critical incident stress debriefing was to mitigate the impact of traumatic events and to accelerate recovery. Critical incident stress debriefing is still widely used among emergency service workers, including emergency healthcare providers, who are exposed to traumatic events during their clinical practice (Smith, 2022).

The evidence for debriefing is contradictory. Research has demonstrated that critical incident stress debriefing for emergency healthcare providers is a cost-effective approach that can reduce the negative impact of traumatic events including compassion fatigue, post-traumatic stress disorder (PTSD) and burnout (Smith, 2022). However, a 2002 Cochrane Review found that single session, individual psychological debriefing following a traumatic event did not prevent the onset of PTSD nor reduce psychological distress (Rose et al., 2002). Moreover, the authors draw the uncompromising conclusion that 'compulsory debriefing of victims of trauma should cease' (Rose et al., 2002). Yet a later Cochrane review identified the benefits of multiple session psychological debriefing, albeit with a low level of certainty due to the high risk of bias in included trials (Roberts et al., 2019).

The evidence surrounding the efficacy of debriefing outside of mental health settings presents a complex picture. Despite mixed findings, it is clear that mental health settings are increasingly integrating post-occurrence practices, or are, at least, are expected to. This shift underscores the importance of adapting and refining interventions to address the unique needs within these environments.

## 5    Post-occurrence Review in Mental Healthcare

In mental health research, most attention has been given to reviews following episodes of seclusion and/or restraint. This is, perhaps, unsurprising given the well-documented, short- and long-term effects for the people involved both psychologically and emotionally. These reviews often have their origins in psychological debriefing and reflect nursing practice (Hammervold et al., 2019). Goulet and Larue (2016, p. 127) define the post-seclusion and/or restraint review as a 'complex intervention… targeting the patient and healthcare team to enhance the care experience and provide meaningful learning for the patient, staff, and organisation'.

Similar to military debriefing, being given the opportunity to process seclusion or restraint experiences is found to be a learning experience, with the potential to improve the quality of care (Hammervold et al., 2020). For healthcare providers, it can provide knowledge about other perspectives and solutions, increase professional and ethical awareness and increase emotional and relational processing. However, there is clear evidence that patients are rarely given the opportunity to participate in debriefing after seclusion or restraint episodes and are therefore not supported in processing experiences. After coercion, patients often suffer silently and must help themselves to prevent negative outcomes (Berring et al., 2024). Both the traumatic experience of being subjected to coercion and its later impact creates an urge to talk to someone, even after a long time with McGuinness et al. (2018) reporting how patients will often talk to their GP or someone else outside the hospital. Providing an opportunity to talk soon after an incident enables patients to recount their narrative and explain their experience of the event. This kind of debriefing can be an opportunity to regain trust (Ling et al., 2015).

Systematic debriefing is a pillar of restraint reduction approaches, and it has been implemented widely, initially in the US in the early 2000s, and later in other western countries, such as Denmark and Norway, as a part of the legislation and often in combinations with other interventions in seclusion and restraint reduction programs. For example, debriefing is one of the 'Six Core Strategies', an evidence-based model to reduce the use of restrictive practices within mental healthcare (Huckshorn, 2004). The goals of debriefing in the Six Core Strategies are twofold. First, to analyse and learn from seclusion and restraint events, then using this learning to inform policies, procedures and practices to avoid future events. Secondly, to mitigate the negative impact of the event for all involved, including witnesses. Similarly, 'Reassurance' is one of the Safewards interventions and describes a low-level opportunity for support after incidents on the ward, including coercive measures, patient violence and conflicts (Bowers, 2014).

## 6     Post-occurrence Review Within Models of Aggression

There is some practical guidance within the aggression management and restraint reduction literature. 'Debriefing' is a pivotal stage across various iterations of 'assault cycle' models (Breakwell, 1997; Kaplan & Wheeler, 1983; Leadbetter & Paterson, 1995). These models provide a structured approach to understanding the dynamics of aggression and outline interventions tailored to each cycle phase. Despite their age, these frameworks remain relevant and continue to offer insights into the processes of recovery and de-escalation.

Kaplan and Wheeler (1983) and Breakwell (1997) focus on a five-stage model, emphasising the critical stages of 'recovery' and 'post-crisis depression', while Leadbetter and Paterson (1995) expand this into a seven-stage model, introducing 'descent', 'transition' and 'resolution'. Notwithstanding the limitation of stage-specific de-escalation models (Hallett & Dickens, 2017), such models collectively address the physiological and psychological shifts post-crisis. In doing so, they highlight the potential need for stage-specific interventions that move from reducing physiological arousal to addressing psychological responses like remorse, shame and hopelessness.

The models advocate a cautious approach to recovery, suggesting a period for physiological de-escalation and warning against premature cognitive engagement that could lead to misinterpreted interactions and provoke re-escalation. They underline the significance of providing space, comfort and a sensitive engagement strategy during the recovery phase to prevent distress and ensure safety. Breakwell (1997) and Leadbetter and Paterson (1995) particularly emphasise the potential for intervention errors during this stage, suggesting careful management to avoid re-escalation.

Leadbetter and Paterson's (1995) concept of 'resolution' offers a more positive outlook than 'post-crisis depression', focusing on re-establishing safety, facilitating physiological de-escalation and supporting individuals in processing their experience and re-establishing connections with others. This stage is crucial for developing insight, appraising responses and considering alternative strategies for future incidents. The importance of reintegration into the community or unit milieu is also stressed, highlighting the comprehensive approach needed to effectively address a crisis's aftermath.

## 7    Post-occurrence Review as an Intervention

The RRN (2019, p. 4) proposes that within practice settings, debriefing is used to describe a 'whole range of different practices and approaches' following distressing incidents, which can be confusing for service users, families, staff and services.

The definitions and components of post-occurrence reviews may vary, but there are commonalities. Most debriefing takes place within a few hours of the incident and is used as an opportunity to allow patients and healthcare providers to reflect on the incident (Baker et al., 2021). Baker and colleagues describe five questions that can lead the reflection:
1. What antecedents had led up to the incident?
2. What specific problems had arisen?
3. Why had they not been solved?
4. What could have been done differently?
5. What would reduce the chances of the same thing happening again?

Recommended debriefing activities in the six core strategies includes an immediate post-event acute analysis and a more formal problem analysis with the treatment team, using root cause analysis (RCA). Six core debriefing seeks to identify why an incident happened, and what can be learnt from it. This is very different to the reassurance intervention within Safewards, which, as the name suggests, seeks to allay the anxieties that patients, including witnesses, may experience following conflict (Safewards, 2023).

## 8    Evidence for Post-occurrence Reviews in Mental Healthcare

Little is known about the effects or effectiveness of post-occurrence review interventions in mental healthcare. At the time of writing, we have found only one randomised controlled trial (RCT) of the intervention (Wullschleger et al., 2021). Wullschleger and colleagues carried out a multicentre, two-armed, RCT with 422 randomised participants, aimed at analysing the effect of debriefing on perceived coercion. People with severe mental disorders, who experienced at least one coercive measure during inpatient treatment, were randomised to an intervention group receiving standardised debriefing intervention, or a control group who received treatment as usual. Interestingly, the subjective perception of coercion was not reduced in the intervention group.

There is a greater body of literature exploring programmes of interventions that include debriefing. Studies of the six core strategies, including at least one RCT, demonstrate that it is effective in reducing coercion (Hirsch & Steinert, 2019). Similarly, Safewards interventions have been found to be effective in reducing conflict, again including one RCT (Finch et al., 2022). However, fidelity to the interventions, in the RCT at least, was low. This, coupled with the number of interventions included in Safewards, means that it is difficult, if not impossible, to unpick the impact of debriefing (reassurance) alone.

The paucity of experimental evidence for, or against, debriefing might be the reason for the numerous scoping, but not systematic, reviews. Scoping reviews have explored staff and patient debriefing after seclusion or restraint (Goulet & Larue, 2016; Sutton et al., 2014) or just restraint (Hammervold et al., 2019), one focused only on staff debriefing after seclusion and restraint (Mangaoil et al., 2020), and one explored factors that influence rates of violence after staff and/or patient debriefing (Asikainen et al., 2020). The one consistent finding is that the evidence for debriefing is limited (Goulet & Larue, 2016; Hammervold et al., 2019), especially as a standalone intervention (Sutton et al., 2014). It appears that service user debriefing is not routinely offered and even where offered, approaches are inconsistent. Nevertheless, service users express a preference for an opportunity to debrief (Sutton et al., 2014), and that post-incident support should include both service users and care providers (Goulet & Larue, 2016).

## 8.1   Summary

When addressing the psychological and emotional aftermath of occurrences that may cause harm within healthcare environments, it is important to take account of the patient's distress, fear and feeling of dehumanisation, and the resultant role conflicts and diminished job satisfaction amongst healthcare staff. Post-incident initiatives are likely to minimise the impact of such occurrences on patients and staff, providing them with an opportunity to make sense of the event and understand its causes, and deliberate on strategies to prevent recurrence. Regulatory frameworks and best practice guidance across healthcare organisations exist in order to mandate post-incident reviews.

Research findings on the efficacy of debriefing in PTSD and psychological distress are mixed for reasons that are not completely clear. Although post-occurrence reviews are widely recommended, there is some literature questioning its prolonged, positive use. Thus, an analytical approach is necessary to how these post-occurrence reviews in mental healthcare could be implemented taking account of the need for learning, understanding and preventing post-coercion, a need for clarity amidst concern over mandatory debriefing, and the ongoing understanding of the post-traumatic situation for the individual in such incidents. The rest of this chapter presents a tentative model of a post-occurrence review intervention.

## 9    Multiaxial Post-occurrence Review

The multiaxial post-occurrence review is proposed as an intervention in line with the World Health Organization's definition of a health intervention as 'an act performed for, with, or on behalf of a person or a population whose purpose is to assess, improve, maintain, promote or modify health, functioning or health conditions', which are constructed on three axes: 'Target'—the intended recipient; 'Action'—the deed undertaken by the actor for the target; and 'Means'—the processes and methodology by which the action is carried out (Fortune et al., 2018, p. 2).

The multiaxial post-occurrence review is a tentative model that aids the facilitation of all debriefing activities in the aftermath of occurrences related to either aggression and violence or the use of restrictive coercive interventions within acute mental health settings. The model proposes that a four-strand post-occurrence review is necessary, with each strand having a distinct target: the service user(s) involved, the staff, those who have witnessed the occurrence and the unit's multidisciplinary team (MDT). While each strand of the review has a distinct purpose and objective that addresses the needs of each target group, the overall outcomes require cohesion between all four. Specific 'actions' and 'means' are tailored to the needs and outcomes of each constituent group. Five core components are crucial: (i) amelioration of distress, (ii) sensitive and effective facilitation of reflection, (iii) collaborative identifying of actionable learning, (iv) preventive strategic planning and (v) the restoration of relationships, with the enactment of these five components responsive to the needs of each constituent group, see Fig. 1.

The term 'multiaxial' describes how each contributory axis (target) is interlinked. The model acknowledges the complex contextual nature of causative/contributory factors within an inpatient milieu, and subsequently attempts to understand

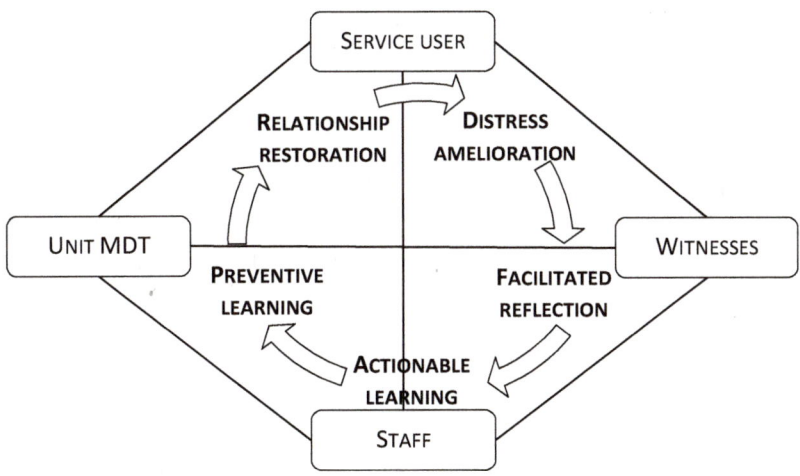

**Fig. 1** Multiaxial post-occurrence review—axes and core components

**Table 1** Multiaxial post-occurrence review: purpose, method and outcome

| Target | Service user | Staff team | Witnesses | Unit MDT |
|---|---|---|---|---|
| Purpose | Process occurrence | Reflective practice | Safety and reassurance | Analysis and prevention |
| Method | Structured engagement [REVIEW] | Supportive review team clinical supervision | Facilitated community meeting | Contextual situational appraisal |
| Outcome | Resolution, preventive plan, and re-engagement | Normative, formative, and restorative supervision | Restoration of therapeutic milieu | Contextual support and preventive adjustments |

an occurrence and proactively prevent future events by fully appreciating each perspective (axis).

The genesis of the model was a multistakeholder collaborative working group through which a national strategy for seclusion and restraint reduction was formulated within the Irish mental health services (Mental Health Commission [MHC], 2014). The strategy proposed a tripartite post-occurrence review of three distinct but associated processes involving service users, staff and the treatment team, all of which aim to effectively use learning from occurrences to prevent future episodes of seclusion or restraint. Notably the strategy, which preceded some of the more recent literature drawn upon in this chapter which brought more prominence to the potential plight of witnesses (Bowers, 2014; DOH, 2014; NICE, 2015), continued to develop iteratively (McKenna, 2015, 2018) and authors of this chapter have collaborated in the proposed expanded model, shown in Table 1.

## 9.1  Strand 1: Service User Review

In health intervention terms, the 'target' is the service user involved, the 'action' is the opportunity provided to process the occurrence, and the 'means' is a structured, purposeful conversation about the occurrence. One practical structure to guide this conversation is using the REVIEW mnemonic provided in Table 2. The simplicity of the structure should neither underestimate the facilitative attentiveness required nor overestimate the skills necessary, many of which are core competencies of practitioners.

The first critical step in assessing a service user's readiness is timing, distinguishing between the 'recovery' or 'descent' and 'resolution' stages (Breakwell, 1997; Leadbetter & Paterson, 1995). Engaging too soon, before normal physiological and emotional regulation is restored, can be counter-productive, causing distress to the service user and possibly compromising staff safety. A reliable indicator of readiness is the individual's response to a respectful invitation to participate in a review, assessing their willingness or voluntary agreement. It is also vital to respect that service user readiness is not subordinated to any procedural timelines, such as the 'end of shift'.

**Table 2**  The REVIEW mnemonic

| R | **Readiness:** Indicators of re-requisite readiness include restoration of normal physiological functioning and return of emotional regulation, as precursors to the cognitive readiness to meaningful engage with the review. |
|---|---|
| E | **Empathic positioning:** Provides the service user with the opportunity to recall their experience of the occurrence unencumbered, using active listening to empathically appreciate their perspective of the occurrence. |
| V | **Verify and validate:** Provides the service user with reassurance that their account is being actively listened to through staff use of paraphrasing, and their responses understood through the use of empathic validation. Open conversational style discussion is used to explore contributory/causative factors, and the effectiveness or otherwise of measures used to support the service user during the occurrence. |
| I | **Innovate:** The conversational style discussion explores alternative strategies that draw upon any successes and remediate any weaknesses identified through the facilitated reflection. Emphasis is placed on generating actionable preventive changes which will avoid recurrence and a plan of preferred support measures in the event of a future difficulty. |
| E | **Engage:** Having established agreed preventive changes to avoid or more effectively respond to any future occurrence, exploration of how best to repair and restore any relationships which may have been compromised, as a pre-requisite to re-engage with staff other service users and the broader therapeutic milieu. |
| W | **What next:** Collaboratively agreed actions are summarised by way of clarifying any final detail required, reaffirming commitment and agreeing specifically on what actions will be undertaken by whom. |

A second consideration involves selecting participants that are agreeable to the service user, balancing their preferences with regulatory requirements. The guidance from the American Psychiatric Association, American Psychiatric Nurses Association and the National Association for Psychiatric Health Systems (APA APNA NAPHS, 2003, p. 7) suggests meeting regulatory requirements without overlooking the patient's individual needs. The final readiness factor is agreeing on a time and place that suits the service user best.

**Empathic positioning** is a core skill of everyday practice. It can be helpful to commence by way of apology that the person has had such an experience, to establish that they feel both safe and comfortable to proceed and to reassure them that you intend to attentively listen, hear and understand their perspective. While apologies can be misunderstood, the context in which it is proposed here is in line with the work of Bennington-Davis (Murphy & Bennington-Davis, 2005) with the apology being for the service's inability to prevent the need for restraint, despite the best efforts of all involved. Although their recollection may differ from others involved, their account is unchallenged at this stage, emphasising the importance of fully appreciating their experience of the event.

Building on the concept of empathetic positioning, active listening extends beyond gaining an appreciation of an individual's perspective and distress, remaining attentive to any revelation of significant, yet previously undisclosed, information such as unnoticed symptoms or past traumas. Additionally, it plays a crucial role in pinpointing crisis moments as critical junctures for individuals to reassess and potentially revise their deeply held views on their functioning or treatment. The importance of recognising and leveraging these opportunities cannot be overstated.

**Verification** is employed, as in everyday practice, through paraphrasing, to establish that the person's account is fully understood, while validation is used to reassure and support the person that their reactions are understood as normal responses to an abnormal event. While the progression is always led by the person's immediate need, a conversational discussion can clarify specific details regarding contributory/causative factors, and the effectiveness, or otherwise, of measures enacted, or not enacted. This step can be closed with a summative account of the occurrence with an acknowledgement of the person's openness in their engagement.

**Innovation** is employed in its literal sense, collaboratively creating new ideas, methods or strategies to enhance future functioning, emphasising learning from past successes and addressing identified weaknesses. Butterworth et al. (2022) found that service users valued contributing to preventive strategies, particularly those that fostered confidence in their coping mechanisms, supported by open communication. The process involves a collaborative ethos, drawing on conflict and learning theories. Danesh (2011) links conflict to unmet universal human needs, as outlined in Maslow's hierarchy, suggesting that fulfilling these needs reduces conflict and supports innovation. Fisher et al. (2011) advocate for principled negotiation, emphasising meeting needs over defending positions, fostering fairness and collaborative problem-solving.

The collaborative approach required for innovation to use creativity and accommodation in generating actionable learning is conducive to Dale's (1972) proposition that deep learning correlates with active participation, emphasising the importance of engaged learning experiences. For individuals who have experienced restrictions, being actively involved is critical. Kahneman and Tversky (1984) discuss cognitive ease in the context of learning, highlighting that easily recalled information requires less effort to process than complex information, which demands more cognitive effort and can increase discomfort and decrease trust. In clinical practice, easily recalled, collaboratively developed strategies are likely to be more effective than more complex interventions in future challenging situations.

**Engage** involves the restoration and repair of relationships which may have been compromised, promoting reconnection with staff, peers and the broader therapeutic milieu, as described by Colton (2004). Following restrictive practices, service users may harbour residual negative feelings about environmental aspects or staff interactions that they believe contributed to their distress. These feelings can range from powerlessness and neglect of basic needs to experiences of inattentive communication, unclear expectations and feeling ridiculed, fostering a perception of an uncaring and unwelcoming environment (Hallett et al., 2023). Not addressing these intense events can leave lingering questions, unresolved emotions and doubts about the fairness of actions taken, potentially reinforcing a divisive 'us versus them' culture (Tingleff et al., 2017).

In response to aggressive incidents, Maier et al. (1987) suggested staff may maintain a 'safe distance' from the service user, characterised by avoidance and minimal interaction. This approach by staff, while intuitively self-protective staff, may be perceived by the service user as distrust or exclusion, possibly exacerbating future incidents. Similarly, Wykes and Whittington (1994) observed a tendency for staff to disengage and reduce availability for interaction after such incidents. Effective reconnection strategies should be customised to the particular situation and needs of the service user, aiming to rebuild relationships. This reconnection process with the service user should be integrated with post-incident reviews involving staff and other witnesses.

**What next** is the final step of the review with service users and involves collaboratively summarising agreed actions, reaffirming commitments made and agreeing specifically on what actions will be undertaken and by whom. A plan for how the progression of agreed actions should be created. Agreed actions should also be recorded collaboratively in line with prevailing regulations. This step also provides the opportunity for closure framed positively by the RRN (2019) as instilling hope, from the collaborative exchange with the service user regarding their challenges and care preferences and having worked through difficult and traumatic emotions. It can help them to move on from the event and to rebuild relationships of therapeutic alliance.

While the REVIEW framework provides a practical guide, the facilitator(s) should remain sensitised in identifying a service user for whom the occurrence has been particularly traumatic and/or requires professional interventions beyond those provided in the review. Notwithstanding the specific tasks to be accomplished, the APA APNA NAPHS (2003) emphasises that the process should be integrated into overall care. If patients are involved in the treatment planning from the start, then debriefing doesn't appear as an isolated task—it becomes an integral part of the treatment planning process.

## 9.2    Strand 2: Staff Review

Whereas the focus on service user review is creating opportunities to process the occurrence, staff needs can be distinguished as either requiring a 'supportive review' or engaging in a collaborative 'occurrence review'. The RRN (2019) differentiates these two distinct needs as 'post-incident support' and 'post-incident reflection'. Irrespective of title, the former addresses the physical and emotional well-being of those involved, while the latter emphasises reflection and learning. What is important is that each has a distinctly different 'target', 'action' and 'means', as shown in Table 3.

**Table 3** Differences between supportive and occurrence reviews

|  | Supportive review | Occurrence review |
|---|---|---|
| Focus | Person[s] | Event[s] |
| Purpose | Facilitated processing | Reflective/educative |
| Attendance | Involved person[s] | Open |
| Approach | Supportive | Detail driven |
| Time focus | Putting 'behind' | 'Future' planning |
| Records | Note of attendance | Agreed specific actions |
| Output | Closure or referral | Preventative plan |

Considering the potential for staff to experience intense physiological arousal and psychological reactions, an initial supportive review may be necessary in instances, particularly when dealing with aggression, which could lead to 'dual escalation' where the safety imperative upon staff's protective or restrictive actions escalates their physiological response. Such recovery for staff parallels the service user's, with the immediate aftermath possibly involving intense cognitive and emotional reactions.

The supportive review is a person-centred, process-oriented intervention for directly involved staff to facilitate reflection, support emotional processing and alleviate distress. While typically involving the individual, it is restricted to those directly involved, focusing on the person's experiences rather than the establishment of data driven fact. Records are limited to invitation and/or attendance, subject to a caveat of disclosure which imposes a professional obligation. Its aim is to assist staff in achieving closure and reintegration into the therapeutic milieu.

In contrast, the occurrence review is an event-focused, facilitated reflective intervention that examines contributory and causative factors, including interventions employed or omitted. It's educative is focused to capture actionable learning for a future-oriented plan to better meet everyone's needs. Unlike the supportive review, it includes all involved and may extend to others to improve practice. The emphasis is on a thorough understanding of the event, with an expectation of attendance, resulting in a detailed plan of agreed actions, specific task allocation, timelines and oversight arrangements.

The post-occurrence review with staff can draw upon existing practices in mental health and medical settings, specifically clinical supervision and debriefing practices. Clinical supervision can be defined as a formal process of professional support and learning, enabling practitioners to develop knowledge and competence, enhancing consumer protection and safety in complex clinical situations (Masamha et al., 2022). This definition reflects Proctor's (1986) framework, which includes normative (oversight and adherence to standards), formative (educative and skill development) and restorative (support for emotional needs) functions.

While clinical supervision offers a foundational approach, the routine retrospective review of occurrences in broader medical contexts also yields valuable insights. Salas et al. (2008) outline a team debriefing framework aimed at enhancing service user safety and boosting both individual and team performance. This structured debriefing allows for reflection on performance, identification of errors and planning for improvement. It starts by defining challenges and outcomes, then thoroughly examines the event, including decisions, alternatives, remediations and successes. This process not only promotes shared learning but also bolsters team cohesion. Salas et al. (2008) emphasise 12 principles for effective debriefings, underlining the need for an organisational culture supportive of learning and the crucial role of a skilled facilitator in fostering a conducive environment for open, constructive dialogue. This approach to critical reflection is pivotal in reinforcing strengths and rectifying weaknesses, ensuring open discussions on team dynamics and adjustments for future strategies.

**Table 4**  The REVIEW mnemonic for staff

| | |
|---|---|
| R | **Readiness:** Indicators of re-requisite readiness include restoration of normal physiological, and emotional regulation, as precursors to the cognitive readiness to meaningful engage with the review. |
| E | **Event reflection:** Provides facilitated critical reflection upon the occurrence with specific attention to contributory/causative factors, and the effectiveness, or otherwise, of measures enacted or not enacted. Discussion is focussed on identifying both interventions that were of particular usefulness, and those which may have been unhelpful. |
| V | **Verify and validate:** Verification is employed by the facilitator to summarise the shared understanding of the event and clarify any remaining detail, and validation acknowledges the complexity of the challenge encountered, as appropriate, and reassures all that each perspective is understood. |
| I | **Innovate:** An open and inclusive discussion explores alternative strategies that draw upon any successes and remediate any weaknesses identified, with emphasis placed on generating actionable preventive changes which will avoid recurrence, and a plan of supportive and safety strategies in the event of future difficulty. |
| E | **Engage:** Exploration of the relationships which may have been compromised, both within and beyond the team, together with the situation and person-specific reparative strategies are agreed upon to facilitate re-engagement to restore a therapeutic milieu. |
| W | **What next:** Collaboratively agreed actions are summarised with clarification of any final details required, reaffirming commitment and agreeing specifically on what actions will be undertaken by whom, and the mechanism of implementation oversight. |

In health intervention terms, the 'target' here is the staff involved, the 'action' is the facilitation of a clinical supervision approach informed by medical debriefing practice and the 'means' is a structured purposeful structured normative, formative and restorative review of the occurrence. The previously explained REVIEW mnemonic with minimal adaptation can guide this process, see Table 4.

Establishing staff **readiness** involves addressing their immediate physical and emotional needs and offering a supportive review as necessary. Just like service users, staff willingness to engage after an invitation is a good indicator of readiness.

**Event reflection** starts with acknowledging the distress associated with the occurrence, reinforcing a moral commitment to the compassionate person-centred recognition of the 'universal humanity' of all involved (Bowers, 2014). The learning and preventive focus of the critical reflection of circumstances surrounding the occurrence is also reinforced, with emphasis on 'fact finding rather than fault finding' (McKenna, 2008).

Guidance from APA APNA NAPHS (2003) underlines the importance of safely encouraging staff to share their feelings honestly, despite potential fears of negative perceptions from supervisors or peers. Although staff and service user perspectives on events can differ (Nolan et al., 2009), acknowledging these varied reactions is crucial, especially following aggressive incidents or the use of restrictive measures. Open discussions allow for a sensitive examination of staff experiences and perceptions. Reflection aims to understand the challenge, intended outcomes and contributory/causative factors. It is important to balance discussions including the 'glad we did' acts with the 'sorry we didn't', and a flip chart can effectively capture this balanced discussion. This process validates staff reactions, promotes a shared understanding and explores alternative strategies for better outcomes in future incidents.

**Verification** is employed to establish that there is a shared understanding of the occurrence with the opportunity to clarify any relevant detail, while validation is used to reassure those present that their reactions are understood within the context of a distressing experience.

**Innovation** involves revisiting reflections to identify alternative strategies that could be more effective, considering physiological responses that may impair communication and decision-making. Discussions focus on creative, actionable strategies for change, supported and agreed upon collaboratively.

**Engagement** focuses on restoring relationships affected by the occurrence, acknowledging and managing the fear that might lead to withdrawal or stricter boundaries (Ezeobele et al., 2020). Recognising the emotional residue within the team is important for maintaining a therapeutic milieu and preventing future conflicts.

Finally, **what next**, as with service users, involves summarising actions and commitments with a detailed plan. This phase allows for constructive dialogue, addressing challenges and reinforcing commitment to therapeutic engagement, helping staff move forward and strengthen professional relationships.

## 9.3    Strand 3: Community Review

The third strand addresses the needs of service users who either witnessed, or have come to learn of, the occurrence. While guidance is inconsistent as to exactly who should be included (DOH, 2014; MHC, 2022; NICE, 2015), it is advisable to consider that within an enclosed milieu, all service users potentially become aware of the occurrence. This approach aligns with Bowers' (2014) warning that exposure to disturbing and distressing occurrences may impact everyone within the treatment milieu. Given the uncertainty surrounding the awareness and impact on service users after an occurrence, along with their concerns for safety and the resultant anxiety and milieu disruption, it is advisable to offer all service users within the unit the chance to participate voluntarily in post-occurrence review processes.

While professional guidance and regulatory mandates require that the post-occurrence needs of 'others' impacted are met, there is limited specific detail as to how 'others' are delineated, how needs are assessed, and the intended outcome of such measures (DOH, 2014; MHC, 2022; NICE, 2015). The imperative, therefore, in this strand is to address the needs of service users within the context of the broader milieu. While the prioritisation of needs will be occurrence and milieu-specific, these broadly align with the five core components of the multiaxial post-occurrence review, see Fig. 1.

In intervention terms, the 'target' group in this strand is the wider 'community', the 'action' is the restoration of the therapeutic milieu and the 'means' is through a structured, purposeful engagement in which all are provided with safety reassurance, a sensitively facilitated opportunity to express any anxiety and concerns, and a collaborative formulated plan to foster mutual respect and support within a community of safety.

This strand highlights the therapeutic community concept, emphasising 'community as method', a common approach in mental health environments (De Leon & Unterrainer, 2020). It underlines the importance of prioritising an individual's overall well-being and the collective potential for improved healing and support through participation in communities that 'teach, heal, and support' (De Leon, 2000, p. 11).

Guiding this strand are two notable frameworks: Bowers' (2014) Safewards model and Lanza's Violence Prevention Community Meetings (VPCMs), which have been extensively applied and researched over two decades (Lanza, 2017; Lanza et al., 2003, 2009). The Safewards model (Bowers, 2014), as stated previously, advocates for 'reassurance' as a method to engage with patients, individually or in small groups, after any anxiety-inducing events, including those indirectly affected. This engagement aims to clarify the event, assess its impact and offer support.

Lanza's (2017) VPCM is a nurse-led group intervention for both service users and staff, fostering a culture of safety and respect and aiming to understand and reduce violence. Lanza (2017) outlines the VPCM as a proactive, preventive intervention, which is also useful post-incident, focusing on collaborative strategies for a safe, respectful community.

The first and primary objective is reassurance of safety, emphasising everyone's well-being and affirming the service's commitment to safety as essential for therapeutic recovery. Bowers (2014) warns of the contagion effect of distressing events, suggesting that unaddressed anxiety from peer behaviour can lead to further conflicts.

Second is providing a clear explanation of the incident respecting privacy, correcting misconceptions and explaining staff actions as in everyone's best interest. This includes differentiating between a person and their behaviour, underscoring that actions taken are non-punitive and aimed at safety (Safewards, 2014). An open discussion follows allowing expression of experiences and feelings, validating diverse perspectives and focusing on issues rather than individuals. This prevents marginalisation and supports reintegration into the therapeutic community. Exploring collaborative strategies to maintain safety is critical, with Lanza (2017) and Bowers' (2014) suggesting proactive management of potential conflicts and enhancing staff visibility as preventative measures. The process concludes with agreements on immediate actions for reassurance and the provision of individual support, summarising commitments and action plans, including follow-up on their effectiveness.

The community review aims to restore a therapeutic environment perceived as safe, enabling service users to progress in their recovery without the anxiety stemming from adverse incidents. Bowers (2014) refers to the Safewards model, which is informed by ethnographic research in mental health settings, underscoring the value of positive recognition, emotional control, expertise and structured approaches to prevent conflicts. Beyond ensuring safety, the review session serves as a platform for demonstrating supportive engagement, fairness and inclusivity, facilitating the resolution of differing viewpoints and adeptly handling possible disputes. This approach not only aids in building positive relationships among service users but also stresses the importance of a meeting's experiential safety, requiring careful attention to those with past trauma and avoiding placing undue blame on individuals. Ideally, sessions would benefit from co-facilitation by someone with direct experience, though this necessitates thoughtful planning and resource allocation.

## 9.4 Strand 4: Unit MDT Review

The fourth and final strand addresses the obligation of treatment units to conduct a structured methodical review in the aftermath of occurrences in order to fully understand all contributory factors which should then inform the implementation of all reasonably practicable remediation and preventive measures to minimise the likelihood of further events. This obligation is explicit in professional guidance and regulatory mandates relating to either the occurrence of aggression and violence or the enactment of restrictive interventions, as previously discussed.

While regulations and guidance broadly share requirements for the critical appraisal of contributory factors and implementation of preventive strategies in general terms, it is less clear how these mandates will be enacted in practice. Therefore, the imperative in this strand of the multiaxial post-occurrence review is to address the needs of the organisation.

In intervention terms, the 'target' in this final strand is the broader 'unit', the 'action' is a critical review of the occurrence and the 'means' is through a contextual consideration of contributory factors, which informs the implementation of preventive measures.

The post-occurrence unit review involves the multidisciplinary treatment team and adopts a contextual approach in the careful situational analysis of each occurrence. For the purposes of this contextual review, occurrences may be considered from four contributory components: the (i) service user, (ii) the staff, (iii) the interaction taking place at the time of the occurrence and (iv) the prevailing environmental circumstances. The primary focus of this critical situational contextual appraisal is to establish, or at least hypothesise as to, the contributory impact of each of the components (McKenna 2008).

Service user considerations include the characteristics and acuity of the person's illness, prior incidents, trauma history, physiological issues (e.g. pain, sleep deprivation, intoxication) and psychological factors (e.g. stress, mental health acuity, cognitive impairment). Staff considerations include age, gender, experience level, training relevance and adequacy, pre-existing relationships with the service user and exposure to past incidents. Broader aspects cover the team's adequacy, experience, cultural competence, cohesion and clear leadership.

Interaction considerations include the nature of the occurrence, whether it was conflictual or aversive, and if service user expectations were met or frustrated. Environmental considerations include intensity and stress factors like crowding, noise, waiting times and frustration. Additionally, safety considerations include the adequacy of preventative measures including safe systems of entry and egress, the presence of panic alarms, clearly communicated response protocols and whether these proved effective. Broader considerations include the availability of comfort measures and access to facilitate simple requests and access to information.

These considerations are indicative rather than prescriptive and will be service-specific. The key objective is to formulate an explanatory hypothesis for acute behavioural distress intense enough to compromise either the person's safety, or that of others. While some behaviours may be clear responses to stress or dissatisfaction, those that are challenging to understand, indicating possible medical or mental health emergencies, require urgent attention. For instance, an involuntarily admitted, acutely unwell service user protesting a smoking ban may be understandable, but unexpected risky behaviour from a usually stable and cooperative service user, without any obvious reason, raises significant concerns. This evaluation is crucial, particularly for individuals with cognitive or communication impairments, who may struggle to articulate their distress, bearing in mind the increased health risks and poorer outcomes commonly associated with mental health conditions.

Irrespective of aetiology, the retrospective situational appraisal also informs the response. This methodical contextual appraisal of contributory illuminates the necessary responses to prevent future occurrences. Identifying actionable changes in response to these incidents is essential, requiring the swift development and implementation of strategies that effectively support the concerned service user, ensure the safety of the broader milieu and staff, and provide the treatment team with appropriate guidance.

The degree to which adjustments can be made to each contributing factor depends on the specific circumstances of the unit. Factors such as the acuity level of the service user, the enforcement of regulations or legal orders and the general acuity of the unit's environment at any given time can pose challenges to even the most dedicated treatment teams. The primary efforts of the treatment team ought therefore to focus on implementing all adjustments that are achievable in the short term, effectively signalling a commitment to safety while meeting the needs of all involved. Possible actions might include enhancing support for service users, increasing unit staffing, implementing low arousal strategies proactively or making feasible adjustments to environmental rules and/or routines. Furthermore, it is important to promptly establish a contingency plan for any adjustments that are beyond the control of the unit.

The immediate implementation of even modest adjustments reinforces the seriousness with which concerns are addressed, fosters trust and a positive perception of a committed team striving to do their best and potentially serves as a model within the wider milieu for the role of compassionate awareness in navigating between conflict and containment.

Finally, it is important to integrate the outputs of the other strands of the multi-axial post-occurrence review which respects the perspectives and commitments of the service user, staff and the broader milieu.

## 10 Conclusion

The strengths of the proposed multiaxial post-occurrence review include its cohesion with a person-centred recovery orientation, supporting the preservation of hope despite temporary difficulties encountered by individuals on their recovery journey, and its emphasis on person-centred care, enabling service users to collaborate with peers and professionals in determining their preferred care and support options.

The proposed model is well aligned with trauma-informed approaches, underpinned in the recognition of potential trauma. It responds by proactively attempting to minimise potential traumatisation and re-traumatisation. Additionally, it promotes safety, trustworthiness, transparency, peer support, collaboration, mutuality, empowerment and choice, the principles underpinning trauma-informed approaches (Substance Abuse and Mental Health Service Administration (SAMHSA), 2014).

It is also well aligned with positive behaviour support approaches in that person-centred facilitated reflections are core elements in the functional assessment of unmet needs. These reflections inform the development of constructive interventions aimed at creating environments that support the mastery of an enriched repertoire of adaptive behaviours and enhancing positive life opportunities.

Apart from the apparent benefit of demonstrating compliance with increasing regulatory professional and regulatory requirements for effective reviews of occurrences, any burden in embracing the proposed model should be modest considering that staff and services are already familiar with, and confident in, the task demands of each strand. The proposed model may assist in achieving greater returns from daily efforts to empathically support and collaboratively empower service users in difficulty, engagement in meaningful reflective practice and fostering a trusting and respectful milieu grounded in our shared humanity.

Finally, the proposed model may contribute to advancing the shift from what has been traditionally framed as a unidimensional obligatory tertiary intervention, to an inclusive, person-centred, needs based preventive intervention that more adequately, equitably and effectively meets the needs of all. An imagined unit in which service users have any untoward occurrence empathically and effectively processed, in which staff are supported both personally and professionally, in which a disturbed milieu is quickly reassured and occurrences are preventively managed is not insurmountable.

## References

American Psychiatric Association American Psychiatric Nurses Association and the National Association for Psychiatric Health Systems. (2003). *Learning from each other: Success stories and ideas for reducing restraint/seclusion in behavioral health*. American Psychiatric Association.

Asikainen, J., Vehviläinen-Julkunen, K., Repo-Tiihonen, E., & Louheranta, O. (2020). Violence factors and debriefing in psychiatric inpatient care: A review. *Journal of Psychosocial Nursing and Mental Health Services, 58*(5), 39–49. https://doi.org/10.3928/02793695-20200306-01

Baker, J., Berzins, K., Canvin, K., Benson, I., Kellar, I., Wright, J., et al. (2021). Non-pharmacological interventions to reduce restrictive practices in adult mental health inpatient settings: The COMPARE systematic mapping review. Health Services and Delivery Research, 9(5). : NIHR Journals Library doi: https://doi.org/10.3310/hsdr09050.

Berring, L. L., Georgaca, E., Hirsch, S., Bilgin, H., Kömürcü Akik, B., Aydin, M., et al. (2024). Factors and processes facilitating recovery from coercion in mental health services—A meta-ethnography [Manuscript in preparation].

Bowers, L. (2014). Safewards: A new model of conflict and containment on psychiatric wards: Safewards: Description of the model. Journal of Psychiatric and Mental Health Nursing, 21(6), 499–508. https://doi.org/10.1111/jpm.12129

Breakwell, G. M. (1997). Coping with aggressive behaviour. BPS Books.

Butterworth, H., Wood, L., & Rowe, S. (2022). Patients' and staff members' experiences of restrictive practices in acute mental health in-patient settings: Systematic review and thematic synthesis. BJPsych Open, 8(6), e178. https://doi.org/10.1192/bjo.2022.574

Care Quality Commission. (2015). Brief guides for inspection teams: Restraint (physical and mechanical). https://www.cqc.org.uk/sites/default/files/20180322_900803_briefguide-restraint_physical_mechanical_v1.pdf

Colton, D. (2004). Checklist for assessing your organization's readiness for reducing seclusion and restraint. Commonwealth Center for Children and Adolescents.

Cusack, P., Cusack, F. P., McAndrew, S., McKeown, M., & Duxbury, J. (2018). An integrative review exploring the physical and psychological harm inherent in using restraint in mental health inpatient settings. International Journal of Mental Health Nursing, 27(3), 1162–1176. https://doi.org/10.1111/inm.12432

Dale, E. (1972). Building a learning environment. Phi Delta Kappa.

Danesh, H. B. (2011). Human needs theory, conflict, and peace. The Encyclopedia of Peace Psychology. https://doi.org/10.1002/9780470672532.wbepp127

De Leon, G. (2000). The therapeutic community: Theory, model, and method. Springer Publishing Company.

De Leon, G., & Unterrainer, H. F. (2020). The therapeutic community: A unique social psychological approach to the treatment of addictions and related disorders. Frontiers in Psychiatry, 11, 786. https://doi.org/10.3389/fpsyt.2020.00786

Department of Health. (2014). Positive and proactive care: Reducing the need for restrictive interventions. Department of Health.

Ezeobele, I. E., Mock, A., McBride, R., Mackey-Godine, A., Harris, D., Russell, C. D., et al. (2020). Patient-on-staff assaults: Perspectives of mental health staff at an acute inpatient psychiatric teaching hospital in the United States. Canadian Journal of Nursing Research, 53(3), 242–253. https://doi.org/10.1177/0844562120904624

Finch, K., Lawrence, D., Williams, M. O., Thompson, A. R., & Hartwright, C. (2022). A systematic review of the effectiveness of Safewards: Has enthusiasm exceeded evidence? Issues in Mental Health Nursing, 43(2), 119–136. https://doi.org/10.1080/01612840.2021.1967533

Fisher, R., Ury, W. L., & Patton, B. (2011). Getting to yes. Penguin.

Fortune, N., Madden, R., & Almborg, A.-H. (2018). Use of a new international classification of health interventions for capturing information on health interventions relevant to people with disabilities. International Journal of Environmental Research and Public Health, 15(1), 145.

Gillespie, G. L., Bresler, S., & Gates, D. M. (2013). Posttraumatic stress symptomatology among emergency department workers following workplace aggression. Workplace Health & Safety, 61(6), 247–254. https://doi.org/10.1177/216507991306100603

Goulet, M.-H., & Larue, C. (2016). Post-seclusion and/or restraint review in psychiatry: A scoping review. Archives of Psychiatric Nursing, 30, 120–128. https://doi.org/10.1016/j.apnu.2015.09.001

Hallett, N., & Dickens, G. L. (2017). De-escalation of aggressive behaviour in healthcare settings: Concept analysis. International Journal of Nursing Studies, 75, 10–20.

Hallett, N., Dickinson, R., Eneje, E., & Dickens, G. L. (2023). Adverse mental health inpatient experiences: Qualitative systematic review of international literature and development of a conceptual framework. *medRxiv*. https://doi.org/10.1101/2023.10.20.23297217

Hammervold, U. E., Norvoll, R., Aas, R. W., & Sagvaag, H. (2019). Post-incident review after restraint in mental health care—A potential for knowledge development, recovery promotion and restraint prevention. A scoping review. *BMC Health Services Research, 19*(1), 235. https://doi.org/10.1186/s12913-019-4060-y

Hammervold, U. E., Norvoll, R., Vevatne, K., & Sagvaag, H. (2020). Post-incident reviews—A gift to the Ward or just another procedure? Care providers' experiences and considerations regarding post-incident reviews after restraint in mental health services. A qualitative study. *BMC Health Services Research, 20*, 1–13.

Hirsch, S., & Steinert, T. (2019). Measures to avoid coercion in psychiatry and their efficacy. *Deutsches Ärzteblatt International, 116*(19), 336–343. https://doi.org/10.3238/arztebl.2019.0336

Huckshorn, K. A. (2004). Reducing seclusion and restraint use in mental health settings: Core strategies for prevention. *Journal of Psychosocial Nursing and Mental Health Services, 42*(9), 22–33.

Iozzino, L., Ferrari, C., Large, M., Nielssen, O., & de Girolamo, G. (2015). Prevalence and risk factors of violence by psychiatric acute inpatients: A systematic review and meta-analysis. *PLoS One, 10*(6), e0128536. https://doi.org/10.1371/journal.pone.0128536

Jansen, T.-L., Hem, M. H., Dambolt, L. J., & Hanssen, I. (2020). Moral distress in acute psychiatric nursing: Multifaceted dilemmas and demands. *Nursing Ethics, 27*(5), 1315–1326. https://doi.org/10.1177/0969733019877526

Johnson, M. E. (2010). Violence and restraint reduction efforts on inpatient psychiatric units. *Issues in Mental Health Nursing, 31*(3), 181–197. https://doi.org/10.3109/01612840903276704

Joint Commission. (2022). Workplace violence prevention standards. *R3 Report: Requirement, Rationale, Reference, 30*, 1–6. https://www.jointcommission.org/standards/r3-report/r3-report-issue-30-workplace-violence-prevention-standards/

Kagee, A. (2002). Concerns about the effectiveness of critical incident stress debriefing in ameliorating stress reactions. *Critical Care, 6*(1), 88. https://doi.org/10.1186/cc1459

Kahneman, D., & Tversky, A. (1984). Choices, values, and frames. *American Psychologist, 39*(4), 341–350.

Kaplan, S. G., & Wheeler, E. G. (1983). Survival skills for working with potentially violent clients. *Social Casework, 64*(6), 339–346.

Krieger, E., Moritz, S., Lincoln, T. M., Fischer, R., & Nagel, M. (2021). Coercion in psychiatry: A cross-sectional study on staff views and emotions. *Journal of Psychiatric and Mental Health Nursing, 28*(2), 149–162. https://doi.org/10.1111/jpm.12643

Lanza, M. L. (2017). Violence prevention community meeting conducted on your unit. *Issues in Mental Health Nursing, 38*(10), 829–836. https://doi.org/10.1080/01612840.2017.1339299

Lanza, M. L., Kazis, L., Lee, A., & Ericsson, A. (2003). A community meeting protocol for assault prevention. *International Journal of Group Psychotherapy, 53*(3), 285–302. https://doi.org/10.1521/ijgp.53.3.285.42819

Lanza, M. L., Rierdan, J., Forester, L., & Zeiss, R. A. (2009). Reducing violence against nurses: The violence prevention community meeting. *Issues in Mental Health Nursing, 30*(12), 745–751.

Leadbetter, D., & Paterson, B. (1995). De-escalating aggressive behaviour. In B. Kidd & C. Stark (Eds.), *Management of violence and aggression in health care* (pp. 49–84). Gaskell/Royal College of Psychiatrists.

Ling, S., Cleverley, K., & Perivolaris, A. (2015). Understanding mental health service user experiences of restraint through debriefing: A qualitative analysis. *The Canadian Journal of Psychiatry, 60*(9), 386–392.

Maier, G. J., Stava, L. J., Morrow, B. R., Van Rybroek, G. J., & Bauman, K. G. (1987). A model for understanding and managing cycles of aggression among psychiatric inpatients. *Psychiatric Services, 38*(5), 520–524. https://doi.org/10.1176/ps.38.5.520

Mangaoil, R. A., Cleverley, K., & Peter, E. (2020). Immediate staff debriefing following seclusion or restraint use in inpatient mental health settings: A scoping review. *Clinical Nursing Research, 29*(7), 479–495. https://doi.org/10.1177/1054773818791085

Masamha, R., Alfred, L., Harris, R., Bassett, S., Burden, S., & Gilmore, A. (2022). Barriers to overcoming the barriers': A scoping review exploring 30 years of clinical supervision literature. *Journal of Advanced Nursing, 78*(9), 2678–2692. https://doi.org/10.1111/jan.15283

McGuinness, D., Murphy, K., Bainbridge, E., Brosnan, L., Keys, M., Felzmann, H., et al. (2018). Individuals' experiences of involuntary admissions and preserving control: Qualitative study. *BJPsych Open, 4*(6), 501–509.

McKenna, K. (2008). *Linking service and safety: Together creating safer places of service: Strategy for managing work-related aggression and violence within the Irish health service.* Health Service Executive. https://www.hse.ie/eng/staff/resources/hrstrategiesreports/linking-service-safety.pdf

McKenna, K. (2015). *Rethinking debriefing: A structure for aligning constituents and process.* Paper presented at the 9th European Congress on Violence in Clinical Psychiatry, Copenhagen, Denmark.

McKenna, K. (2018). *Rethinking debriefing: A structure for integrated post occurrence review.* Paper presented at the Sixth international conference on violence in the health sector: Advancing the delivery of positive practice Toronto, Canada.

Mental Health Commission. (2014). *Seclusion and restraint reduction strategy.* http://hdl.handle.net/10147/627078

Mental Health Commission. (2022). *Code of practice on the use of physical restraint.* https://www.mhcirl.ie/sites/default/files/2023-03/MHC_REVISED%20RULES_Physical%20Restraint.pdf

Mitchell, A. M., Sakraida, T. J., & Kameg, K. (2003). Critical incident stress debriefing: Implications for best practice. *Disaster Management & Response, 1*(2), 46–51. https://doi.org/10.1016/S1540-2487(03)00008-7

Murphy, S. M., Irving, C. B., Adams, C. E., & Waqar, M. (2015). Crisis intervention for people with severe mental illnesses. *Cochrane Database of Systematic Reviews, 2015*(12), CD001087. https://doi.org/10.1002/14651858.CD001087.pub5

Murphy, T., & Bennington-Davis, M. (2005). *Restraint and seclusion. The model for eliminating their use in healthcare.* HCPro.

National Institute for Health and Care Excellence. (2015). *Violence and aggression: Short-term management in mental health, health and community settings (NICE Guideline NG10).* https://www.nice.org.uk/guidance/ng10/evidence/full-guideline-pdf-70830253

National Institute for Mental Health in England. (2004). *Mental health policy implementation guide developing positive practice to support the safe and therapeutic management of aggression and violence in mental health in-patient settings.* National Institute for Mental Health in England.

Needham, I., Abderhalden, C., Halfens, R. J. G., Fischer, J. E., & Dassen, T. (2005). Non-somatic effects of patient aggression on nurses: A systematic review. *Journal of Advanced Nursing, 49*(3), 283–296. https://doi.org/10.1111/j.1365-2648.2004.03286.x

Nolan, K. A., Shope, C. B., Citrome, L., & Volavka, J. (2009). Staff and patient views of the reasons for aggressive incidents: A prospective, incident-based study. *Psychiatric Quarterly, 80*(3), 167–172. https://doi.org/10.1007/s11126-009-9104-8

Nolan, P. (2000). Challenging violence. *Nursing Times, 96*(24), 32–33.

Nyttingnes, O., Ruud, T., & Rugkåsa, J. (2016). 'It's unbelievably humiliating'—Patients' expressions of negative effects of coercion in mental health care. *International Journal of Law and Psychiatry, 49*, 147–153. https://doi.org/10.1016/j.ijlp.2016.08.009

Occupational Safety and Health Administration. (2016). *Guidelines for preventing workplace violence for health care and social service workers.* https://www.osha.gov/sites/default/files/publications/osha3148.pdf

Oxford English Dictionary. (2024). *Review: Verb.* https://www.oed.com/dictionary/review_v?tab=meaning_and_use#25545056

Proctor, B. (1986). Supervision: A co-operative exercise in accountability. In: Enabling and ensuring. M. Marken and M. Payne (eds). Leicester National Youth Bureau and Council for Education and Training in Youth and Community Work, Leicester. p 21–23.

Restraint Reduction Network. (2019). *Post-incident debriefing guidance: For staff working in inpatient settings with children and young people.* https://restraintreductionnetwork.org/wp-content/uploads/2022/06/Post-Incident-Debriefing-Guidance-for-staff-working-in-inpatient-settings.pdf

Roberts, N. P., Kitchiner, N. J., Kenardy, J., Robertson, L., Lewis, C., & Bisson, J. I. (2019). Multiple session early psychological interventions for the prevention of post-traumatic stress disorder. *Cochrane Database of Systematic Reviews, 8,* CD006869. https://doi.org/10.1002/14651858.CD006869.pub3

Rose, S. C., Bisson, J., Churchill, R., & Wessely, S. (2002). Psychological debriefing for preventing post traumatic stress disorder (PTSD). *Cochrane Database of Systematic Reviews, 2,* CD000560. https://doi.org/10.1002/14651858.CD000560

Safewards. (2023). *Reassurance.* https://www.safewards.net/interventions/reassurance

Safewards, B. L. (2014). A new model of conflict and containment on psychiatric wards. J Psychiatr Ment Health Nurs, 21(6):499–508. https://doi.org/10.1111/jpm.12129. Epub 2014 Feb 19. PMID: 24548312; PMCID: PMC4237187.

Salas, E., Klein, C., King, H., Salisbury, M., Augenstein, J. S., Birnbach, D. J., et al. (2008). Debriefing medical teams: 12 evidence-based best practices and tips. *The Joint Commission Journal on Quality and Patient Safety, 34*(9), 518–527. https://doi.org/10.1016/S1553-7250(08)34066-5

Samter, J. R., Fitzgerald, M. L., Braudaway, C. A., Leeks, D. R., Padgett, M. B., Swatz, A. L., et al. (1993). From military origin to therapeutic application. *Journal of Psychosocial Nursing and Mental Health Services, 31*(2), 23–27.

Smith, M. M. (2022). *Critical incident stress debriefing: An integrated review.* DNP, Liberty University.

Substance Abuse and Mental Health Service Administration. (2014). *SAMHSA's concept of trauma and guidance for a trauma-informed approach.* SAMHSA.

Sutton, D., Webster, S., & Wilson, M. (2014). *Debriefing following seclusion and restraint: A summary of the relevant literature.* https://www.tepou.co.nz/uploads/files/resource-assets/debriefing-following-seclusion-and-restraint-281014.pdf

Tingleff, E. B., Bradley, S. K., Gildberg, F. A., Munksgaard, G., & Hounsgaard, L. (2017). "Treat me with respect". A systematic review and thematic analysis of psychiatric patients' reported perceptions of the situations associated with the process of coercion. *Journal of Psychiatric and Mental Health Nursing, 24*(9–10), 681–698. https://doi.org/10.1111/jpm.12410

US Bureau of Labor Statistics. (2022). *Employer-reported workplace injuries and illnesses 2021–2022.* https://www.bls.gov/news.release/pdf/osh.pdf

Wullschleger, A., Vandamme, A., Mielau, J., Stoll, L., Heinz, A., Bermpohl, F., et al. (2021). Effect of standardized post-coercion review on subjective coercion: Results of a randomized-controlled trial. *European Psychiatry, 64*(1), e78.

Wykes, T., & Whittington, R. (1994). Reactions to assault. In T. Wykes (Ed.), *Violence and health care professionals* (pp. 105–126). Springer. https://doi.org/10.1007/978-1-4899-2863-4_7

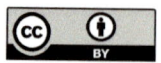

# Final Reflections

Nutmeg Hallett, Richard Whittington, Dirk Richter,
and Emachi Eneje

Emachi Eneje is an expert by experience

This book has presented a rich and diverse exploration of the manifold ways in which coercion and violence are played out within mental health settings. Our book has also documented the extent to which research, policy and practice have shifted from an almost exclusive focus on violence (in the previous 2006 edition) to the problematisation here of coercion as well. Whereas in the previous edition, we tried to gain a better understanding of the origins of violence in order to be able to better

N. Hallett
Risk, Abuse and Violence Research Programme, School of Nursing and Midwifery,
University of Birmingham, Birmingham, UK
e-mail: n.n.hallett@bham.ac.uk

R. Whittington
Research and Education in Security, Prisons and Forensic Psychiatry, St. Olav's hospital,
Trondheim University Hospital, Trondheim, Norway

Department of Mental Health, Norwegian University of Science & Technology (NTNU),
Trondheim, Norway
e-mail: richard.whittington@ntnu.no

D. Richter
Division of Nursing, Department of Health Professions, Bern University of Applied Sciences,
Bern, Switzerland
e-mail: dirk.richter@bfh.ch

E. Eneje
Risk, Abuse and Violence Research Programme, School of Nursing and Midwifery,
University of Birmingham, Birmingham, UK

School of Nursing and Midwifery, University of Birmingham, Birmingham, UK

429

prevent it and—in some circumstances through coercive measures—actively manage it, the use of coercion itself is now being fundamentally questioned. In connection with these changes, the earlier focus on well-being has expanded from employees, then, to now also including service users.

Another change is noteworthy; the 2006 edition ended with a call for an evidence-based approach. Now, through the greater representation of service users at all levels in research and practice development, it is clear there were gaps in that earlier approach. As in other areas of psychiatry, this shows that evidence-based practice alone is not enough; it too often overlooks the unique insights and experiences of those with lived experience. Involving service users in research and the development of mental health practices ensures that the care provided is more holistic, more personalised and more sensitive to the real-world complexities of mental needs. This inclusion helps bridge the gap between clinical evidence and the nuanced, unique needs of individuals, underscoring the necessity of a more integrated approach to mental healthcare.

With these changes in mind, the exploration here has revealed an intricate tapestry of experiences, practices and ethical dilemmas that invites a radical interrogation of traditional psychiatric paradigms and practices. Emerging through the many and varied lenses of personal testimony, empirical research and socio-political critique, it becomes increasingly clear that coercion as a response to violence and self-harm in mental health settings is a complex and subtle phenomenon, deeply embedded within the historical and cultural construction of mental illness and made manifest in myriad ways across individuals, relationships and the mental health system at large.

The personal narratives and empirical examinations collected within this volume have plotted the ubiquity of coercion across a diverse range of mental health settings and geographic locations, challenging the presumption that coercion is a rare or exceptional event. Quite the opposite: coercion, as shown throughout the book, continues to seep into the very grain of global psychiatric care.

The book has also considered how our respect for people compels the ethical interrogation of coercion. It affirms the importance of autonomy, consent and individual rights as central to best practice, while advocating for a thorough re-evaluation of how these concepts are applied, especially in the context of justifying coercion. The discussion of cultural contexts and the demand that cultural competence should become central to mental health care mounts an argument for the necessity of understanding and appreciating the myriad values and norms that ground the varied perceptions and practices of coercion.

The book offers viable and necessary alternatives—focusing on the potential for non-coercive approaches to mental healthcare and patient-centred care—that can move an envisioned 'future', where coercion is no longer the norm, into the present, urging the reader to advocate for changes that would render coercion an oddity, a remnant of an outmoded distant past. An alternative approach grounded in respect for the inherent dignity of the person, and the fostering of genuine recovery, points the way towards a transformation of the very essence of mental health care. This transformation would cast patient autonomy and individual rights as a profound and sustained challenge to the status quo and could serve as a catalyst for a larger politics—the politics of mental health—characterised by a relentless quest for an ethical, effective and compassionate future.

In synthesising the discussions and findings of this book, it is evident that reducing, and ultimately eliminating, coercion in mental health settings is complex and the work that has already begun must continue at pace. It requires a collective effort that encompasses not only service users, mental health professionals, policymakers and researchers but also society at large. By broadening the conversation on coercion and engaging with the perspectives and experiences of those most affected by it, we can begin to forge pathways towards a mental health system that truly respects and upholds the rights and well-being of all individuals.

This book, therefore, stands as a testament to the challenges faced in addressing coercion and violence within mental health care and also, ideally, as a beacon of hope for the future. It calls upon us to persistently and critically reflect on our practices, beliefs and the societal structures that perpetuate coercion and violence, urging us towards a more empathetic, inclusive and rights-based approach to mental health.

There are many voices to be heard from those on all sides with a commitment to this goal but to give a poignant conclusion to our exploration of coercion and violence within mental health settings, we turn to the powerful words of one person with lived experience of mental health services. In the spirit of the interactional ethos that has guided both the original and current edition of this book, we provide the poem not as the final word on the nature of coercion and violence in mental health settings, but rather as the expression of one among many voices that all too often go unheard. It speaks to the necessity for us to listen to the voices and lived experiences of service users and to recognise that we cannot have a conversation about mental healthcare without all perspectives being heeded. It underscores our commitment to broadening the space we hope to have provided here for different perspectives and to fostering an inclusive conversation that grapples with the messiness and complexity of people's real-life experiences whilst reflecting those realities back into mental health practice. In the end, it is our hope that this short testimonial serves as a stark reminder of the necessity for mental health practice which is always underpinned by a compassionate and healing ethos—one that holds the critical importance of our common humanity at its core and that recognises it is ultimately an endeavour that balances individual needs with universal principles.

This poem expresses one viewpoint from the perspective of those who have been often silenced or ignored and offers a reminder of the human cost of many of our current practices. It articulates the resilience and hope of those who have been marginalised, and their plea for understanding, respect and a move towards a more compassionate approach to mental health care. We must listen closely to these voices to ensure humanity stays at the heart of mental health practice in the decades to come:

> The voice of the abused
> Is the softest voice of all
> Even when we cry out
> You do not hear our call
>
> We are drowned out completely
> By your insistence on normality
> Our words you have stolen
> Your promises you have broken
>
> We're used to being humble
> But one day we'll stand tall
> If you'll listen to our whisper
> The softest of them all

Peter Tomlinson